ADVANCES IN

Veterinary Dermatology

Volume 1

ADVANCES IN

Veterinary Dermatology

Volume 1

Proceedings of the First World Congress of Veterinary Dermatology, Dijon, France 27–30 September 1989

EDITED BY

Claudia von Tscharner
Institut für Tierpathologie, Bern, Switzerland

R.E.W. Halliwell
Royal (Dick) School of Veterinary Studies, Edinburgh, UK

Baillière Tindall
London Philadelphia Toronto Sydney Tokyo

This book is printed on acid-free paper

Baillière Tindall 24–28 Oval Road
W.B. Saunders London NW1 7DX, England

The Curtis Center, Independence Square West
Philadelphia, PA 19106–3399, USA

55 Horner Avenue
Toronto, Ontario M8Z 4X6, Canada

Harcourt Brace Jovanovich Group (Australia) Pty Ltd
30–52 Smidmore Street
Marrickville, NSW 2204, Australia

Harcourt Brace Jovanovich Japan Inc.
Ichibancho Central Building, 22–1 Ichibancho
Chiyoda-ku, Tokyo 102, Japan

British Library Cataloguing in Publication Data is available

ISBN 0–7020–1494–X

Printed and bound in Great Britain by Mackays of Chatham PLC, Chatham, Kent

Contributors

Z. Alhaidari *Clinique Vétérinaire, Cidex 248, Route Nationale 85, F–06330 Roquefort Les Pins, France*

R.P. Allaker *Department of Veterinary Medicine & Animal Husbandry, Royal Veterinary College, Hawkshead Lane, North Mymms, Hatfield, Herts AL9 7TA, UK*

F. Ascher *Laboratoires VIRBAC, BP 27, F–06511, Carros Cedex, France*

H.G. Augustin-Voss *Department of Pathology, New York State College of Veterinary Medicine, Cornell University, Ithaca, New York, USA*

K.P. Baker *Faculty of Veterinary Medicine, University College, Ballsbridge, Dublin, Ireland*

N. Barre *Institut d'Elevage et de Medecine des Pays Tropicaux, Craag Domaine de Duclos, BP 1232–97184, Point à Pitre, Cedex, Guadaloupe, French West Indies*

H. Bassett *Department of Veterinary Pathology, University College, Ballsbridge, Dublin, Ireland*

K.M. Beale *Department of Small Animal Clinical Sciences, College of Veterinary Medicine, University of Florida, Gainesville, Florida 32610, USA*

B. Beardi *Tierärztliche Praxis für Hautkrankheiten, Veterinärhistologisches Labor, Kniggestrasse 7, D-3000 Hannover 1, FRG*

D.E. Bevier *Department of Companion Animal and Special Species Medicine, College of Veterinary Medicine, North Carolina State University, Raleigh, North Carolina 27606, USA*

B. Bigler *Kleintierpraxis Laupeneck, Laupenstrasse 33, CH–3008, Bern, Switzerland*

M. Brignac *Veterinary Teaching Hospital, Louisiana State University, Baton Rouge, Louisiana 70803, USA*

A.H.M. van den Broek *Department of Veterinary Clinical Studies, Royal (Dick) School of Veterinary Studies, Summerhall, Edinburgh EH9 1QH, UK*

D.H. Burrell *CSIRO Division of Animal Health, McMaster Laboratory, Private Bag No. 1, PO Glebe, New South Wales 2037, Australia*

J. Bussiéras *Institut de Parasitologie, Ecole Vétérinaire d'Alfort, 7 Ave du General de Gaulle, F–94704 Maison-Alfort Cedex, France*

C.R. Byrne *CSIRO Division of Animal Production, PO Box 239, Blacktown, New South Wales 2148, Australia*

R. Bywater *Beecham Pharmaceuticals, Research Division, Walton Oaks, Tadworth, Surrey, UK*

C.C. Capen *Department of Veterinary Pathobiology, The Ohio State University, 1925 Coffey Road, Columbus, Ohio 43210, USA*

D.N. Carlotti *'Les Places', Sainte Eulalie, F-33560 Carbon-Blanc, France*

J.L. Caswell *Department of Pathology, Ontario Veterinary College, University of Guelph, Guelph, Ontario, Canada N1G 2W1*

A. Chakrabarti *Faculty of Veterinary and Animal Science, Department of Veterinary Medicine and Public Health, Bidhan Chandra Krishi Viswavidyalaya, Mohanpur, Nadia, West Bengal 741252, India*

R. Chermette *Ecole Nationale Vétérinaire d'Alfort, F–94704 Maison-Alfort Cedex, France*

J. Conroy *PO Box Drawer V, College of Veterinary Medicine, Mississippi State University, Mississippi 39762, USA*

J.E. Cooper *The Royal College of Surgeons of England, 35–43 Lincoln's Inn Fields, London WC2A 3PN, UK*

F.M. Crameri *Department of Pathology, New York State College of Veterinary Medicine, Cornell University, Ithaca, New York, USA*

M. Darmon *Centre International de Recherches Dermatologiques (CIRD), Sophia Antipolis, F–06565 Valbonne Cedex, France*

D. Darr *Division of Dermatology, Duke University Medical Center, Durham, North Carolina, USA*

D.J. DeBoer *Department of Medical Sciences, School of Veterinary Medicine, University of Wisconsin-Madison, 2015 Linden Drive West, Madison, Wisconsin 53706, USA*

L. Desplenter *Veterinary Clinic Research, Janssen Research Foundation, B–2340 Beerse, Belgium*

P. Eyre *Virginia-Maryland College of Veterinary Medicine, Virginia-Tech., Blacksburg, Virginia 24061, USA*

V.A. Fadok *National Jewish Center for Immunology and Respiratory Medicine, Goodman 5, 1400 Jackson Street, Denver, Colorado 80206, USA*

L. Ferrer *Facultad de Veterinaria, Dept de Patologia Animal, Universidad Autonoma, E–08193, Bellaterra, Barcelona, Spain*

C.S. Foil *Department of Veterinary Clinical Sciences, School of Veterinary Medicine, Louisiana State University, Baton Rouge, Louisiana 70803–8422, USA*

A.P. Foster *Department of Veterinary Basic Sciences, Royal Veterinary College, Hawkshead Lane, North Mymms, Hatfield, Herts, AL9 7JA, UK*

J.P. Ganiere *Centre National d'Etudes Vétérinaire et Alimentaires, Min. Agriculture et Foret, 22 Rue Pierre Curie, F–94700 Maison-Alfort, France*

B. Goubet *49 Ave du Général de Gaulle, 13160 Chateau Renard, France*

J.M. Gourreau *Laboratoire Central de Recherches Vétérinaire et Alimentaires, Min. Agriculture et Foret, 22 Rue Pierre Curie, F–94700 Maison-Alfort, France*

C.E. Griffin *Animal Dermatology Clinic, 13132 Garden Grove Blvd, Garden Grove, California 92643, USA*

T.L. Gross *California Dermatopathology Service, 3911 West Capitol Avenue, West Sacramento, California 95691, USA*

E. Guaguere *Clinique Vétérinaire Saint-Bernard, 598 Avenue de Dunkerque, F–59160 Lomme, France*

P. Guittin *Department de Pathologie, Centre d'Etudes du Bouchet, F-91710 Vert-le-petit, France*

R.E.W. Halliwell *Department of Veterinary Clinical Studies, Royal (Dick) School of Veterinary Studies, Summerhall, Edinburgh EH9 1QH, UK*

K. Hancock *Regional Burns Unit, St Andrews Hospital, Billericay, Essex, UK*

J.E. Harkness *College of Veterinary Medicine, Drawer V, Mississippi State University, Mississippi 39762, USA*

M.A. Hayes *Department of Pathology, Ontario Veterinary College, University of Guelph, Guelph, Ontario, Canada N1G 2W1*

J.I. Headrick *Royal (Dick) School of Veterinary Studies, Summerhall, Edinburgh EH9 1QH, UK*

D. Horrobin *Efamol Vet, Woodbridge Meadows, Guildford, Surrey GU1 1BA, UK*

S.J. How *Department of Veterinary Medicine and Animal Husbandry, Royal Veterinary College, North Mymms, Hatfield, Herts AL9 7TA, UK*

C.L. Hunt *CSIRO Division of Animal Production, PO Box 239, Blacktown, NSW, 2148 Australia*

D. Bruce Hunter *Department of Pathology, Ontario Veterinary College, University of Guelph, Guelph, Ontario, Canada N1G 2W1*

P.J. Ihrke *Department of Medicine, School of Veterinary Medicine, University of California, Davis, CA c/o T.L. Gross, 3911 West Capitol Avenue, West Sacramento, California 95616, USA*

R. Jayaram *Department of AH and VS, Veterinary College, University of Agricultural Sciences, Hebbal, Bangalore 560 024, India*

D. McEwan Jenkinson *Animal Disease Research Association, Moredun Research Institute, 408 Gilmerton Road, Edinburgh EH17 7JH, UK*

S. Kempson *Department of Preclinical Veterinary Sciences, University of Edinburgh, Summerhall, Edinburgh EH3 1QH, UK*

M. Kietzmann *Institut für Pharmakologie, Toxikologie und Pharmazie, Tierärztliche Hochschule Hannover, Bünteweg 17, D-3000 Hannover 71, FRG*

A.A. Kortt *CSIRO Division of Biotechnology, Parkville, Victoria 3052, Australia*

G.A. Kunkle *Small Animal Clinical Sciences, College of Veterinary Medicine, University of Florida, Box J-126, Health Science Center, Gainesville, Florida 326100–0126, USA*

K.W. Kwochka *Department of Veterinary Clinical Sciences, College of Veterinary Medicine, The Ohio State University, 1935 Coffey Road, Columbus, Ohio 43210, USA*

A.I. Lamport *c/o R.P. Allaker, Department of Veterinary Medicine and Animal Husbandry, Royal Veterinary College, Hawkshead Lane, North Mymms, Hatfield, Herts AL9 7TA, UK*

J. Laurent *64 Rue du Général Mangin, 57500 Saint-Avold, France*

Z. Leish *CSIRO Division of Animal Production, PO Box 239, Blacktown, New South Wales 2148 Australia*

G.G. Lilley *CSIRO Division of Biotechnology, Parkville, Victoria 3052, Australia*

J.D. Littlewood *Animal Health Trust, PO Box 5, Newmarket, Suffolk CB8 7DW, UK*

D.H. Lloyd *Department of Veterinary Medicine and Animal Husbandry, Royal Veterinary College, Hawkshead Lane, North Mymms, Hatfield, Herts AL9 7TA, UK*

D. Lubach *Hautklinik Linden, Medizinische Hochschule, D-3000 Hannover, FRG*

J.M. MacDonald *Small Animal Surgery and Medicine, Auburn University, Auburn, Alabama 36849–5523, USA*

T.O. Manning *Cutaneous Pharmacology and Toxicology Center, College of Veterinary Medicine, North Carolina State University, Raleigh, North Carolina 27606, USA*

C. Marshall *Faculty of Veterinary Science, Department of CAM & S, Medical University of Southern Africa, PO Medunsa 0204, South Africa*

D. Martinez *IEMVT, PB. 1232, 97184 Pointe-à-Pitre, Guadeloupe, Fr. W. Indies*

I.S. Mason *Dermatology Unit, Department of Veterinary Medicine and Animal Husbandry, Royal Veterinary College, North Mymms, Hatfield, Herts AL9 7TA, UK*

K.V. Mason *Albert Animal Hospital, 3331 Pacific Highway, Springwood, Queensland, Australia 4127*

H.-F. Mathes *Sektion Tierproduktion und Veterinaermedizin, Humboldt-Universitaet, Berlin, GDR*

L. Maynard *Laboratoires VIRBAC, BP27, F–06511, Carros Cedex, France*

N.A. McEwan *University of Glasgow Veterinary School, Bearsden Road, Bearsden, Glasgow G61 1QH, UK*

B.J. McEwen *Department of Pathology, Ontario Veterinary College, University of Guelph, Guelph, Ontario, Canada N1G 2W1*

S.R. Merchant *Department of Veterinary Clinical Sciences, School of Veterinary Medicine, Louisiana State University, Baton Rouge, Louisiana 70808, USA*

J.I. Merryman *Department of Veterinary Pathobiology, The Ohio State University, 1925 Coffey Road, Columbus, Ohio 43210, USA*

D.J. Middleton *Pathology Department, Royal Veterinary College, North Mymms, Hatfield, Herts AL9 7TA, UK*

N.A. Monteiro-Riviere *Cutaneous Pharmacology and Toxicology Center, College of Veterinary Medicine, North Carolina State University, Raleigh, North Carolina 27606, USA*

K.A. Moriello *Department of Medical Sciences, School of Veterinary Medicine, University of Wisconsin-Madison, 2015 Linden Drive West, Madison, Wisconsin 53706, USA*

S. Mottier *Institut für Tierpathologie, Laenggasstrasse 122, CH – 3012 Bern, Switzerland*

A. Moussa *Laboratoire de Pathologie Bovine, Min. Agriculture, CNEVA, F-69342 Lyon, Cedex 07, France*

M. Müller *Institut für Tierpathologie, Universität Bern, Laenggasstrasse 122, CH-3012, Bern, Switzerland*

A.C. Mundell *Veterinary Medicine Teaching Hospital, School of Veterinary Medicine, University of California, Davis, California 95616, USA*

J.D. Murray *CSIRO Division of Animal Production, PO Box 239, Blacktown NSW, 2148 Australia*

C.D. Nancarrow *CSIRO Division of Animal Production, PO Box 239, Blacktown, NSW, 2148 Australia*

W.C. Noble *Department of Microbial Diseases, Institute of Dermatology, United Medical and Dental Schools, St Thomas' Hospital, London SE1 7EH, UK*

A. van Oosterwyck *Division of Molecular Neurobiology, Rudolf Magnus Institute and Institute of Molecular Biology and Medical Biotechnology, University of Utrecht, Padualaan 8, 3584 CM Utrecht, The Netherlands*

J.P. Opdebeeck *Department of Parasitology, University of Queensland, St Lucia, Brisbane, Queensland, Australia 4067*

D.M. Pantano *Department of Pathology, New York State College of Veterinary Medicine, Cornell University, Ithaca, New York, USA*

M. Paradis *Faculté de Medecine Vétérinaire, Université de Montreal, CP-5000, St-Hyacinte, Quebec 5S2, Canada*

K. Post *Department of Veterinary Internal Medicine, Western College of Veterinary Medicine, University of Saskatchewan, Saskatoon, Saskatchewan, Canada S7N OWO*

H. Power *School of Veterinary Medicine, University of California, Davis, California 95616, USA*

P. Prelaud *Laboratoire d'Immunologie et d'Allergologie, Department Vétérinaire, 5 Boulevard du Montparnasse, F-75006, Paris, France*

H.W. Radsma *Department of Animal Health, University of Sydney, Private Mailbag 3, Camden, New South Wales 2570, Australia*

R.M. Raisinghani *Department of Parasitology, College of Veterinary and Animal Science, Rajasthan Agriculture University, Bikaner 334001, India*

M. Regnier *Centre International de Recherches Dermatologiques (CIRD), Sophia Antipolis, 06565 Valbonne Cedex, France*

N.W. Rigby *CSIRO Division of Animal Production, PO Box 239, Blacktown, New South Wales 2148 Australia*

J.E. Riviere *Cutaneous Pharmacology and Toxicology Center, College of Veterinary Medicine, North Carolina State University, Raleigh, North Carolina 27606, USA*

T.J. Rosol *Department of Veterinary Pathobiology, The Ohio State University, 1925 Coffey Road, Columbus, Ohio 43210, USA*

E.J. Rosser, Jr. *Department of Small Animal Clinical Sciences, Veterinary Clinical Center, Michigan State University, East Lansing, Michigan 48824-1314, USA*

M. Sahal *Internal Disease Department, University of Ankara, Ankara 66110, Turkey*

A.B. Sanders *Department of Veterinary Medicine and Animal Husbandry, Royal*

Veterinary College, North Mymms, Hatfield, Herts AL9 7TA, UK

D. Scarff *Beaumont Animal Hospital, Camden Town, London, UK*

H. Schaefer *Centre International de Recherches Dermatologiques (CIRD), Sophia Antipolis, 06565 Valbonne Cedex, France*

K.T. Schultz *Department of Pathobiological Sciences, School of Veterinary Medicine, University of Wisconsin-Madison, 2015 Linden Drive West, Madison, Wisconsin 53706, USA*

D.W. Scott *Department of Clinical Sciences, New York State College of Veterinary Medicine, Ithaca, New York 14853, USA*

V.K. Sieber *The Research Institute, (University of Oxford), Churchill Hospital, Oxford OX3 7LJ, UK*

A. Sikdar *Division of Bacteriology and Mycology, Indian Veterinary Research Institute, Izatnagar Up, India*

J.W. Simpson *Department of Veterinary Clinical Studies, Royal (Dick) School of Veterinary Studies, Summerhall, Edinburgh EH9 1QH, UK*

A.N. Sinclair *22 Bligh Crescent, Seaforth 2092, New South Wales, Australia*

D.D. Smeak *Department of Veterinary Clinical Sciences, College of Veterinary Medicine, The Ohio State University, 1935 Coffey Road, Columbus, Ohio 43210, USA*

C.A. Sousa *Elvas Avenue Animal Hospital, 6001 Elvas Avenue, Sacramento, California 95818, USA*

B.M. Spruijt *Division of Molecular Neurobiology, Rudolf Magnus Institute and Institute of Molecular Biology and Medical Biotechnology, University of Utrecht, Padualaan 8, 3584 CM Utrecht, The Netherlands*

D.J. Stewart *CSIRO Division of Animal Health, Parkville, Victoria 3052, Australia*

M.M. Suter *Department of Pathology, New York State College of Veterinary Medicine, Cornell University, Ithaca, New York 14053, USA*

K.L. Thoday *Department of Veterinary Clinical Studies, Royal (Dick) School of Veterinary Studies, Summerhall, Edinburgh EH9 1QH, UK*

C.B. Thomas *Department of Pathobiological Sciences, School of Veterinary Medicine, University of Wisconsin-Madison, 2015 Linden Drive West, Madison, Wisconsin 53706, USA*

M.F. Thorel *Laboratoire Central de Recherches Vétérinaires, Min. Agriculture et Foret, 22 Rue Pierre Curie, F-94703 Maison-Alfort, France*

C.R. Townrow *CSIRO Division of Animal Production, PO Box 239, Blacktown, NSW, 2148 Australia*

C. von Tscharner *Institut für Tierpathologie, Laenggasstrasse 122, CH - 3012 Bern, Switzerland*

M. Varvayanis *Department of Pathology, New York State College of Veterinary Medicine, Cornell University, Ithaca, New York, USA*

K. Vlaminck *Janssen Pharmaceutica N.V., Turnhoutseweg 30, 2340 Beerse, Belgium*

M.W. Vroom *Boxtelsebaan 6, NL-5061 VD Oisterwijk, The Netherlands*

E. Walder *11518 West Pico Blvd, Los Angeles, California 90064, USA*

K.A. Ward *CSIRO Division of Animal Production, PO Box 239, Blacktown, New South Wales 2148 Australia*

S.D. White *Department of Clinical Services, Veterinary Teaching Hospital, Colorado State University, Fort Collins, Colorado 80523, USA*

B.P. Wilcock *Department of Pathology, Ontario Veterinary College, University of Guelph, Guelph, Ontario, Canada N1G 2W1*

J.S. Nimmo Wilkie *Regional Veterinary Laboratory, Benalla, Victoria, Australia*

J.E. Wilkinson *Department of Pathology, New York State College of Veterinary Medicine, Cornell University, Ithaca, NY, USA*

T. Willemse *Department of Clinical Sciences of Companion Animals, Dermatology Section, University of Utrecht, Yalelaan 8, 3584 CM Utrecht, The Netherlands*

B.W. Wilson *CSIRO Division of Animal Production, PO Box 239, Blacktown, NSW, 2148 Australia*

M.A. Wisselink *Department of Clinical Sciences, University of Utrecht, PO Box 80 154, 3508 TD Utrecht, The Netherlands*

J. Woodman *Centre for Tropical Veterinary Medicine, Easter Bush, Roslin, Midlothian EH25 9RG, UK c/o Unité de Recherche Université-INRA d'Immunologie-Parasitaire, Centre INRA de Tours, 37380 Nouzilly, France*

J.A. Yager *Department of Pathology, Ontario Veterinary College, University of Guelph, Guelph, Ontario, Canada N1G 2W1*

Contents

PART 6: WORKSHOP REPORTS

APPENDIX: ABSTRACTS OF POSTERS AND FREE COMMUNICATIONS

The Sponsors of the First World Congress of Dermatology

Principal Sponsor

Allerderm/Virbac

Major Sponsors

Coopers
Dermatologics for Veterinary Medicine Inc (DVM)
Efamol Vet
Friskies Nutrition & Research
Hill's Pet Products
Janssen Animal Health
Leo Laboratories, France
Rhone Merieux
Smith Kline Beecham
Unisabi/Waltham Centre for Pet Nutrition
Vetkem—a Sandoz company

Sponsors

A and M Biosciences
Boehringer
Cavegat
C-Vet
Ciba Geigy
Combe Inc
Delmont Laboratories
Friskies/France
Hoffman La Roche
Proctor and Gamble
Vetoquinol

Preface

The First World Congress of Veterinary Dermatology, held in Dijon, France on 27–30 September 1989, was the culmination of fifteen years of extraordinary progress for the discipline. These years have seen the recognition of dermatology as an independent speciality with examinations to certify the standards and expertise of specialists, the initiation of residency training programmes, the development of special interest groups of practitioners, the publication of a number of textbooks and the launching of the first international journal devoted exclusively to the subject. These advances have emerged in parallel in different parts of the world, with North America, Europe, Australasia and other parts of the world all contributing. However, never before has there been an opportunity to bring together expertise in dermatology of all animal species and from all parts of the globe in one meeting. The Congress truly represented the current state of veterinary dermatology.

The event was attended by some 600 delegates from 35 countries, and five major themes, each consisting of a major review paper supported by four to six scientific papers, were selected. In addition there were workshops, free communications, poster sessions, a special programme on buiatrics and a clinicopathological conference. Full length papers, summaries and abstracts of all of these appear in this publication. In addition to providing a format for the dissemination of the very latest information, it was a forum for the less formal exchange of ideas and experiences, and for the development of links for collaboration in the years ahead. It is planned to hold such conferences every third year, and it is hoped that each one will similarly be a focal point as we advance the discipline into the twenty-first century.

This Congress could not have taken place without the involvement and dedication of many individuals who made up the organizing committees. Their commitment, and the spirit and enthusiasm with which they approached their various tasks was truly remarkable.

Veterinary Dermatology has been fortunate to have enjoyed a close relationship with the manufacturers of pet foods, of pharmaceuticals in general, and in particular the manufacturers of dermatological products, over the years. These companies have recognized that the profession that they serve, the patients that are treated with their products or fed with their foods, the animal owners and the enshrouding economy will all benefit if they contribute to the development of the discipline in both tangible and intangible ways. This philosophy was never more evident than in the magnificent way in which they provided financial support for this Congress. We salute those whose names are listed on page xviii as the true friends of Veterinary Dermatology.

Claudia von Tscharner,
Bern, Switzerland

Richard Halliwell,
Edinburgh, UK

PART 1

HAIR GROWTH AND ITS DISTURBANCES

1.1 The Biology of Hair Growth and its Disturbances

Danny W. Scott

Professor of Medicine, Department of Clinical Sciences, New York State College of Veterinary Medicine, Ithaca, NY, USA

Hair is a characteristic feature of mammals. The factors which control hair growth and replacement have been extensively studied in certain mammals for a variety of motives. Economic pressures have certainly provided a stimulus for research into hair growth in sheep and other species which directly or indirectly serve man's needs (Alexander *et al.*, 1963; Black and Reis, 1979; Goldsmith, 1983; Jarrett, 1977; Kobori and Montagna, 1976; Lyne and Short, 1965; Montagna and Ellis, 1958; Rook and Dawber, 1982; Rook and Walton, 1965; Ryder and Stephenson, 1968; Scott, 1988). In addition, numerous experimental investigations have been carried out on the common laboratory mammals (Goldsmith, 1983; Jarrett, 1977; Kobori and Montagna, 1976; Rook and Dawber, 1982). *In vitro* hair follicle culture systems have been developed (Hardy and Lyne, 1956b; Kobori and Montagna, 1976; Rogers *et al.*, 1988), and will be of enormous benefit for examining: (1) the effects of nutritional factors, hormones, and drugs known to alter hair growth, (2) the biologic and molecular actions of carcinogens, and (3) the tissue-specific expression of isolated keratin genes.

Hair is important in thermal insulation, sensory perception, and as a barrier against chemical, microbial, and physical injury to the skin (Goldsmith, 1983; Jarrett, 1977; Kobori and Montagna, 1976; Lyne and Short 1965; Muller *et al* 1989; Rook and Dawber, 1982; Rook and Walton, 1965; Scott, 1988). In certain goats and in sheep, hair and wool are important economic products. In pet animals, hair is of great aesthetic importance to owners, and a source of great concern when it is not normal. Hair is also a source of many bacteria and fungi, which may contribute to various disease states.

Adaptive changes in the length and density of the pelage related to seasonal variation is an important thermoregulatory device. The ability of the hair coat to regulate body temperature correlates closely with length, thickness, density per unit area, and medullation of individual hair fibres (Dowling and Nay, 1960; Dowling, 1959; Findlay, 1950; Hayman and Nay, 1961; Lyne and Short, 1965; Muller *et al*, 1989; Rook and Walton, 1965; Scott, 1988; Speed, 1960; Wodzicka, 1960; Yeates, 1955, 1957). Together, these factors govern the depth of the layer of still air trapped within the hair coat. Short-term and relatively minor increases in insulation are brought about by piloerection, which increases the depth of the hair coat. In general, hair coats composed of short, thick, medullated fibres are most efficient at high environmental temperatures. Conversely, hair coats composed of long, fine, poorly medullated fibres, with coat depth increased by piloerection, are most efficient for thermal insulation at low environmental temperatures. In addition, coat colour is of some importance in thermal regulation, with light-coloured coats being more efficient in hot, sunny weather (Lyne and Short, 1965; Scott, 1988). Glossiness of the hair coat is important in reflecting sunlight, and tropical breeds of animals tend to have glossy coats which reflect sunlight well, whereas breeds with dull, wooly hair coats show increased body temperature and respiratory rate in the tropics (Hayman and May, 1961; Holmes, 1970; Lyne and Short, 1965).

In all common domestic species, with the exception of the goat, primary (guard, outercoat, kemp) and secondary (down, undercoat) hairs are medullated. Large secondary hairs of the goat are medullated but the small secondary hairs are non-medullated (lanugo) (Muller *et al.*, 1989; Rook and Walton, 1965; Ryder, 1966; Scott, 1988). In sheep and Angora goats, there are three main types of hair fibres (Rook and Walton, 1965; Ryder, 1966; Scott, 1988). *True wool* fibres are fine, tightly crimped, and usually non-medullated. *Kemp* fibres are very coarse, poorly crimped, fairly short in length, and heavily medullated. *Hair* fibres are intermediate between wool and kemp fibres. Kemp fibres are undesirable in good wool because the large medulla causes brittleness and leaves little solid substance to take up dye. The hairs of the cat have also been divided into three types: (1) *guard* hairs (thickest, straight, evenly tapered to a fine tip), (2) *awn* hairs (thinner, possessing subapical swelling below the tip), and (3) *down* hairs (thinnest, evenly crimped or undulating) (Muller *et al.*, 1989).

Disturbances of hair growth in humans are exhaustively detailed (Fitzpatrick *et al.*, 1987; Jarrett, 1977; Kobori and Montagna, 1976; Rook and Dawber, 1982) and, as veterinarians, we draw heavily on this information for own diagnostic, therapeutic, and investigative efforts. However, the information in this article will almost exclusively be taken from studies on our domestic animals. Disorders of hair pigmentation, unless accompanied by growth abnormalities, will not be discussed.

ONTOGENY

The hair follicle is composed primarily of dermal and epidermal tissues that develop from embryonic mesoderm and ectoderm. The embryology of hair follicles and hairs have been studied in cats (Baker, 1974), cattle (Lyne and Heiderman, 1959, 1960; Rook and Walton, 1965) dogs (Conroy, 1968), goats (Margolena, 1959; Wentzel and Vosloo, 1974), pigs (Fowler and Calhoun, 1964; Meyer and Gorgen 1986), sheep (Ahmed *et al.*, 1985; Burns, 1949; Fraser, 1954; Galpin, 1935; Hardy and Lyne, 1956a; Lyne, 1957; Ryder, 1956a; Wildman, 1932), and humans (Fitzpatrick *et al.*, 1987; Goldsmith, 1983; Jarrett, 1977). Primitive hair germs, seen as focal crowding of fetal epidermal basal cells, are first observed during the first trimester of pregnancy. Factors determining the sites of individual hair formations are largely unknown, but follicles and hairs first appear on the face (vibrissae). As the hair germ enlarges and elongates, it becomes assymetrical and grows obliquely downward into the underlying mesoderm. This solid column of cells, now known as the hair peg, carries before it aggregations of mesodermal cells which will form the dermal hair papilla. The lower end of the hair peg becomes progressively more bulbous and concave, and begins to enclose the dermal hair papilla. This lower hair peg-dermal hair papilla union forms the hair bulb. Mesenchymal cells, which are continuous within the dermal hair papilla, surround the length of the hair peg and eventually secrete the connective tissue that becomes the fibrous root sheath. Collections of epithelial cells ('bulges') emerge from the posterior (ental) surface of the hair follicle. The inferior (lower) bulge forms the attachment for downward growing smooth muscle cells which will differentiate into the arrector pili muscle. The middle bulge is the primordium of the sebaceous gland. The superior (upper) bulge is the apocrine sweat gland anlage.

The layer of hair follicle epithelium immediately surrounding the enclosed dermal hair papilla constitutes the hair matrix. Above the hair bulb, a cone of epithelial cells differentiates from the matrix, and will form the hair shaft. A second concentric cone of epithelial cells surrounding the first gives rise to the inner root sheath. Melanocytes appear within the hair matrix. An intraepidermal pathway, the hair tract, is organized and hollowed to allow passage of the hair shaft. No medulla is present in fetal ('lanugo') hairs. Secondary hair follicles arise as separate hair germs from the epidermis, or as buds from the neck of earlier secondary hair follicles.

Numerous experiments have shown that morphogenetic epidermal-dermal interactions occur in embryonal and adult skin, playing an important role in the maintenance and replacement of cutaneous appendages (Goldsmith, 1983; Jarrett, 1977; Lyne and Short, 1965; Rook and Dawber, 1982). Epidermal-dermal recombinations of many kinds have shown that both constituents play determining roles in the morphogenesis of cutaneous appendages, and that informative, as well as permissive messages are exchanged between them. Recent observations indicate that the dermal extracellular matrix plays an essential role, and that, among its various constituents, the collagenous fibrous network may be of primordial importance in constructing the architectural foundations on which to build appendages.

HISTOANATOMY

The microscopic anatomy of hair follicles has been studied in cats (Muller *et al.*, 1989; Schaller and Schwarz, 1972; Schwarz *et al.*, 1976; Strickland and Calhoun, 1963), cattle (Carter and Dowling, 1954; Goldsberry and Calhoun, 1959; Rook and Walton, 1965; Scott, 1988), dogs (Baker, 1966; Creed, 1958; Lovell and Getty, 1957; Muller *et al.*, 1989; Wijeratne *et al.*, 1988), goats (Margolena, 1958, 1959; Rook and Walton, 1965; Sar and Calhoun, 1966; Scott, 1988), horses (Rook and Walton, 1965; Scott, 1988; Talukdar *et al.*, 1972), pigs (Marcarian and Calhoun, 1966; Montagna and Yung, 1964; Rook and Walton, 1965; Scott, 1988; Smith and Calhoun, 1964) and sheep (Kozlowski and Calhoun, 1969; Lyne, 1961; Lyne and Hollis, 1968; Scott, 1988; Stephenson, 1959). In general, no new hair follicles are formed after birth; except in sheep, wherein new hair follicle formation can take place for a short time postnatally. With growth, hair follicle density decreases and hair follicle size increases. All hair follicles grow obliquely (30 - 60°) in relation to the epidermis. The direction of the slope of the hairs, which varies from one region of the body to another, gives rise to the hair tracts (Goldsmith, 1983; Hildebrand, 1952; Jarrett, 1977; Kobori and Montagna, 1976; Lovell and Getty, 1957; Rook and Dawber, 1982; Rook and Walton, 1965). The study of hair tract patterns is called trichoglyphics. The true significance and cause of hair tracts are unknown. With hair slope generally running caudally and ventrally, benefits would include minimal impediment to forward motion, and water flowing off the body onto the ground and not soaking the hair coat, which would reduce its thermal insulating properties. In general, the shape of the hair fibre is determined by the shape of the hair follicle, with straight follicles producing straight hairs. and curly follicles producing curly hairs (Goldsmith, 1983; Jarrett, 1977; Muller *et al.*, 1989; Rook and Dawber, 1982; Rook and Walton, 1965; Ryder and Stephenson, 1968).

The hair shaft is traditionally divided into medulla, cortex, and cuticle (Goldsmith, 1983; Jarrett, 1977; Muller *et al.*, 1989; Rook and Dawber, 1982; Scott, 1988; Wilson and Short, 1979). The *medulla*, the innermost region of the hair, is composed of longitudinal rows of cuboidal cells, or cells flattened from top to bottom. The cells are solid near the hair root, but the rest of the hair shaft contains air and glycogen vacuoles. The *cortex*, the middle layer, consists of completely cornified, spindle-shaped cells, whose long axis is parallel to the hair shaft. These cells contain the pigment that gives the hair its colour. Pigment may also be present in the medulla, but there it has little influence on the colour of the hair shaft. In general, the cortex accounts for about one-sixth to one-third of the width of the hair shaft, and contributes most to the mechanical properties of hair fibres. The *cuticle*, the outermost layer, is formed by flat, cornified, anuclear cells arranged like slates on a roof, the free edge of each cell facing the tip of the hair. Secondary hairs have a narrower medulla and a more prominent cuticle than do primary hairs. The *epicuticle* is an amorphous external layer derived from cuticular cells as an exocellular secretion, or from the outer portion of cuticular cell membranes (Goldsmith, 1983; Jarrett, 1977; King and Bradbury, 1968; Lofts and Truter, 1969).

Hairs usually occur in two basic arrangements: simple or compound (Muller *et al.*, 1989; Rook and Walton, 1965; Scott, 1988). In the simple hair follicle arrangement, characteristic of horses and cattle, hair follicles occur singly and at random, displaying no obvious pattern of distribution (Plate 1A). Each hair emerges from a separate follicular opening, and there are no secondary hair follicles. In the compound hair follicle arrangement, characteristic of cats, dogs, goats and sheep, hair follicles occur in clusters of variable composition (Plate 1B). In general, a cluster consists of two to five large primary hairs surrounded by groups of smaller secondary hairs. One of the primary hairs is the largest (central primary hair), while the remaining primary hairs are smaller (lateral primary hairs). The primary hairs generally emerge independently through separate pores, while the secondary hairs emerge through a common pore. From five to 25 secondary hairs may accompany each primary hair. The hair follicle arrangement of the pig is intermediate between simple and compound, with hairs occurring singly or in clusters of two or three.

The shape and size of hair and wool fibres depends on the size of the follicle, arrangement of cells in the hair bulb, and the arrangement of the inner root sheath (Jarrett, 1977; Lyne and Short, 1965). Large hair follicles produce large hairs, and vice versa. Fibre and hair follicle curling are probably induced by differential growth rates and keratinization on opposite sides of the hair bulb.

The hair follicle has six major components: the dermal hair papilla, the hair matrix, the hair, the inner root sheath, the outer root sheath, and the basement membrane zone (Goldsmith, 1983; Jarrett, 1977; Kobori and Montagna, 1976; Muller *et al.*, 1989; Scott, 1988). The pluripotential cells of the hair matrix give rise to the hair and the inner root sheath. The outer root sheath represents a downward extension of the epidermis. For descriptive purposes, the hair follicle is divided into three anatomic segments: (1) the *infundibulum*, or pilosebaceous region (the upper portion, which consists of the segment from the entrance of the sebaceous duct to the skin surface, (2) the *isthums* (the middle portion, which consists of the segment between the entrance of the sebaceous duct and the attachment of the arrector pili muscle), and (3) the *inferior segment* (the lower portion, which extends from the attachment of the arrector pili muscle to the dermal hair papilla).

The inner root sheath is composed of three concentric layers, which from inside to outside, include: (1) the *inner root sheath cuticle* (a flattened, single layer of overlapping cells that point toward the hair bulb and interlock with the cells of the hair cuticle), (2) *Huxley's layer* (one to three nucleated cells thick), and (3) *Henle's layer* (a single layer of non-nucleated cells) (Black and Reis, 1979; Goldsmith, 1983; Jarrett, 1977; Kobori and Montagna, 1976; Muller *et al.*, 1989; Rook and Dawber, 1982; Scott, 1988). These layers contain eosinophilic cytoplasmic inclusions called trichohyaline granules. The inner root sheath keratinizes and disintegrates when it reaches the level of the isthmus of the hair follicle. The prime function of the inner root sheath is to mold the hair within it, which it effects by hardening in advance of the hair. The amino acid citrulline occurs in high concentrations in hair and inner root sheath, and has been used as a marker for hair follicle differentiation (Goldsmith, 1983; Jarrett, 1977; Muller *et al.*, 1989; Rook and Dawber, 1982).

The outer root sheath is thickest near the epidermis and gradually decreases in thickness toward the hair bulb. In its lower portion (from the isthmus of the hair follicle downward), the outer root sheath is covered by the inner root sheath and does not undergo keratinization, and its cells have a clear, vacuolated cytoplasm (glycogenated). In the middle portion of the hair follicle (isthmus), the outer root sheath is no longer covered by the inner root sheath and undergoes trichilemmal keratinization (keratohyaline granules are not formed). In the upper portion of the hair follicle (infundibulum), the outer root sheath undergoes keratinization in the same fashion as the surface epidermis (keratohyaline granules and orthokeratotic keratin, are formed). The outer root sheath is surrounded by two other prominent structures: a basement membrane zone, or vitreous or 'glassy' membrane (a downward reflection of the epidermal basement membrane zone), and a fibrous root sheath (a layer of dense connective tissue). Perifollicular mineralization of the basement membrane zone has been described in healthy toy poodle bitches (Seaman and Chang, 1984), and may occur as a senile change in other breeds of dogs (Muller *et al.*, 1989), and must be differentiated from the perifollicular mineralization seen in dogs with spontaneous or iatrogenic Cushings' syndrome.

The dermal hair papilla is continuous with the dermal connective tissue and is covered by a thin continuation of the basement membrane zone (Goldsmith, 1983; Jarrett, 1977; Lyne and Short, 1965; Muller *et al.*, 1989; Scott, 1988). The inner root sheath and hair grow from a layer of plump, nucleated epithelial cells that cover the papilla. These cells regularly show mitosis and are called the hair matrix. The size of the dermal papilla and the surrounding hair matrix (the hair bulb) are directly related to the size of the hair produced.

Follicular folds have been described in the hair follicles of animals (Baker 1974; Muller *et al.*, 1989; Scott, 1988). These structures represent multiple (1 to 23) corrugations of the inner sheath which project into the pilary canal immediately below the sebaceous duct opening. These folds are believed to be artifacts of fixation and processing, as they are not seen in unprocessed sections cut by hand.

Two specialized types of tactile hairs are found in mammalian skin: sinus hairs and tylotrich hairs (Muller *et al.*, 1989; Scott, 1988). *Sinus hairs* (vibrissae, whiskers) are found on the muzzle, lips, eyelids, face, throat, and on the palmar aspect of the carpus of cats (pili carpalis, carpal gland). Sinus hairs are thick, stiff, tapered distally, and characterized by an endothelium-lined blood sinus interposed between the follicle and an outer connective tissue capsule. Sinus hairs are thought to function as slow-adapting mechanoreceptors. *Tylotrich hairs* are scattered among ordinary body hairs, are larger than surrounding hair follicles, contain a single stout hair, and are surrounded by an annular complex of neurovascular tissue at the level of the sebaceous glands (Jarrett, 1977; Mann, 1969; Muller *et al.*, 1989; Scott, 1988). Tylotrich hairs are thought to function as rapid-acting mechanoreceptors.

The histologic appearance of hair follicles varies with the stage of the hair cycle, and components of compound follicles may be in different stages (Al-Bagdadi *et al.*, 1977, 1979; Goldsmith, 1983; Jarrett, 1977; Muller *et al.*, 1989; Rook and Dawber, 1982; Scott, 1988). The *anagen* hair follicle is characterized by a well-developed, spindle- or flame-shaped dermal hair papilla, which is completely capped by the hair matrix (the 'ball-and-claw' appearance) to form the hair follicle bulb. Hair matrix cells are often heavily melanized and show mitotic activity. The anagen hair follicle extends into the deep dermis and subcutis. In late anagen, mitosis in the matrix decreases, then stops, and the follicle enters catagen, which is completed in a few days. The melanocytes in the tip of the dermal hair papilla absorb their dendrites. As keratinization of the hair and inner root sheath continues, the terminal portion of the hair, which has become club-shaped, lacks pigment and keratinized fibres extend from it to between surrounding epithelial cells. Since mitosis has ceased, the lower part of the follicle becomes shortened and the connective tissue sheath, particularly the glassy (vitreous) membrane, becomes thickened and corrugated. The inner root sheath disintegrates and disappears. The cells of the external root sheath form a sac in the base of which are the germ cells of the follicle. The club hair is now surrounded by a capsule of partially keratinized cells.

The *catagen* hair follicle is characterized by a thickened, irregular, undulating basement membrane zone at the lower third of the hair follicle, a thickened basement zone between the hair matrix and the dermal hair papilla, a thickened middle third of the outer root sheath, a smaller hair follicle bulb, and a round or ovoid dermal hair papilla. Catagen hair follicles usually account for less than 7% of all hair follicles. The *telogen* hair follicle is characterized by a small dermal papilla which is separated from the hair follicle bulb and no longer capped by the hair matrix, a lack of melanin and mitotic activity, absence of the inner root sheath, a club (brush-like) hair, prominent apoptosis ('dyskeratosis' or 'necrosis' of individual keratinocytes) of the external root sheath, and a basement membrane zone that is thicker than that seen in anagen, but thinner than that seen in catagen.

The hair follicle spontaneously re-enters anagen at the end of telogen, or may be induced to do so prematurely if telogen club hairs are plucked (Goldsmith, 1983; Jarrett, 1977; Rook and Dawber, 1982). Anagen has been divided into six stages: Stages I through IV referred to as proanagen (differentiation), Stage V as mesanagen (transition to rapid growth), and Stage VI as metanagen (post-eruptive hair elongation). In Stage I, cells of the dermal hair papilla increase in size and show increased RNA synthesis, and germinal cells at the base of the epithelial sac simultaneously showing vigorous mitotic activity. In Stage II, the lower part of the follicle grows downward, partially enclosing the dermal papilla. Stage III is characterized by a proliferation of matrix cells which gives rise to the cone of the inner root sheath. Stage IV is characterized by melanocytes which line the dermal hair papilla developing dendrites and beginning to form melanin, hair formation within the cone of the inner root sheath, and formation of the keratogenous zone of the hair just below the level of the sebaceous duct. In Stage V, the tip of the hair has emerged from the cone of the inner root sheath. Stage VI begins as soon as hair emerges at the skin surface.

The density of hair follicles (number of follicles per unit area of skin) varies between species, breeds, individuals, and regions of the body (Goldsmith, 1983; Jarrett, 1977; Rook and Dawber, 1982). For instance, the pig may average 30 hairs/cm^2, the dog 100–600/cm^2, the cow 900/cm^2, the cat 800–1600/cm^2, and the sheep 10 000/cm^2 (Muller *et al.*, 1989; Scott, 1988).

In sheep, the S/P ratio (ratio of the number of secondary hair follicles to each primary hair follicle) has received much study (Rook and Walton, 1965; Ryder, 1956a; Ryder and Stephenson, 1968; Scott, 1988). The greater the S/P ratio, the finer the fleece. Mountain breeds of sheep have mean S/P ratios of 4:1 to 5:1, down breeds 5:1 to 8:1, and Merinos 20:1 to 25:1. The S/P ratio can be a useful indication of fleece type in breeding experiments designed to improve the wool grown. In cats, the S/P ratio was reported to be 10:1 over the back and 24:1 on the abdomen (Baker, 1974). In cattle, S/P ratios of 2:1 to 9:1 have been recorded (Rook and Walton, 1965).

Blood supply to the hair follicle includes blood vessels entering via the dermal hair papilla and others encircling the hair follicle (Goldsmith, 1983; Jarrett, 1977; Lyne and Short, 1965; Muller *et al.*, 1989; Ryder, 1955; Scott, 1988). Hairs will not grow without adequate blood supply to bring essential nutrients to the hair follicle, and larger hair follicles have greater blood supply.

Hair has important tactile functions, and nerve supply arrives via lanceolate nerve endings running parallel to the long axis of the hair follicle, and pilo-Ruffini corpuscles encircling the hair follicle just below the sebaceous gland duct (Goldsmith, 1983; Jarrett, 1977; Kobori and Montagna, 1976). Nerves do not appear to be essential for hair growth. Although unilateral thoracic sympathectomy of sheep resulted in increased wool growth on the operated side, this was thought to be due to increased blood flow (Ferguson *et al.*, 1956).

BIOCHEMISTRY AND PHYSICAL PROPERTIES

Between 90 and 99% of the dry weight of hair and wool is keratin (Goldsmith, 1983; Jarrett, 1977; Ryder and Stephenson, 1968). Because of keratin and disulphide bonding, hairs are among the most durable structures produced by the body, and remain intact for hundreds of years. Hair and wool are composed of hard α-keratin. The major advances since 1950 in our knowledge of hair structural proteins and keratin structure have come largely from the phenomenal effort put into wool research (Black and Reis, 1979; Fraser and Gillespie, 1976; Goldsmith, 1983; Jarrett, 1977; Kobori and Montagna, 1976). Electron microscopy and X-ray diffraction studies have shown that hairs are built in a common arrangement of filaments (microfibrils) of about 7.5 nm diameter embedded in a non-filamentous matrix (Crewther *et al.*, 1980; Fraser *et al.*, 1972; Fraser and Gillespie, 1976; Goldsmith, 1983; Jarrett, 1977; Kobori and Montagna, 1976; Marshall *et al.*, 1980; Rogers, 1959). Filaments are composed of high-sulphur (cystine-rich) proteins and high-tyrosine (glycine- and tyrosine-rich) proteins. Species hairs can show major differences in the type and amount of high-sulphur proteins, whereas the low-sulphur protein microfibrillar fractions are very similar.

Cysteine concentrations are high in the cuticle and cortex, but very low in the root sheaths (Rook and Dawber, 1982). The outer root sheath of anagen hair follicles and hair follicles undergoing repair are rich in *glycogen* (the main carbohydrate reserve for glucose synthesis; glucose being the main energy source for the hair follicle), which disappears in catagen and telogen (Jarrett, 1977; Rook and Dawber, 1982). *Acid mucopolysaccharides* are demonstrable in the perifollicular connective tissue sheath and dermal hair papilla, with small quantities detectable in the outer root sheath (Rook and Dawber, 1982). *Arginine* is in high concentration in trichohyaline granules, and is the precursor of citrulline (Goldsmith, 1983; Jarrett, 1977; Kobori and Montagna, 1976; Rook and Dawber, 1982). The inner root sheath and medulla are rich in citrulline, a unique amino acid not usually found in proteins and virtually devoid of cystine (Goldsmith, 1983; Jarrett, 1977; Kubilus *et al.*, 1980; Kubilus and Baden, 1979; Rook and Dawber, 1982; Sugawara, 1979). Citrulline is formed from the arginine present in trichohyaline granules, and is possibly involved in the aggregation of proteins in cells and in γ-peptide bond cross-linking.

Various enzyme activities have been detected in hair follicles, including phosphorylase, aldolase, succinic dehydrogenase, cytochrome oxidase, alkaline phosphatase, glucose-6-phosphatase, esterases, carbonic anydrase, aminopeptidase, β-glucuronidase, and arginase (Black and Reis, 1979; Goldsmith, 1983; Jarrett, 1977; Kobori and Montagna, 1976; Rook and Dawber, 1982). Enzyme histochemical studies have been performed on the hair follicles of dogs. Schwartzman and Orkin (1962) demonstrated alkaline phosphatase in the connective tissue and capillary endothelial cells of the dermal papilla, and glycogen in the outer root sheath. Conroy and Green (1975) demonstrated alkaline phosphatase in the dermal papilla (regardless of the hair cycle) and Huxley's layer in anagen follicles, and acid phosphatase in the outer and inner root sheaths, the keratogenous zone of the hair shaft, the hair cuticle, and the hair medulla. These results suggested that: (1) alkaline phosphatase was involved in dephosphorylation for the adsorption and transport of chemical substances necessary for the growth of the pilary system, and (2) acid phosphatase was involved in the breakdown of phospholipids and in the necrobiosis of keratinocytes. Al-Bagdadi *et al.* (1978) also demonstrated alkaline phosphatase in the dermal papilla, but reported that it was variably present in anagen follicles and always strongly positive in catagen and telogen follicles, primary and secondary follicles.

Cell proliferation kinetic values were established for the hair follicle epithelium of normal beagles and cocker spaniels (Kwochka and Rademakers, 1989). Values were established by intradermal pulse-labelling injections of [^{3}H] thymidine, examination of cutaneous biopsies, and autoradiography. The basal cell labelling index was 1.46 $\pm$ 0.78% in beagles and 1.07 $\pm$ 0.42% in cocker spaniels.

More is known about the amino acid sequences of the high-sulphur and high-tyrosine proteins of wool than any other type of keratin protein (Alexander *et al.*, 1963; Gillespie *et al.*, 1964; Goldsmith, 1983; Jarrett, 1977; Kobori and Montagna, 1976; Lindley, 1977; Lyne and Short, 1965; Marshall *et al.*, 1980). A number of workers have published electrophoretic patterns of proteins isolated from the keratins of a variety of animals, and on the basis of the observed differences in banding patterns, have suggested that the technique might be of use as an aid to taxonomy, animal classification, and identification (Baden, 1979; Goldsmith, 1983; Kobori and Montagna, 1976; Lindley, 1977; Marshall *et al.*, 1977, 1980). The amino acid composition of hair and wool has been studied and, in general, cystine, serine, and glutamic acid are in the highest concentrations, with smaller quantities of lysine, histidine, arginine, aspartic acid, threonine, proline, glycine, alanine, valine, methionine, isoleucine, leucine, tyrosine, and phenylalanine (Goldsmith, 1983; Jarrett, 1977; Kobori and Montagna, 1976; Lyne and Short, 1965; Rook and Dawber, 1982; Samata and Matsuda, 1988). The epicuticle is rich in cystine, glycine, serine, glutamic acid, and glutamine (Jarrett, 1977; King and Bradbury, 1968; Lofts and Truter, 1969).

Trace elements may be incorporated into hair from several sources, endogenous and exogenous (pollution, cosmetics, environment) (Muller *et al.*, 1989; Rook and Dawber, 1982). In humans, scalp hair has been used in many studies as a sensitive index of environmental pollution (Rook and Dawber, 1982). Recently, attention has focused on the usefulness of hair analyis as a diagnostic tool (Muller *et al.*, 1989). It is well recognized by dermatologists and nutritionists that mineral and trace element analysis of hair samples is *not* a clinically useful tool to assess nutritional status. The reasons for this include environmental effects (topical agents, geographic location, occupational exposures), differing hair growth rates (health, drugs, age, sex), and lack of standardization in analysis techniques.

The most important requirement for follicular protein synthesis is the sulphhydryl-containing animo acid *cysteine*, as it ultimately forms the stable disulphide bonds of hair (Goldsmith, 1983; Jarrett, 1977; Kobori and Montagna, 1976; Rook and Dawber, 1982). Methionine is converted to cysteine in the liver, while cystine is reduced enzymatically to cysteine in the liver and the blood. Inorganic dietary sulphur can be utilized for both methionine and cystine formation in ruminants. but not in human and monogastric mammals. The uptake of radioactive cysteine into follicular cells occurs within hours after injection, firstly in the hair bulb (Black and Reis, 1979; Jarrett, 1977; Lyne and Short, 1965). The availability of sulphur-containing animo acids will affect the rate of synthesis of high-sulphur hair matrix proteins (Gillespie and Reis, 1966; Jarrett, 1977; Lyne and Short, 1965) and a superabundance of cysteine or other sulphur-containing amino acids which can be converted to cystine will increase the amount of sulphur-rich hair matrix proteins (Fraser *et al.*, 1972; Jarrett, 1977).

Within certain limits, the relative proportions of the constituent proteins of wool and hair are susceptible to dietary manipulation. When cysteine, methionine (sulphur-containing amino acids) or proteins rich in these amino acids are infused into the abomasum of sheep to avoid degradation by rumen microorganisms, there is not only a very substantial increase in growth rate of wool, but its cysteine content may increase by 45%. This process is referred to as sulphur-enrichment. Similar, but smaller changes in composition can be induced by changing from a low to a high intake of food.

Air-dried wool retains 16% by weight of water, and by virtue of the hydrophilic properties of keratin, the fibres can absorb up to 35% water before it begins to feel damp (Goldsmith, 1983; Jarrett, 1977). As it absorbs additional water, it gives off heat by an exergonic reaction, a useful property in woollen clothing. Also, the ability of woollen goods to absorb water vapour given off from the skin surface without becoming wet is a valuable property. Other physical properties of hair wool — solubility, tensile strength, elasticity, plasticity, torsional strength — havc been examined, especially in sheep (Alexander *et al.*, 1963; Goldsmith, 1983; Jarrett, 1977; Kobori and Montagna, 1976; Onions, 1962).

HAIR GROWTH AND CYCLE

Hairs do not grow continuously, but in cycles (Goldsmith, 1983; Jarrett, 1977; Kobori and Montagna, 1976; Muller *et al.*, 1989; Rook and Dawber, 1982; Scott, 1980). Each cycle consists of a growing period (anagen), during which the hair follicle is actively producing the hair; a resting period (telogen), when the hair is retained in the hair follicle as a dead or 'club' hair that is subsequently lost; and a transitional pcriod (catagen) between these two stages. From the time it is first formed, each hair follicle undergoes repeated cycles of growth and rest. The relative duration of the phases of the cycle varies with the age of the individual, region of the body, breed, sex, and can be modified by a variety of factors, both physiological and pathological.

The hair cycle and thus, the hair coat, are controlled by photoperiod, ambient temperature, nutrition, other environmental factors, hormones, general state of health, genetics, and poorly understood 'intrinsic factors' (Black and Reis, 1979; Eigenmann *et al.*, 1984; Ferguson, 1979; Ferguson *et al.*, 1949; Goldsmith, 1983; Jarrett, 1977; Gunaratnam and Wilkinson, 1983; Kobori and Montagna, 1976; Lyne and Short, 1965; Muller *et al.*, 1989; Rook and Dawber, 1982; Rook and Walton, 1965; Scott, 1986; Slee and Ryder, 1967). Hair replacement is mosaic in pattern (the activity of a hair follicle is independent of that of its neighbors), is unaffected by castration, and responds predominantly to photoperiod and, to a lesser extent, ambient temperature and nutrition. (Al-Bagdadi *et al.*, 1977; Baker, 1974; Berman, 1960; Berman and Volcani, 1961; Burns, 1943; Comben, 1951; Coop, 1953; Dowling and Nay, 1960; Downes and Hutchinson, 1969; Ebling and Hale, 1970; Goldsmith, 1983; Hart, 1961; Kooistra and Ginther, 1975; Lyne and Short, 1965; Margolena, 1960; Mazak, 1962; Morris, 1961; Muller *et al.*, 1989; Rook and Dawber, 1982; Rook and Walton 1965; Ryder, 1960, 1966, 1970, 1976, 1978; Ryder and Stephenson, 1968; Scott, 1988; Speed, 1960; Thomsett, 1966; Williams, 1964; Wodzicka, 1960; Yeates, 1957). Photoperiod initiates shedding (molt), while temperature, nutrition, and other factors may modify the progress of the molt. Two exceptions to this are (1) the wool follicle of the domestic sheep, in which virtually no cyclic activity occurs (always in anagen), and (2) the course permanent hairs of the equine mane, tail and fetlock ('horsehairs'). Normal cats, dogs, cattle, goats, and horses in temperate latitudes may shed noticeably in the spring and fall. Shedding is, in general, a mechanism of adaptation to changing environmental temperatures and conditions. The increasing photoperiod in spring and the decreasing photoperiod in fall influence the hair cycle through the eyes, hypothalamus, hypophysis, pineal gland, thyroid gland, adrenal gland, and gonads. The shed is usually completed in about 5 weeks. Hair follicle activity is usually maximal in spring and early summer, and minimal in winter. In winter, up to 100% of the primary hair follicles, and 50% of the secondary hair follicles, may be in telogen.

The hair cycle also has an intrinsic or inherent rhythm (Goldsmith, 1983; Jarrett, 1977; Kobori and Montagna, 1976; Lyne and Short, 1965; Rook and Dawber, 1982). Each follicle has an inherent rhythm of cyclical activity, but the timing of the events of this intrinsic system can be influenced by systemic factors, such as hormones. Although many exogenous and endogenous factors can influence the passage of the molt cycle, none alters the sequence.

Because hair is predominantly (65 - 90%) protein, nutrition has a profound effect on its quality and quantity (Goldsmith, 1983; Jarrett, 1977; Kobori and Montagna, 1976; Muller *et al.*, 1989; Scott, 1968; Yeates, 1958). Poor nutrition may produce a dull, dry, brittle, or thin hair coat and may result in retention of the winter coat in cattle and horses.

The hair cycle and hair coat are also affected by hormonal changes (Black and Reis, 1979; Goldsmith, 1983; Jarrett, 1977; Muller *et al.*, 1989; Scott, 1988). Anagen is initiated and advanced and hair growth rate is accelerated by thyroid hormones. Conversely, excessive amounts of glucocorticoids inhibit anagen, suppress hair growth rate, and produce a tender fleece in sheep ('wool-break').

Under conditions of ill health or generalized disease, anagen may be considerably shortened (Muller *et al.*, 1989; Scott, 1988). Accordingly, a large percentage of body hair may be in telogen at one time. Telogen hairs tend to be more easily lost, so the animal may shed excessively. Disease states may also lead to faulty formation of hair cuticle, resulting in a dull, lusterless coat. Severe illnesses (e.g. septicaemia, marked pyrexia) or systemic stress (e.g. pregnancy, parturition) may cause many hair follicles to enter into telogen synchronously and precipitously. Thus, shedding of these hairs (telogen defluxion) occurs simultaneously, often resulting in visible thinning of the hair coat or actual alopecia. In sheep, excessive amounts of glucocorticoids, exogenous or endogenous (e.g. stress associated with injury or disease) are associated with 'tender fleece' and 'wool-break'.

Sheep treated with epidermal growth factor (EGF) develop elevated plasma cortisol and growth hormone concentrations, decreased plasma thyroxine concentrations, periocular and muzzle erythema (presumed to be due to increased cutaneous blood flow and some ruptured blood vessels), decreased wool growth, and often shed the entire fleece (Moore *et al.*, 1985; Panaretto *et al.*, 1984). At the cellular level, these changes are accompanied by reduced mitotic index in hair follicle bulbs, decreased DNA synthesis, weak zones in wool fibres with resultant breaks in the fibres, and telogenization of wool follicles.

The maximum length of hair or wool fibres is genetically determined for each species, and depends on two factors: the rate of hair growth, and the length of anagen (Goldsmith, 1983; Jarrett, 1977; Muller *et al.*, 1989; Rook and Dawber, 1982; Ryder and Stephenson, 1968). The length of anagen is greatly prolonged in domestic sheep, and may last 7 years in merinos, thus eliminating seasonal shedding. Even in sheep, however, there are seasonal changes in wool growth (3 to 12 mm/month), with greatest wool growth occurring in summer and early autumn (Hart *et al.*, 1963; Hart, 1961; Jarrett, 1977; Morris, 1961; Ryder and Stephenson, 1968; Wildman, 1957; Williams, 1964).

The rate of hair growth is genetically preordained, and varies between species, individuals, and regions of the body on the same individual (Goldsmith, 1983; Gunaratnam and Wilkinson, 1983; Jarrett, 1977; Kobori and Montagna, 1976; Muller *et al.*, 1989). The rate of growth seems to be related to the ultimate length of hair in each site. Reported hair growth rates are 0.2 - 0.75 mm/day for sheep (depending on the breed) (Downes and Hutchinson, 1969; Jarrett, 1977; Lyne and Short, 1965; Rook and Walton, 1965; Ryder and Stephenson, 1968), 0.3 mm/day for cats (Baker 1974), 0.04 - 0.71 mm/day for dogs (Al-Bagdadi *et al.*, 1977; Butler and Wright, 1981; Comben, 1951; Gunaratnam, 1986; Gunaratnam and Wilkinson, 1983).

DISTURBANCES IN HAIR GROWTH

Hair growth can be disturbed by numerous disorders (Fitzpatrick *et al.*, 1987; Muller *et al.*, 1989; Rook and Dawber, 1982; Scott, 1988). Although hair loss can occasionally to commonly be associated with virtually all known domestic animal dermatoses (Muller *et al.*, 1989; Scott, 1988) only disorders which directly affect the hair follicle and hair growth will be considered. The most important of these include the inflammatory folliculitides (bacterial, fungal, parasitic, sterile), hormonal imbalances (hypothyroidism, hyperadrenocorticism, hyposomatotropism, gonadal disorders), nutritional disorders (protein, zinc, and Vitamin A deficiencies), certain toxicoses (leucaenosis, selenosis, thallotoxicosis, arsenic toxicosis), certain drugs (glucocorticoids, anticancer agents), and congenitoheriditary problems (hypotrichosis, follicular dysplasia, colour mutant alopecia).

Hypotrichosis and alopecia

Hair loss — hypotrichosis and alopecia — is the most common clinical disturbance of hair growth in domestic animals (Muller *et al.*, 1989; Scott, 1988).

Folliculitis

Folliculitis, regardless of the cause, is characterized by the following primary skin lesions: inflammatory, follicular papules and pustules (hairs emerge from the centre of the lesions, or a pore or 'dimple' is present at the apex of the lesions). Secondary skin lesions include annular areas of erosion, epidermal collarettes, crusting, erythema, hyperpigmentation, and alopecia (Plate 1C). Pruritus varies from intense to non-existent.

Infectious agents are the most common causes of folliculitis, and include bacteria (especially *Staphylococcus* spp. and *Dermatophilus congolensis*), fungi *Microsporum* spp., *Trichophyton* spp.), and parasites (*Demodex* spp., *Stephanofilaria* spp., *Pelodera*, and *Stongyloides*) (Muller *et al.*, 1989; Scott, 1988). Hair loss in these disorders is due to physical and chemical damage to hairs, and toxic and inflammatory damage to hair follicles caused by substances produced by, and directed against, the infectious agents.

Staphylococcal folliculitis (Plate 1D) is: (1) common in dogs (ventral trunk and abdomen, face, feet, pressure points) (Muller *et al.*, 1989) goats (face, pinnae, ventral abdomen, perineum, distal limbs) (Scott, 1988), and horses (saddle-area, posterior pasterns) (Scott, 1988); (2) common in sheep (face, distal limbs, and perineum) (Scott, 1988) and cats (chin, and dorsal neck and back) (Muller *et al.*, 1989) and (3) rare in cattle (tail and perineum) (Scott, 1988) and pigs (trunk) (Scott, 1988).

Dermatophilosis is common in horses, cattle, goats, and sheep (especially dorsal trunk, face, and distal limbs), and rare in dogs, cats, and pigs. *Dermatophytosis* is common in cats (especially head and limbs) (Muller *et al.*, 1989), dogs (especially head and limbs), (Muller *et al.*, 1989) horses (especially saddle-and-tack areas and posterior pasterns) (Scott, 1988), cattle (especially head, neck, escutcheon) (Scott, 1988), goats (especially face, pinnae, neck, and limbs) (Scott, 1988), sheep (face, neck, thorax) (Scott, 1988), and pigs (especially behind ears and trunk) (Scott, 1988).

Demodicosis is common in dogs (especially face and limbs) (Muller *et al.*, 1989), cattle (especially withers) (Scott, 1988), and uncommon to rare in sheep (face, neck, and withers) (Scott, 1988), pigs (snout, ventral chest and abdomen) (Scott, 1988), cats (head and limbs) (Muller *et al.*, 1989), and horses (face and neck) (Scott, 1988). *Stephanofilariasis* is common in cattle (especially ventral chest and abdomen) (Scott, 1988). *Pelodera dermatitis* is uncommon in dogs (Muller *et al.*, 1989), rare in horses, cattle, and sheep (Scott, 1988), and has a contact dermatitis-like distribution.

Sterile folliculitides are uncommon to rare, and include the autoimmune dermatoses pemphigus foliaceus and pemphigus erythematosus, as well as eosinophilic folliculitis, alopecia areata, and alopecia mucinosa. *Pemphigus foliaceus* (Plate 2A) has been reported in dogs (Muller *et al.*, 1989), cats (Muller *et al.*, 1989), horses (Scott, 1988), and goats (Scott, 1988), and typically involves the face, pinnae, distal extremities and trunk. *Pemphigus erythematosus* has been described in dogs and cats (Muller *et al.*, 1989), and involves the face and pinnae. *Sterile eosinophilic folliculitis* has been recognized in dogs ('sterile eosinophilic pustulosis', trunk) (Scott, 1987), cattle (head, neck, and trunk) (Scott *et al.*, 1986), horses ('unilateral papular dermatosis', trunk) (Scott, 1988), and cats (trunk) (Scott *et al.*, 1989). *Alopecia areata* (Plate 2B) is rarely reported in dogs, cats, horses, and cattle (non-inflammatory, head and neck) (Muller *et al.*, 1989; Scott, 1988; Scott and Guard, 1988). *Alopecia mucinosa* (Plate 2C) is extremely rare in cats (non-inflammatory, head) (Muller *et al.*, 1989).

Other infectious causes of alopecia

There are a number of infectious diseases which produce significant alopecia, but not through the process of folliculitis. *White piedra*, caused by the fungus *Trichosporon cutaneum*, is a rare cause of hair loss in horses (Scott, 1988). Hyphae penetrate the hair cuticle (especially the mane and tail), proliferate within the shaft, then break out and surround the shaft to form spongy white nodules through which the hair shaft may break. *Trichomycosis axillaris*, caused by the bacterium *Corynebacterium tenuis*, is a very rare cause of hair loss in dogs (Muller *et al.*, 1989). Bacterial colonies invade and destroy cuticular and cortical keratin, weakening the hair shaft and leading to splitting and breakage.

Leishmaniasis is a common protozoal disease which causes regional (especially the face, pinnae, and limbs) or diffuse alopecia in dogs (Muller *et al.*, 1989; Slappendal, 1988). The pathomechanism of the hair loss is not clear. *Sarcocystosis* is a common protozoal disease which causes alopecia of the tail, pinnae, and distal limbs in cattle (Scott, 1988), and possibly patchy alopecia in goats (Scott, 1988), The pathomechanism of the hair loss is unclear.

Onchocerciasis is a common filarial disease which may cause scarring alopecia (especially the face, neck, and ventral chest and abdomen in horses (Scott, 1988). The alopecia is associated with marked fibrosis and necrosis of hair follicle epithelium.

Hormonal alopecias

Hormonal imbalances are a common cause of alopecia in dogs (Muller *et al.*, 1989; Scott, 1982) but are very uncommon in other domestic species (Muller *et al.*, 1989; Scott, 1988). The pathomechanism(s) of the hair loss is poorly understood in many of these disorders. It appears that hair follicles in different regions of the body vary in their ability to metabolize various hormones, thus helping to explain some of the different patterns of hair loss (Plate 2D) seen in the various hormonal disorders (Goldsmith, 1983; Jarrett, 1977; Kobori and Montagna. 1976; Rook and Dawber, 1982).

Hypothyroidism is by far the most common hormonal alopecia (especially trunk) in dogs (Arslan *et al.*, 1983; Muller *et al.*, 1989; Scott, 1982), but is rarely seen as a naturally occurring disorder in cats (Muller *et al.*, 1989), horses (Lowe *et al.*, 1974; Scott, 1988), cows (Abraham, 1986; Scott, 1988; Zdelar *et al.*, 1981), sheep (Scott, 1988), and goats (Scott, 1988; Sreekumaran and Rajan, 1978). Thyroid hormone is necessary for the initiation of the anagen phase of the hair follicle cycle, and without it there is failure of hair growth and alopecia (Black and Reis, 1979; Chapman *et al.*, 1974; Coop and Clark, 1958; Ferguson *et al.*, 1956, 1960; Godfrey and Tribe, 1959; Goldsmith, 1983; Jarrett, 1977; Kirton *et al.*, 1959; Lyne and Short, 1965; Maddocks *et al.*, 1985; Maqusood, 1950; Muller *et al.*, 1989; Rook and Walton, 1965; Ryder, 1979; Ryder and Stephenson, 1968; Scott, 1988). Thyroid hormone also increases the growth rate of hair and hair fibre length, even in normal animals (Berman, 1960; Black and Reis, 1979; Godfrey and Tribe, 1959; Goldsmith, 1983; Gunaratnam, 1986; Jarrett, 1977; Kobori and Montagna, 1976; Lyne and Short, 1965; Maqusood, 1950; Muller *et al.*, 1989; Rook and Walton, 1965; Ryder and Stephenson, 1968; Scott, 1988). Skin biopsy reveals various combinations of telogenization (Plate 3A) orthokeratosis, atrophy, and excessive trichilemmal keratinization (Plate 3B) of hair follicles (Muller *et al.*, 1989; Scott, 1982, 1988, 1989b).

Hyperadrenocorticism is the second most common hormonal alopecia (especially trunk) in dogs (Muller *et al.*, 1989; Scott, 1982), is rarely diagnosed in cats (Muller *et al.*, 1989; Nelson *et al.*, 1988; Scott *et al.*, 1982) and paradoxically produces hypertrichosis in horses (Scott, 1988). Glucocorticoids inhibit follicular activity, decrease hair growth rate, and decrease fibre diameter (Chapman and Bassett, 1970; Goldsmith, 1983; Jarrett, 1977; Lindner and Ferguson, 1956; Lyne and Short, 1965; Muller *et al.*, 1989; Panaretto and Wallace, 1978a, b; Scott, 1988). In sheep, glucocorticoids also increase the fragility of wool fibres, predisposing to 'wool-break'. Skin biopsies reveal varying combinations of telogenization, orthokeratotic hyperkeratosis, atrophy, mineralization of the basement membrane zone, and excessive trichilemmal keratinization of hair follicles (Muller *et al.*, 1989; Scott, 1988; Scott, 1982, 1989b).

Hyposomatotropism is an uncommon cause of hormonal alopecia (especially trunk) in dogs and has recently been reported to be associated with seasonal flank alopecia in dogs (Muller *et al.*, 1989; Scott and Walton, 1986; Shanley and Miller, 1987). Somatotropin (growth hormone) is important for the initiation of anagen (Ferguson, 1951; Ferguson *et al.*, 1960; Houssay, 1918; Lyne and Short, 1965; Muller *et al.*, 1989) and can increase fibre growth rate and length, even in normal animals (Ferguson *et al.*, 1960; Lyne and Short, 1965; Muller *et al.*, 1989; Scott and Concannon, 1983). Skin biopsies reveal varying combinations of telogenization, orthokeratotic hyperkeratosis, atrophy, and excessive trichilemmal keratinization of hair follicles (Muller *et al.*, 1989; Scott, 1982, 1989b; Scott and Walton, 1986).

Sex hormone imbalances are an uncommon and often poorly understood cause of hormonal alopecia (especially hind quarters, ventrum, neck) in dogs (Carlson, 1985; Fadok *et al.*, 1986; Miller, 1989; Muller *et al.*, 1989; Scott, 1982). Recognized syndromes include hyperoestrogenism in males (functional Sertoli cell neoplasm) and females (functional ovarian neoplasm, polycystic ovaries), testosterone-responsive dermatosis, oestrogen-responsive dermatosis, castration-responsive dermatosis ('woolly syndrome'), and various manifestations of testicular neoplasia (Miller, 1989; Muller *et al.*, 1989). Oestrogens inhibit the initiation of anagen and decrease the growth rate of hair and wool (Dow, 1960; Ferguson *et al.*, 1960; Gardner and DeVita, 1940; Goldsmith, 1983; Jabara, 1962; Jarrett, 1977; Lyne and Short, 1965; Muller *et al.*, 1989; Mulligan, 1943; Rook and Dawber, 1982; Slen and Connell, 1958; Williams *et al.*, 1946). Androgens may delay or accelerate the initiation of anagen, and increase hair and wool fibre diameter and, occasionally length (Fitzpatrick *et al.*, 1987; Goldsmith, 1983; Jarrett, 1977; Kobori and Montagna, 1976; Muller *et al.*, 1989; Rook and Dawber, 1982; Ryder and Stephenson, 1968). Information has been presented which suggests that sex hormone effects on hair follicle are mediated via local receptors and that disturbances in hair growth can be a function of receptor densities or activities in the absence of abnormal blood levels (Fadok *et al.*, 1986; Goldsmith, 1983; Jarrett, 1977; Muller *et al.*, 1989; Rook and Dawber, 1982). Skin biopsies reveal various combinations of telogenization, orthokeratotic hyperkeratosis, atrophy, and excessive trichilemmal keratinization of hair follicles (Muller *et al.*, 1989; Scott, 1982, 1989b).

Telogen defluxion is commonly recognized in cats, dogs, horses and cattle (Muller *et al.*, 1989; Scott, 1988). The pathomechanism of this condition is poorly understood. Various 'stressful' circumstances (high fever, shock, severe illness, pregnancy, lactation, anaesthesia, certain drugs) cause an abrupt, premature cessation of anagen and a sudden synchrony of many hair follicles in telogen (Fitzpatrick *et al.*, 1987; Jarrett, 1977; Kobori and Montagna, 1976; Muller *et al.*, 1989; Scott, 1988). Hairs are then shed profusely 2 - 3 months later as a new wave of hair follicle activity begins. Decreased growth rate of fibres and increased shedding may be seen during oestrus, pregnancy, and lactation (Butler and Wright, 1981; Hale, 1982; Jarrett, 1977; Reid, 1978; Rook and Dawber, 1982).

Nutritional alopecias

Nutritional factors that influence hair growth are very complex (Doney and Smith, 1961; Downes and Sharry, 1971; Fitzpatrick *et al.*, 1987; Goldsmith, 1983; Jarrett, 1977; Kobori and Montagna, 1976; Montagna and Ellis, 1958; Muller *et al.*, 1989; Ryder, 1956b; Rook and Walton, 1965; Scott, 1988; Short, 1955; Yeates, 1958). Hair is about 90% protein with a high percentage of sulphur-containing amino acids, and normal hair growth and skin keratinization requires about 25% of an animal's daily protein requirement (Muller *et al.*, 1989; Rook and Walton, 1965; Scott, 1988). Accordingly, protein deficiency, through starvation, low-protein diets, or chronic catabolic disease, results in abnormal texture and decreased length and diameter of hair and wool fibres, and diffuse thinning of the hair coat or frank alopecia (Black and Reis, 1979; Cabak *et al.*, 1962; Coop, 1953; Downes and Sharry, 1971; Ferguson, 1959; Gillespie and Reis, 1966; Goldsmith, 1983; Hutchinson and Mellor, 1983; Jarrett, 1977; Martin *et al.*, 1969; Montagna and Ellis, 1958; Muller *et al.*, 1989; Scott, 1988; Slen and Whiting, 1952). Histologically, one sees telogenization of hair follicles, orthokeratotic hyperkeratosis, and deformed hair shafts of decreased diameter. Growth rate and strength of hair and wool fibres are particularly sensitive to the amounts and proportions of amino acids available to the air or wool follicle (Black and Reis, 1979; Goldsmith, 1983; Lyne and Short, 1965; Reis and Schinkel, 1963; Reis and Tunks, 1976, 1978; Robards, 1971). Omission of either methionine or lysine results in inhibition of growth and weak fibres (Goldsmith, 1983; Reis and Gillespie, 1985; Reis and Schinkel, 1983; Reis and Tunks, 1976, 1978, 1983, Reis *et al.*, 1975, 1983, 1986; Robards, 1971; Scott, 1988).

The inhibitory effects of certain amino acids and their analogues on wool growth may have application in research aimed at discovering new methods for harvesting wool from sheep (Reis and Gillespie, 1985; Reis and Tunks, 1983; Reis *et al.*, 1983, 1986; Scott, 1988). Many agents that weaken wool are known to inhibit the synthesis of high-tyrosine proteins in wool (Goldsmith, 1983; Jarrett, 1977; Lyne and Short, 1965; Reis and Tunks, 1983; Reis and Gillespie, 1985; Reis *et al.*, 1983). Ethionine, an analogue of methionine, is an inhibitor of wool growth and may cause the shedding of fleece (Reis and Tunks, 1983).

Essential fatty acid deficiency — through low-fat diets or diets depleted through storage, rancidity, and lack of anitioxidants — produces diffuse thinning of hair coat or alopecia, and a dry, brittle hair coat in dogs (Muller *et al.*, 1989; Rook and Walton, 1965), and pigs (Leat, 1962; Scott, 1988). Telogenization and orthokeratotic hyperkeratosis of hair follicles are seen histologically.

Vitamin deficiencies are rare causes of hair loss in domestic animals (Muller *et al.*, 1989; Scott, 1988). The B vitamins serve as cofactors for many enzyme systems as well as amino acid and fatty acid metabolism (Fitzpatrick *et al.*, 1987; Goldsmith, 1983; Jarrett, 1977; Kobori and Montagna, 1976; Muller *et al.*, 1989; Rook and Dawber, 1982; Scott, 1988). *Biotin, pantothenic acid, pyridoxine*, and *riboflavin deficiencies* are known to produce patchy to diffuse alopecia in cats, dogs, and pigs (Cunha *et al.*, 1946; Muller *et al.*, 1989; Scott, 1988). Hypotrichosis in a Charolais calf was reported to respond to folic acid therapy (Bouvet *et al.*, 1988). Vitamin C is important for hair growth and stability through facilitating disulphide links, and a *vitamin C-responsive alopecia* is recognized in calves (Fitzpatrick *et al.*, 1987; Goldsmith, 1983; Scott, 1988). Skin biopsy reveals telogenization and orthokeratotic hyperkeratosis of hair follicles, as well as deformed hair shafts and perifollicular haemorrhage. *Vitamin A deficiency* results in diffuse hair loss and follicular hyperkeratosis in cats, dogs, and cattle (Muller, *et al.*, 1989; Scott, 1988), and a *vitamin A-responsive dermatosis* produces alopecia and seborrhoea, especially in cocker spaniels (Scott, 1986a). Skin biopsies reveal telogenization and orthokeratotic keratosis of hair follicles (Plate 3C). *Vitamin E deficiency* results in diffuse alopecia and seborrhoea in dogs (Scott and Sheffey, 1987).

Mineral imbalances are uncommon causes of alopecia in domestic animals (Muller *et al.*, 1989; Scott, 1988; Underwood, 1977). Zinc is essential to many enzymes and metabolic processes, including keratogenesis (Fitzpatrick *et al.*, 1987; Goldsmith, 1983; Jarrett, 1977; Muller *et al.*, 1989; Scott, 1988). *Zinc deficiency* — through low-zinc diets, diets high in calcium, phytates, or other chelators, or intestinal malabsorption — results in alopecia in dogs (Muller *et al.*, 1989), goats (Miller *et al.*, 1964; Reuter *et al.*, 1987; Scott, 1988), cattle (Ott *et al.*, 1965; Scott, 1988), sheep (Masters *et al.*, 1985; Ott *et al.*, 1964; Scott, 1988) and pigs (Miller *et al.*, 1968; Scott, 1988). Skin biopsy reveals alopecia and follicular parakeratosis. *Iodine deficiency* produces diffuse alopecia with telogenized, hypoplastic hair follicles in all domestic species (Evvard, 1928; Muller *et al.*, 1989; Scott, 1988). Copper is essential in various enzyme systems, including those involved in melanin formation, keratin formation, and disulphide bond linkage (Black and Reis, 1979; Goldsmith, 1983. Jarrett, 1977; Riffard, 1988-1989; Scott, 1988; Underwood, 1977). *Copper deficiency* — through low-copper diets, molybdenum toxicosis, or high dietary levels of substances such as sulphur, zinc, cadmium, iron, lead and calcium — results in fibre depigmentation, and loss of hair or wool fibre tensile strength and elasticity with resultant breakage in cattle and sheep.

Cobalt deficiency produces rough, faded, and brittle hair and wool fibres, as well as decreased fibre production in sheep and cattle (Scott, 1988).

Toxic alopecias

Toxic alopecias are uncommon to rare in domestic animals (Muller *et al.*, 1989; Scott, 1988). Selenium is thought to substitute for sulphur in sulphur-containing amino acids and oxidative enzyme systems (Goldsmith, 1983; Scott, 1988; Underwood, 1977). *Selenosis* — due to high levels of selenium in soil or water, or the presence of selenium-concentrating plants — causes progressive loss of the long hairs of the mane, tail, and fetlock of horses, and occasionally generalized alopecia in horses and pigs (Scott, 1988). It is also a suspected cause of flank alopecia and loss of the beard in goats (Scott, 1988). *Molybdenosis* — due to high levels of dietary molybdenum — interferes with hepatic storage of copper and produces copper deficiency (see previous discussion).

Leucaenosis — due to consumption of the plants of the genera *Leucaena* and *Mimosa* — is a rare cause of acute, generalized alopecia in horses, cattle, sheep and pigs (Gillespie *et al.*, 1980; Hegraty *et al.*, 1964; Kobori and Montagna, 1976; Scott, 1988). These plants contain the toxic animo acid mimosine, which contains a 3-hydroxypyridine-4 moiety that chelates intracellular copper, iron, and zinc, and inhibits DNA synthesis in hair follicle epithelium. Thallium is taken up by anagen hair follicles, resulting in vacuolization of hair matrix cells, nodular enlargements of hair shafts through which breaks occur, and a keratinization defect (parakeratosis) (Plate 3D) (Muller *et al.*, 1988; Rook and Dawber, 1982; Scott, 1988). *Thallotoxicosis* — due to consumption of rodenticides or poisoned rodents — produces alopecia in dogs, cats, and pigs.

Arsenic is a general tissue poison which is localized in hair follicle and hair shaft, and combines with and inactivates enzyme sulphydryl groups. *Arsenic toxicosis* — due to consumption or percutaneous penetration of various arsenic-containing dips, sprays, baits, and medicaments — causes generalized alopecia and seborrhoea in horses, ruminants, swine and dogs. *Mercurialism* — due to the consumption or percutaneous penetration of mercury-containing antifungal agents or medicaments — causes generalized loss of body hair, then the long hairs of the mane and tail in horses and cattle (Rook and Dawber, 1982; Scott, 1988). *Chlorinated naphthalene toxicosis* — caused by consumption and percutaneous penetration of industrial lubricants and wood preservatives — causes generalized alopecia and hyperkeratosis in cattle (Scott, 1988). Chlorinated naphthalenes interfere with the conversion of carotene to vitamin A, and skin biopsy reveals marked orthokeratotic hyperkeratosis of hair follicles.

A variety of circumstances — such as certain drugs, infectious diseases, and metabolic disorders — many inhibit mitotic activity in anagen hair follicles, resulting in hair shaft abnormalities through which breakage occurs (Goldsmith, 1983; Rook and Dawber, 1982; Scott, 1988). The resultant *anagen defluxion* produces the acute loss of dystrophic hairs. *Hypoxia* inhibits development of secondary wool follicles in fetal lambs (Jacobs *et al.*, 1986).

Congenital and hereditary alopecias

The most common types of congenital and hereditary alopecia are the so-called hypotrichoses (Muller *et al.*, 1989; Scott, 1988). *Hypotrichosis* has been reported in all domestic animals (especially cattle, sheep, dogs and cats), takes several symmetrical distribution patterns, may be congenital or tardive in onset, and may be hereditary, infectious, hormonal, or nutritional in origin (Bourdeau *et al.*, 1988; Muller *et al.*, 1989; Scott, 1988; Wijeratne *et al.*, 1988). *In utero* infections with *hog cholera* virus and *bovine virus diarrhoea* virus have been reported to produce hypotrichosis in piglets and calves, respectively (Scott, 1988). Dermatohistopathologic findings are diverse, and usually include various combinations of hair follicle and hair shaft dysplasias, as well as variable abnormalities in sebaceous glands, apocrine glands, arrector pili muscles, vascular supply, and melanogenesis.

Other uncommon to rare causes of congenital and/or hereditary alopecia include *aplasia cutis* (cattle, sheep, horses, pigs, dogs, cats), *ichthyosis* (cattle, dogs), *zinc deficiency* (cattle, dogs), *dermatomyositis* (dogs), and *pili torti* (cats) (Muller *et al.*, 1989; Scott, 1988; Vogt *et al.*, 1988).

Traumatic alopecia

The dictates of fashion and custom impose various physical stresses on canine hair. *Traction alopecia* is seen in dogs who wear various cosmetic devices in their hair coats (Rook and Dawber, 1982). Prolonged traction on hair causes breakage of the shaft, and inflammatory follicular changes which may produce scarring.

Trichorrhexia nodosa and *trichoptilosis* ('split ends') are distinct responses of the hair shaft to physical and chemical injury (Fitzpatrick *et al.*, 1987; Rook and Dawber, 1982; Scott, 1988). They are seen in horses, dogs, and cats subjected to various physical and chemical grooming and topical therapeutic techniques. The hair cuticle and cortex become disrupted and splay out to form nodes, which subsequently fracture transversely, or split longitudinally at the hair tips.

Psychogenic alopecia is seen in cats (Muller *et al.*, 1989), and to somewhat analogous to trichotillomania in humans (Fitzpatrick *et al.*, 1987; Rook and Dawber, 1982). Skin biopsies reveal deformed hairs which may be disconnected from the hair bulb, as well as wrinkled root sheaths and perifollicular haemorrhage.

Miscellaneous alopecias

Alopecia areata is a rare, possibly immune-mediated cause of non-inflammatory, usually annular areas of alopecia, over the head and neck of dogs, cats, horses, and cattle (Muller *et al.*, 1989; Scott, 1988; Scott and Guard, 1988). Skin biopsy reveals early changes of peribulbar lymphocytic perifolliculitis, and late changes of telogenization and atrophy of hair follicles. *Sebaceous adenitis* is an uncommon, possibly immune-mediated cause of focal and annular to diffuse alopecia and hyperkeratosis in dogs and cats (Muller *et al.*, 1989; Scott, 1986c, 1989a). Dermatohistopathologic findings include early granulomatous to pyogranulomatous sebaceous adenitis, and late absence of sebaceous glands. *Discoid lupus* is an uncommon immune-mediated cause of patchy alopecia, especially over the face and neck, in dogs and horses (Muller *et al.*, 1989; Scott, 1988). Skin biopsy reveals hydropic and lichenoid perifolliculitis and dermal fibrosis. *Localized scleroderma (morphea)* is a very rare, possibly immune-mediated cause of patchy, often symmetrical alopecia and sclerosis, especially over the trunk and limbs of dogs (Scott, 1986b). Skin biopsy reveals fibrosing dermatitis, absence of hair follicles, and orphaned glands and arrector pili muscles.

Hypertrichosis

Excessive hair growth is a rare clinical presentation in domestic animals (Muller *et al.*, 1989; Scott, 1988). Hirsutism, which is defined as excessive hair growth in part or all of the male sexual hair pattern, is an inappropriate term in domestic animals (Fitzpatrick *et al.*, 1987; Goldsmith, 1983; Jarrett, 1977; Rook and Dawber, 1982). Hormonal causes of hypertrichosis include *hyperadrenocorticism* in horses (due to elevated blood androgen levels?) (Scott, 1988), *hypothyroidism* in dogs (Muller *et al.*, 1989), *acromegaly* in dogs (due to elevated blood growth hormone levels) (Muller *et al.*, 1989; Scott and Concannon, 1983), and *oestrogen-responsive hypertrichosis* in dogs (Muller *et al.*, 1989). *Inherited hypertrichosis* has been reported in cattle and pigs (Scott, 1988). Hypertrichosis has been seen in association with *maternal hyperthermia* in sheep (Scott, 1988), and *in utero* togavirus infection (*Border disease*) in sheep (Scott, 1988). *Chronic disease states* are reported to cause hypertrichosis in horses (Scott, 1988), and focal hypertrichosis can be seen subsequent to virtually any injury or irritation (Fitzpatrick *et al.*, 1987; Jarrett, 1977; Rook and Dawber, 1982; Scott, 1988). Hypertrichosis has been seen in cattle recovery from foot-and-mouth disease (Bianchi, 1951).

REFERENCES

Abraham, M.J. *et al.* (1986) Clinical features of experimental hypothyroidism in calves. *Kerala Journal of Veterinary Science* **17**:52-70.

Ahmed M.A.A. *et al.* (1985). Micromorphological studies of the epidermis, hair follicles, and skin glands of sheep during prenatal life. *Assiut Veterinary Medical Journal* **14**:19-25.

Al-Bagdadi, F.A. *et al.* (1977). Hair follicle cycle and shedding in male beagle dogs. *American Journal of Veterinary Research* **38**:611-616.

Al-Bagdadi, F.A. *et al.* (1978). Alkaline phosphatase reaction in hair follicles of male beagle dogs during hair cycle stages. *Zentralblatt für Veterinärmedizir* **C 7**:245-252.

Al-Bagdadi, F.A. *et al.* (1979). Histology of the hair cycle in male beagle dogs. *American Journal of Veterinary Research* **40**:1734-1741.

Alexander, P. *et al.* (1963). *Wool: Its Chemistry and Physics* Vol. II. Chapman and Hall, London.

Arslan, S.H. *et al.* (1983). The phase of hair growth in hypothyroidism in the dog. *Veterinary Research Communications* **6**:51-58.

Baden, H.P, (1979). Das Haarkeratin. In: Orfanos, C.E. ed. *Haar und Haarkrankheiten*, p. 23-50. Fischer-Verlag, Stuttgart.

Baker, K.P. (1966). A histological and histopathological study of the skin of the dog. PhD Thesis, University of Dublin.

Baker, K.P. (1974). Hair growth and replacement in the cat. *British Veterinary Journal* **130**:327-384.

Berman, A. (1960). Peripheral effects of 1-thyroxine on hair growth and coloration in cattle. *Journal of Endocrinology* **20**:288-292.
Berman, A. and Volcani, R. (1961). Seasonal and regional variations in coat characteristics of dairy cattle. *Australian Journal of Agricultural Research* **12**:528-538.
Bianchi, C. (1951). Sulla ipertricosi dei bovini. *Profilassi* **24**:5-7.
Black, J.L. and Reis, P.J. (1979). *Physiological and Environmental Limitations to Wool Growth*. University of New England Publishing Unit, Boston.
Bourdeau, P. *et al.* (1988). Alopécie héréditaire généralisée féline. A propos d'un cas observé dans la race Sacré Birmanie. *Recueil de Médicine Vétérinaire* **164**:17-24.
Bouvet, A. *et al.* (1988). Folic acid therapy for alopecia in Charolais calf. *Veterinary Research* **123**:533-535.
Burns, M. (1943). Hair pigmentation and the genetics of color in greyhounds. *Proceedings of the Royal Society of Edinburgh* **61**:31-35.
Burns, M. (1949). The development of the fleece and follicle population in Herdwick sheep. *Journal of Agricultural Science* **44**:443-454.
Butler, W.F. and Wright, A.I. (1981). Hair growth in the greyhound. *Journal of Small Animal Practice* **22**:655-661,
Cabak, V. *et al.* (1962). Severe undernutrition in growing and adult animals. X. The skin and hair of the pigs. *British Journal of Nutrition* **16**:635-639.
Carlson, R.A. (1985). Endocrine alopecia in a dog showing response to FSH administration. *Journal of the American Animal Hospital Association* **21**:735-739.
Carter, H.B. and Dowling, D.F. (1954). The hair follicle and apocrine gland population of cattle skin. *Australian Journal of Agricultural Research* **5**:745-754.
Chapman, R.E. and Bassett, J.M. (1970). The effects of prolonged administration of cortisol on the skin of sheep on different planes of nutrition. *Journal of Endocrinology* **48**:649-664.
Chapman, R.E. *et al.* (1974). The effects of fetal thyroidectomy and thyroxine administration on the development of the skin and wool follicles of sheep fetuses. *Journal of Anatomy* **117**:419-432.
Comben, N. (1951) Observations on the mode of growth of the hair of the dog. *British Veterinary Journal* **107**:231-235.
Conroy, J.D, (1968). Melanoblasts and melanocytes in canine fetal skin and oral mucosa. PhD Thesis, University of Illinois.
Conroy, J.D. and Green, C.A. (1975). Distribution of acid and alkaline phosphatases in canine skin. *American Journal of Veterinary Research* **36**:1697-1703.
Coop, I.E. (1953). Wool growth as affected by nutrition and by climactic factors. *Journal of Agricultural Science* **43**:456-463.
Coop, I.E. and Clark, V.R. (1958). The effect of thyroxine on wool growth and lamb production. *New Zealand Journal of Agricultural Research* **1**:365-381.
Creed, R.F.S. (1958) The histology of mammalian skin, with special reference to the dog and cat. *Veterinary Record* **70**:171-176.
Crewther, W.G. *et al.* (1980) The microfibrillar proteins of α-keratin. In: Parry, D.A.D. ed. *Fibrous Proteins, Scientific, Industrial, and Medical Aspects* Vol. II, pp. 151-160, Academic Press, New York.
Cunha, J.J. *et al.* (1946). Biotin deficiency syndrome in pigs fed desiccated egg white. *Journal of Animal Science* **5**:219-225.
Doney, J.M. and Smith, W.F. (1961). The fleece of Scottish blackface sheep. I. Seasonal changes in wool production and fleece structure. *Journal of Agricultural Science* **56**:365-370.
Dow, C. (1960). Oestrogen-induced atrophy of the skin in dogs. *Journal of Pathology and Bacteriology* **80**:434-435.
Dowling, D.F. (1959). The medullation characteristic of the hair coat as a factor in heat tolerance of cattle. *Australian Journal of Agricultural Research* **10**:736-743.

Dowling, D.F. and Nay, T. (1960). Cyclic changes in the follicles and hair coat in cattle. *Australian Journal of Agricultural Research* **11**:1064-1071.
Downes, A.M. and Hutchinson, J.C.D. (1969). Effect of low skin surface temperature on wool growth. *Journal of Agricultural Science* **72**:155-159.
Downes, A.M. and Sharry, L.F. (1971). Measurement of wool growth and its response to nutritional change. *Australian Journal of Biological Science* **24**:117-123.
Ebling, F.J. and Hale, P.A. (1970). The control of the mammalian moult. *Mem. Soc. Endocrinol.* **18**:215-237.
Eigenmann, J.E. *et al.* (1984). Estrogen-induced flank alopecia in the female dog: Evidence for local rather than systemic hyperestrogenism. *Journal of the American Animal Hospital Association* **20**:621-624.
Evvard, J.M. (1928). Iodine deficiency symptoms and their significance in animal nutrition and pathology. *Endocrinology* **12**:539-581.
Fadok, V.A. *et al.* (1986). Hyperprogesteronemia associated with Sertoli cell tumor and alopecia in a dog. *Journal of the American Veterinary Medical Association* **188**:1058-1059.
Ferguson, K.A. (1951). The effect of hypophysectomy on wool growth. *Journal of Endocrinology* **7**:1xi.
Ferguson, K.A. (1959). Influence of dietary protein percentage on wool growth. *Nature* 184:907.
Ferguson, K.A. (1979). The effect of sympathectomy on wool growth. *Australian Journal of Scientific Research* **B 2**:438-443.
Ferguson, K.A. *et al.* (1949). Studies of comparative fleece growth in sheep. I. The quantitative nature of inherent differences in wool-growth rate. *Journal of Scientific Research B* **2**:42-81.
Ferguson, K.A. *et al.* (1956). The influence of the thyroid on wool follicle development in the lamb. *Australian Journal of Biological Science* **9**:575-585.
Ferguson, K.A. *et al.* (1960). The hormonal regulation of wool growth. *Acta Endocrinologica* **51**:1011-1030.
Findlay, J.D. (1950). The effects of temperature, humidity, air movement, and solar radiation on the behavior and physiology of cattle and other farm animals. *Hannah Dairy Research Institute Bulletin* **9**:1-6.
Fitzpatrick, T.B. *et al.* (1987). *Dermatology in General Medicine* Vol. III. McGraw-Hill Book Company, New York.
Fowler, E.H., Calhoun, M.L. (1964). The microscopic anatomy of developing fetal pig skin. *American Journal of Veterinary Research* **25**:156-164.
Fraser, A.S. (1954). Development of the skin follicle population in Merino sheep. *Australian Journal of Agricultural Research* **5**:737-744.
Fraser, R.D.B. and Gillespie, J.M. (1976). Wool structure and biosynthesis. *Nature* **261**:650-654.
Fraser, R.D.B. *et al.* (1972). *Keratins, Their Consumption, Structure, and Biosynthesis*. Charles C. Thomas Publisher, Springfield, Illinois.
Galpin, N. (1935). The prenatal development of the coat of the New Zealand Romney Lamb. *Journal of Agricultural Science* **25**:344-360.
Gardner, W.U. and DeVita, J. (1940). Inhibition of hair growth in dogs receiving estrogens. *Yale Journal of Biology and Medicine* **13**:213-215.
Gillespie, J.M. and Reis, P.J. (1966). The dietary-regulated biosynthesis of high sulfur wool proteins. *Biochemical Journal* **98**:669-677.
Gillespie, J.M. *et al.* (1964). The isolation and properties of some soluble proteins in wools of increased sulfur content. *Australian Journal of Biological Science* **17**:542-547.
Gillespie, J.M. *et al.* (1980). Changes in matrix proteins of wool and mouse hair following the administration of depilatory compounds. *Australian Journal of Biological Science* **33**:125-136.

Godfrey, N.W. and Tribe, D.E. (1959). The effect of thyroxine implantation on wool growth. *Journal of Agricultural Science* **53**:369.

Goldsberry, S. and Calhoun, M.L. (1959). The comparative histology of the skin of Hereford and Aberdeen Angus cattle. *American Journal of Veterinary Research* **20**:61-63.

Goldsmith, L.A. (1983). *Biochemistry and Physiology of the Skin*. Oxford University Press, Oxford.

Gunaratnam, P. (1986). The effects of thyroxine on hair growth in the dog. *Journal of Small Animal Practice* **27**:17-29.

Gunaratnam, P. and Wilkinson, G.T. (1983). A study of normal hair growth in the dog. *Journal of Small Animal Practice* **24**:445-453.

Hale, P.A. (1982). Periodic hair shedding by a normal bitch. *Journal of Small Animal Practice* **23**:345-350.

Hardy, M.H. and Lyne, A.G. (1956a). The prenatal development of wool follicles in Merino sheep. *Australian Journal of Biological Science* **9**:423-441.

Hardy, M.H. and Lyne, A.G. (1956b). Studies on the development of wool follicles in tissue culture. *Australian Journal of Biological Science* **9**:559-574.

Hart, D.S. (1961). The effect of light-dark sequences on wool growth. *Journal of Agricultural Science* **56**:235-242.

Hart, D.S. *et al.* (1963). Reversed photoperiodic seasons and wool growth. *Nature* **198**:310-311.

Hayman, R.H. and Nay, T. (1961). Observations on hair growth and shedding in cattle. *Australian Journal of Agricultural Research* **12**:513-527.

Hegraty, M.P. *et al.* (1964). Reaction of sheep to the consumption of *Leucaena glauca* to its toxic principle mimosine. *Australian Journal of Agricultural Research* **15**:153-158.

Hildebrand, M. (1952). The integument in Canidae. *Journal of Mammalogy* **33**:419-427.

Holmes, C.W. (1970). Effects of air temperature on body temperatures and sensible heat loss of Friesian and Jersey calves at 12 and 76 days of age. *Animal Production* **12**:493-501.

Houssay, B.A. (1918) Extirpación de la hipófisis en el perro. *Endocrinologia* **2**:497-498.

Hutchinson, G. and Mellor, D.J. (1983). Effects of maternal nutrition on the initiation of secondary wool follicles in foetal sheep. *Journal of Comparative Pathology* **93**:577-581

Jabara, A.G. (1962). Some tissue changes in the dog following stilbestrol administration. *Australian Journal of Experimental Biology and Medical Science* **40**:293-307.

Jacobs, R. *et al.* (1986). Effects of hypoxia on the initiation of secondary wool follicles in the fetus. *Australian Journal of Biological Science* **39**:79-83.

Jarrett, A. (1977). *The Physiology and Pathophysiology of the Skin* Vol. 4. *The Hair Follicle*. London: Academic Press.

King, N.L.B. and Bradbury, J.H. (1968). The chemical composition of wool. V. The epicuticle. *Australian Journal of Biological Science* **21**:375-378.

Kirton, A.H. *et al.* (1959). Some effects of thyroxine on live weight, metabolism, and wool growth of Romney ewes. *New Zealand Journal of Agricultural Research* **2**:1143-1146.

Kobori, T. and Montagna, W. (1976). *Biology and Disease of the Hair*. University of Tokyo Press, Tokyo.

Kooistra, L.H. and Ginther, O.J. (1975). Effects of photoperiod on reproductive activity and hair in mares. *American Journal of Veterinary Research* **36**:1413-1419.

Kozlowski, G.P. and Calhoun, M.L. (1969). Microscopic anatomy of integument of sheep. *American Journal of Veterinary Research* **30**:1267-1279.

Kwochka, K.W. and Rademakers, A.M. (1989). Cell proliferation of epidermis, hair follicles, and sebaceous glands of beagles and cocker spaniels with healthy skin. *American Journal of Veterinary Research* **50**:587-591.

Kubilus, J. and Baden, H.P. (1979). The enzymatic conversation of protein-bound arginine to protein-bound citrulline in epidermis. *Federation Proceedings* **37**:1780.

Kubilus, J. *et al.* (1980). Partial purification and specificity of an arginine converting enzyme from bovine epidermis. *Biochemica et Biophysica Acta* **615**:246-251.

Leat, W.M.F. (1962). Studies on pig diets containing different amounts of linoleic acid. *British Journal of Nutrition* **16**:559-564.

Lindley, H. (1977). The chemical composition and structure of wool. In: Asquith, R.S. ed. *Chemistry of Natural Protein Fibres* pp. 147-162. Plenum, New York.

Lindner, H.R. and Ferguson, K.A. (1956). Influence of the adrenal cortex on wool growth and its relation to break and tenderness of the fleece. *Nature* **177**:188-189.

Lofts, P.F. and Truter, E.V. (1969). The constitution of the epicuticle of wool. *Textile Research Journal* **60**:46-48.

Lovell, J.E. and Getty, R. (1957). The hair follicle, epidermis, dermis, and skin glands of the dog. *American Journal of Veterinary Research* **18**:873-885.

Lowe, J.E. *et al.* (1974). Equine hypothyroidism: the long-term effects of thyroidectomy on metabolism and growth in mares and stallions. *Cornell Veterinarian* **64**:276-295.

Lyne, A.G. (1957). The development of the epidermis and hair canals in the Merino sheep foetus. *Australian Journal of Biological Science* **10**:10-16.

Lyne, A.G. (1961). The post-natal development of wool follicles, shedding, and skin thickness in inbred Merino and Southdown-Merino crossbred sheep. *Australian Journal of Biological Science* **14**:141-156.

Lyne, A.G. and Heiderman, M.J. (1959). The prenatal development of skin and hair in cattle (*Bos taurus* L.). *Australian Journal of Biological Science* **12**:72-95.

Lyne, A.G. and Heiderman, M.J. (1960). The prenatal development of skin and hair in cattle. II. *Bos indicus* X *Bos taurus* L. *Australian Journal of Biological Science* **13**:584-599.

Lyne, A.G. and Hollis, D.E. (1968). The skin of the sheep: A comparison of body regions. *Australian Journal of Biological Science* **21**:499-527.

Lyne, A.G. and Short, B.F. (1965). *Biology of the Skin and Hair Growth*. Angus and Robertson, Sydney.

Maddocks, S. *et al.* (1985). Effect on wool growth of thyroxine replacement in thyroidectomized Merino rams. *Australian Journal of Biological Science* **38**:405-414.

Mann, S.J. (1969). The tylotrich follicle as a marker system in skin. In: Montagna, W. and Dobson, R.L. eds. *Advances in Biology of Skin* Vol 9: Hair Growth, pp. 77-84. Pergamon Press, New York.

Maqusood, M. (1950). Effect of hypo- and mild hyperthyroidism on fleece growth in sheep. *Nature* **166**:647.

Marcarian, N.Q. and Calhoun, M.L. (1966). Microscopic anatomy of the integument of adult swine. *American Journal of Veterinary Research* **27**:765-772.

Margolena, L.A. (1958). Influence of the season on the anatomy of the skin and follicles of wooled sheep and dairy goats. *Virginia Journal of Science* **9**:393-401.

Margolena, L.A. (1959). Skin and hair follicle development in dairy goats. *Virginia Journal of Science* **10**:33-47.

Margolena, L.A. (1960). Season and comparative activity of wool follicles. *Anatomical Record* **138**:368.

Marshall, R.C. *et al.* (1977). High-sulfur proteins in mammalian Keratins: A possible aid in classification. *Australian Journal of Zoology* **25**:121-132.

Marshall, R.C. *et al.* (1980). High-tyrosine proteins of wool, heterogeneity and biosynthetic regulation. *Proc. 6th Int. Wool Test. Res. Conf., Praetoria, 1980*, pp. 147-158.

Martin, Y.G. *et al.* (1969). Wound healing, hair growth, and biochemical measures as affected by subnormal protein and energy intake in young cattle. *American Journal of Veterinary Research* **30**:355-364.

Masters, D.G. *et al.* (1985). Effects of zinc deficiency on the wool growth, skin, and wool follicles of preruminant lambs. *Australian Journal of Biological Science* **38**:355-365.

Mazak, V. (1962). Spring moult in *Equus hemoinus kiang* and a contribution to the phylogenesis of moulting in the subfamily Equinae. *Zoologischer Anzeiger* **168**: 164-167

Meyer, W. and Gorgen, S. (1986). Development of hair coat and skin glands in fetal porcine integument. *Journal of Anatomy* **144**:201-220.

Miller, E.R. *et al.* (1968). Biochemical, skeletal, and allometric changes due to zinc deficiency in the baby pig. *Journal of Nutrition* **95**:278-290.

Miller, W.H. Jr. (1989). Sex hormone-related dermatoses in dogs. In: Kirk, R.W. ed. *Current Veterinary Therapy* Vol. X. pp. 595-602. W.B. Saunders Company, Philadelphia.

Miller, W.J. *et al.* (1964). Experimentally produced zinc deficiency in the goat. *Journal of Dairy Science* **47**:556-561.

Montagna, W. and Ellis, R.A. (1958). *The Biology of Hair Growth*. Academic Press, New York.

Montagna, W. and Yung, J.S. (1964). The skin of the domestic pig. *Journal of Investigative Dermatology* **42**:11-21.

Moore, G.P.M. *et al.* (1985). Epidermal hyperplasia and wool follicle regression in sheep infused with epidermal growth factor. *Journal of Investigative Dermatology* **84**:172-175.

Morris, L.R. (1961). Photoperiodicity of seasonal rhythm of wool growth in sheep. *Nature* **190**:102-103.

Muller, G.H. *et al.* (1989). *Small Animal Dermatology* Vol. IV. W.B. Saunders Company, Philadelphia.

Mulligan, R.M. (1943). Hair loss in male dogs fed stilbestrol. *Proceedings of the Society for Experimental Biology and Medicine* **54**:21-22.

Nelson, R.W. *et al.* (1988). Hyperadrenocorticism in cats: Seven cases (1978-1987). *Journal of the American Veterinary Medical Association* **193**:245-250.

Onions, W.J. (1962). Wool. *An Introduction to Its Properties, Varieties, Uses and Production*. Benn, London.

Ott, E.A. *et al.* (1964). Zinc deficiency syndrome in the young lamb. *Journal of Nutrition* **82**:41-50.

Ott, E.A. *et al.* (1965). Zinc deficiency syndrome in the young calf. *Journal of Animal Science* **24**:735-742.

Panaretto, B.A. and Wallace, A.L.C. (1978a). The administration of flumethasone by three different routes, its measurement in the plasma, and some effects on wool growth in Merino wethers. *Australian Journal of Biological Science* **31**:601-620.

Panaretto, B.A. and Wallace, A.L.C. (1978b). Dexamethasone concentrations in ovine plasma during its intravenous infusion, its relation to production of some endogenous hormones and some of the effects on wool growth. *Australian Journal of Biological Science* **31**:247-256.

Panaretto, B.A. *et al.* (1984): Inhibition of DNA synthesis in dermal tissue of Merino sheep treated with depilatory doses of mouse epidermal growth factors. *Journal of Endocrinology* **100**:24-31.

Reid, R.N.D. (1978). The effects of pregnancy and lactation on wool production and live weight in Polwarth ewes. *Australian Journal of Experimental Agriculture and Animal Husbandry* **18**:58-62.

Reis, P.J. and Gillespie, J.M. (1985). Effects of phenylalanine and analogues of methionine and phenylalanine on the composition of wool and mouse hair.

Australian Journal of Biological Science **38**:151-163.
Reis, P.J. and Schinkel, P.G. (1963). Some effects of sulphur containing amino acids on the growth and composition of wool. *Australian Journal of Biological Science* **16**:218-230.
Reis, P.J. and Tunks, D.A. (1976). The influence of abomasal supplements of zinc and some amino acids on wool growth rate and plasma amino acids. *Journal of Agricultural Science* **86**:475-485.
Reis, P.J. and Tunks, D.A. (1978). Effects on wool growth of the infusion of mixtures of amino acids into the abomasum of sheep. *Journal of Agricultural Science* **90**:173-183.
Reis, P.J. and Tunks, D.A. (1983). Inhibiting effects of ethionine, an analogue of methionine, on wool growth. *Australian Journal of Biological Science* **35**:49-62.
Reis, P.J. *et al.* (1975). Effects of mimosine, a potential chemical defleecing agent on wool growth and the skin of sheep. *Australian Journal of Biological Science* **28**:69-84.
Reis, P.J. *et al.* (1983). Investigations of some amino acid analogues and metabolites as inhibitors of wool and hair growth. *Australian Journal of Biological Science* **36**:157-170.
Reis, P.J. *et al.* (1986). Effects of methoxinine, an analogue of methionine, on the growth and morphology of wool fibres. *Australian Journal of Biological Science* **39**:209-223.
Reuter, R. *et al.* (1987). Zinc responsive alopecia and hyperkeratosis in Angora goats. *Australian Veterinary Journal* **64**:351-352.
Riffard, J. (1988-1989). Le cuivre et les ruminants 1^r e partie: métabolisme, rôle, épidémiologie des carences. *Point Vétérinaire* **20**:905-911.
Robards, G.E. (1971). The wool growth of Merino sheep receiving an exponential pattern methionine infusion into the abomasum. *Australian Journal of Agricultural Research* **22**:261-272.
Rogers, G.E. (1959). Electron microscope studies of hair and wool. *Annals of the New York Academy of Sciences* **83**:378-399.
Rogers, G.E. *et al.* (1988). A procedure for the culture of hair follicles as functionally intact organoids. *Clinical Dermatology* **6**:36-42.
Rook, A. and Dawber, R. (1982). *Diseases of the Hair and Scalp*. Blackwell Scientific Publications, Oxford.
Rook, A.J. and Walton, G.S. (1965). *Comparative Physiology and Pathology of the Skin*, p. 1965. Blackwell Scientific Publications, Oxford.
Ryder, M.L. (1955). Studies on the nutrition of wool follicles in sheep: The anatomy of the general blood supply of the skin. *Journal of Agricultural Science* **45**:311-318.
Ryder, M.L. (1956a). The prenatal development of follicle population in the Romney lamb. *Journal of Agricultural Science* **47**:6-17.
Ryder, M.L. (1956b). Observations of nutritional and seasonal changes in the fleece of some Masham sheep. *Journal of Agricultural Science* **47**:129-136.
Ryder, M.L. (1960). A study of the coat of the mouflon, Ovis musimon, with special reference to seasonal change. *Proceedings of the Zoological Society of London* **135**:387-408.
Ryder, M.L. (1966). Coat structure and seasonal shedding in goats. *Animal Production* **8**:289-302.
Ryder, M.L. (1970). Structure and seasonal change of coat in Scottish wild goats. *Journal of Zoology London* **161**:355-361.
Ryder, M.L. (1976). Seasonal changes in the coat of the cat. *Research of Veterinary Science* **21**:280-283.
Ryder, M.L. (1978) Growth cycles in the coat of ruminants. *International Journal of Chronobiology* **5**:369-394.
Ryder, M.L. (1979). Thyroxine and wool follicle activity. *Animal Production*

28:109-115.

Ryder, M.L. and Stephenson, S.K. (1968). *Wool Growth*. Academic Press, New York.

Samata, T. and Matsuda, M. (1988). Studies on the amino acid compositions of the equine body hair and the hoof. *Japanese Journal of Veterinary Science* **50**:333-340.

Sar, M. and Calhoun, M.L. (1966). Microscopic anatomy of the integument of the common American goat. *American Journal of Veterinary Research* **27**:444-456.

Schaller, R. and Schwarz, R. (1972). Licht-und-elektronenmikroskopische Untersuchungen am Mark Vom Grannenhaar der Katze. *Deutsche Tierärztliche Wochenschrift* **79**:573-577.

Schinckel, P.G. and Short, B.F. (1961): The influence of nutritional level during prenatal and early post-natal life on adult fleece and body characters. *Australian Journal of Agricultural Research* **12**:176-202.

Schwartzman, R.M. and Orkin, M. (1962). *Comparative Study of Skin Diseases in Dog and Man*. Charles C. Thomas Publisher, Springfield, Illinois.

Schwarz, R. *et al.* (1976). Lichtmikroskopische Untersuchungen an der Haut der Katze. *Zentralblatt. für Veterinärmedizin C* **5**:325-341.

Scott, D.W. (1982). Histopathological findings in endocrine skin disorders of the dog. *Journal of the American Animal Hospital Association* **18**:173-183.

Scott, D.W. (1986a). Vitamin A-responsive dermatosis in the cocker spaniel. *Journal of the American Animal Hospital Association* **22**:125-129.

Scott, D.W. (1986b). Localized scleroderma (morphea) in two dogs. *Journal of the American Animal Hospital Association* **22**:207-211.

Scott, D.W. (1986c). Granulomatous sebaceous adenitis in dogs. *Journal of the American Animal Hospital Association* **232**:631-634.

Scott, D.W. (1987). Sterile eosinophilic pustulosis in dog and man: Comparative aspects. *Journal of the American Academy of Dermatology* **16**:1022-1026.

Scott, D.W. (1988). *Large Animal Dermatology*. W.B. Saunders Company, Philadelphia.

Scott, D.W. (1989a). Adénite sébacée pyogranulomateuse stérile chez un chat. *Point Vétérinaire* **21**:107-111.

Scott, D.W. (1989b). Excessive trichilemmal keratinization (flame follicles) in endocrine skin disorders of the dog. *Veterinary Dermatology* **1**:37-40.

Scott, D.W. and Concannon, P.W. (1983). Gross and microscopic changes of the skin of dogs with progestagen-induced acromegaly and elevated growth hormone levels. *Journal of the American Animal Hospital Association* **19**:523-527.

Scott, D.W. and Guard, C.L. (1988). Alopecia areata in a cow. *Agri-Practice* **9**(4):16-19.

Scott, D.W. and Sheffey, B.E. (1987). Dermatosis in dogs caused by Vitamin E deficiency. *Companion Animal Practitioner* **1**(3):42-46.

Scott, D.W. and Walton, D.K. (1986). Hyposomatotropism in the mature dog: A discussion of 22 cases. *Journal of the American Animal Hospital Association* **22**:467-473.

Scott, D.W. *et al.* (1982). Iatrogenic Cushings' syndrome in cats. *Feline Practitioner* **12**:30-36.

Scott, D.W. *et al.* (1986). Sterile eosinophilic folliculitis in cattle. *Agri-Practice.* **7**(3 + 4):8-14.

Scott, D.W. *et al.* (1989). Sterile eosinophilic folliculitis in the cat: An unusual manifestation of feline allergic skin disease? *Companion Animal Practitioner* **19**(8 + 9):6-11

Seaman, W.J. and Chang, S.H. (1984). Dermal perifollicular mineralization of toy poodle bitches. *Veterinary Pathology* **21**:122-123.

Shanley, K.J. and Miller, W.H. (1987). Adult-onset growth hormone deficiency in sibling Airedale terriers. *Compendium for Continuing Education* **9**:1076-1081.

Short, B.F. (1955). Developmental modification of fleece structure by adverse nutrition. *Australian Journal of Agricultural Research* **6**:863-871.
Slappendal, R.J. (1988). Canine leishmaniasis. A review based on 95 cases in the Netherlands. *Tijdschrift voor Diergeneeskunde* **113**:3-18.
Slee, J., and Ryder, M.L. (1967). The effect of cold exposure on wool growth in Scottish blackface and Merino cross Cheviot sheep. *Journal of Agricultural Science* **69**:449-456.
Slen, S.B. and Connell, R. (1958). Wool growth in sheep as affected by the administration of certain sex hormones. *Canadian Journal of Animal Science* **38**:38-47.
Slen, S.B. and Whiting, F. (1952). Wool production as affected by the level of protein in the ration of mature ewes. *Journal of Animal Science* **11**:156-165.
Smith, J.L. and Calhoun, M.L. (1964). The microscopic anatomy of the integument of newborn swine. *American Journal of Veterinary Research* **25**:165-173.
Speed, J.G. (1960). The importance of the coat in Exmoor and other mountain and moorland ponies living out of door. *British Veterinary Journal* **116**:91-98.
Sreekumaran, T. and Rajan, A. (1978). Clinicopathological studies in experimental hypothyroidism in goats. *Veterinary Pathology* **15**:549-555.
Stephenson, S.K. (1959). Wool follicle development in the New Zealand Romney and N-type sheep. V. The prenatal relationships between growth, skin expansion, and primary follicle number. *Journal of Agricultural Research* **10**:453-470.
Strickland, J.H. and Calhoun, M.L. (1963). The integumentary system of the cat. *American Journal of Veterinary Research* **24**:1018-1029.
Sugawara, K. (1979): Presence of citrulline in the membranous protein of stratum corneum of newborn rat and cow snout. *Agricultural and Biological Chemistry* **43**:2215-2217.
Talukdar, A.H. *et al.* (1972). Microscopic anatomy of the skin of the horse. *American Journal of Veterinary Research* **33**:2365-2390.
Thomsett, L.R. (1966). Allergic and endocrine dermatoses in the dog and cat. III. Endocrine disorders and hair loss in the dog. *Journal of Small Animal Practice* **7**:777-780.
Underwood, E.J. (1977): *Trace Elements in Human and Animal Nutrition* Vol. IV. Academic Press, New York.
Vogt, D.W. *et al.* (1988). Hereditary parakeratosis in shorthorn beef calves. *American Journal of Veterinary Research* **49**:120-121.
Webb, A.J. and Calhoun, M.L. (1954). The microscopic anatomy of the skin of mongrel dogs. *American Journal of Veterinary Research* **15**:274-280.
Wentzel, D. and Vosloo, L.P, (1974). Prenatal development of hair follicle groups in Angora goats. *Agroanimalia* **6**:13-24.
Wijeratne, W.V.S. *et al.* (1988). A genetic, pathological, and virological study of congenital hypotrichosis and incisor anodontia in cattle. *Veterinary Record* **122**:149-152.
Wildman, A.B. (1932). Coat and fibre development in some British sheep. *Proceedings of the Zoological Society of London* **79**:257-285.
Wildman, A.B. (1957). Photoperiodicity and wool growth in Romney rams and wethers. *Nature* **180**:296-297.
Williams, A.J. (1964). The effect of daily photoperiods on the wool growth of Merino rams subjected to unrestricted and restricted breeding regimens. *Australian Journal of Experimental Agriculture and Animal Husbandry* **4**:124-128.
Williams, W.L. *et al.* (1946). Local inhibition of hair growth in dogs by percutaneous application of estrone. *Endocrinology* **38**:114-120.
Wilson, P.A. and Short, B.F. (1979). Cell proliferation and cortical cell production in relation to wool growth. *Australian Journal of Biological Science* **32**:317-323.

Wodzicka, M. (1960). Seasonal variations in wool growth and heat tolerance of sheep. 1. Wool growth. *Australian Journal of Agricultural Research* **11**:75-84.

Yeates, N.T.M. (1955). Photoperiodicity in cattle. I. Seasonal changes in coat character and their importance in heat regulation. *Australian Journal of Agricultural Research* **6**:891-902.

Yeates, N.T.M. (1957). Photoperiodicity in cattle. II. The equatorial light environment and its effect on the coat of European cattle. *Australian Journal of Agricultural Research* **8**:733-739.

Yeates, N.T.M. (1958). Observations on the role of nutrition in coat shedding of cattle. *Journal of Agricultural Science* **50**:110-112.

Zdelar, F. *et al.* (1981). Istrazivanja o funkcji stitnjace junadi u tovu s posebnim osvrtom na hipotireozu. I. Eksperimentalna hipotireoza: Klinicka slika, histopatoloske i histokemijske promjene. *Veterinarski Archiv* **51**:243-268.

1.2 Castration Responsive Dermatosis in the Dog

Edmund J. Rosser Jr

Assistant Professor of Dermatology, Michigan State University, Department of Small Animal Clinical Sciences, Veterinary Clinical Center, East Lansing, Michigan, USA

INTRODUCTION

Endocrine-like alopecic disorders that are not due to Cushing's disease or hypothyroidism are often very challenging and frustrating skin diseases. Many of these patients are diagnosed as having a growth hormone responsive dermatosis and after being given a series of growth hormone injections have been returned to normal (Parker and Scott, 1980; Scott and Walton, 1986; Lothrup, 1988). However, many of these patients were not treated with growth hormone to see if they indeed would improve. Also, in my experience, using the current criteria to diagnose growth hormone responsive dermatosis, some of the patients have *not* shown a response to growth hormone injections. It became apparent that some of the dogs that were intact males could be castrated and showed a subsequent complete response to castration (Rosser, 1983, personal observation; Lothrup, 1988). Also, upon reviewing the literature, many of the dogs reported to have growth hormone responsive dermatosis were intact male dogs that had not been castrated (Parker and Scott, 1980; Scott and Walton, 1986). The purpose of this paper is to specify some of the historical, clinical and histopathological features of patients with castration responsive dermatosis as well as to attempt to better understand the pathophysiology of this disease through the evaluation of several endocrine hormones.

MATERIALS AND METHODS

Six, intact, male dogs including one Alaskan malamute, three pomeranians, one chow chow and one miniature poodle were evaluated for a progressive alopecic disorder. Haemograms, serum chemistry profiles, urinalyses and skin biopsies were performed on all six dogs. Skin biopsies were fixed in 10% buffered formalin and examined histologically using a haematoxylin and oeosin stain. Endocrine tests performed included: serum basal thyroid profile (TSH unavailable at the time of this study), combination dexamethasone suppression/ACTH response test on three of the six cases (Zerbe *et al.*, 1988), serum measurement of oestradiol-17 β, testosterone and progesterone, and growth hormone stimulation test. The growth hormone stimulation tests were performed as follows: a basal growth hormone serum sample, followed by the administration of 0.1 mg/kg of xylazine (Rompun^R) given intravenously, followed by 15 and 30 min postinjection growth hormone serum samples (Hampshire and Aaltszuler, 1981). After evaluation of the above data, a recommendation of castration was made for all six dogs and the testicles submitted for histopathological examination. When possible, after the patients hair had regrown, serum samples for measurement of oestradiol-17 β, testosterone, progesterone, and growth hormone stimulation tests were repeated.

RESULTS

Case 1

An 8-year-old, intact, male, Alaskan malamute weighing 54.5 kg, was presented to the hospital for alopecia that first developed at 6 years of age. The alopecia was first noted to develop around the neck, followed by hyperpigmentation and excess scaling. Similar changes developed on the tail, perineal region, flanks and the ventral and lateral chest. Upon physical examination, additional findings included a diffuse thinning of the hair on the trunk and a dull, dry hair coat. Historically, the testicles had descended normally and were palpably normal on physical exam. Results of the haemogram, serum chemistry profile, urinalysis and combination dexamethasone suppression/ACTH response tests were normal. Results of the serum basal thyroid profile, serum measurement of oestradiol-17 β, testosterone, progesterone and growth hormone stimulation tests are shown in Tables 1–5. Abnormalities included: below normal basal serum total T_3 and free T_3, elevated serum oestradiol-17 β, below normal serum testosterone and a low basal serum growth hormone with a poor response to xylazine stimulation. Histopathological examination of skin biopsies revealed atrophy of primary and secondary hair follicles, atrophy of sebaceous and apocrine glands, orthokeratotic hyperkeratosis, hypermelanosis, follicular hyperkeratosis, and hyperoeosinophilic tricholemmal keratinization (Plate 4) (Dunstan, 1986). Eight weeks later, small tufts of hair had grown at the previous skin biopsy sites. The patient was put on sodium levothyroxine (Soloxine^R) at a dosage of 1.2 mg given orally twice daily for 8 weeks and re-

Table 1 Serum basal thyroid profiles

Case No.	Total T_4 ng/ml	Total T_3 ng/ml	Free T_4 pg/ml	Free T_3 pg/ml
1	17.7	0.61	4.80	2.40
2	21.3	0.70	8.60	3.20
3	22.4	0.83	9.10	3.30
4[a]	47.4	1.30	ND	4.00
5	12.6	1.20	6.80	5.10
6	16.6	0.71	6.20	4.40
Normals	10.40	0.75-2.0	3.18	3.2-6.4

[a] Sample was a 6 h postpill evaluation of thyroid hormones.
ND: not done.

Table 2 Serum oestradiol- β

Case No.	Precastration pg/ml	Postcastration pg/ml
1	7.00	0.80
ND	12.0	ND
3	11.0	1.00
Normals	2.0-6.2	
4	107	38[a]
5	40	10
6	95	ND
Normal avg. (Different lab)	24	

[a] Sample taken 6 years postcastration.
ND: not done.

Table 3 Serum testosterone

Case No.	Precastration ng/ml	Postcastration ng/ml
1	0.29	0.02
2	4.36	ND
3	2.26	0.00
4	3.50	0.00[a]
5	5.38	0.10
6	1.82	ND
Normals	0.75-4.0	

[a] Sample taken 6 years postcastration.
ND: not done.

Table 4 Serum progesterone

Case No.	Precastration ng/ml	Postcastration ng/ml
1	0.10	0.80
2	0.00	ND
3	QNS	ND
4	QNS	ND
5	0.38	0.30
6	0.10	ND
Normals	<1.0	

ND: not done.
QNS: quantity not sufficient.

Table 5 Growth hormone stimulation tests.

Case No	Baseline ng/ml	15 min post ng/ml	30 min post ng/ml
1 Pre	0.0	1.00	0.80
Post	0.0	0.60	0.70
2 Pre	6.44	22.17	44.70
Post	ND	ND	ND
3 Pre	0.50	0.50	0.90
Post	0.70	0.70	1.11
4 Pre	ND	ND	ND
Post[a]	1.0	1.0	1.0
5 Pre	1.0	1.0	1.0
Post	1.0	1.0	1.0
6 Pre	0.50	0.70	0.60
Post	ND	ND	ND
Normals	1.0–7.0	5–27	5–27

[a] Sample submitted 6 years postcastration.
ND: not done.

examined. The alopecia had progressed and a 6 h, postpill serum thyroid profile revealed all thyroid values to be well within normal limits. The sodium levothyroxine therapy was discontinued and a recommendation was made that the dog be castrated and the testicles submitted for histopathologic examination. The testicles were histopathologically normal. The skin and hair coat were normal 3 months later, and results of serum oestradiol-17 β, testosterone, progesterone and growth hormone stimulation tests are shown in Tables 2–5. The results of the reproductive hormones measured were within the range expected for a castrated male dog and the growth hormone stimulation test results remained abnormally low.

Case 2

A 2-year-old, intact, male, pomeranian, weighing 1.6 kg, was presented to the hospital for alopecia that was first noted at 1 year old. The alopecia began in the perineal and neck region, followed by hyperpigmentation and excess scaling. Additional findings on physical examination included a patchy alopecia over the trunk and a dull, dry hair coat. Prior to admission the dog had been treated with sodium levothyroxine, 0.1 mg given orally twice daily for 9 months with no improvement. History of testicular development, testicular palpitation, and the results of haemograms, serum chemistry profile and urinalysis were all normal. A combination dexamethasone suppression/ACTH response test was not performed. Remaining endocrine tests are shown in Tables 1-5. Abnormalities included; below normal serum basal total T_3, elevated serum oestradiol-17 β, mildly elevated serum testosterone and low serum progesterone. Results of the growth hormone stimulation test were normal. Examination of skin biopsies revealed the same changes as noted for Case 1. Eight weeks later, small tufts of hair had grown at the previous skin biopsy sites. It was recommended that the dog be castrated and the testicles were examined histologically and were normal. The skin and hair coat were normal 3 months later. Reproductive hormone analysis and growth hormone tests were not repeated.

Case 3

A 2-year-old, intact, male, chow chow, weighing 21.8 kg, was presented to the hospital for alopecia and a change in hair coat colour that was first noted at 1 year old. The alopecia first developed around the neck, perineal region, flanks and ventral trunk, followed by hyperpigmentation, excess scaling and a change in hair coat colour from tan to a rust colour with black streaks. Additional findings on physical examination included a patchy alopecia over the trunk and a dull, dry hair coat. History of testicular development, testicular palpation, results of haemogram, serum chemistry profile and urinalysis were all normal. A combination dexamethasone suppression/ACTH response test was not performed. Remaining endocrine tests are shown in Tables 1-5. Abnormalities included; elevated oestradiol-17 β and a low basal serum growth hormone with a poor response to xylazine stimulation. Examination of skin biopsies revealed the same changes as noted for Case 1. Eight weeks later small tufts of hair had grown at the previous skin biopsy sites. It was recommended that the dog be castrated and the testicles were histologically examined and were normal. There was a complete regrowth of hair 3 months later, and the coat colour returned to normal. The reproductive hormone analyses and growth hormone stimulation test results are shown in Tables 2-5. The results of the reproductive hormones measured were within the range expected for a castrated male dog and the growth hormone stimulation results remained abnormally low.

Case 4

A 5-year-old, intact, male, pomeranian, weighing 4.8 kg, was presented to the hospital for alopecia that was first noted at 3.5 years of age. The alopecia first developed around the neck, tail and perineal region followed by hyperpigmentation and excess scaling. Additional findings on physical examination included a patchy alopecia over the trunk and a dull, dry hair coat. The dog had been treated with sodium levothyroxine at a dosage of 0.1 mg given orally twice daily for 1 year with no response and the medication had been stopped 1 week prior to presentation. History of testicular development, testicular palpation, results of haemogram, serum chemistry profile and urinalysis were all normal. A serum basal thryoid profile, combination dexamethasone suppression/ACTH response test and growth hormone stimulation test were not performed. Remaining endocrine tests are shown in Tables 2–4. Abnormalities included an elevated serum oestradiol-17 β. Examination of skin biopsies revealed the same changes as noted for Case 1. Eight weeks later, small tufts of hair had regrown at the previous skin biopsy sites. The dog was castrated and the testicles were histologically examined and were normal; 3 months later the skin and hair had returned to normal. Shortly after this the owners moved and were temporarily lost to follow-up. The dog represented to the hospital 6 years later because of the redevelopment of alopecia at 11 years of age. This recurrence of alopecia was first noted over the perineal region, medial thighs, tail and around the neck, followed by hyperpigmentation, excess scaling and a change in the hair coat colour from tan to rust coloured. The dog had been placed on sodium levothyroxine at a dosage of 0.1 mg given orally twice daily for the past year with no improvement. A 6 h postpill serum thyroid profile revealed all thyroid values to be well within normal limits. A combination dexamethasone suppression/ACTH response test was normal. The 6-year post-castration reproductive hormone analyses and growth hormone stimulation test are shown in Tables 2–5. Abnormalities included; elevated serum oestradiol-17 β (but lower than before castration), zero testosterone and a low basal serum growth hormone with no response to xylazine stimulation. Skin biopsies revealed the same changes as noted 6 years previously and as noted in Case 1, and 8 weeks later, small tufts of hair had regrown at the skin biopsy sites. The dog was placed on methyltestosterone at a dosage of 0.5 mg given orally every other day for 2 months, followed by the same dosage given only once weekly. After 4 months of treatment there has been a gradual regrowth of hair but not a total regrowth at the time of this most recent evaluation.

Case 5

A 4-year-old, intact, male, pomeranian weighing 2.5 kg, presented to the hospital for alopecia that was first noted at 2 years of age. The alopecia first developed around the neck (Plate 5), perineal region, entire ventral trunk and the medial and posterior thighs, followed by hyperpigmentation (Plate 6), excess scaling and a change in the hair coat colour from tan to rust coloured with black streaks (Plate 7). History of testicular development, testicular palpation, results of haemogram, serum chemistry profile and urinalysis were all normal. The results of a combination dexamethasone suppression/ACTH response test were normal. Remaining endocrine tests are shown in Tables 1–5. Abnormalities included; elevated serum oestradiol-17 β, elevated serum testosterone and low basal serum growth hormone with no response to xylazine stimulation. Examination of skin biopsies revealed the same changes as noted in Case 1. Small tufts of hair had grown at the previous skin biopsy sites 6 weeks later. The dog was castrated and the testicles histologically examined which were normal. The hair had regrown and the hair colour returned to normal 3 months later (Plate 8). The reproductive hormones and the growth hormone stimulation test are shown in Tables 2–5. The results of the reproductive hormones measured were within the range expected for a castrated male dog and the growth hormone stimulation test results remained abnormally low.

Case 6

An 8-year-old, intact, male, miniature poodle, weighing 7.3 kg, presented to the hospital for alopecia that was first noted at 4 years of age. The alopecia first developed in the perineal region, medial and lateral thighs, and ventral trunk followed by hyperpigmentation and excess scaling. At the time of physical examination 80% of the hair on the trunk had been lost and there was concurrent hyperpigmentation and excess scaling. History of testicular development, testicular palpation, results of haemogram, serum chemistry profile and urinalysis were all normal. A combination dexamethasone suppression/ACTH response test was normal. Remaining endocrine tests are shown in Tables 1–5. Abnormalities included; below normal basal serum total T_3, elevated serum oestradiol-17 β and low basal serum growth hormone with a poor response to xylazine stimulation. Examination of skin biopsies revealed the same changes as noted for Case 1. Six weeks later, small tufts of hair had grown at the previous skin biopsy sites. The dog was castrated and the testicles histologically examined which were normal. There was only a partial regrowth of hair 3 months later and the skin was no longer scaly. Follow-up reproductive hormone analysis and growth hormone stimulation tests were not performed. The dog was subsequently placed on sodium levothyroxine at a dosage of 0.2 mg given orally twice daily for the past 1.5 years with no further improvement.

SUMMARY OF ABNORMAL FINDINGS PRIOR TO CASTRATION

Below normal serum basal total T_3 was found in three out of six cases, below normal serum basal free T_3 in one out of six cases, above normal serum oestradiol-17 in six out of six cases, above normal serum testosterone in two out of six cases, below normal serum testosterone in one out of six cases and a low basal serum growth hormone with a poor response to xylazine stimulation in five out of six cases.

Major dermatologic abnormalities included: alopecia, hyperpigmentation and excess scaling of the neck, perineal region, tail, ventral trunk and medial and lateral thighs, with a dull dry hair coat. Some patients also developed changes in the colour of the hair coat.

DISCUSSION

The most consistent abnormalities discovered in this study were an above normal serum oestradiol-17 β and a low basal serum growth hormone with a poor response to xylazine stimulation. However, the only appreciable change in these hormone values postcastration and after there had been regrowth of hair was a decrease in the serum oestradiol-17 β. A similarly abnormal growth hormone stimulation test remained in the patients that it was measured. This suggests that the growth hormone dysfunction documented in these patients is not the primary cause of the alopecic disorder. This can also be supported by the observation that abnormally low serum level basal growth hormone with a poor response to xylazine stimulation may be normal for certain breeds of dogs such as the pomeranian (Schmeitzel and Lothrop, 1988). At least one possible cause for the disorder seems to be a primary reproductive hormone imbalance, possibly an above normal serum oestradiol-17 β. Based on the above noted abnormalities, the following recommendations are made; if the dog is an intact male, that has an elevated serum oestradiol-17 β, that regrows a tuft of hair at previous skin biopsy sites (which is not a change that the author has noticed in patients with either Cushing's disease or hypothyroidism), and has the clinical signs and histophatologic changes in the skin as described in this paper, then the recommended treatment of choice at this time is castration. I have been made aware of cases that fulfil the above criteria and respond to castration, only to later develop a similar alopecic disorder several years later (as observed in one patient in this study (Case 4) which is currently responding to methyltestosterone replacement therapy). Many of these patients have subsequently been treated with various reproductive hormone replacements or growth hormone injections and regrown their hair back in a normal pattern. Certainly, much more investigative work needs to be done to further clarify this disorder.

REFERENCES

Dunstan, R.W. (1986). Selected pathology case reports. *Proceedings of the Annual Meeting of the American Academy of Veterinary Dermatology, New Orleans, 1986*, p. 25.

Hampshire, J. and Aaltszuler, N. (1981). Clonidine or xylazine as provocative tests for growth hormone secretion in the dog. *American Journal of Veterinary Research* **43**:1073-1076.

Lothrup, C.D. (1988). Pathophysiology of canine growth hormone-responsive alopecia. *The Compendium of Continuing Education* **10**:1346-1349.

Parker, W.M. and Scott D.W. (1980). Growth hormone responsive alopecia in the mature dog: a discussion of 13 cases. *Journal of the American Animal Hospital Association* **16**:824-828.

Schmeitzel, L.P. and Lothrup, C.D. (1988). Evaluation of hormonal abnormalities in normal coated pomeranians and pomeranians with growth hormone responsive dermatosis. *Proceedings of the Annual Meeting of the American College of Veterinary Dermatology, Washington DC, 1988*, p. 29.

Scott, D.W. and Walton, D.K. (1986). Hyposomatotropism in the mature dog: a discussion of 22 cases. *Journal of the American Animal Hospital Association* **22**:467-473.

Zerbe, C.A., Refsal, K.R., Schall, W.D., Nachreiner, R.F. and Gossain, V.V. (1988). Adrenal function in 15 dogs with insulin-dependent diabetes mellitus. *Journal of the American Veterinary Medical Association* **193**:454-456.

1.3 Canine Hereditary Black Hair Follicular Dysplasia and Colour Mutant Alopecia: Clinical and Histopathological Aspects

Didier N. Carlotti

Docteur Vétérinaire, Sainte Eulalie, Carbon-Blanc, France

INTRODUCTION

Hereditary alopecias are uncommon in the dog and are very frustrating for the owners, breeders and veterinarians. Colour mutant alopecia (CMA) has been reported since 1975 (Austin, 1975) and black hair follicular dysplasia (BHFD) since 1972 (Selmanowitz *et al.*, 1972).

Colour mutant alopecia is a hereditary tardive alopecia seen in blue and fawn mutants of 11 breeds, whereas hereditary black hair follicular dysplasia has been reported in five pure breeds and mongrels (Table 1) (Austin, 1975; Briggs and Botha, 1986; Ferrer *et al.*, 1988; Foil, 1985; O'Neil, 1981;

Table 1 Reported affected breeds

Colour mutant alopecia	Black hair follicular dysplasia
Doberman pinscher (blue and red and fawn)	Bearded collie
Miniature pinscher (blue)	Dachshund
Irish setter (fawn)	Schipperke
Dachshund (blue)	Bassett hound
Chow-chow (blue)	Papillon
Poodle (blue)	Mongrel
Great dane (blue)	
Whippet (blue)	
Yorkshire terrier (blue)	
Chihuahua (blue)	

Selmanowitz *et al.*, 1977). Colour mutant alopecia usually appears between 3 months and 3 years of age. Black hair follicular dysplasia seems to be less tardive (1 month of age in the original report) (Selmanowitz, 1972), but the puppies do not seem to be affected at birth.

Colour mutant alopecia only appears in the diluted colour areas. In breeds with tan points, these points remain normal and in the one-colour breeds, all the skin is affected. The alopecia is partial and the hair looks dry and dull. Secondary seborrhoea sicca and bacterial folliculitis are common. Black hair follicular dysplasia affects only the black hair coat areas of partially black dogs. The alopecia is partial to subtotal and associated with scaliness.

Diagnosis of both conditions is made by assessment of history, physical examination and histopathology. Follicular keratosis has been described in both diseases, and clumping of melanin was found within hair follicles of dogs affected with CMA and in one case of BHFD (Gosselin *et al.*, 1982). A genetic study of a family of miniature pinschers has shown that the relationship between CMA and the dilute coat colour allele d is not complete (the genotype of blue dogs is dd) (Langeback, 1986). Actually the genetic factors of both diseases are not yet known.

MATERIAL AND METHODS

Colour mutant alopecia was suspected in eight dogs: one blue and tan chihuahua, two blue and tan doberman pinschers, one blue Italian greyhound, one blue standard poodle, two Yorkshire terriers and a miniature pinscher. These dogs were non-pruritic and had suffered from partial seborrhoeic alopecia in the blue areas of the coat since they were several months old. The remaining hair was dry and dull (Plates 9, 11).

Black hair follicular dysplasia was suspected in three dogs: one black and white cocker spaniel, one black and white pointer and one gordon setter. These dogs showed no pruritus and a partial to subtotal seborrhoeic alopecia in the black areas of the coat (Plates 10, 12, 13).

Routine histopathology was performed on all the dogs (haematoxylin and eosin (HE) staining). When bacterial folliculitis and demodicosis were suspected, cutaneous cytology and bacteriology and skin scrapings were performed. The thyrotropin (TSH) response test was performed in four of the 11 dogs.

RESULTS

Histopathology was very similar in the 11 dogs in areas without secondary bacterial infection.

The most important lesions were:

Mild-to-moderate epidermal melanosis; epidermal melanosis;

orthokeratotic hyperkeratosis;
cystic hair follicles and follicular keratosis;
variable follicular atrophy and hair dystrophy;
prominent clumping of melanin both within and around hair follicles with many melanophages surrounding the base of the follicles;
aggregates of melanin in the hair cortex and medulla.

In cases of seborrhoea sicca, mild hyperplastic perivascular dermatitis was noticed. Folliculitis/furunculosis was confirmed by skin biopsies taken in the infected cutaneous areas of the two blue doberman with CMA and the gordon setter with BHFD. One blue doberman pinscher had generalized demodicosis which was controlled after a few months of amitraz therapy.

DISCUSSION

Black hair folllicular dysplasia in gordon setters and pointers has not been reported in the literature. Our cases of CMA were similar to those described previously (Muller *et al.*, 1989). Histopathology showed consistent clumping of melanin both within and around hair follicles. The histopathological findings in our three cases of BHFD were very similar to those seen in CMA, so one cannot differentiate the two diseases by routine histopathology.

Hair loss in CMA could be due to:

hypoactive follicles, producing small dystrophic hairs which do not reach the surface of the skin (Briggs and Botha, 1986);
blockage of follicular orifices by keratin (Briggs and Botha, 1986);
breakage of hair shafts at the site of melanin aggregates (Brignac *et al.*, 1988).

The same mechanisms could lead to alopecia in BHFD, and could be the consequences of defects of epithelialization and melanization identical in both diseases. The manifestation of these defects could be more important in blue or black areas. The abnormal melanization could be due to a melanocyte stimulating hormone (MSH) deficiency, which causes an aggregation of melanin granules into clumps, whereas normal MSH secretion causes dispersion of these granules (Langeback, 1986).

The genetic factors of the two diseases could be the same, since CMA does not seem to be linked to the d allele. The dd genotype could increase the incidence of the disease, possibly by increasing the MSH deficiency. Further studies are needed, particularly in cases of BHFD.

Secondary folliculitis can occur spontaneously in both diseases, although inappropriate steroid therapy, without a clinical diagnosis, could increase the incidence of pyoderma in these diseases. In cases of folliculitis, pruritus can occur but will disappear after antibacterial therapy; in allergic conditions leading to secondary folliculitis, pruritus is still present after such a therapy, alopecia when it exists is mainly due to self-trauma, and histopathology is not comparable.

When CMA or BHFD are suspected, skin biopsies should be performed systematically. Affected dogs should not be used for breeding, particularly when the diagnosis is made early — i.e. when alopecia occurs at a few months of age and the diagnosis is confirmed by histopathology. The same applies even in cases of delayed-onset disease.

REFERENCES

Austin, V. (1975). Blue dog disease. *Modern Veterinary Practice* **36**: 31-34.

Briggs, O.M. and Botha, W.S. (1986). Colour mutant alopecia in a blue Italian greyhound. *Journal of the American Animal Hospital Association* **22**: 611-614.

Brignac, M.M., Foil, C.S., Kareem Al-Bagdadi, F.A. and Kreeger, J. (1988). Microscopy of color mutant alopecia. *Abstracts of the Annual Meeting of the American Academy of Veterinary Dermatology and American College of Veterinary Dermatology, Washington, 1988*, pp. 14-15.

Ferrer, L., Durral, I., Closa, J. and Mascort, J. (1988). Colour mutant alopecia in Yorkshire terriers. *Veterinary Record* **122**: 360-361.

Foil, C.S. (1985). Comparative genodermatoses. *Clinical Dermatology* **3**: 175-181.

Gosselin, Y., Papageorges, M. and Teuscher, E. (1982). Black hair follicular dysplasia in a dog. *Canine Practice* **9**: 8-15.

Langeback, R. (1986). Variation in hair coat and skin texture in blue dogs. *Nordisk Veterinaermedicin* **38**: 383-387.

Muller, G.H., Kirk, R.W. and Scott, D.W. (1989). *Small Animal Dermatology*. W.B. Saunders Company, Philadelphia, 1007 pp.

O'Neil, C.S. (1981). Hereditary skin disease in the dog and in the cat. *The Compendium of Continuing Education* **3**: 791-800.

Selmanowitz, V.J., Kramer, K.M. and Orentreich, N. (1972). Canine hereditary black hair follicular dysplasia. *Journal of Heredity* **63**: 43-44.

Selmanowitz, V.J., Markotsky, J, and Orentreich, N. (1977). Black hair follicular dysplasia in dogs. *Journal of the American Veterinary Association* **171**: 1079-1081.

1.4 Aspects of Feline Symmetric Alopecia

K.L. Thoday

Senior Lecturer in Veterinary Medicine, Department of Veterinary Clinical Studies, Royal (Dick) School of Veterinary Studies, University of Edinburgh, Edinburgh, Scotland

INTRODUCTION

Despite the many endocrine synonyms for the condition, feline symmetric alopecia (FSA) is a condition of multiple aetiology which, when a specific diagnosis cannot be established, may respond well to a number of hormonal regimens. Recently, a number of workers have questioned the existence of any endocrine aetiology suggesting that FSA is usually a manifestation of the psychogenic alopecia and dermatitis complex or hypersensitivity responses. With the exception of a single report, all descriptions of the condition have appeared in review articles/book chapters and have been unsupported by detailed data. This study was therefore carried out to investigate further the possible causes, historical and physical features, biochemical changes, particularly with respect to thyroid function, and the management of FSA.

MATERIALS AND METHODS

The case material comprised 51 consecutive cats referred to me with a diagnosis of FSA. Two cases were lost to follow-up after the first examination and 49 cats were therefore studied in detail.

History, physical and laboratory examinations

Prior to referral, practitioners were directed to instruct owners to discontinue any treatment for a minimum of 6 weeks.

In all cases, a detailed history was taken. This included confirmation of compliance with discontinuing previous drug therapy and questions with respect to grooming behaviour (the presence or absence of excessive licking or scratching or biting and pulling at the hair), whether increased amount of hair was being found in the environment and the possibilities for secret grooming. In addition, owners were questioned on possible alterations in the environment or other potential stress factors which may have occurred around the time of onset of the hair loss.

A full physical examination was then carried out which included assessing the texture of the coat by palpation for stubble, for pruritus by digital stimulation and the ease of epilation of remaining hairs by traction using epilation forceps. In addition, the neck from the larynx to the thoracic inlet was examined meticulously for evidence of goitre.

Subsequently a number of laboratory examinations were carried out in all cats. Animals were evaluated for self-induced hair loss by the microscopic examination of the distal ends of 30 hairs plucked from affected areas. Cats were checked for dermatophytosis using ultraviolet (UV) light and direct microscopic examination and culture, on Sabouraud's dextrose agar and nutrient agar each containing 0.4 mg/ml chloramphenicol and 0.5 mg/ml actidione, of material obtained by dry skin scraping and epilation. Examination for ectoparasites was made macroscopically and microscopically after deep skin scraping.

Faecal samples for examination for endoparasite eggs were obtained by manual removal per rectum or, where this was impossible, were collected by the owners, and subsequently examined in saturated saline in a McMaster counting chamber.

Blood samples were collected from conscious animals by jugular venipuncture after 12 h starvation. Total cholesterol concentrations were determined by a spectrophotometric kit technique (Gilchem). For thyroid hormone determinations, sera were stored at $-40°C$ and samples examined in batch mode. Total thyroxine (T_4) and total triiodothyronine (T_3) concentrations were measured by double antibody radioimmunoassays optimized and validated for use with cat serum as described by Thoday *et al.* (1984). Normal ranges were established by the non-parametric method of percentile estimates using measurements from 318 healthy cats for T_4 and 299 healthy cats for T_3. In addition to the above tests, complete blood counts were carried out on 41 cats.

Further investigations were carried out into the thyroid status of six cats with idiopathic feline symmetric alopecia (IFSA) by using the thyrotropin (TSH) stimulation test previously optimized and validated for use in cats (Thoday, 1986). Only one of these cases had had any thyroid therapy prior to referral (20 μg T_3 three times daily) which resulted in partial hair regrowth. Three cases were totally, and two partially responsive (the latter group including the animal which had partially responded to T_3 treatment by the referring veterinary surgeon) and one was non-responsive to treatment with T_3 (see subsequently). Prior to carrying out the tests, T_3 was discontinued for 8 weeks and serum thyroid hormone concentrations were determined to ensure there was no residual therapeutic suppression and elevation of serum T_4 and T_3 concentrations respectively. For this test, a blood sample was taken between 09.00 and 10.00 h, 0.5 IU/kg bovine TSH (Thyrotropar ®, Armour) was administered intravenously and a second sample taken 6 h later. Sera were assayed as described previously. The results were compared to those obtained from 16 healthy cats using the Mann-Whitney U test.

Diagnostic approaches and treatment protocols

With the exception of the cases of mastocytosis and pediculosis, all other cats were initially treated for fleas at weekly intervals for 6 weeks with topical 0.2% dichlorvos and 0.8% fenitrothion combination (Nuvan Top®, Ciba Geigy) together with routine vacuum-cleaning and subsequent treatment of the environment with a combination of 2.0% iodofenphos and 0.5% dichlorvos (Nuvan Staykil®, Ciba Geigy) and were blood-sampled again at this time. An Elizabethan collar was used on the remaining animals for 6 weeks. A diagnosis of IFSA was based on the history, physical examination, absence of fractured distal hair shafts on microscopic examination, absence of ectoparasites macro- and microscopically, negative UV light examination, failure to demonstrate dermatophytes microscopically or on culture and no response to flea-control measures and the wearing of an Elizabethan collar.

All cases of IFSA were treated with liothyronine sodium (L-T_3, Tertroxin®, Pitman-Moore) at an initial dose of 20 μg/cat twice daily, increasing by 10 μg twice daily every third day, to a maximum of 50 μg twice daily. Cats were re-inspected 3, 8 and 12 weeks after beginning T_3 treatment and intermittently thereafter. Twelve weeks after beginning T_3 treatment, blood samples for serum T_4 and T_3 concentrations were determined 3 h after dosing with 50 μg T_3. The response was subsequently classified as total (hair regrowth complete), partial (either hair regrowth in some sites but not others or general hair regrowth which was not complete) or no response (no change in the condition). Treatment of some cases in the last two groups was by: (i) L-thyroxine sodium (L-T_4, Eltroxin®, Glaxo) at an oral dosage of 50 μg twice daily and subsequently 100 μg twice daily; (ii) depot injections of a preparation containing 21 mg of a combination of four testosterone esters (Durateston®, Intervet Laboratories) administered initially at monthly intervals; (iii) megestrol acetate (Ovarid®, Pitman-Moore) at an initial oral dosage of 5 mg every third day, reducing after 3 weeks to 2.5 mg every third day and subsequently to the lowest possible maintenance dosage (usually 2.5 mg once or twice weekly).

RESULTS

Ultraviolet light examination, direct microscopy and culture for dermatophytes, examination of skin scrapings for ectoparasites and faecal examinations for endoparasite eggs were negative in all 51 cats.

Idiopathic feline symmetric alopecia (IFSA) (Groups 1, 2 and 3)

This was diagnosed in 26 cats.

Historical data

These data are presented in Table 1.

Table 1 Historical data for cases of idiopathic feline symmetric alopecia and definitively diagnosed symmetric alopecia

Group	Breed	Sex (%)	Age at onset (years)
IFSA cases (n = 26)	24 Domestic short-haired 1 Persian cross 1 Burmese cross	15 NF (57.8) 10 NM (38.5) 1 EM (3.7)	1–11 ($\bar{x}$ — 4.5)
Group 1: T_3 totally responsive (n=19)	17 Domestic short-haired 1 Persian cross 1 Burmese cross	9 NF (47.4) 9 NM (47.4) 1 EM (5.2)	1–11 ($\bar{x}$ — 4.3)
Group 2 T_3 partially responsive (n=4)	4 Domestic short-haired	3 NF (75) 1 NM (25)	1.3–6 ($\bar{x}$ — 4.5)
Group 3: T_3 non-responsive (n = 3)	3 Domestic short-haired	3 NF (100)	2.3–8 ($\bar{x}$ — 5.8)
DFSA cases Group 4 (n = 23)	23 Domestic short-haired	10 NF (43.5) 9 NM (39.1) 3 EF (13.0) 1 EM (4.4)	<1–11[a] ($\bar{x}$ — 5.2)

[a] Age at onset based on 22 cases as information unknown for one animal.
DFSA: Definitively diagnosed feline symmetric alopecia.
IFSA: Idiopathic feline symmetric alopecia.
n: Number of observations. $\bar{x}$: Mean.
NF: Neutered female. NM: Neutered male. EM: Entire male. EF: Entire female.

Of the 23 neutered animals where the age at surgery was accurately known, only one had been neutered after 9 months of age. The latent period between neutering and the onset of alopecia ranged from 6 months to 10.5 years with a mean of 4.1 years. The duration of physical signs before referral ranged from 2 weeks to 7 years. No significant variation of onset of alopecia between the months was identified using the Chi-Square (χ^2) test. Seven animals (26.9%) showed symptoms of involvement of other systems in addition to the skin.

These were lethargy (four cases), vomiting of hair (three), and obesity and inappetence (one each).

Seventeen of the cats had received some form of treatment before being referred. These treatments included progestogens (megestrol acetate (12 cats), proligesterone (two)), thyroid hormones (T_3 (three), desiccated thyroid (two)), glucocorticoids (five), methyltestosterone (three) and methyltestosterone and ethinyloestradiol combination (two). In 14 of these, there had been no improvement of the condition. Three cases had shown variable response to a number of drugs (one to T_3, one to each of megestrol acetate, methyltestosterone and to T_3 and one to depot testosterone but not to methyltestosterone/ethinyloestradiol combination, megestrol acetate or proligesterone) but had relapsed at varying intervals after the cessation of treatment.

Physical and laboratory findings

Pretreatment data. The coat changes consisted of bilaterally symmetric alopecia with or without a well-demarcated division between affected and non-affected areas. Generally, there was diffuse thinning of hair over affected sites rather than complete alopecia, although this varied considerably. The remaining primary hairs could be easily epilated. In some cases, secondary hairs could also be easily removed but, in others, epilation could only be achieved with difficulty. Remaining hairs showed no evidence of the distal ends of the shafts being broken when examined microscopically.

The distribution of alopecia was very variable and is shown in Table 2. An example of a severe case is shown in Plate 14A. In general, animals in which the problem was long-standing tended to be more severely affected but this was not universal. In no case were macroscopic skin changes or evidence of pruritus noted.

The mean values and ranges for the other physical and for the laboratory findings of the 26 cats before and after treatment with T_3 are presented in Table 3, divided retrospectively into three groups according to their response to T_3 therapy.

In three cats (one subsequently in each of Groups 1, 2 and 3) the serum T_4 concentration was greater than the upper limit of the reference range. In two, the elevation was marginal (Group 1 cat, 0.2 nmol/1; Group 2 cat, 4.6 nmol/1) while in the Group 3 cat it was 13.6 nmol/1. None of the cats had historical or physical findings suggestive of hyperthyroidism and palpable goitre was not present. A T_3 suppression test using 20 μg T_3 three times daily for seven doses prior to repeat blood sampling 3 h after the last T_3 dose showed reductions of serum T_4 concentrations to 7%, 40% and 6% of the basal concentrations (Groups 1, 2 and 3 cats respectively) suggesting that the raised basal serum T_4 concentrations were not due to thyrotoxicosis. The animals were followed-up for periods of between 2 and 4 years and none developed historical or physical features or laboratory values suggestive of hyperthyroidism.

Table 2 Comparison of distribution of alopecia in cats with idiopathic symmetric alopecia and cats in which the cause of the symmetric alopecia was definitively diagnosed

Site	% Cases affected					
	IFSA Cases				DFSA Cases[a]	
	Groups 1, 2 & 3	Group 1	Group 2	Group 3	Group 4	DFSA with lesions confined to IFSA sites
	(n = 26)	(n = 19)	(n = 4)	(n = 3)	(n = 23)	(n = 16)
Ventral abdomen and medial hind legs	96.2	89.5	100	100	92.0	94.7
Lateral hind legs	57.7	63.2	50.0	33.3	60.0	57.9
Caudal hind legs	50.0	63.2	—	33.3	12.0	5.3
Forelegs	46.2	42.1	75.0	33.3	44.0	42.1
Anogenital region	19.2	15.8	—	33.3	8.0	10.5
Lateral abdomen	19.2	21.1	—	33.3	32.0	36.8
Ventral thorax	11.5	10.5	—	33.3	12.0	15.8
Axillae	7.7	10.5	—	—	8.0	10.5
Lateral thorax	7.7	10.5	—	—	12.0	15.8
Dorsal lumbar region	—	—	—	—	21.7	—
Base of pinnae	—	—	—	—	4.4	—
Median raphé, upper lip	—	—	—	—	4.4	—

[a] Eight cats in the DFSA group had skin lesions (discussed in text) in addition to alopecia.
DFSA: Definitely diagnosed feline symmetric alopecia.
IFSA: Idiopathic feline symmetric alopecia.
n: Number of observations.

Posttreatment data. Historical data for the three response groups are compared in Table 1 and show no obvious difference in the age at onset between them. Both the cross-bred pedigree cats were T_3 totally responsive. While there were equal numbers of neutered males and neutered females in the T_3 totally responsive group, neutered females accounted for 75% and 100% of the T_3 partially and T_3 non-responsive groups respectively.

Liothyronine totally responsive group (Group 1). Initial evidence of regrowth of hair was obvious at a mean of 3.9 weeks (range 3–10 weeks) and was complete by 22 weeks in all but one cat (mean 18.8 weeks; range 12–34 weeks). An example of a typical response is shown in Plate 14B.

Other symptoms associated with IFSA (lethargy, lethargy and inappetence and vomiting of hair) in this group resolved in three cats respectively and one other owner reported that the appetite and activity of her cat had improved although she had not initially reported these as being abnormal.

A Grade II (of V) soft, systolic, cardiac murmur with a split-second sound developed in one cat after 3 weeks of T_3 therapy. The heart rate was 188 beats/min. No evidence of cardiac enlargement was seen radiographically but the ECG revealed evidence of left anterior fascicular block and ventricular premature beats. These abnormalities resolved after the T_3 therapy was stopped. Treatment was changed to monthly injections of depot testosterone. Hair was growing well 3 months later, and no cardiac abnormalities could be detected. This cat is considered in this group because it had previously responded totally to T_3 therapy administered by the referring veterinary surgeon.

In the first three animals treated long-term with T_3, the dosage was reduced every 4 weeks by 10 μg twice daily. In two, hair loss became evident at a dosage of 40 μg twice daily and in one at 20 μg twice daily. The alopecia resolved once the T_3 was increased to 50 μg twice daily. In all but three subsequent cases, the lowest effective maintenance dose of T_3 was determined. In three animals, T_3 was reduced as described and eventually discontinued without recurrence of alopecia. Two animals did not require subsequent treatment. One was treated at a dosage of 50 μg T_3 twice daily when relapses occurred. In the remaining 15 cats, the mean required maintenance dosage of T_3 was 37.5 μg twice daily (range 20–50 μg twice daily).

Liothyronine partially responsive group (Group 2). Initial evidence of regrowth of hair was obvious at a mean of 10 weeks (range 3–22 weeks). Of the four animals, in two the response was acceptable to the owners and the cats were maintained on 50 μg T_3 twice daily. Response to other treatments (testosterone or megestrol acetate) in two was complete.

Liothyronine non-responsive group (Group 3). Three animals failed to show any response to T_3 treatment. One cat also failed to respond to T_4 (50 μg twice daily) and was lost to follow-up. Another was euthanised at the owner's request. The third animal failed to respond to T_4 (50 μg once daily for 8 weeks then 100 μg twice daily for 8 weeks) and treatment was discontinued for a further 8 weeks. A thyroid biopsy was then carried out. No abnormality was noted. The animal subsequently responded completely to depot testosterone.

Eight of the cases on T_3 replacement therapy (six in Group 1 and one in each of Groups 2 and 3) had serum T_3 concentrations greater than the upper limit of the reference range 3 h after dosing with 50 μg T_3. In two of these, this was insignificant (elevations of 0.03 and 0.05 nmol/1) but the elevations in the remainder ranged from 0.52 to 2.30 nmol/1). Only one of the cats had historical or clinical features compatible with iatrogenic hyperthroidism.

Comparison of the pretreatment physical and laboratory findings according to response to liothyronine sodium

There were no obvious differences between the cutaneous lesions in the three groups of IFSA cats. Other physical and the laboratory data were compared using the Kruskal-Wallis test for group differences.

With the exception of the T_4 concentrations there were no significant

Table 3 Physical and laboratory findings in 26 cases of idiopathic feline symmetric alopecia

Ranges	Heart rate (beats/min)	Rectal temp. (°C)	T_4 (nmol/1)	T_3 (nmol/1)	Cholesterol (mmol/1)	RBC ($\times 10^{12}$/1)	PCV (1/1)	ESR mm/h)	Reticulocytes (%)	Eosinophils ($\times 10^{9}$/1)
1) Before T_3 treatment										
Group 1										
Mean	175	38.3	26.2	0.59	5.56	8.74	0.40	6.5	0.2	0.704
Range	148-218	37.4-39.0	7.3-46.4	0.16-1.13	2.49-9.80	7.81-9.41	0.34-0.46	0-24.0	0-1.0	0.228-1.474
Group 2										
Mean	170	38.9	33.4	0.68	5.36	8.69	0.38	2.8	0.1	0.356
Range	150-204	38.2-39.5	20.5-50.8	0.27-0.99	4.59-6.06	8.07-9.02	0.35-0.39	1.0-4.5	0-0.3	0.127-0.588
Group 3										
Mean	158	38.1	45.6	0.66	3.52	9.60	0.45	4.0	0.6	0.896
Range	156-160	38.0-38.2	37.6-59.8	0.58-0.77	3.21-9.81	8.95-10.03	0.40-0.48	0-10.0	0-1.3	0.456-1.700

2) 12 weeks after beginning T_3 treatment										
Group 1										
Mean	172	38.1	7.6	1.31	4.48	9.24	0.41	2.1	0.3	0.763
Range	132-228	37.8-38.5	<1.3-30.2	0.29-3.57	2.95-6.58	7.61-10.48	0.37-0.46	0-7.0	0-1.0	0.054-2.060
Group 2										
Mean	138	38.6	8.5	1.16	4.64	8.66	0.39	0.2	0	0.544
Range	132-143	37.7-39.4	3.8-20.2	0.31-2.56	3.88-5.88	7.93-9.36	0.33-0.44	0-1.0	0-0.3	0.120-0.952
Group 3										
Mean	180	37.6	4.7	1.74	3.69	9.61	0.44	2.0	0.15	0.408
Range	144-216	36.7-38.4	2.8-7.4	0.64 3.34	3.34-4.04	9.50-9.71	0.43-0.45	0-4.0	0-0.3	0.086-0.729
3) Reference range	160-240	37.8-39.2	8.5-46.2	0.13-1.27	1.71 6.68	5.5-10.0	0.24-0.45	4-13	0-0.6	0-1.500

Reference ranges: Heart rate from Tilley (1985); temperature from Kelly (1974); T_4 and T_3 from Thoday *et al*. (1984); ESR from Schappes (1937); other haematological and biochemical parameters from Clinical Laboratory, University of Edinburgh, Department of Veterinary Clinical Studies.
ESR: Erythrocyte sedimentation rate. PCV: Packed cell volume. RBC: Red blood cells. Temp: Temperature.

differences in parameters between the groups. The T_4 concentrations of the three groups (mean values of Groups 1, 2 and 3 were 26.0, 33.4 and 45.5 nmol/l respectively) were significantly different ($p<0.05$), the inference being that the more T_3 responsive an IFSA cat is, the lower is its basal T_4 concentration.

Comparison of pre-and posttreatment clinical and laboratory data for Group 1

Clinical and laboratory values for this group were compared before and 12 weeks after beginning T_3 treatment, by means of Student's paired *t* test.

The serum T_4 and cholesterol concentrations were significantly lower ($t=6.15$; $p<0.001$ and $t=2.80$; $p<0.05$ respectively) and the serum T_3 concentrations significantly higher ($t=2.74$; $p<0.02$) after, compared with before, beginning T_3 therapy. No other parameters studied were significantly altered.

Comparison of pre- and posttreatment physical and laboratory findings for Groups 2 and 3

Because of the small numbers in each, these two groups were considered together. Data were compared before and 12 weeks after beginning T_3 treatment, by means of Student's paired *t* test.

The serum T_4 concentration was significantly lower during T_3 treatment ($t=6.67$; $p<0.001$). No other parameter was significantly altered.

The thyrotropin stimulation test. Clinical and laboratory data for the six cats tested are presented in Table 4. The basal T_4 and T_3 concentrations of the six IFSA cats were within the reference range established for healthy cats. However, the serum T_4 concentration and the absolute increase in serum T_4 concentration, after TSH administration, were all below the mean values for healthy cats. One cat had a T_4 concentration post TSH marginally below the range found in the healthy group. Statistical examination (Mann-Whitney U test) for serum T_4 concentration showed that IFSA cats had significantly lower values than healthy cats for the post TSH concentration ($U=11$, $p=0.006$) and the absolute increase at 6 h ($U=17$, $p=0.022$) but the ratio of post TSH T_4 concentration to pre TSH T_4 concentration, a commonly used index of TSH stimulation in dogs, was not significantly different. For T_3, none of these values was significantly different between the groups.

Definitively diagnosed feline symmetric alopecia (Group 4)

A definitive diagnosis of the cause of the presenting signs was made in 23 of the 51 referred cases (definitively diagnosed feline symmetric alopecia (DFSA)). Two animals lost to follow-up were undiagnosed and are not considered subsequently. One of these had accompanying miliary dermatitis with blood eosinophilia.

Table 4 Clinical and laboratory data of the thyrotropin stimulation test in six cats with idiopathic symmetric alopecia

Cat	Breed	Sex	Age (years)	Previous response to T_3 therapy	T_4 (nmol/1)	T_3 (nmol/1)	Post TSH–basal concentration (nmol/1)		Post TSH ÷ basal concentration	
							T_4	T_3	T_4	T_3
108276	DSH	NF	13	Total	33.0 101.5	0.84 1.22	68.6	0.38	3.08	1.45
130423	DSH	NF	9	Total	13.3 57.0	0.32 0.50	43.6	0.18	4.28	1.56
TSH/FSA/1/84	DSH	NM	12	Total	41.0 65.2	0.62 1.02	24.2	0.40	1.59	1.65
129563	DSH	NF	4	Partial	12.1 79.5	0.61 1.03	67.4	0.42	6.58	1.69
132070	DSH	NF	10	Partial	11.2 54.5	0.72 1.16	43.3	0.44	4.87	1.61
137740	DSH	NM	6	None	17.5 64.3	0.56 1.11	46.7	0.55	3.67	1.98
				Mean (± SD)	21.4 (± 12.6) 70.3 (± 17.6)	0.61 (± 0.17) 1.01 (± 0.26)	49.0 (± 16.8)	0.40 (± 0.12)	4.01 (± 1.69)	1.67 (± 0.18)
				Healthy mean (± SD)	26.1 (± 10.1) 111.8 (± 33.2)	0.69 (± 0.29) 1.33 (± 0.48)	78.7 (± 31.3)	0.60 (± 0.43)	3.4 (± 1.1)	1.93 (± 0.92)
				Healthy range	8.5–46.2 56.8–195.5	0.13–1.27 0.45–2.33	21.6–151.5	0.08–1.33	1.62–6.27	0.95–4.88

For both T_4 and T_3, the first figures are basal concentrations and the second, concentrations six hours after administration of TSH.
DSH: Domestic short-haired. NF: Neutered female. NM: Neutered male.

Historical data

These data are presented in Table 1.

The duration of physical signs before referral ranged from 1 week to 4 years. No significant variation of onset of alopecia between the months was identified using the χ^2 test. In eight cases, pruritus had never been noticed by the owners, ten had been pruritic (usually manifested by licking) from onset and in five others, pruritus had been variable.

Fifteen animals had received some form of treatment before referral. This consisted of megestrol acetate (11 cases), thyroid hormones (T_3 (two); T_4 (one)), parasiticides (two), glucocorticoids (two), stilboestrol implant (one) and systemic antibacterial agents (one).

Dermatological changes

The distribution of the alopecia is shown in Table 2.
In 16 animals, the areas affected were very similar to those seen in IFSA. In seven cases, additional areas to IFSA sites were affected. These were the dorsal trunk (five cases) and the base of the pinnae and median raphé of the upper lip (one case each). The distribution of the alopecia in the IFSA groups taken together is compared with that of the DFSA group in which lesions were confined to IFSA sites in Table 2. This shows the very similar percentage distribution of alopecia over seven of the sites. However, higher percentages of cases with alopecia over the caudal hind legs and the lateral abdomen were seen in the former and the latter groups respectively. Examination of hairs plucked from areas of alopecia showed microscopic evidence of the distal ends of the shafts having been fractured in nine cases (39%) while in the remainder, no such evidence was present suggesting self or spontaneous epilation.

Fifteen cases (69%) showed hair loss unaccompanied by skin changes. Mild miliary dermatitis was present in six cases (26%), mild dorsal seborrhoea sicca in two (9%), focal erythema (at either the pinnal bases or the dorsal lumbar area) in two (9%) and hyperpigmentation and skin thickening in one (4%).

Haematological and biochemical changes

Because a number of conditions were represented in this group, the haematological and biochemical changes within it were not compared.

The most pronounced abnormal laboratory finding was the blood eosinophil count. Ten animals showed an elevated (greater than $1.5 \times 10^9/l$) and three a high normal (greater than $1.1 \times 10^9/l$) total eosinophil count.

Diagnosis, treatment and outcome of the DFSA group

These data are presented in Table 5.

Fleas or their faeces were found on nine animals. One of these animals had kittened 6 weeks before presentation and was diagnosed as having concurrent telogen defluxion. Four of these cats had elevated (greater than $1.5 \times 10^9/l$) total eosinophil counts on first presentation. Flea control produced remission of signs in all cases. In ten animals in which there was no evidence of fleas or

Table 5 Final diagnosis in 23[a] cats in which the cause of symmetric alopecia was determined

Diagnosis	Cases (n = 23)	
	No.	%
Flea infestation	9	39.1
Probable flea infestation (fleas/flea faeces not seen but responded to flea control)	10	43.5
Telogen defluxion	2	8.7
Psychogenic alopecia and dermatitis	1	4.4
Pediculosis	1	4.4
Mastocytosis	1	4.4

[a] One cat had telogen defluxion and fleas.
n: Number of observations.

their faeces on physical examination, flea control as described previously resulted in total remission of signs. An example of such a case is shown in Plates 15A, B. Five of these had elevated (greater than $1.5 \times 10^9/1$) and three high normal (greater than $1.1 \times 10^9/1$) total eosinophil counts on first presentation.

One other cat also showed telogen defluxion which occurred postpartum. In this case, there was no evidence of microscopic damage to the distal ends of plucked hair shafts and hairs for examination were easily epilated. The case of psychogenic alopecia occurred in a domestic short-haired cat and no initiating cause was identified. Many remaining hairs in alopecic areas were fractured as assessed microscopically and could not be easily epilated. During the 6 weeks the cat wore an Elizabethan collar, there was good hair growth. Long-term management was with 1 mg diazepam (Valium®, Roche) twice daily.

The case of pediculosis was confirmed by macroscopic examination and the parasite as *Felicola subrostratus* by microscopic examination. This cat showed alopecia over the lateral and medial hind legs, the ventral abdomen, the forelegs from elbow to carpus and alopecia and erythema at the base of the pinnae. The distal ends of many of the hairs from these sites were fractured as assessed microscopically. The animal responded to weekly sprays with dichlorvos/fenitrothion combination. The case of multiple mast cell tumours showed diffuse partial alopecia over affected areas and over the median raphé of the upper lip. In addition, there was dry scale, hyperpigmentation and small, 2–4 mm, multiple, firm, well-circumscribed yellow papules. The diagnosis was made on skin biopsy and the condition was managed with oral prednisolone.

Comparison of blood eosinophil counts before and 6 weeks after beginning treatment

In 14 cases, blood eosinophil counts were available before and 6 weeks after beginning treatment. In all cases, the posttreatment value was lower than the pretreatment value. However, when these were compared using Student's paired *t* test, the results just failed to be statistically significant ($t = 1.91$; $p > 0.05$).

Comparison of historical, physical and laboratory parameters of the IFSA and the DFSA groups

As, with the exception of T_4 concentrations, there were no significant differences in physical and laboratory parameters of the three IFSA groups; these data were combined and compared by the Wilcoxon Rank Sum Test, to those of the DFSA group in an attempt to identify an effective test for differentiating between them. The serum cholesterol concentration, red blood cell (RBC) count and packed cell volume (PCV) were all significantly lower ($p < 0.05$ in each case) and the eosinophil count significantly higher ($p < 0.001$) in the DFSA group when compared with the IFSA group.

Table 6 compares the eosinophil counts of the IFSA animals with those in the DFSA group. The range in the IFSA cats approximates to, and in the DFSA cats is much greater than, the normal range. The median of the eosinophil count of DFSA animals is more than twice that of the IFSA animals. The predictive values of the total eosinophil count in differentiating IFSA and DFSA are shown in Table 7.

DISCUSSION

Feline symmetric alopecia is a relatively new name for a condition previously termed feline endocrine alopecia (Muller *et al.*, 1989) which itself had numerous hormonal synonyms. FSA is an advance in nomenclature for a

Table 6 Comparison of the total blood eosinophil counts in cats with idiopathic symmetric alopecia and cats in which the cause of the symmetric alopecia was definitively diagnosed

Group	Eosinophil count ($\times 10^9$/1)	
	Median	Range
Idiopathic feline symmetric alopecia ($n = 17$)	0.568	0.127–1.700
Definitively diagnosed feline symmetric alopecia ($n = 23$)	1.365	0.180–14.196
Normal values	0.650[a] (mean)	0–1.500

[a] Mean and range from Schalm *et al.* (1975).
n: Number of observations.

Table 7 Predictive value of the total eosinophil count in differentiating cats with idiopathic symmetric alopecia from cats in which the cause of the symmetric alopecia was definitively diagnosed

Total eosinophil count ($\times 10^9/1$)	Cases		
	IFSA	DFSA	Total
> 1.5	1	10	11
< 1.5	16	13	29
Total	17	23	40

Conclusions: Assuming that the prevalence of IFSA and DFSA cats in this study is the same as in the general population:

(i) A raised eosinophil count ($>1.5 \times 10^9/1$) has a 91% predictive value in excluding IFSA.

(ii) A normal count ($<1.5 \times 10^9/1$) has only a 55% predictive value in indicating IFSA.

DFSA: Definitively diagnosed feline symmetric alopecia.
IFSA: Idiopathic feline symmetric alopecia.

condition which is clearly multifactorial and for which no endocrine aetiology has been proven. However, I believe that where the aetiology is determined, the term feline symmetric alopecia should be used for descriptive purposes only, with the term idiopathic feline symmetric alopecia being reserved for those cases of unknown cause.

Although there are numerous descriptions of the condition, only one (Scott, 1975) has presented detailed clinical and laboratory data. None of his cases appeared to be associated with hypothyroidism. The present study was carried out to assess the varying aetiology of the condition and to investigate further the thyroid function of cats in which a cause for the condition could not be determined.

The presence or absence of pruritus in cats is notoriously difficult to determine but this is crucial in assessing whether FSA is spontaneous or self-induced. Owners may genuinely believe that hair loss in their animal is spontaneous because excessive grooming may only be carried out secretly. Every effort was made in this study to assess, both from the history and the physical examination, whether cases were pruritic. In addition, trichograms were carried out on all cats to determine whether remaining hairs showed evidence of fracture of the distal ends of the shafts. Anagen:telogen ratio studies were not carried out because it was felt that these would be non-contributory as Kunkle (1984) has reported that up to 96% of hairs from healthy cats may be in telogen. Prior to classification as IFSA cases, an Elizabethan collar was used for 6 weeks on any animal in which a definitive diagnosis had not been made to determine whether there was any evidence of hair regrowth when grooming was prevented.

Dermatophytosis and demodicosis may present with symmetric alopecia (Scott, 1980, 1984) and screening tests to eliminate these conditions were carried out on all cases at first presentation but were negative in all 51 cats.

Preliminary observations suggested that the total eosinophil count might be useful in differentiating cases of DFSA from IFSA. As endoparasites may cause a circulating eosinophilia (Schalm *et al.*, 1975), faecal samples from all animals were examined but not identified in any.

Fleas are the most important cause of skin disease in cats in the UK and the signs of infestation vary (Thoday, 1985). Flea control measures were therefore instituted in all cats in which a definitive diagnosis could not be made at the first visit. Environmental flea control measures consisted of vacuum-cleaning of the environment followed by an environmental parasiticidal agent. At the time of this study, insect growth regulators were not available in the UK.

Recently Ihrke (1982), Sousa and Ihrke (1983) and Kunkle (1984) suggested that most cases of FSA were a manifestation of the psychogenic alopecia/dermatitis complex. Thus, prior to classification as IFSA, all cats which failed to respond to other treatments wore an Elizabethan collar for 6 weeks as described above but only one showed evidence of hair regrowth.

Idiopathic feline symmetric alopecia

Because of the multifactorial aetiology of this condition, many of the previous reports of feline 'endocrine' alopecia undoubtedly included animals which would have been classified in the DFSA group in this series. Comparison of this study with the literature is, therefore, complicated.

IFSA was not diagnosed in a pure-bred cat in this study although two pedigree-cross cats were affected. With the exception of Conroy (1964) and Kirk (1980) who described cases in the Siamese breed, all other reports have been in non-pedigree cats. Only one entire cat was affected in this series. Most other authors agree that the condition is seen more commonly in neutered individuals. However, because the majority of mature cats seen at veterinary clinics are neutered, this predisposition may be apparent rather than real. In the present study, 58% of cases were neutered females and 39% neutered males. This is in contrast to the series of 20 cases reported by Scott (1975) in which 90% were neutered males.

In the current series, all but one animal had been neutered before 9 months of age. Premature neutering has been suggested as causal (Scott, 1981) with affected animals producing insufficient androgens and/or oestrogens form their adrenal cortices (Kral, 1959). The latent period between neutering and onset was from 6 months to 10.5 years (mean 4.1 years) which is similar to the range of 1–9 years (mean 5 years) reported by Scott (1975).

The distribution of hair loss in this series was in general agreement with literature reports but while most authors have reported that the condition begins over the anogenital region, this area was affected in only 19% of cases. While four animals were lethargic and one obese, systemic signs suggestive of hypothyroidism were absent in the remainder. Pretreatment laboratory data also did not suggest hypothyroidism as causal. Indeed, three animals had T_4 concentrations above the reference range. Excessive grooming resulting in alopecia may be a feature of hyperthyroidism (Peterson *et al.*, 1983). None of these three cats had historical or physical features suggestive of hyperthyroidism but, prior to beginning T_3 supplementation, a T_3 suppression test was carried out which reduced serum T_4 concentrations to 40% or less of the basal concentrations in all cases. Hyperthyroid cats show little to no decrease in serum T_4 concentrations on T_3 suppression testing (Peterson and Ferguson, 1989) and follow-up of the cases showed no evidence of development of hyperthyroidism in the long term.

In six animals studied, the serum T_4 concentration and the absolute increase in serum T_4 concentration, after TSH administration, were all below the mean values for 16 healthy cats with one cat having a T_4 concentration post TSH marginally below the reference range. Statistical examination of these results showed significant differences.

The TSH stimulation test protocol used in this study was optimized and validated for use in cats. This study (Thoday, 1986) showed that in euthyroid animals, the intravenous administration of TSH at a dose of 0.5 IU/kg bodyweight led to a serum T_4 concentration of greater than 55 nmol/1 6 h after administration and to an increment in the serum T_4 concentration of more than 20 nmol/1. These reference values are similar to those obtained in 19 cats by Hoenig and Ferguson (1983) who, although they recommended using 1 IU/kg TSH, also found peak serum concentrations of T_4 (at least 51.5 nmol/1) at 6 h and a minimum increment in the serum T_4 concentration of 32.3 nmol/1. The only other workers to have investigated TSH stimulation testing in euthyroid cats used an intramuscular route of administration and concluded that a dose of 2.5 IU TSH per cat (which is comparable with my dose per kg) would more than double the basal serum T_4 concentration and give a concentration of greater than 38.6 nmol/1 8 and/or 12 hours later (Kemppainen *et al.*, 1984).

Scott (1975) is the only person to have reported the serum T_4 response to TSH in FSA. Five cats tested showed a normal response to TSH (defined as a doubling or tripling of the basal serum T_4 concentration) 12 h after the subcutaneous administration of 5 IU TSH. Statistical analysis of the results was not carried out. The serum T_3 response to TSH in FSA has not been reported previously. In dogs, this response is not a reliable indicator of thyroid function (Nesbitt, 1983) and these findings were anticipated.

In the present study, the thyroid function of only six animals was investigated using the TSH stimulation test and a considerably larger study is required before drawing any specific conclusions. However, the present data suggest the possibility that IFSA in some cats may be a manifestation of low thyroid reserve. This term was originally used by Jefferies *et al.* (1953) to describe a condition of man characterized by a normal 3-hour thyroidal uptake of ^{131}I and serum protein bound iodine (PBI) concentration but a failure of either to respond to stimulation with TSH. They attributed the condition to the presence of a remnant of thyroid tissue which was being stimulated maximally by endogenous TSH and hence could not respond further to the exogenous hormone. Subsequently, Levy *et al.* (1954) observed that in some circumstances ^{131}I uptake would rise following administration of TSH but the serum PBI concentration would not, whereas in others the reverse occurred. Low thyroid reserve in humans may be a transient phenomenon or may persist indefinitely, as may IFSA. Low thyroid reserve was observed more frequently in patients who had had ^{131}I therapy or subtotal thyroidectomy, but was also seen following thyroiditis and within 3–8 weeks of cessation of prolonged thyroid hormone medication. In the present study, T_3 therapy was discontinued for a minimum of 8 weeks prior to TSH testing in all cats. It is interesting to speculate that, because cases of IFSA may be subdivided retrospectively according to response to T_3, some cases of the syndrome may represent a number of thyroidal and non-thyroidal states.

Because in a preliminary study, the clinical impression gained was that the response to T_3 was better than to T_4, T_3 was used to treat IFSA. An increasing dosage regimen was used to try to prevent possible cardiac or other thyrotoxic problems being brought about by initial slow metabolism of the hormonal supplement or rapid changes in cellular metabolism (Rosychuk, 1982). A maximum total daily dose of 100 μg per cat was used. This is higher than a commonly quoted dose for cats of 13.2 μg/kg/day (Rosychuk, 1982), but compares with the daily dosage of 90 μg T_3 per cat suggested by Holzworth *et al.* (1980) for the treatment of iatrogenic hypothyroidism resulting from the surgical management of hyperthyroidism in animals in which plasma T_3 concentrations remain low despite adequate T_4 concentrations during T_4 supplementation.

In the present study 100 μg T_3 per cat daily appeared to be necessary because a number of cats developed recurrence of alopecia at lower dosages. However, this dosage of T_3 produced serum T_3 concentrations significantly above the reference range in six of the 26 animals. Only one of these showed evidence of iatrogenic thyrotoxicosis which resolved on cessation of therapy but such possible complications should clearly be borne in mind when using this regimen. Where serum T_3 concentrations exceed the reference range, the T_3 dosage should be reduced until reference range values are achieved.

In dogs, the half-life of T_3 is considerably shorter than T_4 and as a result, Nachreiner (1981) has recommended adminstering T_3 on a three-times-daily regimen. However, Rosychuk (1982) has reported successful maintenance of hypothyroid dogs by twice-daily administration of T_3. Reducing the frequency of drug administration is likely to increase owner compliance and in the present series, a twice-daily regimen was found to be satisfactory in the majority of cases.

All IFSA cases were treated with T_3 for 12 weeks before further blood samples were taken to monitor progress. This allowed the establishment of a steady-state situation for thyroid hormones and a clinical assessment of the response to therapy as recommended by Rogers *et al.* (1975) and Muller *et al.* (1983) in dogs.

The serum thyroid hormone concentrations during treatment were assessed from blood samples taken 3 h after the administration of half the daily dose of T_3. While no figures are available for cats, this regimen has been recommended for therapeutic monitoring of hypothyroid dogs treated with T_3 (Rosychuk, 1982).

Retrospectively, the IFSA cases could be divided according to their response to T_3. While equal numbers of neutered females and neutered males were present in Group 1, neutered females predominated in the other two, comprising 75% and 100% of the T_3 partially and non-responsive groups respectively. The significance of these observations is unknown.

Two cats in Group 1 with alopecia at referral of 5 and 11 months' duration respectively did not require long-term T_3 therapy to maintain a normal coat, over follow-up periods of 2 and 4 years respectively. The explanation for these interesting responses is unknown.

When the laboratory findings 12 weeks after beginning T_3 treatment were compared, the T_3 and T_4 concentrations were significantly higher and lower respectively during treatment with T_3 in Group 1 but in Groups 2 and 3 taken together, only the serum T_4 concentrations were significantly different. The low serum T_4 concentration would be expected due to the negative feedback of T_3 on TSH production. Thus, in Groups 2 and 3 taken together, while the exogenous T_3 was at a high enough dose to cause suppression of endogenous T_4 production, it was not sufficient to produce a statistical difference between pre- and during-treatment T_3 concentrations. Similarly, while the serum cholesterol concentration of Group 1 during treatment was significantly lower compared with the pretreatment values, such a difference was not noted for Groups 2 and 3 taken together. Thyroid hormones are known to lower the serum cholesterol concentrations of both hypothyroid and euthyroid humans (Anon., 1951; Kritchevsky, 1958).

The biochemical differences between Groups 1 and Groups 2 and 3 taken together may have a number of explanations. It is possible that owner compliance with the therapeutic regimen or T_3 absorption was poorer in the latter group. Alternatively, it is possible that the aetiology of IFSA is, as in DFSA, multifactorial, thus showing a variable response to T_3 supplementation.

Hair regrowth during T_3 supplementation does not, of course, prove that any of the animals had low thyroid reserve. A thyroid biopsy from one cat in Group 3 showed no histological abnormality suggesting that primary hypothyroidism was not the cause of the condition in this animal. Thyroid biopsies were not carried out on any of the animals in Group 1. In healthy dogs, orally or topically administered T_4 increases the number of hair follicles entering the anagen phase of the hair cycle (Gunaratnam, 1986) and the hair growth in the Group 1 animals may have been the result of a similar mechanism and not to the correction of low thyroid reserve.

Three animals which failed to respond to T_3 responded to other treatment regimens, two to depot testosterone (one in each of Groups 2 and 3) and one to megestrol acetate (Group 2). There are numerous anecdotal reports of these drugs being used successfully to treat FSA (reviews by Scott, 1980; Thoday, 1986). The mechanism of action of these drugs in FSA is unknown although mood modification has been suggested (Ihrke, 1982; Sousa and Ihrke, 1983; Kunkle, 1984). Side-effects of testosterone in cats include aggressiveness and urine spraying in males and overdosage may result in severe hepatobiliary disease and death in both sexes (Scott, 1980). The side-effects of megestrol acetate in cats are legion and include polyuria/polydipsia, increased urinary odour, polyphagia and weight gain, diarrhoea, decreased activity, diabetes mellitus, adrenocortical suppression and atrophy, iatrogenic Cushing's-like syndrome, pyometra, mammary gland hyperplasia and neoplasia and decreased libido and infertility in males (Rosser, 1988). In the present series, only one animal showed side-effects of T_3 therapy (compatible with iatrogenic hyperthyroidism) and these settled rapidly on cessation of treatment. Therefore, T_3 therapy appears a considerably safer alternative for the management of IFSA where treatment is required.

The symptoms of IFSA are primarily aesthetic although seven animals in this series showed symptoms of involvement of other systems in addition to the skin. Three animals in Group 1 showed resolution of these non-cutaneous symptoms in association with regrowth of hair and the appetite and activity of one other cat in this group improved. Where symptoms are confined to the skin, the clinician must always question whether treatment is actually indicated. However, many clients require attempts at management of IFSA and, indeed, the owner of a Group 3 animal in this series requested euthanasia when this was unsuccessful. Provided hair growth can be achieved, free of side-effects and with reference range serum T_3 concentrations 2–4 h post T_3 administration, such attempts at treatment would seem warranted.

Definitively diagnosed feline symmetric alopecia

Of the DFSA cats seen, 16% were entire compared with only 3.7% of the IFSA animals. The age at onset was similar in both groups.

Although seven of the 23 animals showed alopecia at sites other than IFSA predilection areas, the distribution of the major sites of alopecia in the DFSA group was very similar to the former. However, 39% of the DFSA cats showed fractured hairs and 31% accompanying skin changes, whereas these changes were not seen in the IFSA group. Pruritus was observed at some stage in the disease process in 65% of the DFSA group but excessive grooming was presumably taking place in the remainder while the animals were not being observed. Where fractured hairs could not be demonstrated, it must be assumed that hairs were being epilated by the animal.

In this series, fleas or their faeces were found on nine cats. Four of these animals had elevated blood eosinophil counts. In addition ten cats with no macroscopic evidence of flea infestation responded completely to flea control. Of these, five had elevated and three high normal blood eosinophil counts. As all were negative for ectoparasites on skin scrapings and for endoparasites on faecal examination, and as neither dichlorvos nor fenitrothion have known stimulatory action on hair growth, it was concluded that these dermatoses were associated with flea infestation, although skin changes were absent in most.

The pathogenesis of the self-induced alopecia in flea-infested and suspected flea-infested cats is unclear. Although many authors feel that flea bites are capable of inducing significant clinical disease without hypersensitivity being involved (e.g. Nesbitt and Schmitz, 1978), Halliwell (1985) has suggested that clinically significant reactions always involve hypersensitivity. Kunkle (1989) has reported that cats with flea allergy may present with clinically normal skin but self-inflicted symmetric hypotrichosis. Intradermal tests with flea antigen and skin biopsies may have been helpful in determining the pathophysiology of the alopecia in the present cases but these tests were not carried out.

The case of psychogenic alopecia occurred in a domestic short-haired cat and no initiating cause was identified. The distribution of hair loss was symmetric but remaining hairs in affected areas were fractured as assessed clinically and subsequently microscopically and could not be easily epilated. Ihrke (1982) and Sousa and Ihrke (1983) suggested that most cases of feline "endocrine" alopecia were actually manifestations of psychogenic alopecia. Kunkle (1984) agreed and felt that the common feature of the various drugs used to treat the condition was their mood-altering capabilities with some having additional antiinflammatory actions. Both groups suggested that almost all cases of "endocrine" alopecia grew hair when an Elizabethan collar was worn. Only one case in the present series improved with such a collar. Cases of pediculosis and mast cell tumours with symmetric alopecia do not appear to have been reported previously.

Recently, Kunkle (1989) reported that food hypersensitivity and atopy in cats may also result in FSA. This information was not available at the time of the present study and specific diagnostic tests were not carried out for these conditions. However, it is unlikely that they were represented as hair loss in food hypersensitivity and atopy is self-induced, only one cat responded to wearing an Elizabethan collar, and this responded to diazepam alone.

A number of significant differences in laboratory parameters were identified between the IFSA and DFSA groups. The significance of the lower RBC count and PCV in the DFSA groups is unknown because this is the converse of what might have been expected if some cases of IFSA are due to low thyroid reserve. A higher serum cholesterol would be consistent with low thyroid reserve in IFSA but this is a relatively non-specific feature and only four cats in this group were actually hypercholesterolaemic.

The most significant laboratory difference between the two groups was the tendency for elevation of the total eosinophil count in the DFSA group. Eosinophilia in cats may occur in a number of conditions such as flea-bite hypersensitivity (Scott *et al.*, 1986), mast cell disorders (Schalm *et al.*, 1975), and although not represented in this series, food hypersensitivity (White and Sequoia, 1989). It follows from the data presented here that, at present, the most useful screening test for the differentiation of IFSA and DFSA cases is the blood eosinophil count.

REFERENCES

Anon. (1951). Plasma cholesterol and the thyroid. *Lancet* **ii**:578.

Conroy, J.D. (1964). Diseases of the skin. In: Catcott, E.J. (ed.) *Feline Medicine and Surgery* 1st edn, pp. 321-347. American Veterinary Publications, Santa Barbara.

Gunaratnam, P. (1986). The effects of thyroxine on hair growth in the dog. *Journal of Small Animal Practice* **27**:17-29.

Halliwell, R.E.W. (1985). Cited by Kwochka, K.W. and Bevier, D.E. (1987). Flea dermatitis. In: Nesbitt, G.H. (ed.) *Dermatology*, pp. 21-55. Churchill Livingstone, New York.

Hoenig, M. and Ferguson, D.C. (1983). Assessment of thyroid functional reserve in the cat by the thyrotropin-stimulation test. *American Journal of Veterinary Research* **44**:1229-1232.

Holzworth, J., Theran, P., Carpenter, J.L., Harpster, N.K. and Todoroff, R.J. (1980). Hyperthyroidism in the cat: Ten cases. *Journal of the American Veterinary Medical Association* **176**:345-353.

Ihrke, P.J. (1982). Feline alopecia. *Carnation Research Digest* **18**(2):1-4.

Jeffries, W.McK., Levy, R.P., Palmer, W.G., Storaasli, J.P. and Kelly, L.W. (1953). The value of a single injection of thyrotropin in the diagnosis of obscure hypothyroidism. *New England Journal of Medicine* **249**:876-884.

Jefferies, W.McK., Kelly, L.W., Levy, R.P., Cooper, G.W. and Prouty, R.L. (1956). The significance of low thyroid reserve. *Journal of Clinical Endocrinology* 16:1438-1455.

Kelly, W.R. (1974). *Veterinary Clinical Diagnosis* 2nd edn, p. 22. Baillière Tindall, London.

Kemppainen, R.J. Mansfield, P.D. and Sartin, J.L. (1984). Endocrine responses of normal cats to TSH and synthetic ACTH administration. *Journal of the American Animal Hospital Association* **20**:737-740.

Kirk, R.W. (1980). Feline alopecias. In: Kirk, R.W. (ed.) *Current Veterinary Therapy VII — Small Animal Practice*, pp. 490-493. W.B. Saunders Company, Philadelphia.

Kral, F. (1959). *Compendium of Veterinary Dermatology*. Pfizer & Co, New York. Cited by Scott, D.W. (1980). Feline dermatology 1900-1978: A monograph. *Journal of the American Animal Hospital Association* **16**:331-459.

Kritchevsky, D. (1958). *Cholesterol*, pp. 201-202. Chapman & Hall, London.

Kunkle, G.A. (1984). Feline dermatology. *Veterinary Clinics of North America (Small Animal Practice)* **14**:1065-1087.

Kunkle, G.A. (1989). Miliary dermatitis, eosinophilic granuloma complex, and symmetric hypotrichosis as manifestations of feline allergy. In: Kirk, R.W. (ed.) *Current Veterinary Therapy* X — *Small Animal Practice*, pp. 583-586. W.B. Saunders Company, Philadelphia.

Levy, R.P., Kelly, L.W. and Jefferies, W.McK. (1954). The relationship between changes in thyroidal I^{131} uptake and serum protein-bound iodine following thyrotropin. *Journal of Clinical Investigation* **33**:953-954.

Muller, G.H., Kirk, R.W. and Scott, D.W. (1983). *Small Animal Dermatology* 3rd edn, pp. 556-558. W.B. Saunders Company, Philadelphia.

Muller, G. H., Kirk, R.W. and Scott, D.W. (1989). *Small Animal Dermatology* 4th edn, pp. 701-703. W.B. Saunders Company, Philadelphia.

Nachreiner, R.F. (1981). Cited by Rosychuk, R.A.W. (1982). Thyroid hormones and antithyroid drugs. *Veterinary Clinics of North America (Small Animal Practice)* **12**: 111-148.

Nesbitt, G.H. (1983). *Canine and Feline Dermatology: A Systematic Approach*, pp. 99-110. Lea & Febiger, Philadelphia.

Nesbitt, G.H. and Schmitz, J.A. (1978). Fleabite allergic dermatitis: A review and survey of 330 cases. *Journal of the American Veterinary Medical Association* **173**:282-288.

Peterson, M.E. & Ferguson, D.C. (1989). Thyroid diseases. In: Ettinger, S.J. (ed.) *Textbook of Veterinary Internal Medicine* 3rd edn Vol. 2, pp. 1632-1675. W.B. Saunders Company, Philadelphia.

Peterson, M.E., Kintzer, P.P., Cavanagh, P.G. *et al.*, (1983). Feline hyperthyroidism: Pretreatment clinical and laboratory evaluation of 131 cases. *Journal of the American Veterinary Medical Association* **183**:103-110.

Rogers, W.A., Donovan, E.F. & Kociba, G.J. (1975). Lipids and lipoproteins in normal dogs and in dogs with secondary hyperlipidemia. *Journal of the American Veterinary Medical Association* **166**:1092-1100.

Rosser, E.J. (1988). Antipruritic drugs. *Veterinary Clinics of North America (Small Animal Practice)* **18**:1093-1099.

Rosychuk, R.A.W. (1982). Thyroid hormones and antithyroid drugs. *Veterinary Clinics of North America (Small Animal Practice)* **12**:111-148.

Schalm, D.W., Jain, N.C. and Carroll, E.J. (1975). *Veterinary Haematology* 3rd edn, p. 109. Lea & Febiger, Philadelphia.

Schappes, H. (1937). Cited by Altman, P.L. (1961). Blood cells. In: Dittner, D.S. (ed.) *Blood and Other Body Fluids,* p. 122. Federation of American Societies for Experimental Biology, Washington.

Scott, D.W. (1975). Thyroid function in feline endocrine alopecia. *Journal of the American Animal Hospital Association* **11**:798-801.

Scott, D.W. (1980). Feline dermatology 1900-1978. A monograph. *Journal of the American Animal Hospital Association* **16**:390-459.

Scott, D.W. (1981). Refresher Course on Dermatology; Proceedings 57, pp. 1-274. University of Sydney Post-Graduate Committee in Veterinary Science, Sydney.

Scott, D.W. (1984). Feline dermatology 1979-1982: Introspective retrospections. *Journal of the American Animal Hospital Association* **20**:537-564.

Scott, D.W., Walton, D.K. and Slater, M.R. (1986). Miliary dermatitis: A feline cutaneous reaction pattern. *Proceedings Second Annual Kal Kan Symposium* **2**:11-18.

Sousa, C.A. and Ihrke, P.J. (1983). The skin. In: Pratt, P.W. (ed.) *Feline Medicine* pp. 583-584. American Veterinary Publications, California.

Thoday, K.L. (1985). The skin. In: Chandler, E.A., Gaskell, C.J., and Hilbery, A.D.R. (eds), *Feline Medicine*, pp. 3-37. Blackwell Scientific Publications, Oxford.

Thoday, K.L. (1986). Clinical, biochemical and immunological studies of feline thyroid function. Ph.D. Thesis, University of Edinburgh.

Thoday, K.L., Seth, J. and Elton, R.A. (1984). Radioimmunoassay of serum total thyroxine and triiodothyronine in healthy cats: assay methodology and effects of age, sex, breed, heredity and environment. *Journal of Small Animal Practice* **25**:457-472.

Tilley, L.P. (1985). *Essentials of Canine and Feline Electrocardiography* 2nd edn, p. 98. Lea & Febiger, Philadelphia.

White, S.D. and Sequoia, D. (1989). Food hypersensitivity in cats: 14 cases (1982-1987). *Journal of the American Veterinary Medical Association* **194**:692-695.

1.5 The Regulation of Wool Growth in Transgenic Animals

Kevin A. Ward, C.R. Byrne, B.W. Wilson, Z. Leish, N.W. Rigby, C.R. Townrow, C.L. Hunt, J.D. Murray and C.D. Nancarrow

CSIRO Division of Animal Production,
Blacktown, New South Wales,
Australia

INTRODUCTION

Recent developments in the isolation and manipulation of DNA sequences have opened the way for the direct modification of the genetic properties of domestic animals (Palmiter *et al.*, 1982, 1983; Hammer *et al.*, 1985). Using this new technology we are now in position to alter the qualitative and quantitative production of important animal products such as wool, meat and milk (Pursel *et al.*, 1989). One approach to achieving this goal is to identify the rate-limiting components of a production characteristic, and then design a gene combination that can function to overcome the limiting factors. Targets that are particularly attractive for manipulation are circulating hormones (e.g. growth hormone), and essential substrates (e.g. amino acids, carbohydrates).

Wool growth is limited by the availability of the essential amino acid cysteine (Reis and Schinkel, 1963; Reis *et al.*, 1973; Reis, 1979), due to the high frequency of occurrence of this amino acid in fibre keratin proteins (Crewther, 1976). It is not possible to increase the circulating level of cysteine in sheep by a simple feeding regime, however, because the amino acid is rapidly degraded to H_2S by bacteria in the rumen. One approach to overcome this problem is to provide sheep with the enzymes necessary for cysteine biosynthesis, by introducing to the sheep genome the DNA sequences encoding the appropriate proteins.

To achieve this, we have utilized two genes, *cysE* and *cysK*, from the bacterium *Escherichia coli* (Byrne *et al.*, 1987); Denk and Bock, 1987). These genes encode the enzymes serine transacetylase (SAT) (EC.2.3.1.30) and *O*-

acetylserine sulphydrylase (OAS) (EC.4.2.99.8), which catalyse the following reactions.

(1) Serine + Acetyl-CoA $\xrightarrow[\text{serine transacetylase}]{}$ *O*-Acetylserine + CoA-SH

(2) *O*-Acetylserine + H_2S $\xrightarrow[\text{\textit{O}-acetylserine sulphydrylase}]{}$ cysteine + acetate

In this paper we describe our results on the modification of these genes to provide for expression of the genes in eukaryotic cells, and report their transfer to transgenic mice.

MATERIALS AND METHODS

The isolation and characterization of the sheep metallothionein-Ia gene (Peterson and Mercer, 1986), sheep growth hormone gene (Byrne *et al.*, 1987) and *E. coli cysE* (Denk and Bock, 1987) and *cysK* (Byrne *et al.*, 1988) genes have all been reported previously. The manipulation of the sequences that gave rise to the plasmids pMTCE11 and pMTCK11 involved standard recombinant DNA techniques (Maniatis *et al.*, 1982), and will be reported in detail elsewhere (K.A. Ward, and C.R. Byrne, unpublished).

Cell transformation was carried out by the calcium phosphate precipitate method (Wigler *et al.*, 1979). The cells were co-transformed with the plasmid pSV_2neo (Southern and Berg, 1982) and either pMTCE11 or pMTCK11, and stably transformed cells were selected by neomycin resistance.

Transgenic mice were prepared by pronuclear microinjection of one-cell embryos (Brinster *et al.*, 1985; Costantini and Lacy, 1981). About 1–2 pl of DNA (5μg/ml) was injected and surviving embryos were transferred to Quackenbush pseudopregnant female recipients.

To measure SAT and OAS enzyme activities approximately 10^7 cells were homogenized in 50 mM Tris-HC1 buffer, pH 7.5, centrifuged for 20 min at 10 000 × *g* assaying the enzyme activities in the supernatant solution. The method of Kredich and Tomkins (1966) was used to measure SAT activity and a combination of the methods of Becker *et al.* (1969) and Gaitonde 1967), to measure OAS activity.

RESULTS

Modification of the bacterial genes for eukaryotic expression

In order to obtain expression of the bacterial coding sequences in eukaryotic cells, the sheep metallothionein-Ia (MT-Ia) promoter (Peterson and Mercer, 1986) was spliced 5′ to the coding sequence of each bacterial gene, and a polyadenylation signal and four introns were provided by splicing a portion of the sheep growth hormone gene (Byrne *et al.*, 1987) 3′ to each bacterial gene. The structure of the resulting plasmids, pMTCE11 and pMTCK11 are shown in Fig. 1.

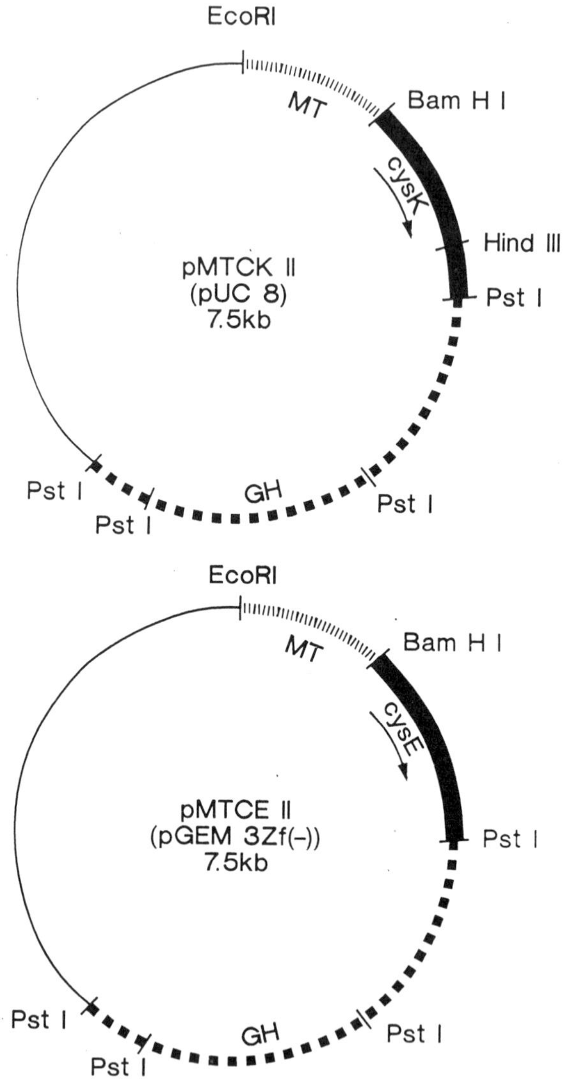

Figure 1 The plasmids pMTCK11 and pMTCE11 were constructed by mutating the bacterial *cysE* or *cysK* gene immediately upstream from the ATG initiation codon, which then allowed the sheep MT-Ia promoter sequence to be inserted in the position shown. The sheep growth hormone gene was joined to the 3′ end of the bacterial coding sequence immediately downstream from the stop codon. The vectors used for the initial cloning are shown in brackets. MT = sheep metallothionein-Ia promoter; GH = sheep growth hormone gene; the direction of transcription of the bacterial genes is shown by arrows.

Expression of MTCE11 and MTCK11 in cells in culture

The two plasmids pMTCE11 and pMTCK11 were introduced into mouse L-cells by the calcium phosphate transformation method (Wigler *et al.*, 1979; Southern and Berg; 1982), and stable transformant cell lines were established for each plasmid. The expression of each of the genes was determined by assaying for the appropriate enzyme activity in cell extracts and by Northern blot analysis of the mRNA produced by the cells.

The enzymic activity of the transformed cell lines are shown in Table 1. Both the pMTCE11 and the pMTCK11 plasmids are expressed in mouse L-cells. In extracts from cells containing pMTCE11, SAT activity was found to be 225 nmol *O*-acetylserine formed/mg protein/30 min, and in extracts from cells containing pMTCK11, OAS activity was measured as 161 nmol cysteine produced/mg protein/30 min. The OAS activity was consistently higher than the SAT activity. The expression of both plasmids is zinc-inducible, although some basal expression is also detectable. The SAT activity increased five-fold and the OAS activity three-fold when cultures were grown overnight in media containing 40 μmol zinc sulphate.

Table 1 Specific activity of serine transacetylase and *O*-acetylserine sulphydrylase in transformed cultures of mouse L-cells

Enzyme source		Specific activity (nmol product/mg protein/30 min)	
		SAT	OAS
E. coli		1.0×10^5	3.9×10^5
MTCE11	+ Zn	225	-
	− Zn	42	-
MTCK11	+ Zn	-	1.5×10^3
	− Zn	-	0.5×10^3

Cells were harvested, homogenized in extraction buffer (50 mM Tris-Cl, pH 7.5) and centrifuged for 20 min at 10 000 x *g*. The supernatant solution was used for the assay of SAT or OAS activity. All values have been corrected for low non-specific activity in cells transformed with vector alone. *E. coli* activity was measured in strain AL509 (SAT) and strain C600 (OAS).

The presence of *cysK*-specific mRNA is readily detected in zinc-induced cultures containing pMTCK11 as shown in Fig. 2. The predicted size of the transcript from the MTCK11 fusion gene is 2.0 kb (see Fig. 1), consisting of 1 kb of this *cysK* gene and 1 kb of the growth hormone gene. An RNA transcript of the size was readily detected in total RNA from cells containing pMTCK11. In addition, a second, smaller transcript (1.6 kb), also of high abundance, was detected in the RNA extracts. The reason for the two different RNA sizes is currently under investigation.

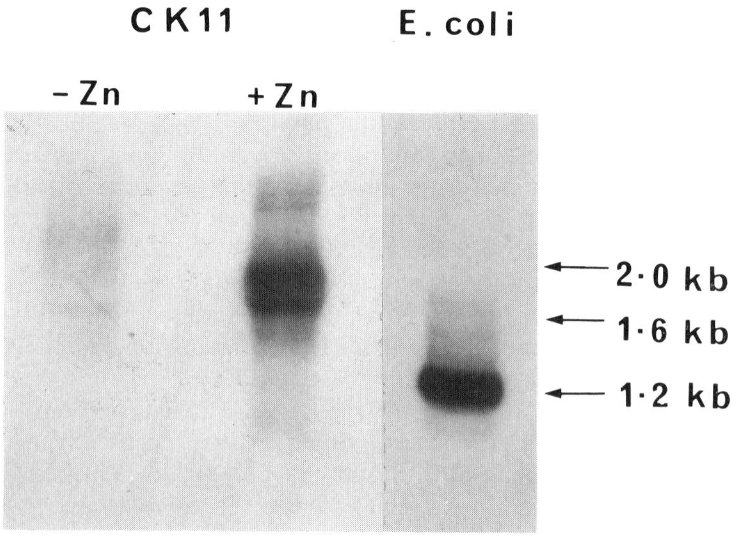

Figure 2 Northern blot analysis of total RNA extracted from mouse L-cells transformed with plasmid pMTCK11. The probe used to detect specific transcripts consisted of an anti-sense RNA to the *cysK* coding sequence. RNA from *E. coli* strain C600 is also shown as a control. Zinc induction of the cells is indicated by (+ Zn).

Production of transgenic mice

The two modified genes have been introduced into mice by microinjection. Six primary mice were obtained, two containing the MTCE11 gene and four containing the MTCK11 gene. Southern blot analysis of three of the transgenic animals is shown in Fig. 3. The number of copies integrated varies between the lines, but in each animal, the intact gene can be excised from the integration site by the restriction enzyme Bam H1, indicating that extensive rearrangement of the genes has not taken place. Progeny of these mice are currently being produced to enable the expression of the genes to be measured.

DISCUSSION

The use of gene transfer for the introduction of new metabolic pathways to animals opens up an area of great potential for increasing domestic animal productivity. Bacteria are a rich source of functional gene sequences, and the main difficulty in the approach resides in making the appropriate modifications to the genes to ensure adequate levels of regulated expression in the host animal. In the project described in this paper, regulation is provided by the use of the sheep MT-Ia promoter, which has shown remarkable regulation of the sheep growth hormone gene in transgenic mice (Shanahan *et al.*, 1989). Our results in cell culture show that the sheep MT-Ia promoter can regulate

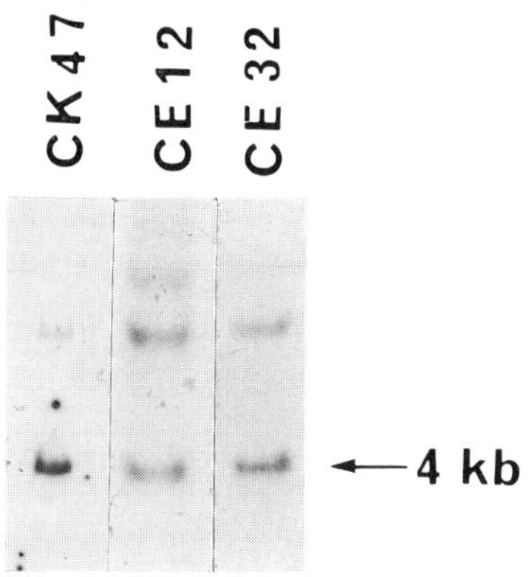

Figure 3 Southern blot analysis of three transgenic mice; CK47 contains the fusion gene insert of plasmid pMTCK11, while CE12 and CE32 contain the insert from pMTCE11. DNA was extracted from tail tissue and digested with the restriction enzyme Bam H1, which has a unique site in both fusion genes. The probes used consisted of DNA encoding the *cysE* or *cysK* genes. A tandem array of the insert arranged head-to-tail produces a DNA fragment of size 4 kb for each gene. Head-to-head or tail-to-tail arrangements produce bands of larger size.

bacterial genes in eukaryotic cells in much the same way as it regulates the sheep growth hormone gene in cell culture. Whether the same regulation can be obtained in transgenic animals remains to be seen.

Regulation and appropriate tissue-specific expression of the bacterial genes in this project is necessary for several reasons. Tissue-specific expression is required because the complete pathway can only operate if a supply of H_2S is available, and this substrate is only present in significant amounts in the sheep's digestive tract. Thus, the enzymes encoding the pathway must be produced in the rumen and intestinal epithelia. The sheep MT-Ia promoter drives the transcription of genes in the intestine of transgenic mice in response to zinc induction (Shanahan *et al.*, 1989), and therefore is a particularly attractive choice for this work. The promoter should also provide zinc-induced regulation of the genes. Such regulation is likely to be important because the first reaction of the pathway utilizes the co-enzyme acetyl-CoA, whose depletion in tissues such as the liver would likely be deleterious to the transgenic animal.

ACKNOWLEDGEMENTS

The authors gratefully acknowledge the expert technical assistance of Mrs Gina Hardwicke, Mrs Astrid Dafter and Ms Kathy Lewis.

REFERENCES

Becker, M.A., Kredich, N.M. and Tomkins, G.M. (1969). The purification and characterization of *O*-acetylserine sulfhydrylase-A from *Salmonella typhimurium*. *Journal of Biological Chemistry* **244**: 2418–2427.

Brinster, R.L., Chen, H.Y., Trumbauer, M.E., Yagle, M.K. and Palmiter, R.D. (1985). Factors affecting the efficiency of introducing foreign DNA into mice by microinjecting eggs. *Proceedings of the National Academy of Science, USA* **82**: 4438–4442.

Byrne, C.R., Wilson, B.W. and Ward, K.A. (1987). The isolation and characterization of the ovine growth hormone gene. *Australian Journal of Biological Science* **40**: 459-468.

Byrne, C.R., Monroe, R.S. Ward, K.A. and Kredich, N.M. (1988). DNA sequences of the *cysK* regions of *S. typhimurium* and *E. coli* and linkage of the *cysK* regions to *ptsH*. *Journal of Bacteriology* **170**:3150-3157.

Costantini, F. and Lacy, E. (1981). Introduction of a rabbit beta-globin gene into the mouse germ line. *Nature* **294**: 92-94.

Crewther, W.G. (1976). Primary structure and chemical properties of wool. In: Ziegler, K. (ed.) *Fifth International Wool Textile Research Conference* Vol. 1, pp. 1-101. German Wool Research Institute, Aachen.

Denk, D. and Bock, A. (1987). L-Cysteine biosynthesis in *Escherichia coli*: nucleotide sequence and expression of the serine acetyltransferase (*cysE*) gene from the wild-type and a cysteine-excreting mutant. *Journal of General Microbiology* **133**: 515-525.

Gaitonde, M.K. (1967). A spectrophotometric method for the direct determination of cysteine in the presence of other naturally occurring amino acids. *Biochemical Journal* **104**: 627-633.

Hammer, R.E., Pursel, V.G., Rexroad, C.E., Jr., *et al.* (1985). Production of transgenic rabbits, sheep and pigs by microinjection. *Nature* **315**: 680-683.

Kredich, N.M. and Tomkins, G.M. (1966). The enzymic synthesis of L-cysteine in *Escherichia coli* and *Salmonella typhimurium*. *Journal of Biological Chemistry* **241**: 4955-4965.

Maniatis, T., Fritsch, E.F. and Sambrook, J. (1982). *Molecular cloning*: *A laboratory manual*. Cold Spring Harbor Laboratory, Cold Spring Harbor, New York.

Palmiter, R.D., Brinster, R.L., Hammer, R.E., *et al.* (1982). Dramatic growth of mice that develop from eggs microinjected with metallothionein-growth hormone GH fusion genes stimulate growth in mice. *Nature* **300**: 611-615.

Palmiter, R.D., Norstedt, R.E., Gelinas, R.E., Hammer, R.E. and Brinster, R.L. (1983). Metallothionoin human GH fusion genes stimulate growth in mice. *Science* **222**: 809-814.

Peterson, M.G. and Mercer, J.F.B. (1986). Structure and regulation of the sheep metallothionein-Ia gene. *European Journal Biochemistry* **160**: 579-585.

Pursel, V.G., Pnkert, C.A., Miller, K.F., *et al.* (1989). Genetic engineering of livestock. *Science* **244**: 1281-1288.

Reis, P.J. (1979). In: Black, J.L. and Reis, P.J. (eds.) Effect of amino acids on the growth and properties of wool. *Physiological and Environmental Limitations to Wool Growth*, pp. 223-242. University of New England Publishing Unit, Armidale, Australia.

Reis, P.J. and Schinkel, P.G. (1963). Some effects of sulphur-containing amino acids on the growth and composition of wool. *Australian Journal of Biological Science* **16**: 218-230.

Reis, P.J., Tunks, D.A. & Downes, A.M. (1973). The influence of abomasal and intravenous supplements of sulphur-containing amino acids on wool growth rate. *Australian Journal of Biological Science* **26**: 249-258.

Shanahan, C.M., Rigby, N.W., Murray, J.D., *et al.* (1989). Regulation of expression of a sheep growth hormone fusion gene in transgenic mice. *Molecular and Cell Biology* **9**: 5473-5479.

Southern, P.J. and Berg, P. (1982). Transformation of mammalian cells to antibiotic resistance with a bacterial gene under control of the SV40 early region promoter. *Journal of Molecular and Applied Genetics* **1**: 327-341.

Wigler, M., Pellicer, A., Silverstein, S., Axel, R., Urlaub, G., *et al.* (1979). DNA-mediated transfer of the adenine phosphoril osyltransferase ions into mammalian cells. *Proceedings of the National Academy of Science, USA* **76**: 1373-1376.

1.6 The Histologic Analysis of Endocrine-related Alopecia in the Dog

Thelma Lee Gross and Peter J. Ihrke

Consultant in Dermatopathology and General Pathology, California Dermatopathology Service, West Sacramento; and Professor of Dermatology, Department of Medicine, School of Veterinary Medicine, University of California, Davis, California, USA

INTRODUCTION

Endocrine alopecia has been broadly characterized as a non-inflammatory atrophy of hair follicles that is presumably the result of the hormonal influences on hair growth and maturation. Hyperadrenocorticism, hypothyroidism, Sertoli cell tumour, and growth hormone/castration-responsive alopecia are the most commonly recognized canine endocrine-related skin diseases (Muller *et al.*, 1989). The latter syndrome is poorly understood and may constitute a disease complex with increased prevalence in specific breeds.

Alopecia is a characteristic clinical feature of most canine endocrine-related skin diseases. Bilaterally symmetrical truncal alopecia may be due to multiple aetiologies, including endocrinopathy, hereditary follicular dysplasia, and pruritic skin disease with self trauma. Consequently, the veterinary clinician commonly utilizes the skin biopsy as a diagnostic tool in assessing the presence of endocrine-related skin disease in dogs.

In the past, endocrine skin diseases commonly have been grouped together histologically. It has been reported that follicular changes in the various forms of endocrine alopecia are similar and consist of atrophy with a preponderance of telogen hairs (Scott, 1982). Techniques to distinguish the specific endocrinopathy often have involved special staining to detect changes in mucin or elastin levels in the dermis, the latter requiring comparison with matched controls (Scott, 1982; Scott and Walton, 1986). Endocrine-induced changes in other adnexal structures such as hypertrophy of arrector pili muscles (Scott, 1982), or atrophy of adnexal glands (Barsanti *et al.*, 1983; Nesbitt *et al.*, 1980; Scott, 1982; Watson 1985) have been reported; however, these structures vary normally depending on location in the skin and thus usually are not reliable indicators of endocrine disease on routine skin biopsy.

Reports of epidermal changes seen with endocrine-related skin disease have varied. Epidermal atrophy has been described in hyperadrenocorticism (Carlotti *et al.*, 1987; Scott, 1982; White, 1986), hypothyroidism (Martin and Capen, 1979; Scott, 1982), hypoandrogenism (Scott, 1982), and growth hormone- responsive alopecia (Scott and Walton, 1986). Acanthosis has been reported in hyperadrenocorticism (Scott, 1982), hypothyroidism (Fadok and Gross, 1982; Martin and Capen, 1979; Scott 1982), Sertoli cell tumour (Scott, 1982), and hyperstrogenism (ovarian imbalance type I) (Scott, 1982). Normal epidermal thickness has been reported in diethylstilbestrol (DES)-induced alopecia (Barsanti *et al.*, 1983).

A specific diagnosis beyond 'compatible with endocrine skin disease' is not made routinely in the practice of diagnostic surgical pathology. This is the likely result of a tendency to view follicular and adnexal changes as similar among the various types of endocrine disorders. Recent observation and personal communication with others have suggested that some distinctive and consistent histologic lesions are present on routine light microscopic examination of haematoxylin and eosin (HE)-stained sections of skin biopsy speciments from dogs with various forms of endocrine-related skin disease. These findings include the presence of catagen in addition to telogen follicles, particularly abnormal catagen follicles termed 'flame follicles' (R.W. Dunstan, personal communication), and an increase (A.A. Stannard, personal communication) or decrease in epithelial thickness of the epidermis and follicular infundibulum.

An expanded use for the skin biopsy in the diagnosis of endocrine-related alopecia could be advantageous, as results could indicate the most expeditious direction for laboratory evaluation. The purposes of this study were to characterize the histologic features of each of the principle subtypes of canine endocrine alopecia and subsequently to determine whether histologic examination of skin biopsy specimens from dogs with clinically confirmed endocrine-related skin disease might be used to predict the specific underlying skin disease.

MATERIALS AND METHODS

Skin biopsy specimens were obtained from 43 dogs with endocrine-related skin disease. All diagnoses were confirmed by clinical findings, laboratory evaluation, and response to appropriate endocrine manipulation (Table 1). All of the routine HE-stained sections were examined by the pathologist in the study (Gross) in single blinded fashion. The pathologist received no data as to the signalment or clinical history on any dog. The study included 14 dogs with hypothyroidism, nine with hyperadrenocorticism, ten with growth hormone-responsive alopecia, five with Sertoli cell tumour, and five with iatrogenic

Table 1 Criteria used for confirmation of canine endocrine skin disease

Hypothyroidism	TSH stimulation test—abnormal; Response to thyroid hormone replacement (after confirmatory testing)
Hyperadrenocorticism	Elevated serum alkaline phosphatase; ACTH stimulation test—abnormal; Low dose dexamethasone suppression test—abnormal; Endogenous ACTH—abnormal; Reponse to therapy with O'P'DDD (after confirmatory testing)
Growth hormone/castration responsive alopecia	Breed specificity; TSH and ACHTH stimulation tests—normal; Xylazine response test—abnormal; Response to exogenous growth hormone or response to castration
Sertoli cell tumour	Presence of testicular tumour (histology); Response to castration
Iatrogenic hyperoestrogenism/alopecia	ACTH and TSH stimulation tests—normal; Response to termination of DES therapy, or response to ovariohysterectomy

hyperoestrogenism due to DES administration or ovariohysterectomy-responsive alopecia (ovarian imbalance Type I). Ovariohysterectomy-responsive and iatrogenic hyperoestrogenism cases were examined together, due to the small number of total cases (five) and the suspected similarity in aetiopathogenesis.

Skin biopsy specimens from affected dogs were obtained from areas of alopecia and processed for routine histopathology. Dogs with biopsy specimens indicating calcinosis cutis or active pyoderma were excluded from the study, since calcinosis cutis would lend an obvious bias towards hyperadrenocorticism and pyoderma might have an effect on epidermal or follicular epithelial thickness, or follicular cycles.

Epidermal thickness, follicular infundibular thickness (thickening of the superficial portion of the hair follicle above the level of the adnexal appendages), type of follicular atrophy present (telogen or catagen), and the presence or absence of flame follicles were noted. For clarity and simplicity, only primary hairs were examined for stage of hair growth cycle and other morphologic characteristics. Telogen phase, the phase of physiological inactivity, was defined by a shortening and narrowing of the follicle with loss of visible hair shafts. Often, only a thin remnant of follicular sheath remained, terminating at the level of adnexal glands, above a cord of dense collagen, which represented the residual connective tissue support structure for the follicle. Catagen phase, the resting phase immediately preceding telogen, was characterized by prominence of the external root sheath of the hair follicle, a thickened glassy membrane, and prominent tricholemmal keratinization. Hair shafts were often still present within the infundibulum of the follicle.

The term flame follicle was used in this study to describe a follicular aberration resembling the catagen hair follicle. Flame follicles had exaggerated tricholemmal keratinization. Spike of keratin extended through the follicular wall to the outer root sheath, creating a flame-like configuration within the follicle. Hair shafts were not observed.

Hyperplasia (acanthosis) or atrophy of the epidermis and follicular infundibulum was defined as an increase or decrease in thickness from the normal three to four cell layers characteristic of both epithelial sites.

RESULTS

The results of histologic evaluation of specimens from 43 dogs are presented in Table 2. All dogs had follicular growth cycle arrest of telogen type, catagen type, or both. The proportion of catagen versus telogen hairs was variable and not consistent for individual types of endocrine skin disease. Flame follicles were observed with greatest prominence and abundance in growth hormone/castration-responsive alopecia. Epidermal and follicular infundibular epithelial atrophy and hyperplasia were both seen, the former most consistently in hyperadrenocorticism and the latter most consistently in hypothyroidism and Sertoli cell tumour. Many dogs, notably those with growth

Table 2 The histologic evaluation of skin biopsy specimens from dogs with endocrine-related alopecia

Clinical diagnosis	Epidermal thickness	Follicular thickness	Flame follicles
Hypothyroidism	Acanthosis 14/14	Acanthosis 14/14	0/14
Hyperadrenocorticism	Atrophy (6/9)	Atrophy (6/9)	1/9
Growth hormone	Atrophy (3/10)	Atrophy (3/10)	5/10
	Acanthosis (3/10)	Acanthosis (3/10)	
Sertoli cell tumour	Atrophy (1/5)	Atrophy (1/5)	2/5
	Acanthosis (4/5)	Acanthosis (4/5)	
Hyperoestrogenism	Acanthosis (2/5)	Acanthosis (2/5)	0/5

hormone-responsive alopecia, had no change in either epidermal or follicular infundibular thickness.

Hypothyroidism

Specimens examined from the 14 dogs with hypothyroidism showed mild-to-moderate acanthosis of the epidermis, as well as thickening of the follicular infundibulum (Fig. 1). Epidermal atrophy was not observed. Mild dermal and periadnexal inflammation consisting of mixtures of lymphocytes, neutrophils, macrophages and plasma cells was present in 12 of 14 dogs.

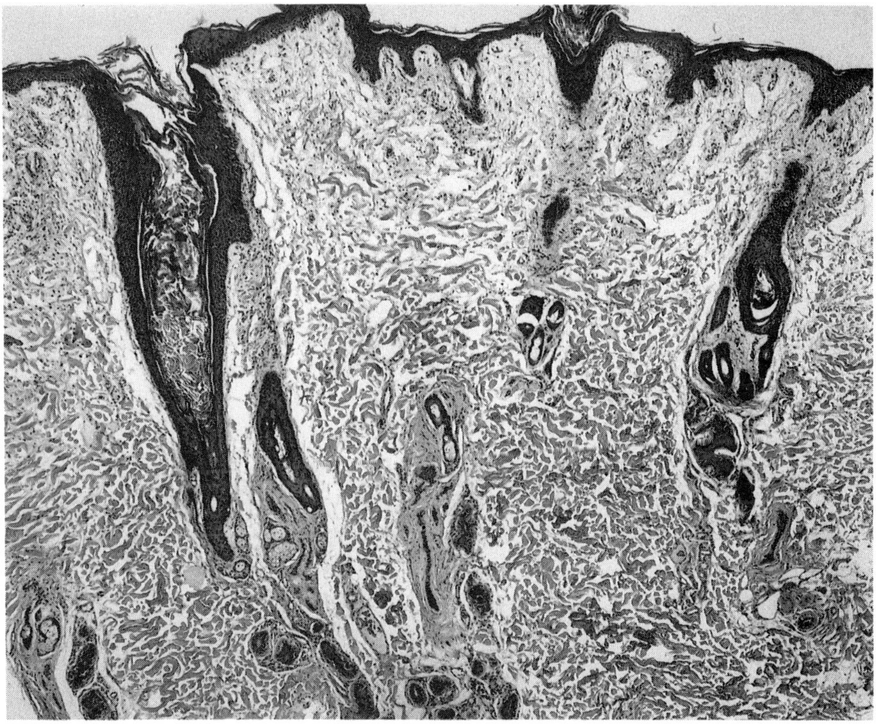

Figure 1 Hypothyroidism. Increase in thickness of epidermis and follicular epithelium; note thin epithelial remnant characteristic of telogen follicle x100.

Telogen was the predominant phase of the follicular growth cycle observed in 11 of 14 dogs (Fig. 1). Catagen hairs were predominant or present in equal proportion with telogen hairs in three dogs. Flame follicles were not observed.

Hyperadrenocorticism

Epidermal and follicular infundibular atrophy were present in specimens from six of nine dogs (Fig. 2). Biopsy specimens from the remaining three dogs showed no change in epidermal or follicular infundibular thickness. Telogen follicles predominated in specimens from seven of nine dogs. Catagen hairs were predominant in two dogs and in one of these cases, rudimentary flame follicles were observed.

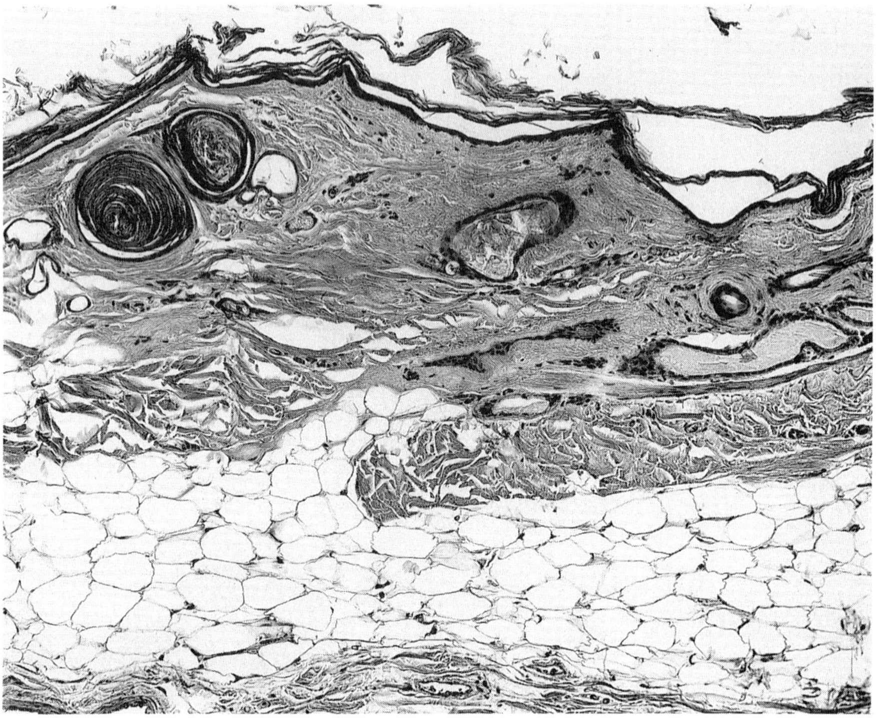

Figure 2 Hyperadrenocorticism. Epidermal and follicular indundibular atrophy. Dermal atrophy is also present. x100.

Growth hormone/castration-responsive alopecia

Epidermal and follicular infundibular thickness was variable but did not diverge from normal to any substantial degree. Epidermal and follicular infundibular atrophy were mild and multifocal in specimens from three of ten dogs. Increased thickness of the epidermis and superficial hair follicles was similarly not severe but was seen as a slight increase of one or two cell layers over normal in scattered foci in three dogs.

Catagen hairs were present in equal proportion with telogen hairs or were predominant in seven of ten dogs. In one dog, hair follicles were distorted and dysplastic in appearance and could not be definitively identified as either catagen or telogen phase. Striking and numerous flame follicles were seen in five dogs (Fig. 3), all of which had mostly catagen hairs. Flame follicles were absent in five dogs, three of which had few catagen hairs.

Sertoli cell tumour

In specimens from the five dogs examined, four dogs had mild-to-moderate epidermal and follicular infundibular thickening (Fig. 4), and one dog had

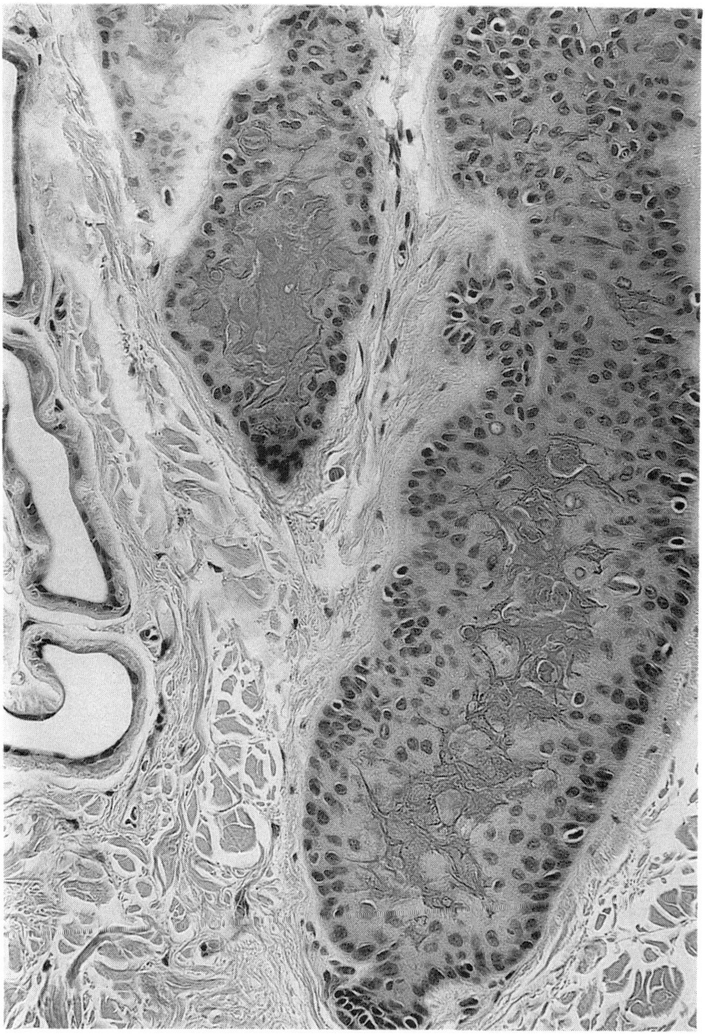

Figure 3 Growth hormone/castration-responsive alopecia: flame follicles. Note prominent tricholemmal keratinization which creates a flame-like configuration within the follicular wall. x248.

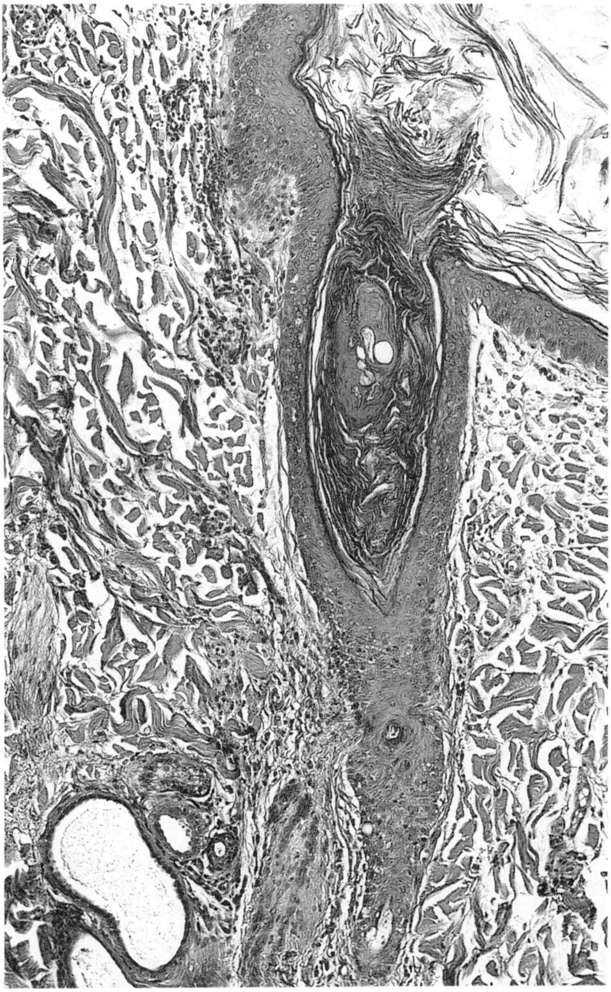

Figure 4 Sertoli cell associated alopecia. Thickening of the epidermis and follicular infundibulum. Chronic mixed inflammatory infiltrates are present in the superficial and perifollicular dermis. x100.

mild, scattered foci of atrophy at both sites. Mild chronic inflammation was seen superficially and periadnexally in specimens from two dogs (Fig. 4).

Telogen hairs predominated in three dogs and catagen hairs predominated in two dogs. Rudimentary flame follicles were observed occasionally in two dogs in which catagen hairs were prominent.

Iatrogenic hyperoestrogenism/ovariohysterectomy responsive alopecia

Epidermal and follicular epithelium showed mild thickening in specimens from two of five dogs. In one of these two dogs, there was focal moderate thickening of the epidermis. The three remaining dogs were normal at these epithelial sites (Fig. 5). Epidermal atrophy was not observed.

The proportion of catagen and telogen hairs was highly variable but telogen predominated in three of five dogs (Fig. 5). Catagen hairs were present in equal numbers or predominated in two dogs. Flame follicles were not observed.

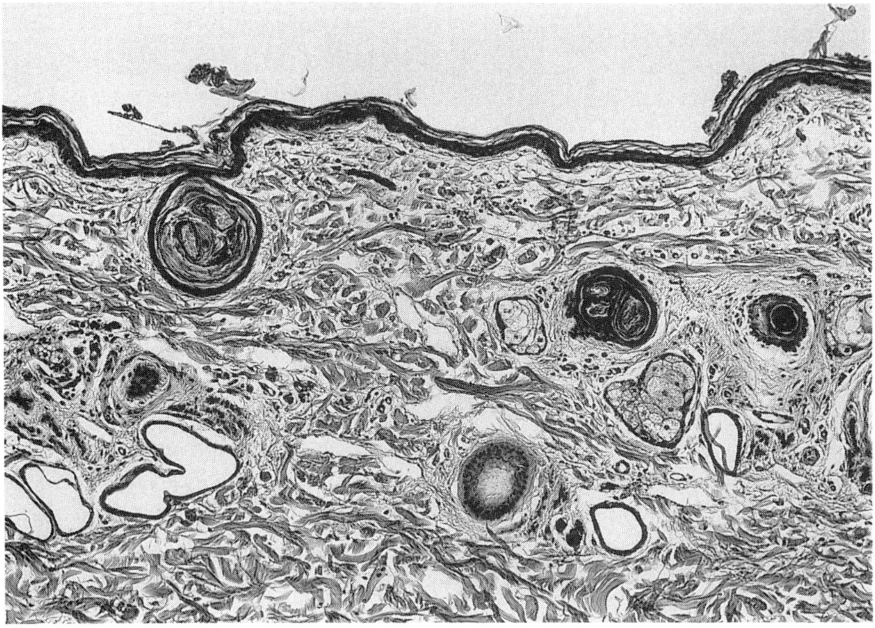

Figure 5 Ovariohysterectomy-responsive alopecia. Normal epidermis and follicular infundibulum. Thin, cord-like remnants of telogen follicles are observed. x 87.5.

DISCUSSION

Diagnostically useful histologic features suggested in this study included epidermal and follicular infundibular acanthosis in hypothyroidism, epidermal and follicular infundibular atrophy in hyperadrenocorticism, and the presence of numerous, prominent flame follicles in growth hormone/castration-responsive alopecia. Follicular atrophy, characterized by the presence of catagen or telogen hairs, was present in specimens from all dogs.

Epidermal and follicular infundibular acanthosis was present in all dogs with hypothyroidism. Epidermal atrophy was not observed. Acanthosis was also a feature of specimens from four of five dogs with Sertoli cell tumour; however, the overall numbers are too few to make any accurate assessment. It should be noted that inflammation was a feature of specimens from 12 of 14 dogs with hypothyroidism and two of five dogs with Sertoli cell tumour. It is likely that inflammation, probably associated with chronic pyoderma, contributed to the thickening of the skin in these diseases (Scott, 1982). However, since mild acanthosis was present in non-inflamed specimens from dogs with hypothyroidism and Sertoli cell tumour, this may be a primary feature. Whether or not acanthosis is a primary or secondary manifestation of endocrine-related skin disease does not diminish its diagnostic usefulness in interpreting skin biopsies if random sampling of alopecic areas of affected dogs consistently reveals this change.

Hyperadrenocorticism was the only endocrine skin disease characterized by diffuse epidermal and follicular infundibular atrophy, seen in specimens from six of nine dogs studied. The remaining three dogs had normal thickness of epidermis and follicular infundibulum; acanthosis was not seen. Epidermal atrophy in hyperadrenocorticism corresponds to findings of previous reports (Muller *et al*, 1989; Watson, 1985); however, atrophy of the follicular infundibulum previously has not been described. Epidermal atrophy has been attributed to an antianabolic effect suppressing epidermal growth as a result of the influence of cortisol (Lever and Schaumburg-Lever, 1983). Mild multifocal epidermal and follicular infundibular atrophy was seen in three dogs with growth hormone/castration responsive alopecia and in a single dog with Sertoli cell tumour.

The most significant histologic feature of growth hormone/castration responsive alopecia was the frequent prominence of catagen hairs (seven of ten dogs) and the presence of flame follicles. Only dogs with growth hormone responsive alopecia had numerous, prominent, well developed flame follicles within a single biopsy specimen (five of ten dogs). Therefore, skin biospy specimens demonstrating prominent flame follicle formation may be suggestive of growth hormone/castration responsive alopecia, particularly if the affected dog is of one of the breeds at increased risk: chow chow, keeshound or pomeranian. However, recent evidence obtained by one author (Gross), suggested that flame follicle formation may be a feature of follicular growth abnormality in general in these breeds. One pomeranian with hyperadrenocorticism and one pomeranian with DES-induced alopecia had prominent flame follicle formation in skin biospy specimens.

A recently recognized follicular dysplasia in Siberian husky dogs also is characterized by flame follicles (Post *et al.*, 1988). The significance of this finding is as yet unkown, but the histologic diagnosis of alopecia in the Siberian Husky may be problematical if flame follicles are present. In addition, postclipping alopecia in plush-coated breeds may be manifested as catagen predominance with flame follicle formation.

In this study, follicular atrophy was documented in all dogs; however, the overall proportion of catagen versus telogen hairs was variable and diagnostically useful trends were not discovered. This variability may depend on the stage of the disease at the time of biopsy, or other factors such as breed and individual differences in the expression of the hormonal imbalance in the skin. Follicular atrophy, as it occurs in endocrine skin disease, is actually an arrest of the hair growth cycle. Thus affected hairs are in catagen or telogen phase. Over time, the hair follicles also may be reduced in height and thickness and can appear much smaller than hairs that are cycling normally.

Other syndromes to consider in the differential diagnosis of hair growth cycle arrest include follicular dysplasia, telogen effluvium, and postclipping alopecia. Follicular dysplasia is a poorly understood syndrome with marked breed predilection suggesting an inheritable basis. In follicular dysplasia, there may be tologen or catagen arrest in conjunction with follicular distortion (dysplasia), follicular atrophy, or melanin pigment disturbances of the hair follicle. An early age of onset generally is observed. Telogen effluvium can cause precipitous loss of hair following stress from disease or physiologic causes, such as whelping and heavy lactation. Histologically, diffuse telogen arrest is seen, but follicles are not as diminished in size as are the telogen hairs of endocrine-related skin disease. Postclipping alopecia is characterized by a lack of hair regrowth after clipping or shaving, and is most common in thick-coated breeds, such as malamutes, samoyeds, chow chows, and Siberian husky dogs. Histologically, as stated above, there is diffuse catagen arrest, and flame follicles occasionally may be observed. Knowledge of the clinical features is useful in distinguishing endocrine-related alopecia from these three syndromes.

Routine histopathologic evaluation of dogs with suspected endocrine-related skin disease may be more rewarding than previously recognized. Biopsy of skin from areas of alopecia may reveal histologic features that will direct the clinician more effectively and economically towards conclusive diagnostic laboratory testing and therapy.

REFERENCES

Barsanti, J.A., Medleau, L. and Latimer, K. (1983). Diethlystilbesterol-induced alopecia in a dog. *Journal of the American Veterinary Medical Association* **182**: 63–64.

Carlotti, D., Legeay, Y. and Audry, A. (1987). Syndrome de Cushing spontane et d'origine iatrogene chez le chien: Clinique et etiopathogenie. *Le Point Veterinaire* **18**: 671–676.

Fadok, V.A. and Gross, T.L. (1982). Hypothyroidism in a Borzoi secondary to lymphocytic thyroiditis. *Dermatology Reports* **1**: 1–2.

Lever, W.F. and Schaumburg-Lever, G. (1983). *Histopathology of the Skin* 4th edn, p. 285. J.B. Lippincott, Philadelphia.

Martin, S.L. and Capen, C.C. (1979). Hypothyroidism and the skin. In: Muller, G.H. (ed.) *Veterinary Clinics of North America* **9**(1): 29–39.

Muller, G.H., Kirk, R.W. and Scott, D.W. (1989). *Small Animal Dermatology* 4th ed, pp. 595–658. W.B. Saunders Company, Philadelphia.

Nesbitt, G.H., Izzo, J., Peterson, L. and Wilkins, R.J. (1980). Canine hypothyroidism: A retrospective study of 108 cases. *Journal of the American Veterinary Medical Association* **177**: 1117–1122.

Post, K., Dignean, M.A. and Clark, E.G. (1988). Hair follicle dysplasia in a Siberian Husky. *Journal of the American Animal Hospital Association* **24**: 659–662.

Scott, D.W. (1982). Histopathologic findings in endocrine skin disorders of the dog. *Journal of the American Animal Hospital Association* **18**: 173–183.

Scott, D.W., and Walton, D.K. (1986). Hyposomatotropism in the mature dog: A discussion of 22 cases. *Journal of the American Animal Hospital Association* **22**: 467–473.

Watson, A.D.J. (1985). Oestrogen-induced alopecia in a bitch. *Journal of Small Animal Practice* **26**: 17–21.

White, S.D. (1986). Facial dermatosis in four dogs with hyperadrenocorticism. *Journal of the American Veterinary Medical Association* **188**: 1441–1444.

PART 2

ALLERGIC SKIN DISEASES

2.1 Clinical and Immunological Aspects of Allergic Skin Diseases in Domestic Animals

Richard E.W. Halliwell

Department of Veterinary Clinical Studies, Royal (Dick) School of Veterinary Studies, University of Edinburgh, Edinburgh, Scotland

INTRODUCTION

The diagnosis and therapy of allergic skin diseases of domestic animals forms a major part of the total effort in companion animal practice. Although great strides have been made in our understanding of certain facets of the pathogenesis of these diseases in the past two decades, a great many aspects remain unclear. This paper will review the current knowledge of the clinical and immunological aspects of the major disease entities, and will compare and contrast them with those believed to be operative in man.

THE ATOPIC DISEASES

Definition

The term atopy was introduced by Coca and Cooke (1923) to describe three familial diseases of man that appeared to have many features in common, namely atopic dermatitis, allergic asthma and hay fever. Although environmental allergens were implicated in all of them, the antibody involved was unusual in that it was not demonstrable by the standard precipitation reactions, and was termed reagin (Coca and Grove, 1925). An appropriate working definition of atopy is thus 'the inherited predisposition to develop reaginic antibodies to environmental allergens that results in allergic disease' (Halliwell and Gorman, 1989a).

The nature of the reagin, and its role in the diseases

The landmark studies of Prausnitz and Küstner (1921) showed that the antibody was heat labile and that it could be transfered to the skin of normal individuals by intradermal injection. The antibody fixed to the skin at the site of injection, and a wheal and flare reaction could be elicited at that site by the same allergens to which the donor was allergic. That the transference of antibody could cause disease was shown previously following an anecdotal observation by Ramirez (1919). One of his patients who had no previous history of allergic disease, was hospitalized for a blood transfusion. Shortly after returning home, he went for a ride in a horse-drawn carriage and suffered an acute attack of asthma. It was subsequently determined that the donor of the blood that he had received was allergic to horse dander, and thus the sensitive state had been transferred to the patient by the transfusion.

Little progress was made on further elucidating the nature of the reagin until the late 1960s. At that time the leading candidate was IgA, but Ishizaka and his colleagues showed unequivocally that the reaginic activity was associated with a hitherto undescribed immunoglobulin class that they termed IgE (Ishizaka *et al.*, 1966). The antibody fixes to mast cells and basophils via the Fc portion, and bridging of two adjacent molecules by bivalent or multivalent allergen initiates degranulation and release of not only performed mediators, but also the membrane derived mediators of the arachidonic acid cascade.

Although it is clear that the manifestations of the atopic diseases result largely from the effects of IgE, there is evidence that IgG antibody may be pathogenic in some instances. The latter antibody is heat stable, and remains at the site of passive sensitization for 2–4 h only (Parish, 1970). Patients with disease resultant from this type of antibody will still have positive skin tests, although larger amounts of antigen are required to elicit a response. The subclass IgG_4 has been implicated (Vijay and Perelmutter, 1977) — the subclass which paradoxically is increased in patients who have undergone successful hyposensitization. The contrasting features of the two types of homocytotropic antibody are summarized in Table 1.

In many patients with asthma, bronchial provocation produces a biphasic response. The immediate response is believed to involved mast cells, whereas

Table 1 Contrasting features of IgE and IgG homocytotropic antibody

	IgE	IgG
Amount of antigen required to elicit a positive skin test	Very little	Greater amount
Heat labile	Yes	No
Persistance at site after intradermal injection	48 h+	2–12 h

the late phase reaction which occurs some 4–6 h after provocation apparently involves basophils. The latter response is increasingly viewed as important in the pathogenesis of asthma. A similar biphasic response can be induced in some allergic patients by intradermal injection of allergen, although higher doses are required to produce the late phase reaction than those necessary to produce an immediate response. IgE is implicated in the cutaneous and the respiratory responses of both types, and all are ameliorated following successful immunotherapy (Solley *et al.*, 1976; Frew and Kay, 1988).

In the atopic diseases of man, IgE antibody is implicated in most cases of hay fever and allergic asthma but its association with atopic dermatitis is less clear. Positive intradermal skin tests, and elevated levels of total and allergen-specific IgE are commonplace; however, there is usually little clinical association of the antibody with the disease, and many regard it as an epiphenomenon. On the other hand, there are cases where the removal of the allergen(s) implicated results in dramatic resolution (Adkinson and Platts-Mills, 1988).

Factors predisposing to an IgE response

All normal individuals have low levels of IgE antibody, and there are a number of factors known to modify positively or negatively, the likelihood that an immune response to a given antigen will include the IgE isotype.

The dose of antigen

Low dose antigenic stimulation favours an IgE response, particularly when administered repeatedly. In contrast higher doses favour the usual IgM response followed by IgG but without detectable IgE. In this context it is noteworthy that the amount of ragweed pollen inhaled by a human patient with hay fever is of the order of 1 μg/season (Marsh, 1975).

The molecular structure

In general, allergens responsible for allergic diseases tend to be relatively large and complex. However the chemical nature that specifically predisposes to the IgE isotype response remains obscure. Berrens (1971) has suggested that it is a function of the number of reactive lysine–sugar residues. It would be intriguing to examine the antigens from parasites such as *Ascaris* for this feature. These not only are potent allergens in their own right, but also they tend to prime the host to an IgE response to any unrelated allergen administered at the same time.

Particulate size and solubility of the antigen

Larger pollens, spores or other allergenic particles are deposited in the upper airway of man, and thus cause symptoms of allergic rhinitis. Smaller particles may reach the lower airway and induce asthma in sensitive individuals. However oral breathing can alter this, and favour access of large pollens to the lower airway. The solubility of the antigen contained in the pollen or spore is also relevant.

Genetic makeup of the individual

Studies in man have shown that the total level of IgE is subject to genetic control that is not linked to genes of the major histocompatibility or HLA complex (Meyers and Marsh, 1981). In contrast, there are a number of instances in which an IgE response to a particular allergen has been shown to be HLA linked (Marsh *et al.*, 1987).

Concomitant infections

Parasite infections enhance the IgE response to any allergen administered at the same time. It is intriguing to postulate that this could be relevant to animals, in which such infections are commonplace. Also, there is evidence that concommitant virus infections may help trigger an IgE response, and controlled studies in dogs have similarly shown that immunization with live, attenuated vaccines at the time of antigenic presentation can potentiate this isotype (Frick and Brooks, 1983).

Other factors relating to the pathogenesis

It has become clear over the years that there are factors other than the level of allergen-specific IgE antibody that account for the symptomatology of the atopic diseases. Atopic people have abnormal dermal and pulmonary responses to agents such as histamine and methacholine, and multiple observations suggest a rather poor relationship between the level of antibody, access of allergen and the severity of the disease. Also, the amount of histamine release from basophils of different individuals following an identical challenge varies, and is subject to genetic control (Marone *et al.*, 1986), with similar findings being noted in dogs (Schwartzman *et al.*, 1971). Two major theories have been proposed to account for these and other similar observations.

The β-adrenergic theory of atopy

Szentivanyi (1968) suggested that many of the abnormalities seen in atopy could be the result of an imbalance of adrenergic and cholinergic regulatory influences due to a blockade of β-adrenergic receptors. It was further suggested that this was a reflection of lowered cyclic AMP levels which could be due to increased cyclic AMP phosphodiesterase activity. It is, indeed, possible to ascribe the beneficial effects of many of the therapeutic agents that ameliorate the clinical signs of the atopic diseases to their effects on cyclic AMP levels.

Histamine releasing factors and IgE heterogeneity

More recently, important observations have been made regarding a group of cytokines termed histamine releasing factors, or HRFs (Lichtenstein, 1988). These substances are heterogeneous, and can be derived from lymphocytes macrophages and platelets. They have affinity for IgE from atopic individuals, and when they bind to this antibody on the surface of basophils from either atopic or normal individuals, they cause spontaneous histamine release in an antigen non-specific manner. In contrast, they have no effect on basophils sensitized with IgE from normal individuals. Mast cells are apparently less susceptible to these effects, but the implications for these cells have not been evaluated in such detail. This has led to the proposal that IgE is heterogeneous, and that atopics have a special type of IgE, termed IgE + . Non-atopics possess IgE −, which can still give a positive skin test and a positive radioallergosorbent test (RAST), but which causes only mild disease or no disease. The concept is indicated diagramatically in Fig. 1.

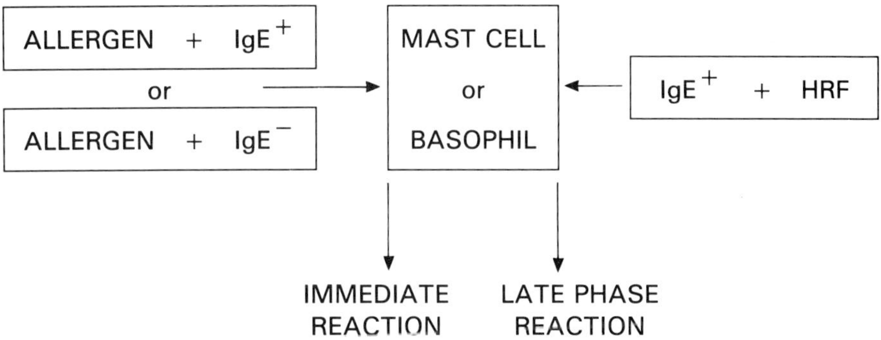

Note: It appears that
* Mast cells are involved in immediate reactions
* Basophils are involved in late phase reactions

Figure 1 Postulated interaction of IgE^{+}, IgE^{-} and histamine releasing factors with basophils and mast cells. The interaction appears more significant in the case of basophils. After Lichtenstein (1988).

Spontaneous production of HRF in seasonally allergic individuals increases during the season of involvement, and in food allergic patients when eating the offending food (Kuna *et al.*, 1989; Sampson *et al.*, 1989). Successful immunotherapy is associated with reduced spontaneous HRF production (Kuna *et al.*, 1989). It is intriguing to postulate that it might also be associated with a conversion from IgE + to IgE −, experiments that have yet to be undertaken.

CANINE ATOPIC DISEASE

The first reported diagnosis of canine atopy was made by a medical allergist (Wittich, 1941), and the condition is now recognized as one of the more common causes of puritic skin disease in the dog (Halliwell and Schwartzman, 1971; Scott, 1981). Terms employed to describe the condition include atopy, atopic disease, atopic dermatitis and allergic inhalent dermatitis. I prefer the first two. The use of the term atopic dermatitis implies that it is the same entity as atopic dermatitis of man. There are, in fact, a number of important differences, which are listed in Table 2. Most significant of these is the fact that the specific allergic management of the condition (i.e. allergy testing and hyposensitization), is generally accepted in veterinary medicine and is highly effective whereas such approaches are rarely employed in man as they are believed to be of little if any value.

Table 2 Contrasting features of canine atopic disease and atopic dermatitis of man

	Canine atopic disease	Atopic dermatitis of man
Positive skin tests	+ + +	+ + +
Correlation of skin tests with disease	+ +	+/−
Peak age of onset	6 months–3 years	3–6 months
Response to firm stroking	?	Paradoxical blanching
Response to methacholine	?	Delayed blanching
Response to histamine	Reduced[a]	Reduced
Histopathology	Perivascular mononuclear infiltrate	Similar
Elevated cyclic AMP phosphodiesterase	Yes[a]	Yes
Therapeutic response to hyposensitization	Yes	No

[a] Only shown in an experimental model

Regarding the last term (allergic inhalant dermatitis), it is unclear whether the respiratory tract is in fact the route of access of allergen. Implicating that route is the observation that when experimentally bred atopic dogs are nebulized with ascaris antigen, not only do they undergo bronchoconstriction, but also they develop dermatitis (Butler *et al.*, 1983). As evidence against that route, it would seem unlikely that inhaled allergen could avoid being bound by both mucosal and systemic antibody before reaching the site of fixation of IgE antibody on dermal mast cells. Support for the theory that percutaneous penetration of allergen could be responsible has recently been derived from studies in man. Patch tests performed on uninvolved skin of patients with atopic dermatitis using allergens to which they were positive by prick test, produced positive reactions indicating that percutaneous penetration of allergen through the relatively thicker human epidermis was readily achieved (Adinoff *et al.*, 1988). The contrasting evidence regarding the potential role of these two routes is summarized in Table 3.

Table 3 Route of access of allergen in canine atopic disease: evidence in favour of the cutaneous and respiratory routes

In favour of the percutaneous route	In favour of the respiratory route
1. Patch tests on normal skin of humans with atopic dermatitis are often positive.[a]	1. Basenji-greyhound 'atopic' dogs develop dermatitis when nebulized with ascaris antigen.[b]
2. Circulating antibody and local (respiratory tract) antibody would prevent inhaled allergen from reaching the skin.	2. Some dogs develop signs of atopic disease in situations in which percutaneous penetration would be unlikely, e.g. high-rise appartments.
3. The distribution is more consistant with percutaneous penetration.	
4. The thinner canine epidermis would facilitate percutaneous penetration as compared with man.	

[a] Adinoff *et al.* (1988).
[b] Butler *et al.* (1983).

The immunopathogenesis of canine atopy

Canine IgE was identified shortly after the antibody was described in man. It was shown to share common antigenicity with the human antibody (Halliwell *et al.*, 1972) and to be exclusively associated with mast cells in canine skin (Halliwell, 1973). Levels of the immunoglobulin are very much higher in the dog with levels of around 200 μg/ml frequently found in normal dogs (Vriesendorp *et al.*, 1975) which contrasts to a range of around 20–200ng/ml in man (Zetterstrom and Johansson, 1981). This is probably reflective of the much higher incidence of endoparasite infection in dogs. Indeed in a recent survey of sera from heavily parasitized Florida 'pound' dogs, some animals had levels of the order of 1mg/ml (Halliwell, 1987, unpublished data). Thus although allergic humans tend to have higher levels of IgE, this is not true for the dog (Vriesendorp *et al.*, 1975) due to the high level of parasite induced IgE and the relatively low level of allergen-specific IgE.

The detection of allergen-specific IgE in canine sera by means of the RAST has been described (Halliwell and Kunkle, 1978). Antibody was detected in the sera of most dogs suffering from atopic disease, and was absent from sera of normal dogs. Correlation between positive RAST and positive skin tests varied with the antigen, and was good for ragweed, but poor for house dust. However, the study provided support for the role of IgE in the immunopathogenesis of the canine disease.

More recently, Willemse *et al* (1985a) induced homocytotropic antibodies in normal dogs which were heat-stable, resistant to reduction by 2-mercaptoethanol, and fixed to skin for 2–4 h. The implication was that these were of the IgG_1 (or $_d$) subclass, but the critical experiment of removing IgG_1 from sera by passage through an immunoabsorbent column to show removal of skin-sensitizing antibody was not reported. In further studies, allergen-specific IgG_1 antibodies were detected in the sera of dogs with signs of atopy (Willemse *et al.*, 1985b). It was proposed that this antibody could be involved in the pathogenesis of canine atopy, and particularly that it might be responsible for disease in patients with negative immediate skin tests. However, one would still expect that animals with disease due to such an antibody would show positive skin tests, although it might be necessary to employ extracts of higher strength. Also, one would expect that allergen-specific antibodies of the IgG class would be found in association with IgE, for in atopic people the levels of the two classes tend to be correlated (Platts-Mills *et al.*, 1980).

In summary, it is likely that there exists in dogs a short-term sensitizing antibody of the IgG class. Its precise definition, and its role, if any, in allergic diseases remains to be elucidated.

Experimental models of canine atopy

A number of attempts have been made to develop colonies of atopic dogs in order to better study the pathogenesis of the condition. In one study, the progeny of atopic/atopic matings were followed for 2–3 years. By 24 months, 18 out of 27 showed positive skin tests, and 13 had dermatological signs compatible with atopy (Schwartzman, 1984). Interesting data have emerged from a study of a colony of basenji-greyhound crosses that manifest clinical signs of atopic disease upon repeated nebulization with ascaris antigen and also have heightened airway reactivity and a blunted leukocyte cyclic AMP response to β-adrenergic agents (Butler *et al.*, 1983). This was shown to be associated with elevated mononuclear leukocyte cyclic AMP phosphodiesterase (Hirshman *et al.*, 1987). Similar biochemical changes were found in unrelated atopic basenjis, but the latter did not show airway hyperresponsiveness. This suggested that the skin changes and the airway abnormalities are not linked, and do not result from the same underlying biochemical defect, as summarized in Table 4.

Table 4 Clinical, biochemical and functional abnormalities in the basenji–greyhound atopic dog model

	Basenji–Greyhound	Basenjis	Greyhounds
Skin test reactivity	Yes	Yes	No
Airway hyperreactivity	Yes	No	No
Leucocyte cAMP phosphodiesterase	Elevated	Elevated	Normal
Clinical signs of atopic disease	Yes	Yes	No

Data from Hirshman *et al.* (1987).

Clinical features

Atopic disease has a peak age of onset between 1 and 3 years of age, and most studies reveal a slight female sex predisposition. There are marked breed predispositions which will vary with the geographic variations in the genetic pool (Schick and Fadok, 1986).

The hallmark of the clinical signs is pruritus, which often has a characteristic distribution involving the feet, the face and the ventrum. It is questionable if there is a primary eruption, but a variety of secondary changes resulting from self-trauma are seen. Chronic cases show seborrhoea, lichenification and hyperpigmentation, and a secondary staphylococcal infection is frequently observed. It is possible that the latter results from impaired cell-mediated immune responses and/or from an increased adherence of staphylococci to the stratum corneum cells of the atopic dog, as discussed in papers elsewhere in this publication (Nimmo-Wilkie, Ch. 2.5; McEwan, p. 449).

Diagnosis

Willemse (1986) has recently suggested the adoption of diagnostic criteria to aid in the diagnosis based to some extent upon those applied to the diagnosis of atopic dermatitis in man. A controversial point is the relegation of the demonstration of the presence of IgE or of IgG_1 antibody to environmental allergens as a minor criterion. This seems inappropriate in a disease in which there appears to be a strong aetiological association with skin sensitizing antibody, of whichever class, and in a disease which responds well to hyposensitization.

I make a diagnosis of atopy using the following three criteria:

1. Compatible clinical signs.

2. Evidence of IgE antibody to environmental allergens assessed either by skin tests or *in vitro* tests.
3. A positive correlation between the presence of IgE antibody to an allergen and the presence of that allergen in the environment at a time coincident with the clinical signs.

Skin tests

A full discussion regarding skin test techniques is beyond the scope of this paper, and the reader is referred to a recent text (Halliwell and Gorman, 1989b). However two recent publications on the topic deserve mention.

It is known that corticosteroids profoundly inhibit the skin test response, and it is important in this context to consider not only parenterally administered agents but also those applied topically which are readily absorbed percutaneously. Additionally, it has recently been shown that antihistamines will interfere with the response for up to 10 days after withdrawal (Barbet and Halliwell, 1989). Another important consideration is the use of tranquilizers, which must obviously not be antihistaminic. It is a common clinical observation that animals that struggle unduly during skin testing tend to have suppressed tests. Kunkle (1989) has shown that some dogs skin tested without tranquillization, show markedly increased plasma cortisol. The mean plasma cortisol level in 30 dogs increased from 3.43μg/dl to 6.04μg/dl during the procedure. Whereas some dogs were not greatly affected (e.g. 1.15μg/dl), the levels in one Lhasa apso increased from 1.72μg/dl to 11.42μg/dl. This suggests that it could be prudent to use tranquilizers routinely in an attempt to limit such responses which clearly could affect the skin test results.

In vitro *tests*

Both RAST and an enzyme linked immunosorbent assay (ELISA) are commercially available in the USA, and are likely to become available in other parts of the world shortly. Both tests measure the same allergen-specific IgE antibody, and would be expected to be equivalent in value. One problem in dogs is the much higher background level of IgE antibody than that found in man. Presumably this is directed against parasite antigens. Such high levels might be expected to interfere with the assay, and this is the subject of another paper in this symposium (Griffin *et al.*, Ch. 2.4). The relative merits of RAST and skin tests are compared in Table 5. The possibility that corticosteroids could have an inhibitory effect in the ELISA is controversial. It has been claimed that they interfere, but there is no published controlled study which addresses this question.

Dipstick technology has advanced rapidly in recent years, and the commercial availability of a product for canine use has recently been announced (Bioproducts, Phoenix, Arizona). Reports of its value in the field are awaited with interest. A similar product marketed for use in man has been shown to give results which correlate well with results of RAST (Twiggs *et al.*,

Table 5 Relative advantages of intradermal skin tests and RAST in the diagnosis of canine atopic disease

Skin tests	RAST
More sensitive	More specific
Cheap	More expensive
Quick	Takes 2–4 days including mail time
Assesses mast cell function as well as antibody level	Assesses antibody level alone
Inhibited by corticosteroids	Corticosteroids should have no effect
Inhibited by antihistamines	Antihistamines have no effect

1989), and it is hoped that similar correlative studies will be undertaken in dogs. Attention should also be drawn to the basophil degranulation test discussed elsewhere (Prelaud, Ch. 2.2), although the requirement for fresh blood and access to a specialized laboratory limits its widespread application.

Therapy

The clinician has a number of therapeutic approaches. Corticosteroids have for long been popular in practice, but their side-effects following long-term use means that alternative therapy must be used for animals that are affected for other than short seasons each year. Antihistamines are efficacious in a small number of cases, and some patients respond better to one preparation than another. The use of essential fatty acids has been described (Lloyd, 1989), and represents an exciting new therapeutic approach. Also, a number of non-steroidal mast cell stabilizers are entering the clinical trial stage in dogs, and some are showing encouraging results.

However, the mainstay in terms of efficacy and cost is hyposensitization, which was recently the subject of a placebo controlled trial (Willemse *et al.*, 1984). The median symptom score of 27 allergen-treated atopic dogs improved 61.5%, whereas that of 24 placebo treated animals was unchanged. In 59% of treated animals there was at least a 51% improvement in clinical signs compared with 21% of control animals (Table 6). The critical time appeared to be 9 months in that a response was unlikely to occur if there had been no improvement by then.

Hyposensitization is a generally safe form of treatment, with the incidence of anaphylactic reactions being <1%. In a few cases adverse reactions take the form of a worsening of the clinical signs for 12–48 h following the injection. These are more likely to occur in highly sensitive individuals, and it is prudent to employ lower doses of allergen in such animals. Improvement is either gradual, or it may be cyclical following each injection, with some exacerbation

Table 6 Results of hyposensitization in canine atopic disease

	Placebo treated (%) ($n = 24$)	Allergen treated (%) ($n = 27$)
Median of improvement in symptom scores	0.0	61.5
Percentage of dogs improving >51%	21	59

Data from Willemse *et al.* (1984).

occuring after 10–15 days. Most patients will require maintenance therapy indefinitely, although in the long term, injections can often be given at increasing intervals or just preseasonally as appropriate.

Finally, it is important to emphasize that combination therapy often represents the very best approach. Essential fatty acids, antihistamines and hyposensitization have varying effects in different cases, and any or all of them can have a 'steroid-sparing' effect. Shampoo therapy also has a place, not only in cases of secondary pyoderma or seborrhoea, but also for a direct antipruritic effect, e.g. coal tar. Each case is different, and a careful and thoughtful approach is the key to success.

ATOPIC DISEASE IN OTHER SPECIES

Canine atopy fulfills the accepted criteria for an atopic disease, but the situation in other species is less clear.

Cats show both respiratory and cutaneous disease in response to environmental allergens, but a genetic predisposition has yet to be demonstrated. Atopic rhinitis of cattle is more convincing in that breed predispositions and an association with environmental allegens are clearly demonstrated (Pemberton and White, 1976), and bovine IgE has been well characterized (Gershwin and Dygert, 1983). It is not clear whether the recently described familial allergic rhinitis of cattle is a manifestation of the same entity (Krahwinkel *et al.*, 1988). A recent report documents a seasonal pruritic dermatitis in sheep which the authors believed had features of an atopic disease (Scott and Campbell, 1987). Further characterization is awaited with interest.

FOOD ALLERGY

Immunopathogenesis

Adverse reactions to food are not always immune mediated. Idiosyncratic reactions, toxicity, and pharmacologic or metabolic reactions may also be involved (Anderson and Sogu, 1984).

It is well established that macromolecular antigens are capable of penetrating the normal, intact gastrointestinal tract. Most antigens implicated are heat and acid stable glycoproteins with molecular weights of 18 000–36 000 daltons. Milk, fish, shellfish, soya and wheat are most often implicated in man.

Although antibodies to dietary allergens of all the major immunoglobulin classes and also immune complexes are found in sera of patients with food hypersensitivity, the main distinction between findings in affected and normal individuals is in the level of allergen-specific IgE. Cell-mediated responses to food allergens are also found, but such reactions are also commonly demonstrable in normals. The conclusions are that type 1 hypersensitivity is responsible for most, if not all immune mediated adverse reactions to food (Johansson *et al.*, 1984).

The immunopathogenesis in domestic animals is unknown. Although positive immediate skin test reactivity is often shown, and the presence of allergen-specific IgE antibody in the sera of affected dogs is sometimes demonstrable by the use of commercially available laboratory assays, there have been no controlled trials documenting the restriction of either positive test to affected animals.

Clinical signs

In man, the skin, gastrointestinal tract and respiratory systems are most often affected, but a wide range of additional signs are sometimes ascribed to food hypersensitivity.

In veterinary medicine, the condition appears to affect dogs and cats with approximately equal frequency, but with a somewhat differing clinical picture.

Cutaneous signs in cats are always pruritic, and have a predilection for the head and neck in some 50% of cases (White and Sequoia, 1989). Miliary dermatitis, varying manifestations of self-trauma and eosinophilic plaques may be seen. Signs seen in dogs include pruritus that may be generalized or localized to particular areas of the body, recurrent moist dermatitis, allergic otitis externa, urticaria or predisposition to recurrent staphylococcal folliculitis (White, 1986). Response to corticosteroids in both species is quite variable. Food hypersensitivity may also cause diarrhoea (Walton, 1967), and a number of chronic gastrointestinal conditions affecting both dogs and cats may respond to dietary manipulation which suggests the possibility of an allergic aetiology.

Diagnosis and therapy

Therapy should involve elimination of the offending allergen from the diet, and thus the correct diagnosis is imperative.

The diagnostic value of skin tests in man has long been controversial. The predictive value of a negative prick test is good, and approximates to 90–100%. However the predictive value of a positive test is much lower, and has been estimated as 5–76% dependent upon the frequency with which the allergen is implicated as a cause of hypersensitivity (Sampson and Albergo, 1984). It appears that RAST is little better. In one recent carefully controlled study in children, the predictive value of RAST and prick tests was similar at 80%, but both showed around 30% of false positives (Sampson and Albergo, 1984). An interesting recent report described the use of patch tests using allergen and dimethyl sulphoxide (DMSO) (Breneman *et al.*, 1989).

In animals, there is currently no good alternative to the use of selected prepared diets formulated to exclude any of the original constituents fed to the patient. Lamb and rice is generally preferred for dogs, and unfortunately it does not appear that commercial preparations are acceptable as diagnostic aids. In one study some 20% of dogs that were asymptomatic on lamb and rice suffered a relapse with the introduction of the commercial substitute (White, 1986). Such diets are, however, frequently acceptable for maintenance purposes. Although most dogs show a substantial improvement within 3 weeks of institution of the hypoallergenic diet, data elsewhere in this publication suggests that in rare cases much longer is required (White and Mason, Workshop Report 6). The diagnosis is confirmed if the patient relapses upon reintroduction of the original diet within 10–14 days.

ALLERGIC CONTACT DERMATITIS

Immunopathogenesis

Classically, a rigid distinction between irritant contact and allergic contact dermatitis is made, but more recent understanding of the pathophysiology of the two conditions suggests that this may be inappropriate. Detailed ultrastructural and immunohistochemical studies reveal a similar admixture of suppressor/cytotoxic T cells in both types of condition (Ranki *et al.*, 1983). Also, it is recognized that the most potent contact sensitizers often have irritant properties. Thus although 'true' reactions of either type are certainly encountered, many cases of contact dermatitis probably contain facets of both entities. Another confusing situation is that although mononuclear cells predominate in early lesions, in some cases appreciable numbers of basophils are revealed with the use of special fixative and staining conditions (Dvorak and Mihm, 1972). This suggests that cutaneous basophil hypersensitivity may contribute to the pathogenesis in many instances.

Potent cutaneous sensitizers are usually haptens of low molecular weight (<500 daltons) that are lipid soluble and bind covalently to skin proteins. Propensity to induce sensitivity is enhanced by increasing concentrations, by moisture, by close contact (e.g. absence of hair) and by preexistant cutaneous inflammation or abrasions. Induction of the immune response follows presentation of the antigen by Langerhans la positive cells to T-lymphocytes. An additional trigger is required for the induction of the immune response in the form of interleukin 1. This role can also be assumed by epidermal cell-derived thymocyte-activating factor (ETAF) which can be produced by both keratinocytes and Langerhans cells and is similar, if not identical to interleukin 1. It is not clear whether the cellular interaction which generates the immune response occurs in the skin, or the local lymph node.

Clinical signs

Allergic contact dermatitis is uncommon in the dog, and is rarely diagnosed in the cat and other domestic animals. In large part this may be due to the excellent protection afforded by the haircoat. Substances implicated have included dyes, mordants and finishes used in the manufacture of carpets, wood resins, preservatives, polishes, cleansing agents and weeds (Walton, 1977; Nesbitt and Schmitz, 1977; Kunkle and Gross, 1984). The condition is variably pruritic but always exhibits a primary eruptive process which is papular or macular. A secondary staphylococcal infection is frequently superimposed. Chronic changes of hyperpigmentation and lichenification may ensue.

Diagnosis and therapy

The optimum therapy is clearly the exclusion of the allergen from the environment, with corticosteroid therapy being the only viable alternative.

Recent years have provided little in the way of improved diagnostic aids. It is customary to approach the diagnosis in two parts. Firstly, confirmation of a diagnosis of allergic contact dermatitis, and secondly implication of the allergen. The first is most readily achieved by noting improvement following a complete change of environment. Implication of the allergen is achieved by selective environmental challenge or by patch testing with commercially available patch tests or with selected items from the environment.

HYPERSENSITIVITY TO PARASITES

Introduction

Both endo- and ectoparasites can engender interesting allergic responses which on the one hand can cause host damage, but which may also lead to varying degrees of immunity. Insect hypersensitivity is a frequent cause of skin disease in domestic animals, and the clinical signs can range from the chronic and mild to the acute and life-threatening. Anaphylactic shock can result from hymenoptera sensitivity, and it has also been recorded following bites of the imported fire ant, *Solenopsis invicta* (Halliwell and Gorman, 1989c). In other instances, the response is less severe, but adds to the pathogenicity of the parasitic disease. An example is hypersensitivity to the ear mite *Otodectes cynotis* which has been documented in cats (Powell *et al.*, 1985), and on clinical grounds it seems likely that it also occurs in dogs. Of great interest is the hypersensitivity response in porcine scabies (Cargill and Dobson, 1979) which can apparently lead to spontaneous resolution of the condition. In the case of canine scabies it appears that the immune response is less effective, in that although antiinflammatory therapy with corticosteroids can lead to a great increase in the number of viable mites recoverable upon skin scraping, the disease does not resolve without parasiticidal therapy. However, the best example of hypersensitivity leading not only to recovery but to a high degree of subsequent immunity is tick hypersensitivity which is a subject of another report in this publication (Opdebeck and Merchant, Workshop Report 5).

Flea hypersensitivity

Flea hypersensitivity is the most common non-routine reason for presentation of dogs and cats to veterinarians in the South, Southeast and Western parts of the USA, and in Western Europe. The species of flea most commonly found upon dogs and cats in Florida is *Ctenocephalides felis*, with *Pulex irritans* also sometimes involved (Harman *et al.*, 1987). This condition has been the subject of research in our laboratory for the past decade. The work has involved only dogs, and although many of the features may also apply to cats, this has yet to be established.

The flea allergen

The flea allergen(s) are present in saliva, and are injected when the flea takes a protein meal. Although early work employing the guinea pig as an experimental model suggested that the major flea allergen was a hapten (Young *et al.*, 1963), a number of protein antigens have recently been identified as being allergenic in dogs. Molecular weights ranged from 18 000–45 000 daltons, and a major allergen was noted of between 30 000 and 32 000 daltons (Halliwell *et al.*, 1987; Preston and Halliwell, unpublished data). Activity was not detectable in low molecular weight fractions of flea allergen in the animals examined.

Immunopathogenesis

Observation of the sites on hypersensitive dogs at which fleas feed, reveals visible reactions that persist in some cases for up to 5–6 days. Similar responses are noted to injected allergenic extract. Skin biopsies taken 15–20 min after the fleas bite show a histopathological picture consistant with an IgE mediated reaction (Gross and Halliwell, 1985), and allergen specific IgE antibody is detectable in the majority of sera from animals with flea allergy dermatitis (Halliwell and Longino, 1985). Biopsies taken 24–48 h after biting reveal evidence of cell-mediated hypersensitivity (Gross and Halliwell, 1985). Most clinically affected dogs show both immediate and delayed reactions, but in 10–20% of patients delayed reactions only are noted, with somewhat fewer showing visible immediate reactions alone.

Of great interest was the demonstration that basophils accounted for up to 20% of the cellular infiltrate in biopsies taken from 4–18 h after biting, implying involvement of cutaneous basophil hypersensitivity (Halliwell and Schemmer, 1987). It is also likely that late-phase IgE reactions are involved, and the finding that affected animals sometimes have quite high levels of IgG antibody, indicates the potential for the involvement of Arthus reactions. The immunopathogenesis is thus multifaceted.

Induction of hypersensitivity

Flea allergy was induced experimentally, in our laboratory, in 24 flea-naive dogs of random and mixed breeds, and both sexes, obtained from Cheyenne, Wyoming through the Department of Animal Resources, Colorado State University. Prior to exposure to fleas, all showed negative intradermal skin tests to 1/1000 W/V *Ct. felis* allergen (Greer Laboratories, Lenoir, North Carolina, USA). The dogs were assigned to three groups of eight. Two groups were exposed to the bites of 25 *Ct. felis* for 15 min either once or three times weekly, and a viable flea population was maintained continually on the third group. All animals were skin tested with flea allergen weekly, and the reactions were recorded at 15 min using a scale of +1, +2 and +3. A negative response was no greater than the diluent control, and a +3 reaction approximated the size of an injection of 1/100 000 weight per volume (w/v) of histamine phosphate. Reactions were also similarly graded at 24 h by reference to the size of the previous immediate histaminc wheal.

All animals that were intermittantly exposed developed positive immediate and delayed skin tests within 3–8 weeks, whereas the animals that were continually exposed either failed to develop positive skin tests, or developed them later and to a lesser degree (Figs 2a, b). After 24 weeks, half of the animals that were initially continually exposed were changed to once or three times weekly exposure. Similarly, half of those that were intermittantly exposed were changed to continual exposure. In the latter case, strongly positive immediate and delayed skin tests developed within 8 weeks, but changing animals from intermittent to continual exposure had no effect upon the skin tests. It thus appears that the relative or total lack of skin test reactivity resulting from continual exposure persists only as long as continual exposure is maintained.

Early studies on the induction of hypersensitivity to flea antigen in guinea pigs, showed that a state of delayed hypersensitivity commenced first to be followed by coexistant immediate and delayed hypersensitivity and then immediate reactivity alone. With continuing antigenic exposure, all animals became non-reactive by 140 days (Benjamini *et al.*, 1961). This same orderly sequence was not observed in the canine studies, with visible immediate and delayed reactions apparently commencing in random sequence (Table 7).

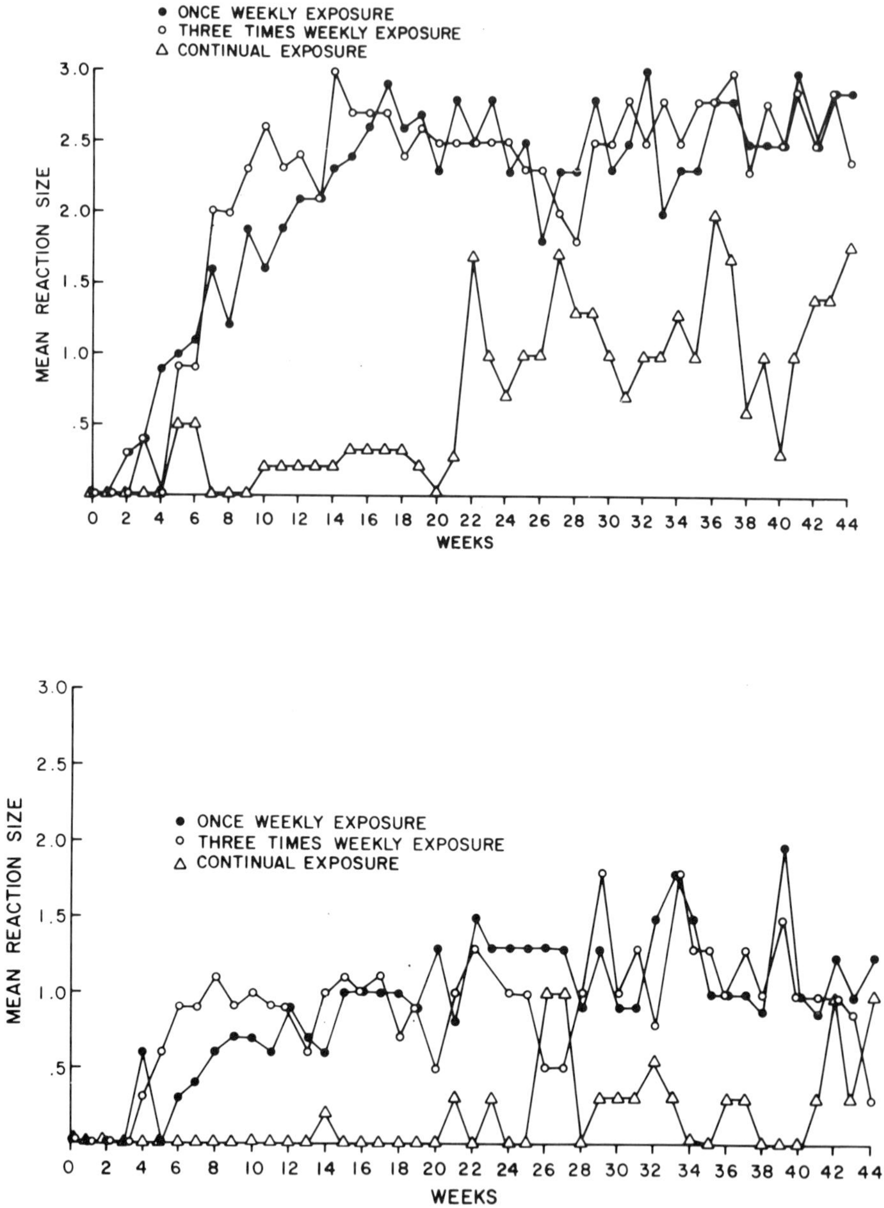

Figure 2a,b Immediate (a) and delayed (b) skin test responses to intradermal injection of flea allergen during induction of hypersensitivity in flea-naive dogs employing differing exposure regimens.

Table 7 Onset of visible immediate and delayed skin reactivity during the induction of flea bite hypersensitivity in 20 flea-naive dogs

	No. of dogs
Immediate reactivity first	6
Immediate and delayed reactivity commenced the same week	5
Delayed reactivity first	9

Further studies have revealed the following additional information concerning the development of flea hypersensitivity (Halliwell *et al.*, 1987).

1. Atopic dogs are predisposed to the development of flea allergy.
2. Animals raised in environments in which fleas are endemic year round (e.g. Florida) are less likely to develop severe flea allergy than those whose early years are spent in the North of the USA and who move to flea endemic areas at an older age.
3. The degree of hypersensitivity tends to wane with age in some animals with continued exposure, although many animals maintain their hypersensitive state indefinitely.

Serological response during induction of hypersensitivity

Antibody to flea allergen was measured in sera from the 24 dogs during the induction of hypersensitivity using previously described methods (Halliwell and Longino, 1985). Animals that developed positive skin tests generally showed increasing levels of both IgE and IgG antibody at or about the time that positive skin test reactivity was demonstrable. In contrast, antibody of both classes was low or absent in sera from the continually exposed dogs. The possibility that antibody might have been rendered undetectable due to the antigen persisting from the continued exposure was examined, but samples taken 1–2 weeks after removal of the fleas remained at the same level.

Antibody levels to flea allergen in normal and affected dogs

The finding that dogs continually exposed to fleas appeared to have little or no detectable immune response prompted an investigation into the antibody levels to flea allergen in dog populations with varying clinical responses to flea exposure. Florida stray (pound) dogs can be assumed to be continually and massively exposed to fleas, and yet RAST revealed little or no IgE or IgG antibody to flea allergen in such animals (Halliwell and Longino, 1985). In many cases the levels of resultant radioactivity were no greater than those found in the preliminary samples taken from the flea naive dogs from Cheyenne, Wyoming. In contrast, high levels of both IgE and IgG were demonstrable in most sera from flea-allergic dogs presented for therapy to the Dermatology Clinic of the University of Florida.

A further study was undertaken to confirm these findings using a better defined population and an ELISA technique (Halliwell *et al.*, 1985), employing the same antigen and antisera used in the above study. Sera were obtained from dogs owned by clients of the Veterinary Medical Teaching Hospital of the University of Florida on which heavy persistant populations of fleas had been noted for the past 6 months, and yet who suffered no clinically evident dermatitis. Control sera from flea-naive dogs were obtained from the humane society in Calgary, Alberta (courtesy of Dr J. Stone) at the time of routine examination, and sera were examined from a further 35 dogs presented with flea allergy dermatitis. The results (Fig. 3a,b) were similar to the study cited above. The mean level of IgG anti-flea antibody in the 26 sera from continually exposed dogs was 329 relative antibody units (RAU), which was significantly lower than the mean value of 929 RAU in 35 sera from dogs clinically allergic to fleas ($p = <0.001$).

The data from these two studies is supportive of the inferences drawn from the experimental induction of hypersensitivity, namely that persistant antigenic stimulation from a continual flea population leads to a state of partial or complete immunological tolerance.

Clinical signs and diagnosis

In canine flea allergy there is always a primary papular eruption which may initially be urticarial. A variety of secondary changes resulting from self-trauma and chronic inflammation ensue, and the sites of predilection include the lower back and posterior thighs.

In the cat the distribution is quite variable, and miliary dermatitis, eosinophilic plaques or merely hair loss from excessive licking may be seen.

Diagnosis in both species requires all of the following:

1. Compatible clinical signs.
2. Evidence of the presence of fleas or of flea dirt.
3. A positive immediate or delayed reaction to intradermal injection of 1/1000 w/v flea allergen.

Therapy

Unfortunately, there is no evidence that flea hypersensitivity is amenable to hyposensitization. Results of double-blind studies in both dogs and cats have failed to show efficacy (Halliwell, 1981; Kunkle and Milcarsky, 1985). Flea control and antiinflammatory therapy alone are of value.

Parasite hypersensitivity in other species

These are important causes of skin disease in both domesticated and in non-domesticated animals and caused by both endo- and ectoparasites. Many are the subject of reports elsewhere in this publication.

Dermatitis in horses resulting from infection with the filarid parasite

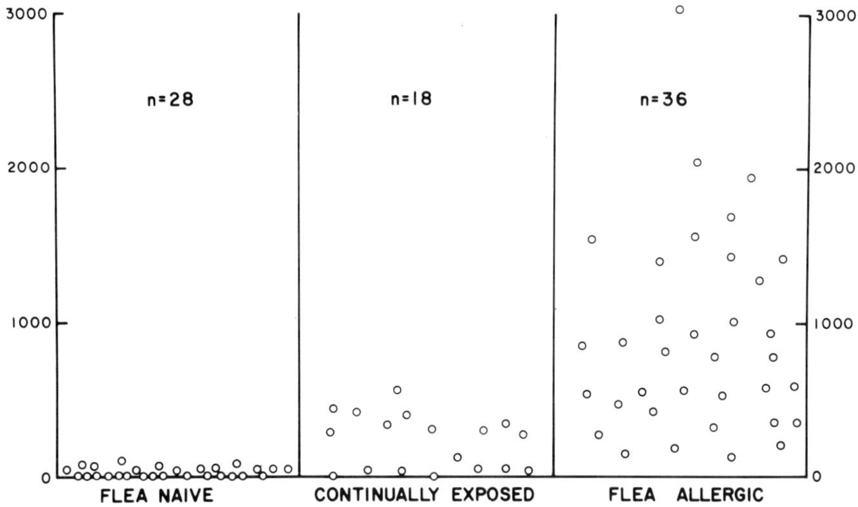

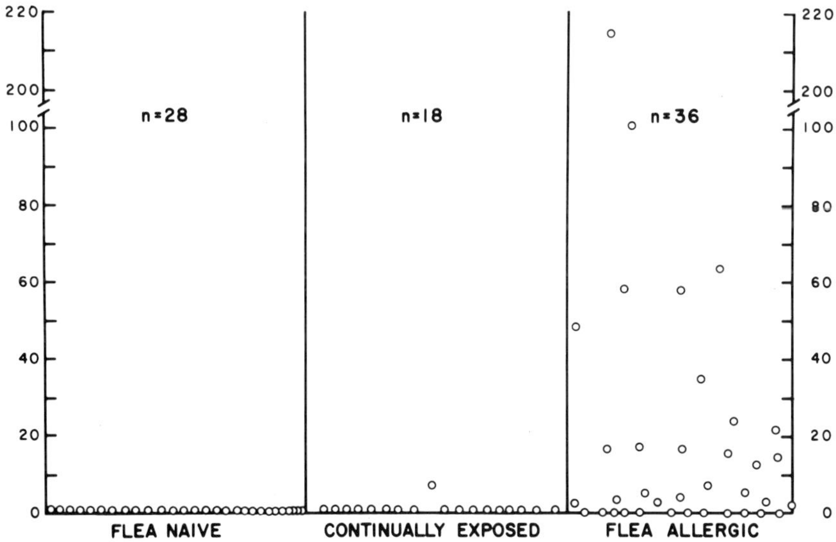

Figure 3a,b Levels of IgG (a) and of IgE (b) antibodies to flea allergen in relative antibody units in differing dog populations.

Onchercerca cervicalis, was until recently a very common entity in many parts of the world. Many infected animals are asymptomatic, and yet the parasite is readily demonstrable in the skin. This implies that hypersensitivity reactions are responsible for the clinical signs. However the advent of ivermectin has placed this parasite on the endangered species list, and a number of interesting questions regarding the immune responses to the parasite are likely to remain unanswered.

Hypersensitivity of horses to the bites of *Culicoides* spp has been likened to flea allergy in the dog. It is the cause of sweet itch (or Queensland itch), and may be responsible for other dermatoses of the horse. There are clearly demonstrable immediate and delayed hypersensitivity components, and reaginic antibody has been demonstrated by passive transfer tests (Matthews *et al.*, 1983). It also seems likely that late-phase IgE mediated reactions are contributory, but attempts in our laboratory to demonstrate features consistant with cutaneous basophil hypersensitivity were unsuccessful.

Of great interest is the fact that early exposure of horses to *Culicoides* tends to be protective in a manner analogous to that seen in flea hypersensitivity in dogs (Brostrom *et al.*, 1987). In contrast, first exposure to the parasite later in life tends to favour the development of a severe allergic response.

Evidence of the existence of *Culicoides* hypersensitivity in sheep in Britain has recently been reported (Connan and Lloyd, 1988). Affected animals had pruritic, scaling and crusted lesions affecting particularly the ears, inner elbows, thighs and the udder region (Plates 16A, B). Positive immediate and delayed intradermal skin tests resulted from injections of an antigen prepared from *Culicoides obsoletus*.

CONCLUSIONS

This paper has reviewed the current state of knowledge regarding allergic skin disease of animals. In some areas considerable advances have been made over the past two decades, but in others our state of knowledge is quite rudimentary. Continued collaboration between clinicians, immunologists and pharmacologists will be required to enable ongoing progress. Furthermore, the funding agencies must remain convinced that these diseases are not only very important in the context of health and welfare of animals, but also that they offer important models for the counterpart diseases of man.

REFERENCES

Adinoff, A.D., Tellez, P. and Clark, R.A.F. (1988). Atopic dermatitis and aeroallergen contact sensitivity. *Journal of Allergy and Clinical Immunology* **81**: 736–742.

Adkinson, N.F. and Platts-Mills, T.A.E. (1988). IgE and atopic disease. In: Samter M. *et al.* (eds) *Immunological Diseases* p. 120. Little, Brown and Company, Boston.

Anderson, J.A. and Sogu, D.D. (eds) (1984). *Adverse reactions to foods.* NIH publication No. 84: 2442.

Barbet, J.L. and Halliwell, R.E.W. (1989). Duration of inhibition of immediate skin test reactivity by hydroxyzine hydrochloride in dogs. *Journal of the American Veterinary Medical Association* **194**: 1565–1569.

Benjamini, E., Feingold, B.F. and Kartman, L. (1961). Skin reactivity in guinea pigs sensitized to flea bites: The sequence of reactions. *Proceedings of the Society for Experimental Biology and Medicine* **108**: 700–702.

Berrens, L. (1971). The chemical classification of the atopic allergens: an attempt at interpretation. *International Archives of Allergy and Applied Immunology* **41**: 186–198.

Breneman, J.C., Sweeney, M. and Robert, A. (1989). Patch testing demonstrating immune (antibody and cell-mediated) reactions to foods. *Annals of Allergy* **62**: 461–469.

Brostrom, H., Larsson, A. and Troedsson, M. (1987). Allergic dermatitis of Icelandic horses in Sweden: an epidemiological study. *Equine Veterinary Journal* **19**: 229–236.

Butler, J.M., Peters, J.E., Hirshman, C.A. *et al.* (1983). Pruritic dermatitis in asthmatic basenji-greyhound dogs: a model for human atopic dermatitis. *Journal of the American Academy of Dermatology* **8**: 33–38.

Cargill, C.F. and Dobson, K.J. (1979). Experimental *Sarcoptes scabei* infestation in pigs. (1) Pathogenesis. *Veterinary Record* **104**: 11–14.

Coca, A.F. and Cooke, R.A. (1923). On the classification of the phenomena of hypersensitiveness. *Journal of Immunology* **8**: 163–182.

Coca, A.F. and Grove, E.F. (1925). Studies in hypersensitiveness X111. A study of the atopic reagins. *Journal of Immunology* **10**: 445–464.

Connan, R.M. and Lloyd, S. (1988). Seasonal allergic dermatitis in sheep. *Veterinary Record* **123**: 335–337.

Dvorak, H.F. and Mihm, M.C. (1972). Basophil leucocytes in allergic contact dermatitis. *Journal of Experimental Medicine* **135**: 235–242.

Frew, A.J. and Kay, A.B. (1988). The pattern of human late-phase skin reactions to extracts of aeroallergens. *Journal of Allergy and Clinical Immunology* **81**: 1117–1121.

Frick, O.L. and Brooks, D.L. (1983). Immunoglobulin E antibodies to pollens augmented in dogs by virus vaccines. *American Journal of Veterinary Research* **44**: 440–445.

Gershwin, L.J. and Dygert, B.S. (1983). Development of a semi-automated assay for bovine immunoglobulin in E: Definition and standardization. *American Journal of Veterinary Research* **44**: 891–895.

Gross, T.L. and Halliwell, R.E.W. (1985). The histopathology of experimental flea allergy dermatitis in dogs. *Veterinary Pathology* **22**: 78–81.

Halliwell, R.E.W. (1973). The localisation of IgE in canine skin: an immunofluorescent study. *Journal of Immunology* **110**: 422–430.

Halliwell, R.E.W. (1981). Hyposensitization in the treatment of flea bite hypersensitivity: Results of a double-blind study. *Journal of the American Animal Hospital Association.* **17**: 249–253.

Halliwell, R.E.W. and Gorman, N.T. (1989a). In: *Veterinary Clinical Immunology*, W.B. Saunders Company, pp. 213–214, Philadelphia.

Halliwell, R.E.W. and Gorman, N.T. (1989b). In: *Veterinary Clinical Immunology*, W.B. Saunders Company, pp. 238–242, Philadelphia.

Halliwell, R.E.W. and Gorman, N.T. (1989c). In: *Veterinary Clinical Immunology*, W.B. Saunders Company, p. 270. Philadelphia.

Halliwell, R.E.W. and Kunkle, G.A. (1978). The radioallergosorbent test in the diagnosis of canine atopic disease. *Journal of Allergy and Clinical Immunology* **62**: 236–242.

Halliwell, R.E.W. and Longino, S.L. (1985). IgE and IgG antibodies to flea allergen in differing dog populations. *Veterinary Immunology and Immunopathology* **8**: 215–133.

Halliwell, R.E.W. and Schemmer, K.R. (1987). The role of basophils in the immunopathogenesis of hypersensitivity to fleas (*Ctenocephalides felis*) in dogs. *Veterinary Immunology and Immunopathology* **15**: 283–29.

Halliwell, R.E.W. and Schwartzman, R.M. (1971). Atopic disease in the dog. *Veterinary Record* **89**: 209–214.

Halliwell, R.E.W., Schwartzman, R.M. and Rockey, J.H. (1972). Antigenic relationship between human IgE and canine IgE. *Clinical and Experimental Immunology* **10**: 399–407.

Halliwell, R.E.W., Hines, M.T. and Brim, T. (1985) Studies on equine recurrent uveitis. II. The role of infection with *Leptospira interrogans* serovar *pomona*. *Current Eye Research* **4**: 1033–1040.

Halliwell, R.E.W., Preston, J.F. and Nesbitt, J.G. (1987) Aspects of the immunopathogenesis of flea allergy dermatitis in dogs. *Veterinary Immunology and Immunopathology* **17**: 483–494.

Harman, D., Halliwell, R.E.W. and Greiner, E.C. (1987). Flea species infesting dogs and cats in North Central Florida. *Veterinary Parasitology* **23**: 135–140.

Hirshman, C.A., Leu, D.B., Austin, D.R. *et al.* (1987). Elevated mononuclear leukocyte phosphodiesterase in allergic dogs with and without airway hyperresponsiveness. *Journal of Allergy and Clinical Immunology* **79**: 46–53.

Ishizaka, K., Ishizaka, T. and Hornbrook, M.M. (1966). Physicochemical properties of reaginic antibody. V. Correlation of reaginic activity with yE-globulin antibody. *Journal of Immunology* **97**: 840–853.

Johansson, S.G.O., Dannalus, A. and Lilja, G. (1984). The relevance of anti-food antibodies for the diagnosis of food allergy. *Annals of Allergy* **53**: 665–670.

Krahwinkel, D.J., Schmeitzel, L.P., Fadok, V.A. and Kitchen, H. (1988). Familial allergic rhinitis in cattle. *Journal of the American Veterinary Medical Association* **192**: 1593–1596.

Kuna, P., Alam, R., Kuzminska, B. and Rozniecki, J. (1989). The effect of preseasonal immunotherapy on the production of histamine-releasing factor (HRF) by mononuclear cells from patients with seasonal asthma: results of a double-blind, placebo-controlled randomized study. *Journal of Allergy and Clinical Immunology* **83**: 816–825.

Kunkle, G.A. (1989). Atopy in pet animals. *Journal of Small Animal Practice* **30**: 219–223.

Kunkle, G.A. and Gross, T.L. (1984). Allergic contact dermatitis to *Tradescantia fluminensis* (wandering Jew) in a dog. *Compendium of Continuing Education for the Practicing Veterinarian* **5**: 925–930.

Kunkle, G.A. and Milcarsky, J.A. (1985). Double-blind flea hyposensitization in cats. *Journal of the American Veterinary Medical Association* **186**: 677–680.

Lichtenstein, L.M. (1988). Histamine releasing factors and IgE heterogeneity. *Journal of Allergy and Clinical Immunology* **81**: 814–820.

Lloyd, D.H. (1989). Essential fatty acids and skin disease. *Journal of Small Animal Practice* **30**: 207–212.

Marone, G., Poto, S., Celestino, D. and Bonini, S. (1986). Human basophil releasibility. III. Genetic control of human basophil releasibility. *Journal of Immunology* **137**: 3588–3592.

Marsh, D.G. (1975). Allergens and the genetics of allergy. In: Sela, M. (ed.) *The Antigens* Vol. 3, pp. 271–359. Academic Press, New York.

Marsh, D.G., Freidhoff, L.R., Ehrlich-Kautzky, E., Bias, W.B. and Roebber, M. (1987). Immune responsiveness to *Ambrosia artemisifolia* (short ragweed) pollen allergen *Amb aVI* (Ra6) is associated with HLA-DR5 in allergic humans. *Immunogenetics* **26**: 230–236.

Matthews, A.G., McPherson, E.A. and Imlah, P,I, (1983). A reagin-like antibody in equine serum. I. Occurence and some biological properties. *Veterinary Research*

Communications **6**: 13–23.
Meyers, D.A. and Marsh, D.G. (1981). Report of an NIAID-sponsored workshop on the genetics of toal IgE levels in man. *Journal of Allergy and Clinical Immunology* **67**: 167–170.
Nesbitt, G.H. and Schmitz, J.A. (1977). Contact dermatitis in the dog. A review of 35 cases. *Journal of the American Hospital Association* **13**: 155–163.
Parish, W.E. (1970). Short-term anaphylactic antibodies in human sera. *Lancet i*, 591–592.
Pemberton, D.H. and White, W.E. (1976). Bovine nasal granuloma in Victoria: A search for the causative allergens. *Australian Verterinary Journal* **53**: 155–157.
Platts-Mills, T.A.E., Chapman, M.D. and Marsh, D.G. (1980). Human IgE and IgG antibody responses to the "minor" ragweed allergen Ra3. Correlation with skin tests and comparison with other allergens. *Journal of Allergy and Clinical Immunology* **120**: 129–134.
Powell, M.B., Weisbroth, S.H., Roth, L. and Wilhelmson, C. (1985). Reaginic hypersensitivity in *Otodectes cynotis* infestation of cats and the mode of mite feeding. *American Journal of Veterinary Research* **41**: 877–822.
Prausnitz, C. and Küstner, H. (1921). Studien über die Uberimfindlichkeit. *Zentralblatt für Bakteriologie* **86**: 160–169.
Ramirez, M.A. (1919). Horse asthma following blood transfusion: report of a case. *Journal of the American Medical Association* **73**: 984–985.
Ranki, A., Kanerva, L., Forstrom, L., Konttinen, Y. and Mustakallio, K.K. (1983). T and B lymphocytes, macrophages, and Langerhans cells during the course of contact allergic and irritant reactions in man. *Acta Dermato-Venereologica (Stockholm)* **63**: 376–383.
Sampson, H.A. and Albergo, R. (1984). Comparison of results of skin tests, RAST and double-blind placebo-controlled food challenges in children with atopic dermatitis. *Journal of Allergy and Clinical Immunology* **74: 26**–33.
Sampson, H.A., Broadbent, K.R. and Bernhill-Broadbent, J. (1989). Spontaneous release of histamine from basophils and histamine-releasing factor in patients with atopic dermatitis and food hypersensitivity. *New England Journal of Medicine* **321**: 228–232.
Schick, R.O. and Fadok, V.A. (1986). Responses of atopic dogs to regional allergens: 268 cases 1981–1984. *Journal of the American Veterinary Medical Association* **189**: 1493–1496.
Schwartzman, R.M. (1984). Immunologic studies of progeny of atopic dogs. *American Journal of Veterinary Research* **45**: 375–378.
Schwartzman, R.M., Rockey, J.H. and Halliwell, R.E.W. (1971). Canine reaginic antibody. Characterisation of the spontaneous anti-ragweed and the induced anti-dinitrophenyl reaginic antibodies of the atopic dog. *Clinical and Experimental Immunology* **9**: 549–569.
Scott, D.W. (1981). Observations on canine atopy. *Journal of the American Animal Hospital Association* **17**: 91–100.
Scott, D.W. and Campbell, S.G. (1987). A seasonal pruritic dermatitis resembling atopy in sheep. *Agricultural Pracrice* **8**: 46 49.
Solley, G., Gleich, G.J., Jordan, R.E. and Schroeter, A.L. (1976). The late phase of the immediate wheal and flare reaction: its dependence upon IgE antibodies. *Journal of Clinical Investigation* **58**: 408–420.
Szentivanyi, A. (1968). The beta-adrenergic theory of the atopic abnormality in bronchial asthma. *Journal of Allergy* **42**: 203–232.
Twiggs, J.T., Gray, R.L., Pichler, K. and Weiner, R. (1989). Evaluation of multi-allergen dipstick screening test. *Annals of Allergy* **63**: 225–228.
Vijay, H.M. and Perelmutter, L. (1977). Inhibition of reagin mediated PCA reactions in monkeys and histamine release from human leucocytes by human IgG_4 subclass.

International Archives of Allergy and Applied Immunology **53**: 78–87.

Vriesendorp, H., Schmidt-Mercz, B.M.J., Visser, T.P., Halliwell, R.E.W. and Schwartzman, R.M. (1975). Serological DL-A typing of atopic and normal North American dogs. *Transplantation Proceedings* **7**: 375–377.

Walton, G.S. (1967) Skin responses in the dog and cat due to ingested allergens. Observations on 100 confirmed cases. *Veterinary Record* **81**: 709–713.

Walton, G.S. (1977) Allergic contact dermatitis. In: Kirk, R.W. (ed.) *Current Veterinary Therapy*, p. 571. W.B. Saunders Company, Philadelphia.

White, S.D. (1986). Food hypersensitivity in 30 dogs. *Journal of the American Veterinary Medical Association* **188**: 695–698.

White, S. and Sequoia, D. (1989). Food hypersensitivity in cats: 14 cases 1982–1987. *Journal of the American Veterinary Medical Association* **194**: 692–695.

Willemse, A. (1986). Atopic skin disease: a review and a reconsideration of diagnostic criteria. *Journal of Small Animal Practice* **27**: 771–778.

Willemse, A., van den Brom, W.E. and Rijnberk, A. (1984). Effect of hyposensitization on atopic dermatitis in dogs. *Journal of the American Veterinary Medical Association* **184**: 1277–1280.

Willemse, A., Noordzij, A., Rutten, VPGM and Bernadina, W.E. (1985a). Induction of non-IgE anaphylactic antibodies in dogs. *Clinical and Experimental Immunology* **59**: 351–358.

Willemse, A., Noordzij, A., van den Brom, W.E. and Rutten, V.P.G.M. (1985b). Allergen specific IgG_d antibodies in dogs with atopic dermatitis as determined by the enzyme linked immunosorbent assay (ELISA). *Clinical and Experimental Immunology* **59**: 359–363.

Wittich, F.W. (1941). Spontaneous allergy (atopy) in the lower animal. *Journal of Allergy* **12**: 247–251.

Young, J.D., Benjamini, E., Feingold, B.F. and Noller, H. (1963). Allergy to flea bites. V. Preliminary results of fractionation and assay for allergenic activity of material derived from the oral secretion of the cat flea *Ctenocephalides felis felis*. *Experimental Parasitology* **13**: 155–166.

Zetterstrom, O. and Johansson, S.G.O. (1981). IgE concentrations measured by PRIST in serum of healthy adults and in patients with respiratory allergy. A diagnostic approach. *Allergy* **36**: 537–547.

2.2 Basophil Degranulation Test in the Diagnosis of Canine Allergic Skin Diseases

Pascal Prelaud

Laboratoire d'Immunologie et d'Allergologie, Department Veterinaire, Paris, France

INTRODUCTION

Atopy is a common pruritic dermatitis in the dog. In addition to a careful history and examination of the clinical signs, the diagnosis is made by the use of intradermal skin testing to aeroallergens and interpretation of results at 15–20 min (Willemse, 1983; Muller *et al.*, 1989). The purpose of intradermal skin testing is to identify the specific allergens which are involved in the allergic reaction. After that a specific immunotherapy can be attempted to control the disease. However, practitioners can be disappointed by the results of skin tests in dogs presumed to be atopic (Vollset, 1985). The unreliable results could be due to poor quality allergenic extracts in some veterinary kits and to a lack of experience in skin testing. The commercialization of allergen specific IgE *in vitro* tests promised an aid in the diagnosis of atopy. However, the results of allergen specific IgE, IgGd and IgG determination give some contradictory results (Halliwell and Kunkle, 1978); Schwartzman *et al.*, 1983; Willemse *et al.*, 1985b; Griffin, 1989; Prélaud and Sainte Laudy, in press). For these reasons, we tried to set up a cellular test, for *in vitro* exploration of hypersensitivities in the dog.

Basophils, like mast cells, are target cells of anaphylaxis and have been studied much more extensively in the past few years. It is no longer considered a secondary cell and its role in major allergic reactions is now widely accepted. Mast cells and basophils are characterized by cytoplasmic granules whose stroma is composed of glycosilaminoglycans. These granules contain preformed mediators such as histamine, enzymes and particularly proteases, hydrolases, such as succinyl dehydrogenase, and chemotactic substances.

To study basophils, it is necessary to set up staining methods (Shelley and

Juhlin, 1961; Shelley, 1974), or to measure preformed mediator release, such as histamine in man, in the incubation medium (Sainte Laudy, 1988). The histamine release test has been used in the dog (Schwartzman *et al.*, 1971; Peters *et at.*, 1982; Prélaud, 1986). However, it cannot be routinely performed because blood histamine levels in the dog are too low.

We set up a cellular test comparable to the human basophil degranulation test, to explore canine immediate hypersensitivity. The basophil degranulation test was developed by Shelley and Juhlin (1961) on human and rabbit basophils. The principle of the test is the loss of affinity for cationic dyes of sensitized basophil granules after an antigenic stimulation.

In the dog and cat, cationic dyes, such as toluidine blue and alcian blue, either fail to stain basophils or stain too few of them, to be useful (Jain, 1986; Prélaud and Sainte Laudy, 1988). This is probably due to a lack of sulphated glycosilaminoglycans in the granule stroma of mature basophils in these two species.

Shelley (1974) described an enzymatic method to stain basophil granules. It uses the transformation of iodonitrotetrazolium (INT) by succinyldhydrogenase in a dark purple formazan. We used this technique to stain canine basophil granules. We applied this test to the diagnosis of canine atopy, food and hormonal hypersensitivity, and compared our results with those obtained by skin testing.

MATERIAL AND METHODS

Selection of dogs

The animals from the control group ($n = 50$) are adult dogs (age ranging from 1 to 10 years, 25 German shepherds, five poodles, 2 labradors, one collie and 17 mongrels), who had not suffered from any pruritc dermatitis for at least 1 year. These dogs were not skin tested and have never shown any clinical signs of atopy as described by Willemse (1986).

The atopic dogs, used ($n = 99$) had a clinical diagnosis of atopy according to Willemse's criteria (Willemse, 1986b). All of them presented at least three major and two minor criteria of atopy, excluding biological and skin tests.

Skin tests

Skin tests were performed with standardized aqueous extracts (Dome-Hollister-Stier Laboratories) of the most common aeroallergens encountered in Paris (*Dermatophagoïdes farinae*, *D. pteronyssinus* cat dander, *Alternaria* sp., *Aspergillus* sp. *Cladosporium* sp., *Penicillium* sp. (molds mixed 1), grasses, alder, English plantain, birch, hazel, plane tree, ash, mugwort). One-twentieth ml of a four activity unit by RAST (AUR)/ml or 1/1000 w/v allergen saline solution was injected intracutaneously. Assessments of tests were made between 15 and 20 min, after injection. All erythematous wheals of a mean diameter over 10 mm and greater than the mean diameter of positive (histamine dichlorhydrate 1/10 000 w/v) and negative controls were considered as positive.

All the dogs were tested prior to specific immunotherapy, and at least 2 months after steroid or antihistamine therapy.

Basophil degranulation test

Preparation of sensitized cells

As described by Sainte Laudy (1987), blood was taken with heparin (5 IU/ml) and EDTA (5mM). The whole blood was centrifuged at 500 *g* for 10 min and the buffy coat was then collected and washed in a washing buffer (NaCl 130mM, Hepes 20mM, pH 7.4).

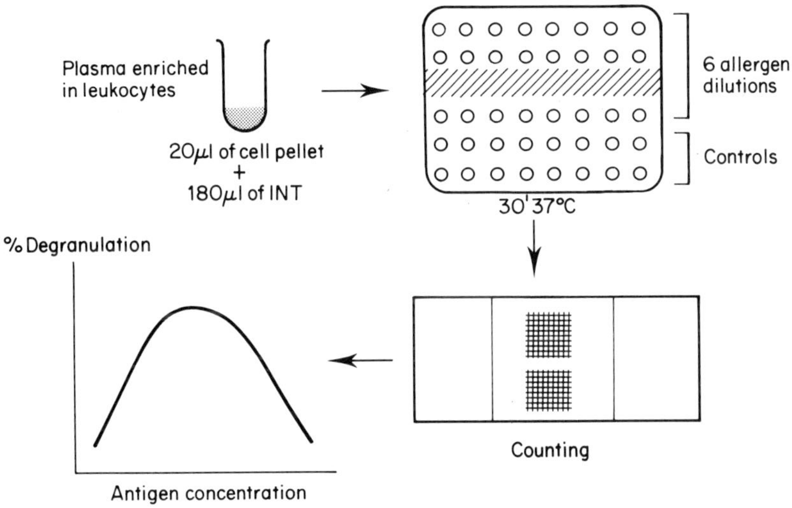

Figure 1 Principle of canine basophil degranulation test.

Measurement of basophil reactivity

Allergen extracts (Dome-Hollister-Stier) were provided freeze dried. A 10 mg/ml stock solution was kept at −80°C.

For the measurement of basophil reactivity, washed leukocytes were resuspended and centrifuged (500 *g* for 10 min) in a Hepes calcium buffer (washing buffer plus Ca^{++} 5mM).

An aliquot of the cell pellet was mixed (v/v) with the allergen dilutions (from 10^{-8} mg/ml) and incubated at 37°C for 20 min. For each experiment, a minimum of six allergen dilutions were simultaneously tested versus two allergen-free controls. Leukocytes were then stained.

Staining of basophils

Iodonitrotetrazolium staining was performed according to Shelley (1974); 10µl of the cell pellet were mixed with 140µl of freshly dissolved INT (0.1%) (Sigma) in 0.1 M PBS containing 0.5 M sodium succinate pH 7.4 at 37°C for 30 min.

Cells were counted between 30 min and 2 h. For this purpose, cell suspensions were allowed to sediment in Fuchs Rosenthal haemocytometer. Stained cells were counted for each allergen dilution. The basophil reactivity, for each allergen dilution was expressed as the percentage of unstained basophils compared with the controls. Only the basophils which did not degranulate were stained. By the use of the Poisson's law, the statistical threshold of positivity of the maximum percentage of degranulation was calculated according to Petiot *et al.* (1981): the more cells that are counted in the control, the less the threshold of significance. For example if 30 stained cells are counted in the control, the threshold of significance of the test is a maximum percentage of degranulation of 33%. If the number of cells counted is 100, this threshold decreases to 20%.

In this study we were limited in the number of basophil degranulation tests to 1-3 allergens per dog. This is why these allergens were chosen according to the season of pruritus and/or skin tests results.

RESULTS

Skin tests

Skin tests were positive in 75 of the 99 atopic dogs tested (76%). The most common allergen giving positive reactions was the house dust mite. *Dermatophagoides farinae* (Df) (62%); other non-seasonal allergens seemed to be less common: *D. pteronyssinus* (Dpt) 15%, cat dander 3%, molds 1%. Pollen allergies were also uncommon: grass 11%, Artemisia 6%, tress O. In ten cases with a positive skin test to grass pollen, the pruritus appeared during late spring, the grass pollen season in Paris.

Basophil Degranulation Test (BDT)

In the control group, all the dogs were tested for house dust mites (Df, Dpt), grass pollen and flea. We never observed any significant basophil degranulation (Tables 1 to 4). The choice of allergen in atopic dogs was made according to the season of pruritus and sometimes to skin test results. The results are shown in Tables 1 to 4. In six cases we were unable to do the test because of the small number of stained cells. In the other cases, the number of stained cells in the controls, varied from 20 to 71. In all positive cases

Table 1 Basophil degranulation to *Dermatophagoides farinae* in atopic and non-atopic dogs

	No. of dogs with		
	BDT+	NS BDT	Total
Atopic dermatitis with positive skin tests to *D. farinae*	47	14	61
Atopic dermatitis with negative skin tests to *D. farinae*	3	24	27
Control	0	50	50

BDT+: Significant basophil degranulation.
NS BDT: Non-significant basophil degranulation.

Table 2 Basophil degranulation to *Dermatophagoides pteronyssinus* in atopic and non-atopic dogs

	No. of dogs with		
	BDT+	NS BDT	Total
Atopic dermatitis with positive skin tests to *D. pteronyssinus*	10	5	15
Atopic dermatitis with negative skin tests to *D. pteronyssinus*	9	28	37
Control	0	47	47

BDT+: Significant basophil degranulation.
NS BDT: Non-significant basophil degranulation.

Table 3 Basophil degranulation to *Ctenocephalides felis* in atopic and non-atopic dogs

	No. of dogs with		
	BDT+	NS BDT	Total
Atopic dogs with positive skin tests to flea extracts	12	5	17
Atopic dogs with negative skin tests to flea extracts	2	5	7
Control dogs	0	50	50

BDT+: Significant basophil degranulation.
NS BDT: Non-significant basophil degranulation.

Table 4 Basophil degranulation to grass pollen in atopic and non-atopic dogs

	No. of dogs with		
	BDT+	NS BDT	Total
Atopic dermatitis with positive skin tests to grass pollen	9	2	11
Atopic dermatitis with negative skin tests to grass pollen	0	4	4
Control	0	50	50

BDT+: Significant basophil degranulation.
NS BDT: Non-significant basophil degranulation.

(significant degranulation), we obtained a dose-dependent bell-shaped curve. We obtained positive basophil degranulation test in 68 of the 99 dogs tested, and, once more, Df was the more frequent allergen encountered, with positive basophil degranulation test in 50% of the atopic dogs tested. Basophil degranulation tests in dogs with non-seasonal atopy were positive to Dpt in 36% and to cat dander in two of the three cases with positive skin tests.

In the cases of pollen allergy basophil degranulation tests to grass were positive in 9/11 dogs with spring pruritus (Table 4) and to Artemisia in 2/3 dogs with positive skin tests to the latter pollen.

The correlation between positive skin tests and positive basophil degranulation test was: 75% to all allergens, 57/76 (75%) of Df and Dpt together, 47/61 (77%) for Df, 10/15 (67%) for Dpt, 2/3 for cat, 2/3 for Artemisia and 9/11 for grass pollen.

In 20 atopic dogs we did the test with a mixture of meat (lamb, pork, beef) (Laboratoires des Stallergénes). In five cases we obtained a significant basophil degranulation. Four of these five dogs responded dramatically to an elimination diet (chicken and rice). We also did this test in 20 healthy dogs and we never observed any significant basophil degranulation.

Six female dogs showing pruritic papular dermatitis during each pseudopregnancy were also tested with progesterone. They had negative skin tests to flea and aerollaergens. In four cases the basophil degranulation was positive to progesterone (Fig. 2). All these dogs were spayed and did not suffer from any pruritic dermatitis for 1 year after surgery.

DISCUSSION

Positive skin tests were obtained in 76% of the atopic dogs tested. The most common allergen reactions in Paris are to house dust mites. Surprisingly,

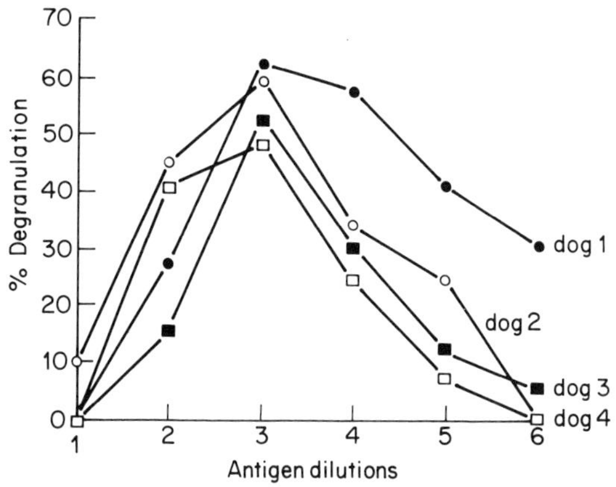

Figure 2 Significant basophil degranulation to progesterone in four cases of suspected progesterone hypersensitivity.

sensitivity to Dpt is uncommon. Similar results have also been described in the dog by Vollset (1985). This is different from the results obtained in man: humans are often allergic to both mites, Df and Dpt. However, in the dog, monosensitization to Df is the most common case. Such results could be explained by a higher incidence of Df in the bedding of dogs or by the recognition by the canine immune system of specific antigenic fraction of D, which are different from Dpt. This hypothesis needs to be confirmed.

Within the limits of the study, the basophil degranulation test can be considered a good aid in the diagnosis of atopic dermatitis because none of the control dogs had positive basophil degranulation tests and 68% of atopic dogs had positive basophil degranulation tests.

The correlation between the skin test and the basophil degranulation test is very high for house dust mites and in the few cases of pollen allergy tested. The correlation has probably been enhanced by the fact that we used allergenic extracts of the same origin for both *in vivo* and *in vitro* tests.

In man, cellular tests seem to be preferable for *in vitro* diagnosis of allergy than serological tests (allergen specific IgG or IgE determination), (Lichtenstein and McGlashan, 1986). In the dog, these data are also in favour of cellular tests and these preliminary results have to be confirmed and compared to serological tests (allergen specific IgE, IgG and IgGd determination).

The basophil degranulation test could be used as an aid in the diagnosis of atopy when skin tests cannot be performed or when they give negative or unexpected results. The role of the basophil degranulation test in the diagnosis of food and progresterone hypersensitivity cannot be determined because of the small number of cases studied.

A few technical problems limit the routine use of the basophil degranulation test in the dog. The first is the collection of the sample. At least 7–10 ml of blood are needed and such a volume is often difficult to obtain from small animals. As basophils are fragile, the test must be done within 24 h of collection. Another drawback for the routine use of the basophil degranulation test is that it is time consuming and stained cells must be counted within a few hours after staining. Because only a few allergens can be tested, it can be considered as a reference test and not a screening test.

SUMMARY

The basophil degranulation test, using iodonitrotetrazolium staining, has been applied for the diagnosis of canine atopy. The correlation between positive skin tests and basophil degranulation is over 70% for aeroallergens. The test has also been used with food allergens, progesterone and flea extracts. Some signficant degranulation has been observed. However, the small number of dogs tested does not permit any conclusion. In the diagnosis of atopy the basophil degranulation test can be considered as a reference test, but its use in practice is limited.

REFERENCES

Griffin, C. (1989). RAST and ELISA testing in canine atopy. In: Kirk, R.W. (ed.) *Current Veterinary Therapy* Vol. X, pp. 592–595., W.B. Saunders Company, Philadelphia.

Halliwell, R.E.W. and Kunkle, G.A. (1978). The radioallergosorbent test in the diagnosis of canine atopic disease. *Journal of Allergy and Clinical Immunology* **62** 236–242.

Jain, N.C. (1986). The basophil and the mast cell. In: Jain, N.C. (ed.) *Schalm's Veterinary Hematology*, p. 757. Lea & Febiger, Philadelphia.

Lichtenstein, L.M. and MacGlashan, D.W. (1986). The concept of basophil relesability. *Journal of Allergy and Clinical Immunity* **77**: 291–294.

Mulller, G.H., Kirk, R.W. and Scott, D.W. (1989). *Small Animal Dermatology* 4th edn, 1007pp. W.B. Saunders Company, Philadephia.

Peters, J.E., Hirshman, C.A. and Malley, A. (1982). The Basenji-Greyhound dog model of asthma: leukocyte histamine release, serum IgE and airway response to inhaled antigen. *Journal of Immunology* **129**: 1245–1249.

Petiot, J.F. Sainte Laudy, J. and Benvéniste, J. (1981). Interpretation du résultat d'un test de dégranulation des basophiles humains. *Annales de Biologie Clinique* **39**: 355–358.

Prélaud P. (1986). Exploration *in vitro* de l'hypersensibilité immédiate chez le chien. *Free communications of the XIth WSAVA Congress, Paris, 1986*, C47.

Prélaud, P. and Sainte Laudy, J. (1988). Set up of a canine basophil degranulation test: Correlation with two major allergens (*Dermatophagoïdes & Ctenocephalides felis*) *Proceedings of the XIIIth WSAVA Congress, Barcelona, 1988*, p. 121.

Prélaud, P. and Sainte Laudy, J. IgG spécifiques de l'acarien de la poussière *Dermatophagoïdes farinae* chez les chiens atopiques et non-atopiques *Revue de Médecine Vétérinaire* (in press).

Sainte Laudy, J. (1987). Standardization of basophil degranulation for

pharmacological studies. *Journal of Immunological Methods* **98**: 279-285.
Sainte Laudy, J. (1988). Place de l'étude "*in vitro*" du basophile human parmi les techniques d'exploration de l'hypersensibilité immédiate. *Le Biologiste* **177**: 303-309.
Schwartzman, R.M., Rockey, J.H. and Halliwell, R.E.W. (1971). Canine reaginic antibody characterizarion of the spontaneous antiragweed and induced antidinitrophenyl reaginic antibodies of the atopic dog. *Clinical and Experimental Immunology* **9**: 549-569.
Schwartzman, R.M., Massicot, J.G., Sogn, D.D. and Cohen, S.G. (1983). The atopic dog model. Report of an attempt to establish a colony. *International Archives of Allergy and Applied Immunology* **72**: 97-101.
Shelley, W. (1974). Immune basophil degranulation. Detection by iodonitrotetrazolium stain. *International Archives of Allergy* **47**: 810-817.
Shelley, W. and Juhlin, L. (1961). A new test for detecting anaphylactic sensitivity: the basophil reaction. *Nature* **191**: 1056-1058.
Vollset, I. (1985). Atopic dermatitis in norwegian dogs. *Nord. Vet-Med.* **37**: 97-106.
Willemse, A. (1983). Investigation of symptomatology and the significance of immediate skin test reactivity in canine atopic dermatitis. *Research in Veterinary Science* : 262-265.
Willemse, A. (1986). Atopic skin disease: a review and reconsideration of diagnostic criteria. *Journal of Small Animal Practice* **27**: 771-778.
Willemse, A., Noordzij, A., Van den Brom, W.E. and Rutten, V.P.M.G. (1985a). Allergen specific IgGd antibodies in dogs with atopic dermatitis. *Clinical and Experimental Immunology* **59**: 359-363.
Willemse, A., Noordzij. A., Rutten, V.P.M.G. and Bernadina, W.G. (1985b). Introduction of non-IgE anaphylactic antibodies in dogs. *Clinical and Experimental Immunology* **59**: 351-358.

2.3 The Reaction of Feline Skin to the Intradermal Injection of Allergenic Extracts and Passive Cutaneous Anaphylaxis Using Serum From Skin Test Positive Cats

Diane E. Bevier

Assistant Professor of Dermatology, Department of Companion Animal and Special Studies Medicine, College of Veterinary Medicine, North Carolina State University, Raleigh, North Carolina, USA

INTRODUCTION

Skin testing to produce localized immediate hypersensitivity reactions for diagnosis of allergic disorders in man was originally described by Blackley in 1873 and led to immunotherapy as treatment first used by Noon in 1911. Since that time the question of standardization of methods and interpretation of skin testing results has continued to challenge doctors interested in allergy in all species.

The presence of the immunglobulin IgE and atopy has been well documented in the dog (Patterson *et al.*, 1963; Schwartzman, 1968). Several studies have evaluated skin test reactivity in the normal canine population (August, 1982; Baker, 1971; Scott, 1981). Reports of positive skin test reactivity varied from 0% reactivity (Scott, 1981) to 86.7% positive reactions in 90 normal dogs to house dust at 1000 protein nitrogen units (PNU) concentration (August, 1982).

Feline atopy is becoming increasingly recognized (Halliwell, 1983; 1985; Reedy, 1983, 1985a,b,c; Scott, 1987; Kunkle, 1984). Intradermal skin testing is a useful diagnostic tool in feline allergic disease (Halliwell, 1985; Reedy, 1983, 1985a,c; Kunkle, 1984). Protocols for both feline intradermal skin testing and hyposensitization have been directly transposed from the dog to the cat, and are as variable as in the canine atopy literature (Reedy, 1985b; Kunkle, 1984).

The purpose of this study was to determine the response of clinically normal cats to varying dilutions of allergen extracts and recommend an appropriate skin test protocol for the cat.

MATERIALS AND METHODS

Cats

Fifty cats were selected for the study. Prior to skin testing, a physical examination was performed. Cats with evidence of systemic disease, inflammatory skin disease or alopecia were excluded. The following variables were recorded for each cat: sex, breed (where applicable), age (estimated by dentition), body weight, coat pigmentation (light, medium or dark), and evidence of ectoparasites.

Cats used in the study had a negative feline leukaemia virus tests (FELV) status within 2 months of skin testing.

Allergens

Twenty-four aqueous allergen extracts (Greer Laboratories Inc., Lenoir, NC 28645, USA) preserved with 0.4% phenol, were used for intradermal skin testing (Table 1). These 24 allergens were chosen from the standard battery of 53 allergens used to skin test dogs at the University of Wisconsin and accounted for the greatest number of positive skin test responses in dogs diagnosed as having atopy.

Allergenic extracts were supplied in strengths measurable by PNU/ml or on a basis of weight/volume (w/v). Each 10 000 PNU equals one mg of protein nitrogen. The weight/volume measure is a standard based on the weight of the dried extract in a known volume of extracting fluid.

Six dilutions of each allergen were made using sterile normal saline. Allergens known to have high potential for irritant reactions were tested at a seventh dilution. Allergens were diluted to the following PNU/ml: 1500, 1250, 1000, 750, 500, 250, and 25. Those allergens supplied on a weight/volume basis were diluted as follows: 1:500, 1:1000, 1:2000, 1:3000, and 1:4000. Allergen dilutions were prepared the day before each cat was skin tested.

Histamine phosphate (Eli Lilly and Company, Indianpolis, IN 46206, USA) was prepared as a 1:100,000 solution to be used as a positive control.

INTRADERMAL SKIN TESTING

Experiment 1

Cats were anaesthetized with ketamine hydrochloride (20 mg/kg) intramuscularly. The hair was clipped bilaterally on the thorax using a number 40 blade in a 24 by 20 cm rectangle. Prepared histamine solution (0.05 ml) as a

Table 1 Allergens used in intradermal skin testing

Experiment 1	Presently used skin test strength (PNU) in clinical patients	Experiment 2
1. House dust	250, 25, 2.5	1. House dust
2. Cottonseed	1000	2. Mixed feathers
3. Kapok	1000	3. Brome grass
4. Mixed feathers	500	4. Cocklebur
5. Sheep wool	1000	5. Firebush
6. Brome grass	1000	6. Ragweed mix
7. Timothy — Orchard grass mix	1000	7. Maple mix
8. Cocklebur	1000	8. Alternaria
9. Firebush	1000	9. Aspergillus
10. Lamb's quarter	1000	10. Flea
11. Marsh elder	1000	
12. English plantain	1000	
13. Ragweed mix	1000	
14. Sheep and red sorrel	1000	
15. Yellow dock	1000	
16. Black willow	1000	
17. Maple mix	1000	
18. Oak	1000	
19. Grass smut mix	1000	
20. Alternaria tenus	1000	
21. Asperigillus mix	1000	
22. Helminthosporum	1000	
23. Penicillium	1000	
24. Flea	1:1000, 1:4000 wt vol	

positive control and an equal amount of sterile saline as a negative control were injected intradermally at the beginning and completion of both sides. One millilitre (ml) tuberculin syringes with 27 gauge 3/8 inch needles were used for the intradermal injections of 0.05 ml of each dilution of allergen. Cats were skin tested with 13 allergens on the right side and 12 allergens on the left side. The dilutions of each allergen were injected intradermally in horizontal rows with the injection sites of the increasing dilutions of each allergen spaced approximately 1.5 cm apart. The horizontal rows were approximately 1.5 cm apart. The numerical order of the allergens was reversed after the initial 25 cats in order to avoid bias due to location. Reactions were read at 15 min. The right side was read before the left side injections were done. The wheals were evaluated by visual observation, digital palpation and direct measurement of the reactions using calipers. Positive reactions were those which had an average diameter greater than or equal to the halfway point between the average diameter of the saline and histamine controls on that side or those with turgidity, and/or erythema, detected by digital palpation and visual examination. I performed all injections and measurements, and recorded skin test reactions.

After wheals were evaluated on the right side, the cat was then placed in right lateral recumbency and the procedures were repeated on the left side for the remaining 12 allergens. No further examination of wheals was made after the initial readings at 15 min.

Experiment 2

One month after the initial skin testing, 10 cats with negative intradermal skin test results were retested using 10 allergens (Table 1). These allergens were selected from the initial study results as those which yielded the highest percentage positive skin test responses. Allergens were diluted to the following PNU/ml: 10 000, 4000, 3000, 2500, 2000, and wt/vol: 1:100, 1:200, 1:300, 1:400. The controls, intradermal skin testing and wheal evaluation were carried out in the same manner as the first experiment.

Statistical methods

Positive reactions to each allergen were reported as the percentage of cats showing reactivity. The effects of sex, age and coat pigmentation on intradermal skin test reactivity of each allergen were tested using analysis of variance. Fisher's least significant difference was used to compare any two means of significant components when the analysis of variance indicated valid mean differences. A stepwide multiple regression procedure was used to indicate factors affecting the size of the histamine control wheal: $p \leq 0.05$ was considered significant (Bruning and Kintz, 1977).

RESULTS

Experiment 1

The percentage of animals showing positive reactions to six or seven dilutions of each allergen is shown in Table 2. Twenty-one allergens showed a reactivity of 10% or less positive reactions at the lowest dilution. Firebush and flea showed intermediate reactivity with 22% of cats having positive reactions at 1500 PNU/ml. One allergen, house dust, produced a higher number of positive reactions (30%), at 1500 PNU/ml.

Five allergens, house dust, kapok, firebush, lamb's quarter and oak, produced significant differences in reactivity between male and female cats (Table 3). Three of these allergens showed greater reactivity in female cats and two in male cats.

Significant differences in reactivity between the three age groups were noted

Table 2 Percentage of normal cats ($n = 50$) with positive skin test responses

Allergen	1500	1250	1000	750	500	250	25	PNU/ml
1. House dust	30	30	30	28	28	22	18	
2. Cottonseed	6	4	0	2	0	0	0	
3. Kapok	8	6	6	4	4	0	0	
4. Mixed feathers	10	8	8	8	6	0	0	
5. Sheep wool	0	0	0	0	0	0	0	
6. Brome grass	2	0	0	0	0	0		
7. Timothy — Orchard grass mix	4	2	0	0	0	0		
8. Cocklebur	2	0	0	0	0	0		
9. Firebush	22	22	20	18	12	10		
10. Lambs quarter	2	2	2	2	2	2	2	
11. Marsh Elder	10	8	8	6	0	0		
12. English Plantain	2	0	2	0	0	0		
13. Ragweed mix	0	0	0	0				
14. Sheep and Red Sorrel	0	0	0	0	0			
15. Yellow Dock	4	0	0	0	0	0		
16. Ash	4	2	2	2	2	0		
17. Maple Mix	2	0	0	0	0			
18. Oak	4	4	4	4	4	4		
19. Smut mix	0	0	0	0	0	0		
20. Alternaria tenus	0	0	0	0	0	0		
21. Asperigillus mix	2	2	2	2	2	2		
22. Helminthosporum	0	0	0	0	0	0		
23. Penicillium	0	0	0	0	0	0		
24. Flea	22	20	20	18	12			
	1:500	1:1000	1:2000	1:3000	1:4000			Wt. Vol.[a]

[a]Flea

Table 3 Allergens showing significantly different responses in male and female cats

Allergen	Percentage of cats reacting positively: Female	Male
1. House Dust	26.43	6.30
3. Kapok	6.16	0.00
9. Firebush	10.21	21.54
10. Lamb's Quarter	0.00	6.42
18. Oak	7.04	0.00

for seven allergens (Table 4). These included house dust, mixed feathers, timothy-orchard grass mix, firebush, ash, oak and fleas. A higher level of reactivity was seen for six of these allergens in young cats and three in aged cats. A lower level of reactivity was seen for one and two allergens in adult and aged cats, respectively.

Table 4 Allergens showing significantly different responses between cats of different ages

Allergen	Percentage of cats reacting positively		
	Young Less than 1½ years	Adult 1½ - 7 years	Aged Older than 7 years
1. House dust	33.78[a]	13.95	37.31[a]
4. Feather	10.91	0.38[b]	20.75[a]
7. Timothy — Orchard grass mix	4.55[a]	0.45	0.00
9. Firebush	26.32[a]	13.95	0.00[b]
16. Ash	12.50[a]	0.45	0.00
18. Oak	14.29[a]	3.06	0.00[b]
24. Flea	22.22[a]	11.90	28.57[a]

[a] Significantly higher level of reactivity.
[b] Significantly lower level of reactivity.

Eight allergens showed significant differences between animals with varying degrees of coat pigmentation (Table 5). These included house dust, kapok, firebush, lamb's quarter, marsh elder, ash, oak and aspergillus. A higher level of reactivity was seen for six of the allergens in cats with dark coat pigmentation and two allergens in light coat colour cats. A lower level of reactivity was seen for one allergen in cats with a medium coat colour.

Mean histamine wheal diameter was calculated for male and female cats, each age group, and cats of varying coat pigmentation (Table 6).

Table 5 Allergens showing significantly different responses between cats of different coat colours

Allergen	Light	Medium	Dark
1. House dust	13.48	12.39	28.21[a]
3. Kapok	8.33	0.53[b]	11.11
9. Firebush	14.29	8.82	30.43[a]
10. Lamb's quarter	0.00	0.00	12.73[a]
11. Marsh elder	0.00	1.59	18.64[a]
16. Ash	8.30[a]	0.53	0.00
18. Oak	9.59[a]	0.00	12.73[a]
21. Aspergillus	0.00	0.00	12.73[a]

[a] Significantly higher level of reactivity.
[b] Significantly lower level of reactivity.

Table 6 Mean histamine wheal diameter (MHWD) (mm)

Sex	MHWD	Coat pigmentation	MHWD	Age	MHWD
Male ($n = 17$)	11.15	Light ($n = 11$)	10.66	Young ($n = 7$)	10.71
Female ($n = 33$)	10.52	Medium ($n = 31$)	10.63	Adult ($n = 37$)	10.71
		Dark ($n = 8$)	11.50	Old ($n = 6$)	10.63

Experiment 2

The percentage of animals showing positive reactions at four or five dilutions of the 'high concentration' allergens is shown in Table 7. Eight allergens continued to show reactivity of 10% or less positive reactions at the lowest dilution. Flea showed intermediate reactivity with 20% of cats having positive reactions at dilution 1. Firebush produced the highest number of positive reactions (50%).

Table 7 Percentage of cats ($n = 10$) with positive skin test reactions to 'high concentration' allergens

Allergen	10 000	4000	3000	2500	2000	PNU/ml
1. House dust	10	10	10	10	10	
2. Mixed feather	10	10	0	0	0	
3. Brome grass	0	10	0	0	0	
4. Cocklebur	0	0	0	0	0	
5. Firebush	50	50	40	40	40	
6. Ragweed mix	0	0	0	0	0	
7. Maple mix	0	10	0	0	0	
8. Alternaria	0	0	0	0	0	
9. Aspergillus	0	10	10	10	10	
10. Flea	20	30	40	20		
	1:100	1:200	1:300	1:400		wt/vol.[a]

[a] Flea

DISCUSSION

The function of a skin test antigen and intradermal skin testing is to measure skin reactivity, safely indicating the presence or absence of specific immunologic sensitivity. The ideal skin test antigen should identify all individuals with specific immunologic experience (sensitivity) and identify only those individuals with that experience (specificity) (Sbarbaro, 1978).

Unfortunately, positive intradermal skin test reactivity to an allergen does not always indicate a clinically relevant hypersensitive state (Barbee, 1976, 1981; Fontana *et al.*, 1976; Lessof and Barnetson, 1984). There are numerous reasons for false positive skin tests. These include improper preparation and administration of the allergen solution (Sheldon *et al.*, 1976), skin testing with substances which non-specifically release histamine or contain histamine themselves (Doeglas and Nater, 1968), dermographic subjects (Johnson and Cazort, 1959), remnants of past sensitivity or harbinger of future sensitivity (Hagy and Settipane, 1971), and dissociation of positive skin reactivity and clinical sensitivity (Slavin, 1974).

Studies evaluating the non-allergic human population have shown at least one positive intradermal reaction in 9–50% of normal subjects (Barbee *et al.*, 1981; Hagy and Settipane, 1971; Curran and Goldman, 1961; Grow and

Herman, 1936; Rackemann and Simon, 1935; Lindbladd and Farr, 1961). In different reports the incidence of positive skin tests to at least one antigen in normal dogs has ranged from 0 to 60% using currently accepted skin testing protocols (August, 1982; Baker, 1971; Scott, 1981; Reedy, 1985a,c).

The normal cats in this study in Experiment 1 showed 30% positive reactions to house dust at the lowest testing dilution (1500 PNU). Looking at our currently used house dust skin testing dilutions, 250 and 25 PNU, reactivity levels were 22% and 18%, respectively, of cats tested. This certainly falls comfortably within the range of accepted positive skin test incidence reported for normal subjects of other species.

Of the reasons listed for false positive reactions on intradermal skin testing the two that have the broadest application to our cat population are improper preparation and dissociation of positive skin test reactivity and clinical sensitivity. Whether a skin test reaction is a non-specific response to an irritant or a true reflection of IgE bound to mast cells in the skin can be evaluated through the use of the Prausnitz-Kustner test (passive cutaneous anaphylaxis) (Ovary, 1958). This test was performed using serum from our normal skin test positive cats (Bevier, unpublished data, 1985).

Dissociation of positive skin reactivity and clinical sensitivity occurs (Barbee *et al.*, 1976, 1981; Fontana *et al.*, 1976; Lessof and Barnetson, 1984; Slavin, 1974; Peshkin, 1955). There is evidence that the appearance of clinical signs in those individuals with skin-test-positive subclinical hypersensitivities may in part depend on the number of allergens which a patient becomes sensitized to, the so-called 'hypersensitivity threshold' (Fontana *et al.*, 1976; Hagy and Settipane, 1971).

Of the 31 cats showing positive reactions on skin testing, 16 showed only one positive reaction (Table 8). The normal cats in this study reacted to an average of 2.3 allergens. A group of 15 cats diagnosed as having allergic inhalant dermatitis reacted to an average of 5.6 allergens in a comparable battery of 24 allergens.

Experiment 2 evaluated the potential for 10 allergens (showing the greatest

Table 8 Number of allergens reacted to/cat

No. of allergens Reacted to	No. of cats ($n = 50$)
0	19
1	16
2	4
3	6
4	1
5	0
6	3
7	0
8	1

reactivity in experiment 1), to induce irritant reactions: 10 000 PNU is 10–40 times the normal concentration currently used in intradermal skin testing. Of the allergens tested, firebush and flea seemed to have the greatest potential to be irritant, as increasing concentrations showed increased numbers of reactive cats. The other eight allergens did not show this tendency.

Feingold (1973) noted that the softer, more glabrous skin of human females showed an abnormal flaring response and increased sensitivity to certain allergens. The most recent study of allergen reactivity in 90 normal dogs (August, 1982) showed a significantly higher level of reactivity for four of 25 allergens in female dogs. The cats in this study showed differing reactions related to the sex of the cat for five allergens; three in females, two in males. This difference (showing no preference for positive reactions in male versus female cats) may be due to many cats being neutered at a young age and thus lacking long-term effects of sex hormones on their skin.

In human studies, positive skin test reactions were more commonly seen in children who reacted more often and to more dilute solutions of allergens (Barbee *et al.*, 1981; Peshkin, 1955). Feingold (1973) observed occasional reduced reactivity in infants and geriatric patients. It is generally agreed that skin reactivity in humans is reduced with advancing age (Tuft *et al.*, 1955). In a group of 90 clinically normal dogs (August, 1982) tested with 25 allergenic extracts, overall reactivity was less in adult dogs age 1–4 years. Seven allergens showed differing reactivity between the three age groups of cats. The reactivity of cats to these particular allergens was greater for young (< $1\frac{1}{2}$ years) and older (> 7 years) cats for six and three of the allergens, respectively. Adult cats ($1\frac{1}{2}$ to 7 years) were less reactive overall when compared with the other two age groups (Table 4).

Humans with naturally pigmented skin have lower levels of skin test reactivity than those with fair skin (Feingold, 1973). In one study in the dog (August, 1982), an overall reduction in reactivity was noted for seven of 25 allergens tested as the degree of coat pigmentation increased. No such tendency was seen in the cats tested. In fact, a higher level of reactivity was seen in cats with dark coat colour for six of 24 allergens. The difference between cats versus humans and dogs may be explained by the fact that the haired skin of cats is virtually devoid of melanocytes and pigment and their coat colour does not correspond to skin pigmentation as in many canine breeds (Scott, 1980).

Reactivity of human skin to histamine is greatest during the first decade of life, decreases throughout life and falls markedly after the age of 60 (Stuckey *et al.*, 1985). Mean histamine wheal diameter (MHWD) tended to increase significantly as the age of one group of 90 dogs increased, although the effect of age alone contributed only about 2.7% of the variation of the MHWD between three age groups examined (August, 1982). In the cats, MHWD showed no significant differences related to the sex, age or coat pigmentation of the cats tested. Differences may have been noticed if histamine was tested at varying dilutions and end point reactions recorded (Stuckey *et al.*, 1985).

In summary, currently used allergen concentrations listed in Table 1 appear to be optimal for intradermal skin testing in the cat with the exception of firebush and flea antigen. Although minor differences in skin test reactivity related to sex, age and coat pigmentation of the cats tested, these were not consistent enough to recommend variations in testing protocols based on these factors.

Lastly, this study reemphasizes the importance and necessity of interpreting the intradermal skin test, as any other diagnostic test, in terms of the history, physical examination and thorough knowledge of the patient being treated.

REFERENCES

August, J.R. (1982). The reaction of canine skin to the intradermal injection of allergenic extracts. *Journal of the American Animal Hospital Association* **18**:157-163.

Baker, K.P. (1971). Intradermal tests as an aid to the diagnosis of skin disease in dogs. *Journal of Small Animal Practice* **12**:445-452.

Barbee, R.A., Leibowitz, M.D., Thompson, H.C., *et al.* (1976). Immediate skin test reactivity in a general population sample. *Annals of Internal Medicine* **84**:129-133.

Barbee, R.A., Brown, W.G., Kaltenborn, M.S. *et al.* (1981). Allergen skin test reactivity in a community population sample: Correlation with age, histamine skin reaction, and total serum immunoglobulin E. *Journal of Allergy and Clinical Immunology* **68**:15.

Blackley, C.H. (1873). *Experimental Researches on the Causes and Nature of Catarrhus Aestivus (Hay fever and Asthma).* Balliere, Tindall and Cox, London.

Bruning, J.L. and Kintz, B.L. (1977). *Computational Handbook of Statistics* 2nd ed, pp. 107-142. Scott, Foresman and Company, Glenview, Illinois.

Curran, W.S., Goldman, G. (1961). The incidence of immediately reacting allergy skin tests in a 'normal' adult population. *Annals of Internal Medicine* **55**:777-783.

Doeglas, H.M.G. and Nater, J.P. (1968). Histamine in foods causing false-positive scratch tests. *Journal of Allergy* **42**:164.

Feingold, B.F. (1973). Introduction to clinical allergy. Charles C. Thomas Publisher, Springfield, Illinois.

Fontana, V.J., Wittig, H., Holt, L.E. Jr. (1976). Observations on the specificity of the skin test. The incidence of positive skin tests in allergic and non-allergic children. *Journal of Allergy* **34**:348-353.

Grow, M.H., Herman, W.B. (1936). Intracutaneous tests in normal individuals. *Journal of Allergy* **7**:108-111.

Hagy, G.W. and Settipane, G.A. (1971). Prognosis of positive allergy skin tests in an asymptomatic population. *Journal of Allergy and Clinical Immunology* **48**:200.

Halliwell, R.E.W. (1983). Immunology and Dermatology. *Australian Veterinary Practice* 1983; **13**:177.

Halliwell, R.E.W. (1985). Alopecia and pruritus in the cat. *Proceedings of the American Animal Hospital Association* **52**:150.

Johnson, T.J. and Cazort, A.G. (1959). Dermographia — clinical observations. *Journal of the American Medical Association* **23**:169-172.

Kunkle, G.A. (1984). Feline dermatology. *Veterinary Clinics of North America (Small Animal Practice)* **14**:1065.

Lessof, M.H., Barnetson, R.S.T.C. (1984). Diagnostic methods — skin tests. In: Lessof M.H. (ed.) *Allergy: Immunologic and Clinical Aspects* pp. 73-92. John

Wiley and Sons, Chichester.

Lindbladd, J.H., Farr, R.P. (1961). The incidence of positive intradermal reactions in humans without history of rhinitis or asthma. *Journal of Allergy* **32**:392-401.

Ovary, Z. (1958). Passive cutaneous anaphylaxis in the mouse. *Journal of Immunology* **81**:355-357.

Peshkin, M.M. (1955). Pitfalls of the skin tests in allergy. *Journal of the American Medical Association* **157**:820-823.

Patterson, R. Pruzansky, J.J. and Chung, W.W.V. (1963). Spontaneous canine hypersensitivity of ragweed. Characterization of the serum factor transferring skin, bronchial and anaphylactic sensitivity. *Journal of Immunology* **90**:35-42.

Rackemann, F.M. and Simon, P.A. (1935). Technic on intracutaneous tests and results of routine tests in normal persons. *Journal of Allergy* **6**: 184–188.

Reedy, L.M. (1983). Feline dermatology. *Proceedings of the American Animal Hospital Association* **50**:145.

Reedy, L.M. (1985a). Canine and feline atopy: Diagnosis. *Proceedings of the American Animal Hospital Association* **52**:105.

Reedy, L.M. (1985b). Canine and feline atopy: Treatment. *Proceedings of the American Animal Hospital Association* **52**:110.

Reedy, L.M. (1985c). Allergy testing — canine and feline. *Proceedings of the American Animal Hospital Association* **52**:147.

Sbarbaro, J.A. (1978). Skin test antigens: An evaluation whose time has come. *American Review of Respiratory Diseases* **118**:1-5.

Schwartzman, R.M. (1968). Clinical manifestations and treatment of atopy in the dog. *Veterinary Medicine Small Animal Clinics* **63**:1131-1136.

Scott, D.W. (1980). Feline Dermatology 1900-1978: A Monograph. *Journal of the American Animal Hospital Association* **16**:334-335.

Scott, D.W. (1981). Observations on canine atopy. *Journal of the American Animal Hospital Association* **17**:91-100.

Scott, D.W. (1987). Feline dermatology. *Journal of the American Hospital Association* **23**:255-274.

Sheldon, J.M., Lovell, R.G., and Matthews, K.P. (1976). *A Manual of Clinical Allergy* Appendix 1, pp. 507-532. W.B. Saunders Company, Philadelphia.

Slavin, R.G. (1974). Skin tests in the diagnosis of allergens of the immediate type. In: *Medical Clinics of North America* Vol 58, pp. 65-69. W.B. Saunders Company, Philadelphia.

Stuckey, M.S., Witt, C.S., Schmitt, L.H. *et al.* (1985). Histamine sensitivity influences reactivity to allergens. *Journal of Allergy and Clinical Immunology* **75**:373-376.

Tuft, L., Heck, V.M. and Gregory, D.C. (1955). Studies in sensitization as applied to skin test reactions. III. Influence of age upon skin reactivity. *Journal of Allergy* **26**:359-366.

2.4 The Effect of Serum IgE on an *in vitro* ELISA test in the Normal Canine

C.E. Griffin,[1] K.A. Moriello,[2] and D.J. DeBoer[2]

[1] *Director, Animal Dermatology Clinic;*
[1] *Clinical Instructor, College of Medicine*
University of California, Irvine, California, USA

[2] *Assistant Professor, School of Veterinary Medicine, University of Wisconsin, Madison, Wisconsin, USA*

INTRODUCTION

Two commercial *in vitro* tests for the diagnosis of canine atopic disease are being offered in the USA. The tests are based on the principles of the radioallergosorbent test (RAST) for the detection of antigen-specific IgE. One test utilizes an enzyme linked immunoassay (ELISA), while the other utilizes radiolabelled anti-IgE (RAST). Preliminary independent studies revealed a potential problem with false positive results. Normal dogs and dogs with scabies that were intradermal test negative had multiple strong positive results on these *in vitro* tests. (Griffin, 1989).

Normally in human atopics the RAST tests correlate with intradermal tests about 8% of the time. When they do not correlate typically the intradermal test is positive and the RAST is negative. However, in the atopic patients that are intradermal test negative and RAST positive there usually is a high serum IgE level (Caprio *et al.*, 1983). These findings suggest that high serum IgE levels may lead to a higher incidence of false positive RASTs, as defined by negative intradermal testing.

It is our hypothesis that the false positive results seen in clinically normal dogs that are intradermal test negative could be explained by high serum IgE levels, since normal dogs can have serum IgE levels 100 times that seen in normal humans. It is believed this high IgE level reflects the parasite infestations to which normal dogs are frequently exposed (Halliwell 1989).

The purpose of this study is to determine the effects of ascarid infection on ELISA testing. In addition we will determine if the serum IgE level correlates with the development of false positive ELISA tests.

MATERIALS AND METHODS

Fifteen dogs were purchased from a commerical laboratory. The dogs were taken by Caesarian section from bitches on a routine worming programme to minimize the potential for ascarid infection. The dogs were divided into three groups. All 15 dogs were intradermal tested negative on study days 0 and 90 to the antigens listed in Table 1. On study days 0, 30, 60, 90 serum samples were collected, randomized and coded, then submitted for ELISA testing; in one

Table 1 Intradermal skin test with individual antigens [a]

Controls	Grasses	Weeds	Trees
Saline	Kentucky blue grass	Cocklebur	Ash
Histamine	Brome grass	Firebush	Aspen
	Meadow fescue grass	lamb's quarter	Birch
	Timothy-Orchard grass mix	Marsh elder	Box elder
		Mugwort	Elm
	Rye perenial grass	Pigweed	Maple mix
		English plantain	Oak
		Raweed mix	Sycamore
		Sheep and red sorrel	Blue willow
		Yellow dock	

Housedust	Epithelia	Molds
House dust 250 PNU	Cat epithelia 500 PNU	Smut mix
House dust 25 PNU	Mixed feathers	Grass smut
House dust 2.5 PNU	Sheep wool	Alternaria tenuis
Mixed HMRU dust 250 PNU		Aspergillus
Mixed HMRU dust 25 PNU		Cladosporium
		Helminthosporum
		Hormodendrum
		Penicillium

Insects	Miscellaneous
Flea 1:1000	Cottonseed
Flea 1:4000	Grain dust mix 250 PNU
Black fly	Grain dust mix 25 PNU
Black fly	Kapok
Mosquito	Nylon
Mosquito	Pyrethrum
Deer fly	tobacco 500 PNU
Deer fly	
Horse fly	
Horse fly	
Red ant	
Red ant	
Black ant	
Black ant	

[a] Greer Laboratories, Lenoir, North Carolina, USA

batch to the antigens listed in Table 2. The samples were also submitted to an immunology research laboratory directed by R.E.W. Halliwell for the determination of serum IgE.

Group 1 consisted of six dogs intradermally injected with 0.1 mg of ascarid 1 antigen at study days 1 and 16. Group 2 consisted of six dogs orally inoculated with 135–140 *Toxocara canis* ova at days 1 and 31. Group 3 consisted of three control dogs.

False positive ELISA scores were defined as the scores that were ≥ 101 ELISA antibody units (eau) or ≥ 211 eau in dogs that were clinically normal and intradermal test negative. The value of 101 eau is the level that the commercial laboratory uses for determining a significant positive (2 plus) reaction. A 3 plus or greater reaction is any test result above 210 eau.

Table 2 ELISA Midwest regional screen

Group I grasses	Group II grasses	Group III grasses	Group IV ragweed	Group V herb/shrub
Blue	Bermuda	Brome	Ambrosia	Dock/Sorrel
Redtop	Johnson	Rye		Marsh-elder
Timothy	Orchard	Fescue		Plantain
	Quack	Canary		Cocklebur

Group VI herb/shrub	Group VII trees	Group VIII trees	Group I trees	Group X trees
Lambs quarter	Birch	Ash	Cedar	Pine
Pigweed	Box-elder	Elm	Alder	Mulberry
Mexican firebush	Cottonwood	Hickory	Hazelnut	Walnut
Russian thistle	Oak	Sycamore		

Group XI house dust mite	Group XII epidermals	Group XIII fungi
Dermatophagoides	Dog hair	Alternaria
	Cat hair	Aspergillus
	Feathers	Hormodendrum
	Horse hair	Helminthosporium

Group XIV fungi	Group XV flea
Penicillium	Flea
Rhizopus	
Sphacelothea holci	
Stemphylium	

RESULTS

There was no statistically significant difference between the three groups for the development of false positives over time or related to ascarid infection. However, of the total ELISA test results, there were 457 false postive results at 101 eau and 324 false positive results at 211.

All 60 samples (100%) had at least one of the 15 ELISA test groups reported as a false positive using the recommended 101 eau cut-off. There were marked differences depending on the type of group being tested as shown in Table 3. Linear regression analysis of the 60 samples by SYSTAT statistical programme is shown in Fig.1 for false positive ≥ 101. Figure 2 is for false positive greater

Table 3 Percentage of samples with at least one ELISA group positive

ELISA Group	% Positive (≥ 101 eau)	% Positive (≥ 211 eau)
Any pollen	59	47
Housedust mite	78	75
Epidermal	2	0
Mold 13	82	42
Mold 14	69	34
Any groups	100	99

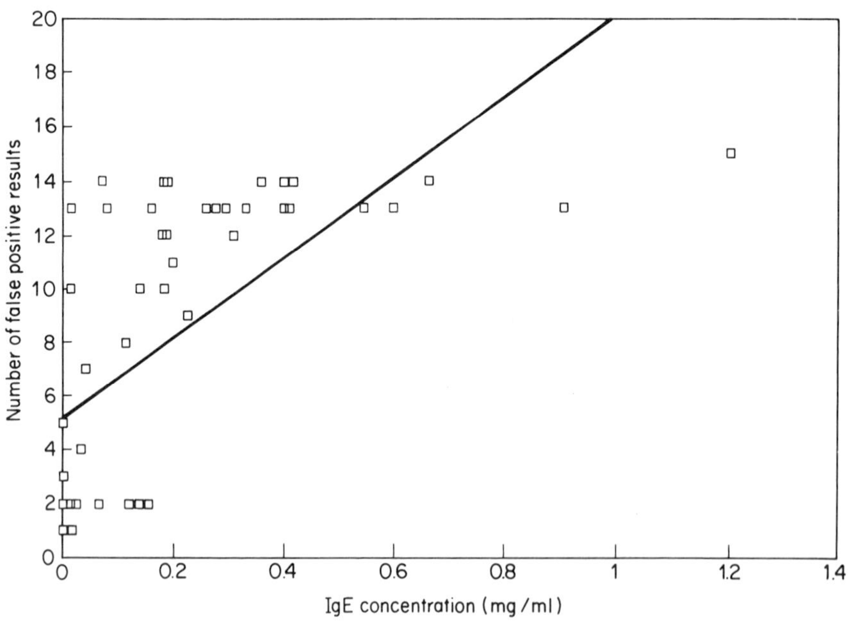

Figure 1 False positives vs IgE concentration (y=0.015x+5.2 R2=0.45 *p*=0.00).

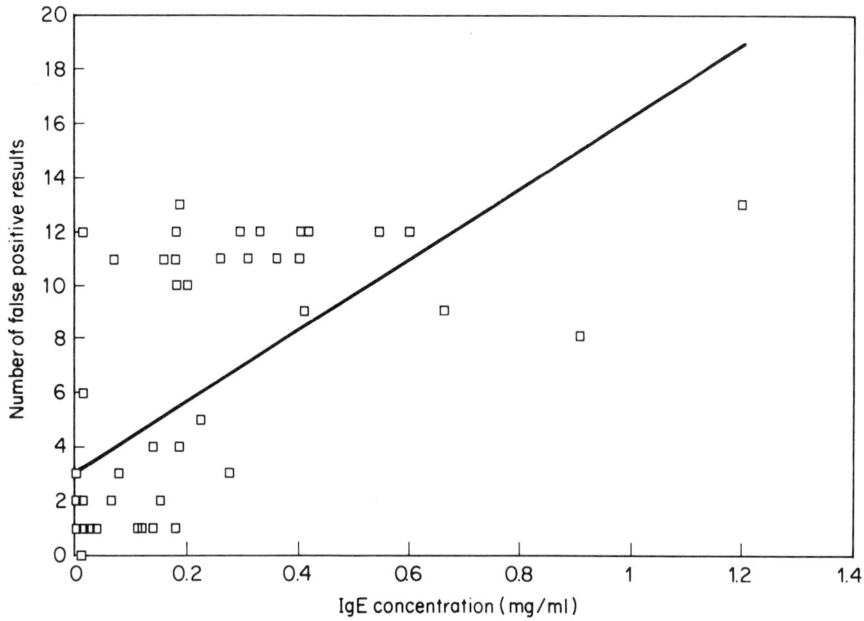

Figure 2 False positives vs IgE concentration (y=0.013x+3.1 R2=0.43 *p*=0.00).

than 210 eau. There is a statistically significant correlation between false positive results and serum IgE levels. The squared multiple R determined by linear regression analysis is the coefficient of determination. The coefficient of determination multiplied by 100 indicates the percentage of the variability of false positive that can be explained by variation in serum IgE concentration. Linear regression analysis was done for each ELISA test group and the coefficient of determination (R^2) and p value are shown in Table 4.

The 60 samples were also divided into four groups based on the serum IgE

Table 4 Results of linear regression analysis comparing IgE concentration on X axis to number of false positives (101 eau cut-off) on Y axis for each ELISA test group

ELISA group	R2	*p*	ELISA group	R2	*p*
I	0.400	0.000	IX	0.293	0.000
II	0.383	0.000	X	0.363	0.000
III	0.382	0.000	XI	0.234	0.000
IV	0.519	0.000	XII	0.517	0.000
V	0.369	0.000	XIII	0.059	0.06
VI	0.409	0.000	XIV	0.002	0.74
VII	0.376	0.000	XV	0.387	0.000
VIII	0.228	0.000			

levels shown in Tables 5 and 6; χ^2 analysis showed there is a statistically significant difference between all four groups for the pollen reactions and flea at both the 101 eau and 211 eau cut-offs. The difference was not statistically significant for house-dust mite, molds or epidermals at both the 101 and 211 eau cut-off utilized. The epidermals are not affected by serum IgE and do not give false positive results. House-dust mite was significantly different for false

Table 5 Four groups of samples based on serum IgE concentration with the corresponding number of false positives at 101 cut-off for each ELISA test group

IgE μg/ml	ELISA Test group false positives (101)														
	I	II	III	IV	V	VI	VII	VIII	IX	X	XI	XII	XIII	XIV	XV
3 OR < $n=16$	1	0	1	0	1	1	0	0	0	0	9	0	15	12	0
12–80 $n=14$	6	7	6	5	4	7	5	4	3	5	9	0	14	7	1
114–260 $n=15$	10	12	12	7	10	11	9	10	7	11	12	0	10	9	5
> 275 $n=16$	15	15	15	15	15	15	15	15	14	15	15	1	8	13	13
χ^2 $p=$	Groups 1–10, 15<10^{-5}								0.020.380.0021						

The bottom row shows the p value for χ^2 analysis between the four groups.
n: Number of samples.

Table 6 Four groups of samples based on serum IgE concentration with the corresponding number of false positives at 211 cut-off for each ELISA test group

IgE μg/ml	ELISA Test group false positives (101)														
	I	II	III	IV	V	VI	VII	VIII	IX	X	XI	XII	XIII	XIV	XV
3 OR < $n=16$	0	0	0	0	0	0	0	0	0	0	9	0	14	8	0
12–80 $n=14$	4	3	4	2	2	3	4	1	1	2	7	0	6	1	1
114–260 $n=15$	9	9	9	7	7	7	7	6	5	8	12	0	4	4	2
> 275 $n=16$	15	14	14	14	13	14	12	8	8	12	15	0	4	7	6
χ^2 $p=$	Groups 1–7, 10<10^{-5}							0.000.00		0.01	NC	0.12		0.11	0.01

The bottom row shows the p value for χ^2 analysis between the four groups.
n: Number of samples.

positive at the 211 eau cut-off. This probably reflects that though false positives are very common there is still a relationship as was shown by linear regression analysis. The molds had the most interesting results. False positives are very common and linear regression did not show significant results however the slope was showing an inverse relationship with IgE concentration. For mold mix XIII there was a significant ($p = 0.003$) difference between the four groups at the 101 eau cut-off for false positive but not at 211 eau. As Table 5 shows this is an inverse relationship with serum IgE. Mold mix XIV had no significant difference.

DISCUSSION

The inability to detect a relationship between ascarid inoculation and its effect on false positive ELISA and serum IgE concentration could reflect several problems. It is possible that no ascarid infection occurred following the oral inoculation. Many of the dogs at day 0 already had high serum IgE levels and numerous false positive ELISA results. It is possible that they were already resistant to ascarid infection. These dogs may already have been ascarid exposed as this parasite can infect fetuses *in utero*. Since we saw no rise in serum IgE over time we could not see significant changes in number of false positives. However by looking at the 60 samples as separate tests and comparing serum IgE concentration to false positive ELISA scores we did find a significant relationship.

It is interesting that different types of antigens were affected differently by the serum IgE concentration. The relationship between pollen scores and serum IgE concentration was expected. The lack of false positives to the epidermals and the high incidence of false positive results to house-dust mite and mold antigens was an unexpected finding.

The increased incidence of false positives as serum IgE increases could be explained by an increase in binding to non-antigen specific IgE. This would not explain why there is such a difference between group unless different antigens have variation in their ability to bind to non-specific IgE. The results with molds which show a tendency towards an inverse relationship would not be compatible with this explanation.

It is also possible that the ELISA test is measuring something other than IgE. This possibility could be determined by heat inactivating the high serum IgE samples and repeating the tests.

It is also possible that the ELISA tests and intradermal tests were both correct in their measurements. Our results could also be explained if there were two types of IgE present. One type of antigen specific IgE that binds to mast cells and is associated with the clinical symptoms of atopic disease, and another that is produced in normal animals. This normal IgE could be found in the serum but not attached to mast cells. Our variation in positive ELISA tests might reflect that the samples with high serum IgE came from animals that were exposed to the antigens and produced more normal IgE. This could be evaluated by doing Prausnitz-Küstner (PK) tests from atopic intradermal test positive dogs and normal dogs with high serum IgE and positive ELISA tests, before and after heat inactivation.

CONCLUSION

Our results have shown that normal dogs with high serum IgE levels do have an increased number of positive ELISA test results. It also showed that for most of the antigens tested there was a direct significant relationship between the two. The exact cause for these findings is unknown and awaits further studies.

ACKNOWLEDGEMENT

Special thanks to R.E.W. Halliwell for determining serum IgE levels, and to Bioproducts for Medicine Inc., for the ELISA tests.

REFERENCES

Caprio, R.E., Furth, K., Rosner, I. and Rappaport, I. (1983). Predicitive value of serum IgE on the correlation of RAST and intradermal testing in an atopic population. *Immunology and Allergy Practice* **5**:234–242.

Griffin, C.E. (1989). RAST and ELISA testing in canine atopy. In: Kirk, R.W. (ed.) *Current Veterinary Therapy X. Small Animal Practice*, pp. 592–595. W.B. Saunders Company, Philadelphia.

Halliwell, R.E.W. (1989). Atopic disease. In: Halliwell, R.E.W. and Gorman, N.T. (eds) *Veterinary Clinical Immunology*, pp. 232–252. W.B. Saunders Company, Philadelphia.

All p values in this paper, less than 0.000 were rounded off to 0.000.

2.5 Cell-mediated Immune Function in Dogs with Atopic Dermatitis

Judith S. Nimmo Wilkie

Regional Veterinary Laboratory, Benalla, Victoria, Australia

INTRODUCTION

Since an association between inhaled allergens and skin disease in dogs was first recognized in the 1930s (Burns, 1933); the entity known as canine allergic inhalant dermatitis, or canine atopic dermatitis has become a widely diagnosed condition (Nesbitt, 1978).

Canine atopic dermatitis is believed to be a Type I hypersensitivity in susceptible individuals which leads to the formation of skin-sensitizing antibodies to inhaled allergens which, in turn, results in pruritic skin disease (Halliwell and Schwartzman, 1971). However, the reason certain dogs are susceptible, and the pathogenesis of atopic disease is not known. Neither is it known if it is a similar mechanism to that causing human atopic dermatitis, although there are similarities between the two diseases (Rhodes *et al.*, 1987). It has been known for some time, that certain abnormal immune responses to viruses and to contact allergens occur in persons with atopic dermatitis (Krafchik, 1983). Furthermore, deficiencies in number and function of suppressor T-cell populations have been identified in people with atopic dermatitis (Strannegard *et al.*, 1976; Leung *et al.*, 1981; Stingl *et al.*, 1981). This led to the hypothesis that abnormal suppressor T-cell function in atopic people allows excessive IgE production by B-cells (Strannegard *et al.*, 1976; Beer *et al.*, 1982). Further work with respect to the interaction of lymphocytes and histamine, as one of the major mediators of Type 1 hypersensitivity, had identified an increased susceptibility of human atopic lymphocytes to histamine (Strannegard and Strannegard, 1977) and decreased histamine-induced suppression by atopic suppressor T-lymphocytes (Beer *et al.*, 1982).

In this study, some of the functions of the cell-mediated immune system, especially with regard to suppressor T-cell function, have been examined in dogs with atopic dermatitis. By comparing these with those of normal dogs in whom experimental Type 1 hypersensitivity had been induced, it was hoped to identify which, if any, of the alterations observed in the atopic dogs were not a result of the Type 1 hypersensitivity and may, therefore, be intrinsic to the atopic state.

MATERIALS AND METHODS

Throughout this study the following animals were used. Since not every animal was used in every assay, the number of animals participating in each experiment is given in the results of that experiment.

Dogs

These were 22 normal dogs and 20 dogs with atopic dermatitis, including dogs of both sexes, and of various ages and breeds. Atopic dogs had a clinical history and clinical signs appropriate to atopy (Scott, 1981), absence of any other dermatological disease, a skin biospy sample with histopathological findings typical of atopic dermatitis (Scott, 1981), a positive skin reaction to at least one of fifteen standard test allergens. Details were as previously described (Nimmo Wilkie, 1986).

Separation of peripheral blood mononuclear cells

Peripheral blood was obtained by venipuncture into evacuated tubes containing EDTA. The buffy coat was harvested into Hank's buffered salt solution (HBSS) and the mononuclear cell layer was harvested by density centrifugation as previously described, before being resuspended in a complete medium (Nimmo Wilkie, 1986).

Lymphocyte stimulation

Peripheral blood mononuclear cells (pbmc) were stimulated with 1μg/ml or 5μg/ml of Concanavalin A (Con A) and incubated for 72 h. Tritiated thymidine uptake was used to measure the resultant blastogenesis, as described (Nimmo Wilkie, 1986). The stimulation index (SI) was calculated by counts per minute (cpm) Con A stimulated cells divided by cpm unstimulated cells, where cpm were counts per minute for tritium.

The 24 h preincubated cells were stored at room temperature in whole blood (plus EDTA) for 24 h before being separated and stimulated with Con A, as above (Nimmo Wilkie 1986); The % enhancement was calculated as 100 x [(cpm Con A stimulated, 24 preincubated, cells divided by cpm Con A stimulated fresh cells) – 1)].

Histamine comitogenesis

Histamine dihydrochloride at 10^{-6}M was added together with 5μg/ml of Con A to pbmc and the percentage enhancement of blastogenesis was calculated as above (Nimmo Wilkie, 1986).

Autologous lymphocyte co-culture assay

Pbmc were separated as described and incubated for 24 h without additives, with 10^{-5}M histamine, or 1,5, or 20μg/ml of Con A. These were then called effector cells (E) which were prevented from being further stimulated and added to freshly separated, autologous pbmc, designated responder cells (R), and then stimulated with 5μg/ml of Con A (Nimmo Wilkie, 1986). The percentage suppression was calculated as 100x [(cpm Con A stimulated, R plus E divided by cpm Con A stimulated fresh R plus unstimulated E)] (Nimmo Wilkie, 1986).

Cutaneous mitogens

The dogs were injected intradermally with 50μg of phytohaemagglutinin (PHA) or Con A. Sterile saline was used as a control. Skin thickness at the injection site was recorded preinjection and at 24 h postinjection. The difference in thickness was recorded in millimetres (Nimmo Wilkie, 1986).

Contact sensitant

Dogs were sensitized with a topical application of 2% solution of dinitrochlorobenzene (DNCB). Two weeks later at a different skin site 0.5 ml of a 0.01% solution of DNCB was applied topically. The skin thickness of the site was measured preapplication and at 24 h postapplication (Nimmo Wilkie, 1986).

Experimental Type 1 hypersensitivity

Five non-atopic dogs were sensitized to ascaris antigen by three subcutaneous injections of 10μg of antigen at 3-day intervals (Nimmo Wilkie, 1986). Anaphylaxis was induced by intravenous administration of ascaris antigen to anaesthetized dogs, until a dramatic fall in blood pressure occurred. Recovery was induced by injecting epinephrine intravenously (Nimmo Wilkie, 1986). *In vitro* and *in vivo* immunological tests were performed before, and 24 h after, anaphylaxis (Nimmo Wilkie, 1986).

Statistical analysis

Means of results for atopic dog group were compared to means for the normal dog group using Students' *t* test. Probabilities of less than 0.5 were considered significant. For the experimental hypersensitivity experiment means of results for the group before and after anaphylaxis were compared using Students' t test.

RESULTS

Lymphocyte stimulation

There was no statistically significant difference between the normal and atopic dog groups with respect to stimulation index following stimulation of pbmc *in vitro* with either 1 or 5μg/ml of Con A (Nimmo Wilkie, 1986).

24 h Preincubation assay

The percentage enhancement of Con A mitogenesis was decreased for atopic dogs especially at suboptimal (1μg/ml) levels of mitogen ($p \leq 0.001$), (Nimmo Wilkie, 1986). Values are given in Fig. 1.

Histamine comitogenesis

Mitogenesis due to optimal (5μg/ml) levels of Con A was enhanced by the addition of 10^{-6}M histamine for normal dogs but not for atopic dogs ($p \leq 0.001$), (Nimmo Wilkie, 1986) values are given in Fig. 1.

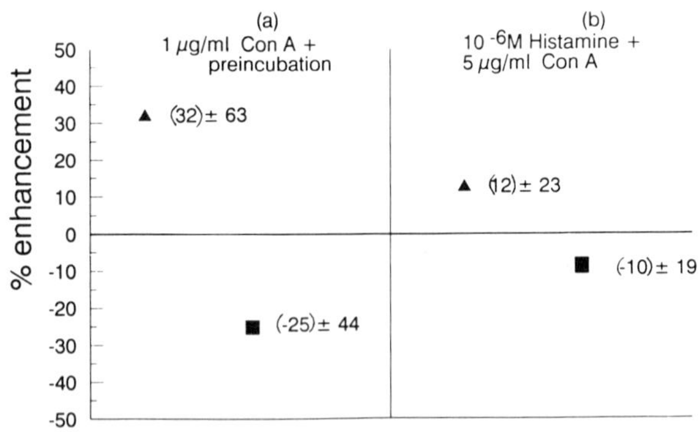

Figure 1 Enhancement of Con A mitogenesis by 24 h preincubation (a) or 10^{-6}M histamine (b). ▲ = mean of 21 normal dogs ■ = mean of 13 atopic dogs ± = standard deviations.

Autologous lymphocyte co-culture assay

Con A-induced suppression: The percentage suppression was statistically significantly lower for atopic dogs than normal only at supraoptimal levels of

Con A (20µg/ml) ($p \leq 0.001$), (Nimmo Wilkie, 1986). Values are given in Fig. 2.

Histamine induced suppression

The percentage suppression induced by 10^{-5}M histamine was much lower for atopic dogs ($p \leq 0.001$). Values are given in Fig. 2.

Spontaneous suppression

The percentage supression produced by untreated effector cells was very significantly higher ($p \leq 0.001$) for atopic dogs (Nimmo Wilkie, 1986). Values are given in Fig. 2.

Cutaneous mitogens

For both Con A and PHA, the change in skin thickness was significantly greater ($p \leq 0.001$) for atopic dogs (Nimmo Wilkie, 1986). Values are given in Fig. 3.

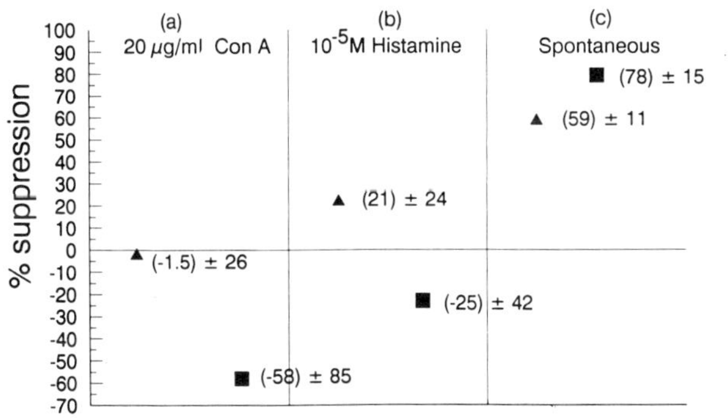

Figure 2 Percentage suppression in the autologous lymphocyte coculture assay, induced by 20µg/ml Con A (a), 10^{-6}M histamine (b) or untreated cultures (spontaneous) (c). ▲ = mean of 21 normal dogs ■ = mean of 18 atopic dogs ± = standard deviations.

Contact sensitant

The response to DNCB was significantly smaller ($p \leq 0.001$) for atopic dogs (Nimmo Wilkie, 1986). Values are given in Fig. 3.

Experimental Type 1 hypersensitivity

For the five dogs at 24 h postanaphylaxis the lymphocyte stimulation index was not significantly different, but the percentage enhancement due to 24 h

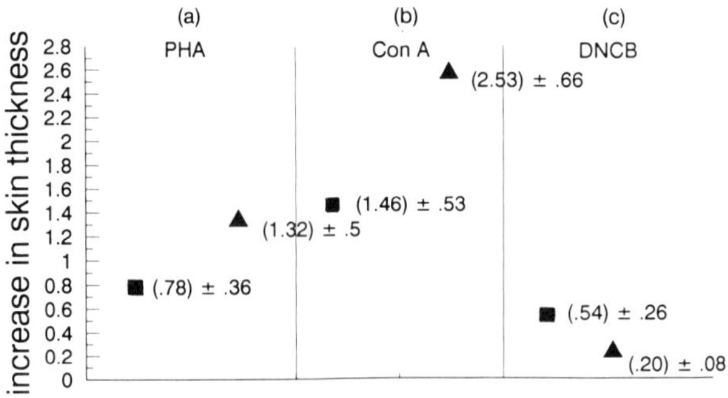

Figure 3 Cutaneous response to intradermally injected mitogens (a) PHA (a) or Con A (b) or the contact sensitant DNCB (c) ■ = mean of 21 normal dogs, ▲ = mean of 17 atopic dogs (a + b) or mean of 8 atopic dogs (c) ± = standard deviations.

preincubation was decreased ($p \leq 0.1$). Values are as follows: presentitization, % enchancement mean (x) = 2.76 and standard deviation (sx) = 52.5; postanaphylaxi x = −57.8, sx = 29.1. The percentage enhancement of Con A mitogenesis due to 10^{-4}M histamine declined ($p \leq 0.05$). Presentization x = 10.66, sx = 13.49 postanaphylaxis x = 9.76, sx = 12.04. (Nimmo Wilkie, 1986).

In the autologous lymphocyte coculture assay, Con A-induced suppression was not significantly different postanaphylaxis but histamine-induced supression declined ($p \leq 0.01$). Percentage suppression induced by 10^{-5}M histamine presentitization; x = 13.98, sx = 28.3, postanaphylaxis, x = 45, sx = 20.45. Spontaneous suppression increased significantly ($p \leq 0.01$) from presentitization level of x = 50, sx = 5.09 to a postanaphylaxis-level of x = 66.1 sx = 7.48 (Nimmo Wilkie, 1986).

The response to cutaneous mitogens decreased significantly for PHA ($p \leq 0.05$) and Con A ($p \leq 0.01$) postanaphylaxis from presentatitization levels of x = 1.06, sx = 0.57 for PHA and x = 26, sx = 0.87 for Con A to postanaphylaxis levels of x = 0.42, sx = 0.88 (PHA) and x = 0.78, sx = 0.82 (Con A). For the contact allergen DNCB there was a decline from x = 0.5, sx = 0.12 to x = 0.38, sx = 0.18 but no statistical significance was shown (Nimmo Wilkie, 1986).

DISCUSSION

Although it is still not certain that human and canine atopy share a common pathogenesis, *in vitro* cell-mediated immune function was found to be altered in the atopic dogs in this study, as it is in atopic people. Although Con A-induced blastogenesis of pbmc was not different from normal, the pbmc of atopic dogs that had been preincubated for 2 h failed to show the enhancement of Con A mitogenesis that the normal canine cells did. This lack of enhancement has been reported in people with SLE and was suggested to have been the result of a deficiency in a subpopulation of short-lived suppressor cells (Bresnihan and Jasin, 1977). Furthermore, histamine added simultaneously with the mitogen (Con A) failed to enhance the mitogenesis of atopic dog pbmc, although normal canine pbmc did respond. Histamine is believed to enhance Con A mitogenesis by acting via H_1 receptors and to suppress by acting via H_2 receptors (Suzuki and Huchet, 1981; Beaulieu *et al.*, 1986). Human atopic lymphocytes appear to be most susceptible to the suppressive effects of histamine (Strannegard and Strannegard, 1977). Similarly canine atopic lymphocytes may be more susceptible to the suppressive effects of histamine or, alternatively, may simply be failing to respond to its enhancing effects because of occupation of histamine receptor sites by endogenous histamine.

Histamine or Con A, when used to pretreat pbmc in the autologous co-culture assay, induce suppressor cell activity. Atopic human lymphocytes show decreased ability to generate histamine-induced suppression (Beer *et al.*, 1982). Similarly atopic dog pbmc showed decreased histamine-induced suppression, in this study. Con A-induced suppression was decreased for atopic dogs only at supraoptimal levels of mitogen. Since histamine and Con A are believed to act on a different subset of suppressor T cells (Suzuki and Huchet, 1981) different results for each assay might be expected. Con A-induced suppression has been shown to be normal (Beer *et al.*, 1982) or decreased (Stingl *et al.*, 1981) or, as for the atopic dogs, decreased only at supraoptimal levels of mitogen (Rola-Pleszcynski and Blanchard, 1981). Decreased Con A-induced suppression was, however, shown to precede the onset of atopic dermatitis in a group of children (Stingl *et al.*, 1981), suggesting a possible role in the pathogenesis of the disease. Spontaneous suppression, generated by untreated cells has not been examined for human atopics but, in this study, was very significantly increased for the atopic dogs. The significance of this is unknown but one must consider the possibility that this represents histamine-induced suppression due to to autologous, circulating histamine resulting from the type 1 hypersensitivity reaction in the atopic dogs. This might also explain the failure of these cells to be further stimulated by pretreatment with histamine *in vitro*.

The presence of skin-sensitizing antibodies alone does not cause atopic dermatitis, since infection with ascarids causes production of IgE antibodies, but is not routinely manifested as a dermatitis. Consequently, it seemed appropriate to examine cell-mediated immune function at the cutaneous level in atopic dogs, especially as people with atopic dermatitis are known to have abnormal cutaneous responses to certain viruses and fungi (Krafchik, 1983). Furthermore, human atopic dermatitis patients have been shown to have a diminished response to contact sensitants (Palacios *et al.*, 1966). In this study, atopic dogs also have a very significantly decreased response to a contact sensitant, although inducing contact hypersensitivty was difficult even in normal dogs. The cutaneous response to mitogens injected intradermally was, by contrast, markedly greater than normal in the atopic dogs. The reason for the apparently conflicting results of these two tests of cutaneous delayed hypersensitivity is unknown. However the tests do differ in that the contact sensitant must work through the Langerhan's cell, whilst the mitogen can act directly on cutaneous lymphocytes. Despite the apparent contradictory nature of the results, both tests show alterations in cell-mediated immune function before and after induction of anaphylaxis, it was hoped to distinguish functions that were altered as a result of the pharmaco-physiological events occurring during a Type 1 hypersensitivity reaction. As might be expected, histamine-modulated lymphocyte functions were altered. Histamine-induced suppression in the autologous lymphocyte co-culture assay was reduced, as was the enhancing effect of histamine as a comitogen. Spontaneous suppression in the autologous lymphocyte co-culture assay was, however, increased. Con A blastogenesis was not significantly altered but enhancement by preincubation of cells for 24 h, declined. The cutaneous reponse to intradermally injected mitogens declined significantly postanaphylaxis. The response to the contact allergen also declined but not significantly. Failure to show a significant difference was most likely due to the small initial response making any small differences beyond the capabilities of the measuring instrument to detect.

Thus, almost all the alterations in cell-mediated immune function detected in atopic dogs were reproduced in normal dogs by inducing Type 1 hypersensitivity and an episode of anaphylaxis. In particular, the histamine-modulated functions were altered, presumably due to release of endogenous histamine during anaphylaxis. Histamine has also been shown to diminish the delayed hypersensitivity reponse to intradermally injected antigen (Rocklin, 1976), which explains the decrease in the cutaneous reponse to the mitogens. These alterations in cell-mediated immune function are most likely, the result of Type 1 hypersensitivity rather than changes intrinsic to the atopic state.

The two alterations in cell-mediated immune function that were not reproduced by experimental Type 1 hypersensitivity were the reduction in Con A-induced suppression, at supraoptimal levels of the mitogen, in the autologous lymphocyte assay and the increased response to intradermally injected mitogens. The diminution of the Con A-induced suppression in this study, albeit only at supraoptimal levels, as has been reported in man (Rola-Pleszcynski and Blanchard, 1981) and the report of this alteration preceding onset of dermatitis in atopic children (Chandra and Baker, 1983), together with the present evidence that this change is unrelated to the release of pharmacological mediators of anaphylaxis, point to a possible significant role in the pathogenesis of atopy.

The increased response of atopic dogs to cutaneous mitogens was unexpected in view of the diminished response to the contact allergen and a similarly decreased response in human atopics (Palacios *et al.*, 1966). Experimental production of Type 1 hypersensitivity and anaphylaxis in the normal dogs failed to reproduce the increase in cutaneous response but rather caused the decline in response that might be expected following massive endogenous histamine release (Rocklin, 1976). It seems possible that this altered cutaneous response is evidence of an immunological abnormality at the cutaneous level that may well be important in understanding how and why the skin becomes the target organ for Type 1 hypersensitivity when it manifests as atopic dermatitis. Furthermore the response to cutaneous mitogens, particularly Con A, was so much greater, and so significantly different than in normal dogs, that it is possible this test could be used as simple, rapid screening test for atopy.

REFERENCE

Beaulieu, L. Beaudoin, J., Jobin, M. and Hebert, J. (1986). Effects of H_1 and H_2 receptor agonists on nonspecific proliferative response of human peripheral blood lymphocytes. *International Archives of Allergy and Applied Immunology* **79**: 249–252.

Beer, D.J., Osband, M.E., McCaffrey, R.P., Soter, N.A. and Rocklin, R.E. (1982). Abnormal histamine-induced suppressor cell function in atopic subjects. *New England Journal of Medicine* **306**: 454–458.

Bresnihan, B. and Jasin, H.E. (1977). Suppressor function of peripheral blood mononuclear cells in normal individuals and in patients with systemic lupus erythematosus. *Journal of Clinical Investigation* **59**: 106–116.

Burns, P.W. (1933). Allergic reaction in dogs. *Journal of the American Veterinary Medical Association* **83 (NS36)**: 627–634.

Chandra, R.K. and Baker, M. (1983). Numerical and functional deficiency of suppressor T cells precedes development of atopic eczema. *Lancet ii*: 1393–1394.

Halliwell, R.E.W. and Schwartzman, R.M. (1971). Atopic disease in the dog *Veterinary Record* **89**: 209–214.

Kratchik, B.R. (1983). Atopic dermatitis. *Pediatric Clinics of North America* **30**: 669–685.

Leung, D.Y.M., Rhodes, A.R. and Geha, R.S. (1981). Enumeration of T cell subsets in atopic dermatitis using monoclonal antibodies. *Journal of Allergy and Clinical Immunology* **67**: 450–455.

Nesbitt, G.H. (1978). Canine allergic inhalant dermatitis: A review of 230 cases. *Journal of the American Veterinary Medical Association* **172**: 55–60.

Nimmo Wilkie, J.S. (1986). Studies on Cell-mediated immune function in dogs with atopic dermatitis. Ph D thesis, University of Guelph, Canada.

Palacios, J. Fuller, E.W. and Blaylock, W.K. (1966). Immunological capabilities of patient with atopic dermatitis. *Journal of Investigative Dermatology* **47**: 484–491.

Rocklin, R.E. (1976). Modulation of cellular-immune responses *in vivo* and *in vitro* by histamine receptor-bearing lymphocytes. *Journal of Clinical Investigation* **57**: 1051–1058.

Rhodes, K.H., Kerdel, F. and Sotger, N.A. (1987). Comparative aspects of canine and human atopic dermatitis. *Seminars in Veterinary Medicine and Surgery (Small Animal)* **2**: 166–172.

Rola-Pleszczynski, M. and Blanchard, R. (1981). Abnormal suppressor cell function in atopic dermatitis. *Journal of Investigative Dermatology* **76**: 279–283.

Scott, D.W. (1981). Observations on canine atopy. *Journal of the American Animal Hospital Association* **17**: 91–100.

Stingl, G., Gazze, L.A., Czarneki, N. and Wolff, K. (1981). T cell abnormalities in atopic dermatitis patients: imbalances in T cell subpopulations and impaired generation of Con A-induced suppressor cells. *Journal of Investigative Dermatology* **76**: 468–473.

Strannegard, I.L. and Strannegard, O. (1977). Increased sensitivity of lymphocytes from atopic individuals to histamine-induced suppression. *Scandinavian Journal of Immunology* **6**: 1225–1231.

Strannegard, I.L., Lindholm, L. and Strannegard, O. (1976). T lymphocytes in atopic children. *International Archives of Allergy and Applied Immunology* **50**: 684–692.

Suzuki, S. and Huchet, R. (1981). Mechanisms of histamine-induced inhibition of lymphocyte response to mitogens in mice. *Cellular Immunology* **62**: 396–405.

2.6 Fat Absorption in Dogs with Atopic Dermatitis

A.H.M. van den Broek and J.W. Simpson

Department of Veterinary Clinical Studies, Royal (Dick) School of Veterinary Studies, University of Edinburgh, Edinburgh, Scotland

INTRODUCTION

Canine atopy and human atopic dermatitis, though not strictly analogous, (Halliwell and Gorman, 1989) are both cutaneous manifestations of atopic disease.

Dietary supplementation with essential fatty acids (EFA), particularly evening primrose oil (EPO), has been associated with significant clinical improvement in cases of human atopic eczema (Hansen, 1933; Lovell *et al.*, 1981; Wright and Burton, 1982) and canine atopy (Lloyd, 1989; Miller *et al.*, 1989).

Although it is recognised that dietary EFA deficiency, maldigestion and malabsorption (Rivers and Frankel, 1981; Sherertz, 1986; Simpson, 1987) may compromise EFA intake, studies of plasma concentrations of EFA and their metabolites have provided putative evidence that human atopic eczema is associated with impaired EFA metabolism rather than deficient EFA intake (Wright, 1985; Manku *et al.*, 1984). It has been proposed (Manku *et al.*, 1984) that the gammalinolenic acid (GLA) component of EPO bypasses this defect. However, in some cases of human atopic eczema (Morse *et al.*, 1989) and canine atopy (Lloyd, 1989) oral EPO administration fails to produce any clinical improvement. This may be associated with impaired absorption of dietary EFA and GLA.

In this present study quantitative absorption of long chain triglyceride was determined in clinically normal dogs and dogs with confirmed atopic dermatitis.

MATERIALS AND METHODS

Animals

Group 1

These were 14 clinically normal dogs, domestic pets, aged between 2 and 12 years (mean age 6 years 3 months) and comprised entire male and female and neutered animals of several breeds including the German shepherd dog, Labrador retriever, boxer, setter and spaniel.

Group 2

These were 20 dogs with confirmed atopic dermatitis, domestic pets, aged between 1 and 9 years (mean age 3 years 10 months) and comprised entire male and female animals of several breeds including the German shepherd dog, Labrador retriever, golden retriever, boxer, setter, spaniel, pointer, West Highland white terrier and Jack Russell terrier.

Parasitosis was ruled out by examination of skin scrapings, none of the dogs had positive reactions to the intradermal injection of flea antigens. A diagnosis of atopic disease was made on the criteria proposed by Willemse (1986) together with one or more positive immediate reactions to intradermal tests. In 11 cases the possibility of concurrent food allergy was ruled out by dietary restriction (van den Broek, 1989). None of the dogs manifested clinical evidence of hormone imbalance.

Method

Quantitative fat absorption was assessed using the method described by Simpson and Doxey (1983) as modified by Simpson and van den Broek (1990).

None of the dogs had received medication for at least 3 weeks prior to investigation. Each dog was fasted for 12 hours, weighed and fed corn oil (3 ml/kg) to a maximum of 90 ml. Immediately before and at 60, 120, 180 and 240 min after feeding the corn-oil 2 ml venous blood samples were collected in anticoagulant free Vacutainer tubes (Becton Dickinson). The serum was harvested and the triglyceride concentration determined by a Technicon RA500 auto-analyser, using a commercial test kit (Technicon, Basingstoke).

Statistics

The mean, standard deviation was calculated at each time of sampling for each group. The area under the curve at 3 and 4 h was determined for each group. Differences between the groups were compared by the Student's two sample t test using separate variance estimations for each group.

RESULTS

The number of dogs in each group together with the mean, standard deviation, maximum and minimum values and number of dogs outside the normal range at each sampling time are shown in Table 1.

The mean concentrations of serum triglyceride and the standard error of the mean, for each group, at each sampling time are shown graphically in Fig. 1.

At 0, 60 and 240 min no significant difference was detected between the mean concentration of triglyceride in the serum of normal and atopic dogs.

Table 1 Concentration (mmol/litre) of serum trigylceride in 14 normal dogs and 20 dogs with atopic dermatitis at each sampling time

Time (min)	Parameter	Normal	Atopic
Zero	Mean	0.55	0.52
	Range	0.38–0.77	0.31–0.81
	SD	0.09	0.16
	No <NR		5
	No >NR		1
60	Mean	0.84	0.70
	Range	0.44–1.89	0.32–1.36
	SD	0.37	0.29
	No <NR		4
	No >NR		0
120	Mean	1.34*	0.98*
	Range	0.62–2.26	0.31–2.45
	SD	0.49	0.49
	No <NR		5
	No >NR		1
180	Mean	1.78**	1.02**
	Range	0.72–3.05	0.44–2.19
	SD	0.69	0.50
	No <NR		4
	No >NR		0
240	Mean	1.47	1.10
	Range	0.67–2.71	0.47–2.25
	SD	0.63	0.50
	No <NR		4
	No >NR		0

SD: Standard deviation
No <NR: number of dogs with values less than the normal range
No >NR: number of dogs with values greater than the normal range
Mean = with same superscript are significantly different
* = $p<0.05$; ** = $p<0.001$.

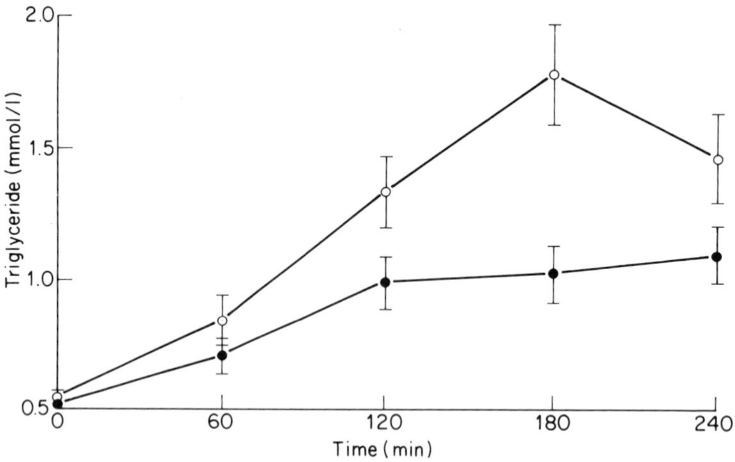

Figure 1 Fat absorption in normal (o ——— o) and atopic (• ——— •) dogs. Points are mean ± SEM.

The mean concentration of triglyceride in the serum of dogs with atopic dermatitis at 120 and 180 min (0.98 mmol/l and 1.02 mmol/l) was significantly lower ($p<0.05$ and $p<0.001$, respectively) than that of normal dogs (1.34 mmol/l and 1.78 mmol/l, respectively).

The area under the curve at 180 and 240 min for dogs with atopic dermatitis (3.23 and 4.32 units, respectively) was significantly lower ($p<0.01$ and $p<0.05$, respectively) than that for normal dogs (4.50 and 5.96, respectively).

DISCUSSION

In this present study the peak serum triglyceride concentration recorded after feeding corn-oil was significantly lower ($p<0.001$) in atopic than normal dogs. This may be indicative of impaired fat absorption or increased plasma triglyceride clearance in atopic dogs. Further studies are necessary to clarify this and to investigate whether EFA absorption is particularly affected.

Impaired intestinal fat absorption may explain the dose-clinical response relationship observed in patients receiving oral EPO (Wright and Burton, 1982) and the reported absence of an increase in plasma dihomo-gammalinolenic acid concentration in some patients receiving oral EPO (Morse *et al.*, 1989) which contains its precursor gammalinolenic acid.

However, in this present study no significant difference was detected in the resting concentration of serum triglyceride though in five atopic dogs (25%) the serum triglyceride concentration was below the normal range. Similarly, studies of plasma phospholipids have demonstrated normal (Schalin-Karrila *et al.*, 1987) or raised (Manku *et al.*, 1984; Wright, 1985) EFA concentrations in human atopic eczema. Although these observations provide no supportive evidence for compromised intestinal absorption of fatty acids it is possible that the plasma concentration is maintained while reserves are depleted and non-essential utilization is depressed.

The observation of reduced intestinal fat absorption and plasma clearance in rats injected with interleukin-1 (Lopez-Soriano, 1988) has demonstrated the susceptibility of both processes to mediators of the inflammatory response. Therefore, though reduced intestinal fat absorption or increased triglyceride clearance may be involved in the genesis of canine atopic dermatitis it is also possible that they are influenced by the various mediators released in the inflammatory reaction.

Studies of the plasma concentration of EFA and their metabolites in cases of human atopic eczema have focused attention on an apparent disturbance in EFA metabolism, possibly due to impaired delta-6-desaturase activity (Manku *et al.*, 1984). While a similar defect may occur in canine atopy, observations made in this present study suggest that impaired absorption or clearance of triglycerides may be associated with the development of this condition.

ACKNOWLEDGEMENTS

The authors would like to thank The Waltham Centre for Pet Nutrition, Melton Mowbray for its financial support.

REFERENCES

Halliwell, R.E.W. and Gorman, N.F. (1989). Atopic diseases. In: Halliwell, R.E.W. and Gorman, N.F. (eds) *Veterinary Clinical Immunology*, pp. 232-252. W.B. Saunders Company, Philadelphia.

Hansen, A.E. (1933). Serum lipid changes and therapeutic effects of various oils in infantile eczema. *Proceedings of the Society of Experimental Biology and Medicine* **31**: 160-161.

Lloyd, D.H. (1989). Essential fatty acids and skin disease. *Journal of Small Animal Practice* **30**: 207-212.

Lovell, C.R., Burton, J.C. and Horrobin, D.F. (1981). Treatment of atopic eczema with evening primrose oil. *Lancet* **i**: 278.

Lopez-Soriano, F.J. (1988). Effects of Interleukin-1 on lipid metabolism in the rat. *The Biochemist* **10**: 14-15.

Manku, M.S., Horrobin, D.F., Morse, N.L. Wright, S. and Burton, J.L. (1984). Essential fatty acids in the plasma phospholids of patients with atopic eczema. *British Journal of Dermatology* **110**: 643-648.

Miller, W.H., Griffin, C.E., Scott, D.W., Angarano, D.K. and Norton, A.C. (1989). Clinical trial of DVM derm caps in the treatment of allergic disease in dogs: a nonblind study. *Journal of the American Animal Hospital Association* **25**: 163-168.

Morse, P.F., Horrobin, D.F., Manku, M.S., Stewart, J.C., Allen, R. *et al.* (1989). Meta-analysis of placebo-controlled studies of the efficacy of gamma-linolenic acid in the treatment of atopic eczema. Relationship between plasma essential fatty acid changes and clinical response. *British Journal of Dermatology* **121**: 75-90.

Rivers, J.P.W. and Frankel, T.C. (1981). Essential fatty acid deficiency. *British Medical Bulletin* **37**: 59-64.

Schalin-Karrila, M., Mattila, L., Jansen, C.F. & Uotila, P. (1987). Evening primrose oil in the treatment of atopic eczema: effect on clinical status, plasma phospholipid fatty acids and circulating blood prostaglandins. *British Journal of Dermatology* **117**:11-19.

Sherertz, E.F. (1986). The skin in essential fatty acid deficiency. In: Roe, A. (ed.) *Nutrition and the Skin*, pp. 117-130. A.R. Liss, New York.

Simpson, J.W. (1987). In: Grunsell, C.S.G., Hill, F.W.G. and Raw, M.E. (eds) *The Veterinary Annual*, pp. 319-323. Scientechnica, Bristol.

Simpson, J.W. & Doxey, D.L. (1983). Quantitative assessment of fat absorption and its diagnostic value in exocrine pancreatic insufficiency. *Research in Veterinary Science* **35**:249-251.

Simpson, J.W. and van den Broek, A.H.M. (1990). Assessment of fat absorption in normal dogs and in dogs with hyperadrenocorticalism. *Research in Veterinary Science* **48**: 38–42.

Van den Broek A.H.M. (1989). Cutaneous hypersensitivity (allergy) in dogs. In: Grunsell, C.S.G., Raw, M.E. and Hill, F.W.G. (eds) *The Veterinary Annual* pp. 245-250. 29th issue, Butterworth, London.

Willemse, T. (1986). Atopic skin disease: a review and reconsideration of diagnostic criteria. *Journal of Small Animal Practice* **127**: 771-778.

Wright, S. (1985). Atopic dermatitis and essential fatty acids: a biochemical basis for atopy; *Acta Dermato-Venereologica (Stockholm) 114*: 143-145.

Wright, S. and Burton, J.C. (1982). Oral evening primrose seed oil improves atopic eczema. *Lancet* **ii**: 1120-1122.

PART 3

INFLAMMATORY MEDIATORS AND THEIR CONTROL

3.1 Inflammatory Mediators and Skin Disease

D.H. Lloyd

Senior Lecturer in Veterinary Medicine (Dermatology), Department of Veterinary. Medicine and Animal Husbandry, Royal Veterinary College, Hatfield, Herts, UK

INTRODUCTION

Inflammation involves the complex interaction of many soluble substances (Table 1), cells and other structural components leading in skin to the classical signs and symptoms of warmth, redness, swelling, pain and pruritus. The soluble substances involved in these processes are termed mediators. They are

Table 1 Some mediators of inflammation

Chemotactic factors, ECF-A, NCF-A
Coagulation and fibrinolysis products
Collagen fragments
Complement
Cytokines
Eicosanoids
Eosinophil products
Histamine
Insulin
Interferons
Kinins and kallikrein
Neurohumoral agents e.g. Substance P, Sensory nerve permeability factor, Calcitonin gene-related peptide
Oxygen radicals
Plasminogen activator
Platelet activating factor
Proteases
Serotonin

ECF: eosinophil chemotactic factor.
NCF: neutrophil chemotactic factor.

derived from cells or plasma precursors and generally have diverse effects, not only promoting inflammation but also limiting it to maintain homoeostasis once the primary inflammatory stimuli have been contained (Garcia Leme, 1981; Besedovsky and del Rey, 1987; Greaves and Camp, 1988; Nossal, 1989). Our increasing knowledge of inflammatory mediators shows that, in most cases, multiple pathways towards the different manifestations of inflammation exist. This has greatly complicated studies of the mediators which have generally relied on purified tissue fluid extracts or recombinant preparations and on the use of specific inhibitors to investigate their effects. As yet, little is known of the tissue levels of these substances and thus it is uncertain whether the effects obtained under experimental conditions represent conditions which obtain *in vivo*. These uncertainties have also limited the use of inhibitors of these substances as therapeutic agents and it is clear that a much more detailed understanding of inflammatory processes will be needed before antiinflammatory drugs can be developed which will be effective and free from undesirable side-effects.

A review of mediators of inflammation has little relevance unless the interaction with the immune system is considered. The range of compounds involved is large and a comprehensive analysis is beyond the scope of this chapter. This review will thus concentrate on factors involved in inflammation in the skin with particular reference to the defensive role of the epidermis and recent developments in our knowledge of an emerging group of potent mediators with a broad spectrum of activities, the cytokines.

INFLAMMATION, IMMUNITY AND THE SKIN

The skin surface forms a barrier zone which must resist the infectious, traumatic and toxic challenges of the environment. In doing this it continually undergoes inflammatory reactions designed to promote its defensive and repair processes. It has been known for some time that the epidermis in both animals and man contains humoral factors such as immunoglobulins, complement and transferrin (Page and Remington, 1967; Forstrom *et al.*, 1975; Lloyd *et al.*, 1977; Jenkinson *et al.*, 1979). In man, antitoxin production has been demonstrated in sweat (Page and Remington, 1967). In cattle production at the skin surface of different classes of immunoglobulins in response to vaccination and challenge has been reported (Lloyd *et al.*, 1987). Thus antitoxic and antimicrobial activity, including complement fixing reactions, are potentially possible both in the living epidermis and in the stratum corneum although evidence of the function of these substances *in vivo* is lacking (Jenkinson *et al.*, 1989). More recently it has been recognized that the epidermis is an important arm of the immune system involved in antigen recognition and the generation of not only cell-mediated and humoral responses but also of potent inflammatory mediators and modulators capable of inducing changes both in the skin and in the body as a whole.

The epidermis as an immunocompetent tissue

The living epidermis is composed of three main types of cells, the keratinocyte, the Langerhans' cells and the melanocyte. It is now apparent that the Langerhans' cells are derived from bone marrow precursors of macrophage/monocyte lineage which constantly repopulate the epidermis. They can express Class II MHC products (Ia, HLA-/DR in man) and are capable of antigen processing and presentation to sensitized T-cells. They can act as both inducers and accessory cells in the generation of cytotoxic T-cell responses. Such reactions may be involved in the pathogenesis of allergic contact dermatitis, in which the role of Langerhans' cells is well established, and in other inflammatory skin diseases (Stingl *et al.*, 1978; Choi and Sauder, 1986). As yet most of the work on Langerhans' cell function has been carried out in laboratory animals and man but these cells are known to be present at the skin surface in cattle and sheep both in the epidermis and in the sweat gland duct (Jenkinson *et al.*, 1966; Jenkinson and Blackburn, 1967; Hollis and Lyne, 1972; Montgomery *et al.*, 1982) and recent studies have demonstrated the presence of Class II MHC positive, acetyl cholinesterase positive dendritic cells, probably Langerhans' cells, in the epidermis of the sheep (Jenkinson, personal communication).

The keratinocytes also play an active role in epidermal inflammatory and immune responses. They are an important source of the cytokines, interleukins 1 and 2 (IL–1, IL–2), which amplify the process of antigen presentation between Langerhans' cells and T-cells and the subsequent clonal expansion of the T-cells (Edelson and Fink, 1985; Dreno *et al.*, 1989) but also have other important effects on inflammation. Indeed, it is increasingly apparent that the epidermis is also an important source of a variety of other cytokines with both local and distant effects (Table 2). Current knowledge of this rapidly changing field is summarized below.

Activities of the cytokines in inflammation and immunity

The cytokines form a rapidly growing family of glycoproteins which are produced by leukocytes and a range of other cells. The diversity of their sources and functions is illustrated in Table 2 which summarizes knowledge from studies *in vitro* and *in vivo* using material from a variety of species. Their actions are concerned principally with activation of T- and B- lymphocytes, haematopoeisis, cytotoxic and antimicrobial effects, and other inflammatory reactions which enable the regulation of local and systemic responses to infection, neoplasia and degenerative changes (Billingham, 1987; Hamblin, 1988).

Action on T-cells

The principal cytokines acting on T-cells are IL–1 and IL–2 (Williams *et al.*, 1985; reviewed by: Dinarello, 1988a; Hamblin, 1988; Sauder, 1989). When

Table 2 Some sources and actions of cytokines involved in inflammation

Substance	Sources	Actions
IL-1	Many types of cell (Table 3)	Wide variety of local and systemic actions (Tables 4, 5 and 6)
IL-2	T-Cells, keratinocytes	Stimulates T-cell proliferation, activity of cytolytic T- and NK cells, production of LAK and murine epidermal Thy-1 positive cells; promotes growth and differentiation of B-cells; increases macrophage cytotoxicity.
IL-3	T-Cells, keratinocytes	Stimulates formation of neutrophils, eosinophils, monocytes, megakaryocytes, mast cells and erythroid cells by bone marrow cells; promotes growth and differentiation of B-cells; can activate NK cells.
IL-4	T-Cells	Promotes growth, differentiation and immunoglobulin isotype regulation of B-cells; blocks production of TNF-α, IL-1 and PGE_2 by monocytes; stimulates monocyte differentiation and induction of MHC class I and II antigens; stimulates T-cell growth.
IL-5	T-Cells	Promotes growth and differentiation of activated B-cells; involved, with IL-4, in isotype switching.
IL-6	T-, B-Cells, monocytes, fibroblasts, keratinocytes, endothelial cells, astrocytes, mesangial cells, bone marrow stroma	Promotes B-cell differentiation and immunoglobulin synthesis; stimulates growth and induces IL-2 receptors on T-cells and thymocytes; induces cytotoxic T-cells; is a haematopoetic growth factor; stimulates hepatic acute phase protein synthesis; induces ACTH secretion; weak antiviral activity

IL-7	Murine bone marrow stroma,	Stimulates lymphoid progenitor cells.
IL-8	Monocytes, human psoriatic skin fibroblasts	Elicits granule exocytosis and production of superoxide and hydrogen peroxide by neutrophils; induces neutrophil migration *in vivo*, lymphocyte migration *in vitro*; activity profile similar to C5a.
GM-CSF	T-Cell, fibroblast, endothelial cell, keratinocyte	Stimulates neutrophil, eosinophil and monocyte or macrophage precursor proliferation; also affects activities of the mature cells, promotes cytokine production (e.g. IL-1, TNF)
M-CSF	Monocyte, fibroblast, endothelial cell	Stimulates monocyte or macrophage precursor proliferation; also affects activities of the mature cells.
G-CSF	Macrophage, fibroblast	Stimulates neutrophil precursor proliferation; also affects activities of the mature cells.
TNF-α TNF-β	Leukocytes, fibroblast	Antitumour activity including efficacy against hairy cell leukaemia and cutaneous T-cell lymphoma; share a wide variety of activities with IL-1 (see Table 4)
IFN-γ	T-Cell	Promotes monocyte and macrophage antitumour and antimicrobial effects, HLA-DR and Fc receptor expression and stimulates production of IL-1, TNF, PGE_2; augments NK cell function; activates B-cells; regulates immunoglobulin and collagen metabolism.

IL: interleukin; G: granulccyte; M: macrophage; CSF: colony stimulating factor; TNF: tumour necrosis factor; IFN: interferon; PG: prostaglandin.

antigen presenting cells process and present antigen to T-cells they release IL–1 which stimulates the production of IL–2 and expression of IL–2 receptors by T helper cells. Interaction of the IL–2 and its receptors then stimulates clonal expansion of the T-cells; IL–1 also protects T helper cells from the effects of T suppressor cells. The IL–2 activity is principally directed at T- and other closely related lymphocytes (Table 2) but it also has effects on B-cells and macrophages. In contrast, IL–1 acts on a broad variety of cells and tissues.

Action on B-cells

B-Cell growth and differentiation is influenced by interleukins 1, 2, 3, 4, 5 and 6 and by interferon gamma; IL–4 also regulates immunoglobulin isotype production. The final differentiation of B-cells into antibody producing cells is promoted by IL–6 (Table 2) (Kirnbauer *et al.*, 1989; Nossal, 1989) and it has been suggested that abnormal expression of IL–6 may be a factor in the development of generalized autoimmune disease (Kishimoto, 1989).

The colony stimulating factors

These cytokines serve to control the proliferation and development of haematopoetic progenitor cells and are also able to upgrade the functions of the mature granulocytes and macrophages or monocytes. Similar properties are seen in IL–3 and, together with GM-CSF, it displays a much broader range of actions than M- and G-CSF (Table 2) (Clark, 1988; Klingemann and Eaves, 1988; Klingemann, 1989). The potent neutrophil activating effects of IL–8 (neutrophil activating factor) (Colditz *et al.*, 1989) have been likened to those exerted by complement component C5a (Walz *et al.*, 1987).

Interferons

The interferons comprise three groups of cytokines designated alpha, beta and gamma (α, β, γ). Interferons α and β are produced principally by leukocytes and fibroblasts in response to virus or double-stranded ribonucleic acid. Interferon α has antitumour and antiviral effects (Spiegel, 1987). Recombinant preparations have proved effective in the treatment of skin diseases including hairy cell leukaemia, cutaneous T-cell lymphoma, herpes and papilloma virus infections. Interferon β appears to have similar antitumour and antiviral properties but studies of its activity have been limited by difficulties in its production (Jaffe and Sherwin, 1989).

Interferon γ shares many of the antiviral and antitumour activities of the α and β groups but also has distinct immunomodulatory effects (Table 2) which are being exploited in clinical medicine in man (Jaffe and Sherwin, 1989). Demonstration of inhibitory activity towards procollagen mRNA transcription (Granstein *et al.*, 1987) and IL–4-mediated IgE synthesis (Snapper and Paul, 1987) suggests that interferon γ may be of use in the therapy of diseases such as rheumatoid arthritis, scleroderma and atopic dermatitis.

Interleukin 1 and tumour necrosis factor

Originally IL–1 was purified from activated macrophages but is now known to be synthesized by a variety of cells following stimulation with physical, chemical or immunogenic agents (Table 3). Two forms have been cloned, IL-1 β from human monocytes and IL-1 α from a murine macrophage cell line.

Table 3 Sources of interleukin 1

Keratinocytes
Dendritic cells
Langerhans' cells
Macrophages and monocytes
Natural killer cells
B-Cells
Neutrophils
Fibroblasts
Blood vessel endothelium
Blood vessel smooth muscle
Gingival epithelium
Mesangial cells
Astroglia
Microglia
Osteoblasts

Studies with these products confirm most of the results obtained previously which demonstrated the multiple biological properties of IL-1 (Tables 4, 5 and 6) (Dinarello, 1988a; Sauder, 1989). Although chemically dissimilar, the α and β forms of IL-1 appear to share the same spectrum of biological activities. However, IL-1 beta is readily oxidized and may thus appear to be less potent than IL-1 α which is very stable.

The wide range of biological activities induced by IL-1 are mediated via the central nervous system, changes in metabolism, effects on the cardiovascular system and blood vessel endothelia, and effects on leukocyte activity (Tables 4, 5 and 6). These activities can be divided into two categories (Dinarello, 1988a): 1) the acute phase changes including fever, sleep, ACTH release, vascular effects, hepatic protein synthesis, decreased plasma iron and zinc levels, increases in neutrophils and increased production of interferon and colony stimulating factors, and 2) systemic immunostimulation, with the development of specific antibodies or specific cytotoxic T-cells. These changes provide less favourable conditions for the survival of pathogens and promote the activity of both cellular and humoral defence systems (see Dinarello, 1988a). Recent evidence shows that IL-6 also has a wide range of activity and is a potent inducer of the acute phase responses and ACTH production. Production of this cytokine is also induced in bone marrow stroma by IL-1 and so the haematopoetic effects of IL-1 are caused, at least in part, by IL-6. Thus the relative roles of these two cytokines may need to be re-evaluated (Kishimoto, 1989). Recently IL-4 has been shown to be a potent inhibitor of IL-1 release by human monocytes, mimicking the action of the glucocorticoid, dexamethasone (Hart *et al.*, 1989).

Table 4 Actions induced by interleukin 1 systematically

CNS effects
Endogenous pyrogen fever
Promotion of slow wave sleep
Increased ACTH and corticosteroid levels
Metabolic effects
Production of acute phase proteins
Reduced albumin synthesis
Depressed cytochrome P-450 activity
Reduced serum iron and zinc levels
Reduced lipoprotein lipase
Changes in insulin production
Cardiovascular effects
Hypotension
Reduced central venous pressure
Reduced vascular resistance
Increased heart rate and cardiac output
Fall in blood pH
Effects on vascular endothelia
Synthesis and release of PGE_2 and PGI_2
Promotes adherence of leukocytes
Promotes procoagulation of activity
Increases release of platelet activating factor
Production of plasminogen activator inhibitor
Effects on leukocytes
Lymphopenia
Neutrophilia
Stimulates bone marrow precursors
Increased thromboxane A_2 synthesis
Promotes antitumour activity

CNS: central nervous system.
PG: prostaglandin.
ACTH: adrenocorticotrophic hormone.

Tumour necrosis factor (TNF), which is derived from T-cells, has properties which are closely similar to those of IL–1 and the two cytokines have marked synergistic effects (Dinarello, 1988b). However, TNF does not degranulate basophils and is a poor activator of T- and B- cells; it induces neutrophil superoxide production in contrast to IL–1.

MEDIATOR INTERACTING AND THE CONTROL OF INFLAMMATION

The picture is emerging of an integrated system of self-regulating mechanisms

Table 5 Effects of interleukin 1 on leukocytes

Cell	Effects
Neutrophils	Chemotaxis; increase bone marrow release, increased thromboxane synthesis, release of hydrolytic enzymes, antimicrobial activity
Eosinophils	Degranulation
Basophils	Histamine release
Macrophages or monocytes	Increased antimicrobial and cytotoxic activity, IL-1 and thromboxane production; prostaglandin and enzyme release
T-Cells	Proliferation; IL-2 production and increased IL-2 receptor expression; release of other cytokines
B-Cells	Proliferation; production of IL-4, interferon β_2 and immunoglobulin
NK Cells	Increased binding to tumour cells; synergism with interferon and IL-2 in antitumour effects; production of IL-1.

in which powerful proinflammatory substances are balanced by others with antiinflammatory action. It appears that IL–1 is a key substance which is of particular importance to the skin. It exerts its effects both directly and indirectly through the actions of other mediators. Its interaction with two other potent proinflammatory systems, the eicosanoids and platelet activating factor (PAF) is of particular importance (Greaves and Camp, 1988; Cunningham 1990). Activation of phospholipase A_2 leads to the synthesis of PAF and of prostaglandins and leukotrienes (Fig. 1). Prostaglandin E_2 can potentiate the action of PAF but inhibits the synthesis of IL–1 whilst the leukotrienes can promote IL–1 synthesis (Rola-Pleszczynski and Lemaire, 1985; Kunkel *et al.*, 1986); IL–1 can promote the synthesis of PAF (Bussolino *et al.*, 1986). The importance of PAF and prostaglandin E_2 as dual mediators of IL–1 induced inflammation has been demonstrated in an ocular model by

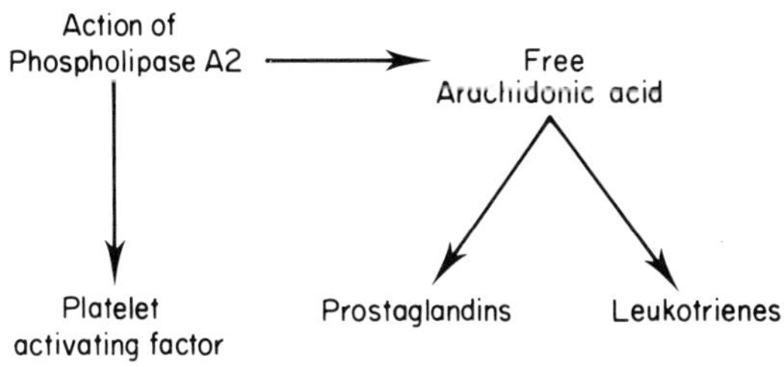

Figure 1 Role of phospholipase A_2 in the generation of platelet activating factor and the eicosanoids.

Table 6 Effects of interleukin 1 on other cells

Cell	Effects
Epithelial cells	Proliferation; collagen synthesis
Endothelial cells	Proliferation; promotion of procoagulant activity, leukocyte adhesion, prostaglandin synthesis and release; release of GM-CSF; inhibition of plasminogen activator
Fibroblasts	Proliferation; release of proteolytic enzymes, plasminogen activator, GM-CSF; production of PGE_2, interferon β
Synovial cells	Proliferation; release of proteolytic enzymes, prostaglandins, plasminogen activator
Chondrocytes	Proliferation; release of proteolytic enzymes, prostaglandins, plasminogen activator; inhibition of proteoglycan synthesis; resorption of cartilage
Osteoblasts and osteoclasts	Bone resorption via osteoclast activating factor; matrix synthesis inhibition; plasminogen activator release
Muscle	Release of prostaglandin; proteolysis and release of amino acids
Adipocyte	Inhibition of lipoprotein lipase, fatty acid synthesis; hyperlipidaemia; cachexia
Brain	Prostaglandin release; fever; slow wave sleep; anorexia
Hepatocyte	Production of acute phase proteins; decreased production of albumin and transferrin; depression of cytochrome P-450 activity
Various tumour cells	Cytotoxicity; growth inhibition
Thyrocytes and pancreatic islet cells	Cytotoxicity
A variety of cytokine secreting cells	Increases production of IL-1, IL-2, GM-CSF, interferons, leukocyte inhibitory migration factor

GM-CSF: granulocyte-macrophage colony stimulating factor: PG: prostaglandin.

Rubin and Rosenbaum (1988) who showed that increases in vascular permeability and cellular infiltration could be almost completely inhibited when combined treatment with a PAF antagonist and an inhibitor of prostaglandin synthesis was used.

All of these inflammatory reactions depend on the action of phospholipase A_2 (Fig. 1). Inhibition of this enzyme by lipocortin (macrocortin) (Blackwell *et al.*, 1980) explains the efficacy of glucocorticoid antiinflammatory action although this may not apply to all species and has been questioned in studies of equine inflammation (Lees *et al.*, 1987). Essential fatty acids which are now being used to treat atopy in both animals and man (Horrobin, 1989; Lloyd, 1990) are also believed to act at this point by raising cyclic adenosine monophosphate levels and thereby inhibiting phospholipase activity.

The search is on for compounds which can mimic the action of the glucocorticoids without their undesirable side-effects. As yet, no suitable candidates are available for clinical use, but it is questionable whether potent chemicals capable of comprehensively blocking inflammation are appropriate therapeutic agents for the majority of inflammatory diseases. We should perhaps devote more attention to the development of modes of therapy which reinforce the natural homoeostatic systems of the body. This will however depend on a much better understanding of the processes of inflammation.

REFERENCES

Besedovsky, H. and del Rey, A. (1987). Neuroendocrine and metabolic responses induced by interleukin-1. *Journal of Neurosciences Research* **18**: 172–178.

Billingham, M.E.J. (1987). Cytokines as inflammatory mediators. *British Medical Bulletin* **43**: 350–370.

Bussolino, F., Breviario, F., Tetta, C. *et al.* (1986). *Journal of Clinical Investigation* **77**: 2027–2033.

Blackwell, G.J., Carnuccio, R., Di Rosea, M. *et al.* (1980). Macrocortin: a polypeptide causing the anti-phospholipase effect of glucocorticoids. *Nature* **287**: 147–149.

Choi, K.L. and Sauder, D.N. (1986). The role of Langerhans cells and keratinocytes in epidermal immunity. *Journal of Leukocyte Biology* **39**: 343–358.

Clark, S.C. (1988). Biological activities of human granulocyte-macrophage colony-stimulating factor. *International Journal of Cell Cloning* **6**: 365–377.

Colditz, I., Zwahlen, R., Dewald, B. and Baggiolini, M. (1989). *In vivo* inflammatory activity of neutrophil activating factor, a novel chemotactic peptide derived from human monocytes. *American Journal of Pathology* **134**: 755–760.

Cunningham, F.M. (1990). Pro-inflammatory mediators and human skin disease. In: Hensby, C. N. and Galli, C. (eds) *Skin Pharmacology and Toxicology*. Plenum, New York. (in press).

Dinarello, C.A. (1988a). Cytokines: interleukin-1 and tumour necrosis factor (cachectin). In: Gallin, J.I., Goldstein, I.M. and Snyderman, R. (eds) *Inflammation: Basic Principles and Clinical Correlates*, pp. 195–208. Raven Press, New York.

Dinarello, C.A. (1988b). The biology of interleukin 1, comparison to tumour necrosis factor and the effect of the combination of these cytokines. In: Bonavida, B., Gifford, G.E., Kirchner, H, and Old, L.J. (eds) *Tumour Necrosis Factor/Cachectin and Related Cytokines*, pp. 154–159. Karger, Basel.

Dreno, B., Hallett, M.M., Moisan, J.P., Soulillou, J.P. and Jacques, Y. (1989). Interleukin 2-like material in human epidermis: a ligand for the human interleukin 2-receptor 55 kD alpha chain. *Journal of Investigative Dermatology* **93**: 78–82.

Edelson, R.L. and Fink, J.M. (1985). The immunologic function of skin. *Scientific American* **252**: 46–53.

Forstrom, L., Goldyne, M.E. and Winkelmann, R.K. (1975). IgE in human eccrine sweat. *Journal of Investigative Dermatology* **64**: 156–157.

Garcia Leme, J. (1981). Regulatory mechanisms in inflammation: new aspects of

autopharmacology. *General Pharmacology* **12**: 15–24.
Granstein, R.D., Murphy, G.F., Margolis, R.J. *et al.* (1987). Gamma-interferon inhibits collagen synthesis *in vivo* in the mouse. *Journal of Clinical Investigation* **79**: 1254–1258.
Greaves, M.W. and Camp, R.D.R. (1988). Prostaglandins, leukotrienes, phospholipase, platelet activating factor and cytokines: an integrated approach to inflammation of human skin. *Archives for Dermatological Research* **280** (Suppl.) S33–41.
Hamblin, A.S. (1988). Lymphokines and interleukins. *Immunology* (Suppl. 1), 39–41.
Hart, P.H., Vitti, G.F., Burgess, D.R. *et al.* (1989). Potential anti-inflammatory effects of interleukin 4: suppression of human monocyte tumour necrosis factor alpha, interleukin 1 and prostglandin E2. *Proceedings of the National Academy of Science of the USA* **86**: 3803–3807.
Hollis, D.E. and Lyne, A.G. (1972). Acetylcholinesterase-positive Langerhans' cells in the epidermis and woold follicles of the sheep. *Journal of Investigative Dermatology* **58**: 211–217.
Horrobin, D.F. (1989). Essential fatty acids in clinical dermatology. *Journal of the American Academy of Dermatology* **20**: 1045–1053.
Jaffe, H.S. and Sherwin, S.A. (1989). Current status of recombinant cytokines as clinical therapeutics. *Drugs of Today* **25**: 311–320.
Jenkinson, D.M. and Blackburn, P.S. (1967). The distribution of nerves, monoamine oxidase and cholinesterase in the skin of the sheep and goat. *Journal of Anatomy* **101**: 333–341.
Jenkinson, D.M., Sengupta, B.P. and Blackburn, P.S. (1966). The distribution of nerves, monoamine oxidase and cholinesterase in the skin of cattle. *Journal of Anatomy* **100**: 593–613.
Jenkinson, D.M., Lloyd, D.H. and Mabon, R.M. (1979). The antigenic composition and source of soluble proteins on the surface of the skin of sheep. *Journal of Comparative Pathology* **89**: 43–50.
Jenkinson, D.M., Menzies, J.D., Pow, I.A. *et al* (1989). Actions of bovine skin washings and sera on the motile zoospores of *Dermatophilus congolensis*. *Research in Veterinary Science* **47**: 241–246.
Kirnbauer, R., Kock, A., Schwartz, T. *et al.* (1989). IFN-beta2, B cell differentiation factor 2, or hybridoma growth factor (IL-6) is expressed and released by human epidermal cells and epidermoid carcinoma cell lines. *Journal of Immunology* **142**: 1922–1928.
Kishimoto, T. (1989). The biology of interleukin-6. *Journal of the American Society for Hematology* **74**: 1–10.
Klingemann, H.G. (1989). Clinical applications of recombinant human colony-stimulating factors. *Canadian Medical Association Journal* **140**: 137–142.
Klingemann, H.G. and Eaves, C.J. (1988). Colony stimulating factors. *Bone Marrow Transplantation* **3**: 177–184.
Kunkel, S.L., Chensue, S.W. and Phan, S.H. (1986). Prostaglandins as endogenous mediators of inteleukin-1 production. *Journal of Immunology* **136**: 186–192.
Lees, P., Higgins, A.J., Sedgwick, A.D. and Daniel, M.J. (1987). Actions of betamethasone in models of acute non-immune inflammation. *British Veterinary Journal* **143**: 158.
Lloyd, D.H. (1990). Essential fatty acids in dermatological disorders of dogs and cats. In: Horrobin, D.F. (ed.) *Omega-6 Essential Fatty Acids: Pathophysiology and Roles in Clinical Medicine*. Alan R. Liss, New York. (in press).
Lloyd, D.H., Mabon, R.M. and Jenkinson, D.M. (1977). The antigenic constituents of cattle skin washings. *Journal of Comparative Pathology* **87**: 75–82.
Lloyd, D.H., Jenkinson, D.M., Miller, P.N. and Sykes, T.J. (1987). Sequential

production of specific antibodies in serum and at the skin surface following intradermal vaccination with *Dermatophilus congolensis*. *Veterinary Immunology and Immunopathology* **16**: 247-251.

Montgomery, I. Jenkinson, D.M. and Elder, H.Y. (1982). The ultrastructure of the sweat gland duct of the ox, sheep and goat before and during sweating. *Journal of Anatomy* **134**: 741-755.

Nossal, G.J.V. (1989). Immunologic tolerance: collaboration between antigen and lymphokines. *Science* **245**: 147-153.

Page, C.O. and Remington, J.S. (1967). Immunologic studies in normal human sweat. *Journal of Laboratory and Clinical Medicine* **69**: 634-650.

Rola-Pleszczynski, M. and Lemaire, I. (1985). Leukotrienes augment interleukin 1 production by human monocytes. *Journal of Immunology* **135**: 3958-3961.

Rubin, R.M. and Rosenbaum, J.T. (1988). A platelet activating factor antagonist inhibits interleukin 1- induced inflammation. *Biochemical and Biophysical Research Communications* **154**: 429-436.

Sauder, D.N. (1989). Interleukin 1. *Archives of Dermatology* **125**: 679-682.

Snapper, C.M. and Paul, W.E. (1987). Interferon gamma and B cell stimulatory factor-1 reciprocally regulate IgE isotype production. *Science* **236**: 944-946.

Spiegel, R.J. (1987). The alpha interferons: clinical overview. *Seminars in Oncology* **14,** 1-5.

Stingl, G., Katz, S.I., Clement, L., Green, I. and Shevach, E.M. (1978). Immunologic function of Ia-bearing epidermal Langerhans' cells. *Journal of Immunology* **121**: 2005-2013.

Walz, A., Peveri, P., Aschauer, H. and Baggiolini, M. (1987). Purification and amino acid sequencing of NAF, a novel neutrophil-activating factor produced by monocytes. *Biochemical and Biophysical Research Communications* **149**: 755-761.

Williams, J.M., Deloria, D., Hansen, J.A. *et al.* (1985). The events of primary T-cell activation can be staged by use of Sepharose-bound anti-T3 (64.1) monoclonal antibody and purified interleukin-1. *Journal of Immunology* **135**: 2249-2255.

3.2 The Response of the Eosinophil in Acute Inflammation in the Horse

B.J. McEwen[1], B.P. Wilcock[1], J.A. Yager[1], and P. Eyre[2]

[1]*Department of Pathology, Ontario Veterinary College, University of Guelph, Guelph, Ontario, Canada; and* [2]*Dean, Virginia-Maryland College of Veterinary Medicine, Blacksburg, Virginia, USA*

INTRODUCTION

Eosinophils are traditionally viewed as significant cellular participants in allergic reactions and parasitic infestations (Butterworth and David, 1981; Kay, 1985). Both reactions involve IgE-dependent hypersensitivity and are consequently mediated by products liberated during non-cytolytic mast cell degranulation (Butterworth and David, 1981). Peptides, lipids and amines derived from mast cells are presumably responsible for recruiting eosinophils to the sites of inflammation (Schwartz and Austen, 1984; Clark *et al.*, 1975; Turnbull and Kay, 1976). In parasitic infestations, eosinophils function as killer-effector cells (Butterworth and David, 1981) whereas in allergic reactions, they supposedly fulfill a palliative function by virtue of their reserve of antiinflammatory products (Goetz *et al.*, 1975).

In contrast to what is known of the response and function of the eosinophil in parasitic and allergic reactions, a relative paucity of information exists regarding the response of the eosinophil in other types of acute inflammation. The behaviour of the eosinophil leukocyte in acute inflammation is typified by an abrupt decrease in the number of circulating cells (Duncan and Prasse, 1986; Jain, 1986; Bass *et al.*, 1980). This initially occurs because eosinophils are sequestered in the inflammatory focus and reticuloendothelial system and persists because their emigration from bone marrow is inhibited (Bass, 1975; Runge *et al.*, 1985). Bacteria, phlogistins (Bass, 1975; Runge *et al.*, 1985; Fechter *et al.*, 1986) and the complement fragment C5a (Bass *et al.*, 1980) cause a decrease in the numbers of circulating eosinophils and a notable infiltrate about the inflammatory focus. The latter is observed only in animals in which a peripheral eosinophilia has been induced by a parasitic infestation (Bass, 1975; Bass *et al.*, 1980; Runge *et al.*, 1985; Fechter *et al.*, 1986).

In the classical laboratory animal models of inflammation, the eosinophil is not considered to be an integral component of the inflammatory reaction. Yet in a retrospective, histological study of equine dermatitis we found that eosinophils formed the predominant leukocyte infiltrate in over half of the skin biopsies examined (McEwen *et al.*, 1989). This finding could have been interpreted as allergy to ectoparasites or other agents, based on the unverified assumption that the leukocyte infiltrates seen in equine skin share the same pathogenic mechanisms and aetiological implications as they do in other species, but because species differences in the biology of inflammation do exist, perhaps the equine inflammatory process is not accurately reflected in the existing models in other species.

Investigations of equine inflammation *in vivo* have primarily addressed the pharmacological and biochemical responses of the horse to the phlogistins carrageenan or turpentine (Higgins and Lees, 1983; Higgins and Lees, 1984a, b; Higgins *et al.*, 1984; Lees and Higgins, 1984, 1986; Sedgwick *et al.*, 1986; Smith and Cipriano, 1987). Biochemical analyses of the inflammatory exudate recovered from subcutaneous tissue cages or sponges yielded prostaglandin E_2, leukotriene B_4 and the metabolites of prostacylin and thromboxane A_2 (Higgins and Lees, 1984a, b; Sedgwick *et al.*, 1986). Neutrophils, but not eosinophils, were aspirated from the exudate (Higgins and Lees, 1984a, b). Other than the observation that significant numbers of eosinophils accumulate at sites of histamine injection (Archer, 1959, 1960), there is sparse documentation of the histological response of equine skin to known phlogistins or inflammatory mediators.

The objective of this study was to investigate the histology of the acute inflammatory reaction in horses to a variety of inflammatory mediators and phlogistins, and specifically examine the response of the equine eosinophil leukocyte. The leukocyte infiltration was also monitored using the skin window technique (Rebuck and Crowley, 1955) to assess its value as a possible replacement for skin biopsy in experimental protocols.

MATERIALS AND METHODS

Animals

Five horses (one stallion, two mares and two geldings) were used in this study. These included three standardbreds, one Appaloosa and one quarterhorse-Arab cross. The horses were fed grain and hay twice daily with unrestricted access to a salt block and water. Animals were stabled in box stalls at the Ontario Veterinary College and were exercised regularly. One month prior to the experiment, all horses were vaccinated against rabies (Trimune, Fort Dodge Laboratories Inc., Fort Dodge, Iowa), tetanus (Tetnogen toxoid, MTC Pharmaceuticals, Cambridge, Ontario), equine influenza A (Fluvac, Fort Dodge Laboratories Inc., Fort Dodge, Iowa), equine viral rhinopneumonitis

(Pneumabort, Fort Dodge Laboratories Inc., Fort Dodge, Iowa) and Eastern and Western encephalitis (Haver-Lockehart, Shawnee, Kansas). They were also given ivermectin paste (Eqvalan, Merck & Co. Inc., Rahaway, New Jersey) *per os* to control helminth parasites.

Intradermal injections

The following agents were injected intradermally: 10^{-5}M histamine diphosphate (Sigma Chemical Co., St Louis, Missouri); 3×10^{-7}M leukotriene B_4 (LTB_4) and 4×10^{-5}M leukotriene C_4 (LTC_4) (LTB_4 and LTC_4 were kindly provided by Dr J.D. Rokach, Merck-Frosst Canada Inc., Montreal, Quebec); zymosan activated serum (ZAS); 1000 protein nitrogen units (PNU)/ml tabanid extract (horsefly extract, Hollister-Stier, Division of Miles Laboratories, Rexdale, Ontario) and 0.5% carrageenan (Sigma). Sterile physiological pyrogen-free saline (Astra Pharmaceuticals, Mississauga, Ontario) was used as the negative control.

Zymosan activated serum was made by adding 25 mg of washed zymosan (Sigma) to each ml of autologous fresh equine serum. This mixture was placed in a shaking water bath (37°C, 120 oscillations/min) for 60 min. The mixture was centrifuged at 1500 ***g*** for 20 min and the ZAS was aspirated by sterile pasteur pipette. All agents except the leukotrienes were passed through sterile 0.2 μm filters (Acrodisc filters, Gelman Sciences Inc., Ann Arbor, Michigan) prior to use.

Prior to each series of biopsies, differential leukocyte counts were determined from Wright's stained smears made of peripheral blood. Because multiple biopsies were obtained from each animal, a minimum of 7 days separated each series of injections. The hair on the lateral neck was shaved 24 h prior to the intradermal injections. Immediately preceding the injections, the skin was cleansed with hibitane soap and rinsed with 70% alcohol and chlorhexidine. For each agent a total of seven 0.1 ml intradermal injections, 10 cm apart, were made in the lateral neck in each horse. Following measurement of skin fold thickness by spring-loaded calipers at 0.25, 0.5, 1, 2, 4, 8 and 24 h, the subcutis was infiltrated with Lidocaine (Xylocaine 2%, Astra Pharmaceuticals, Mississauga, Ontario). Punch biopsies, 6 mm in diameter (Baker's Biopsy Punch, Dormer Laboratories Inc., Pointe-Claire, Quebec) were then obtained and the skin wound was sutured. The skin biopsy was fixed by immersion in 10% neutral buffered formalin. It was then bisected, embedded in paraffin, sectioned 6 μm thick and stained routinely with haematoxylin and eosin (HE).

The slides were evaluated without knowledge of the identity of the horse, treatment or time of biopsy. The number of eosinophils, neutrophils and mononuclear cells (lymphocytes, macrophages) were counted in six high power (40×) fields defined by a lattice squared grid inserted into one eyepiece of the microscope.

Skin windows

The dorsal mid-thoracic skin was prepared as described above. A 1 cm^2area, as defined by a template, was abraded using a sterile scalpel blade until slightly bleeding. Following direct application of 0.1 ml of the phlogistin or mediator onto the abraded surface, a sterile round 18 mm glass coverslip (Fisher Scientific, Whitby, Ontario) was applied to the area and held in place by sterile surgical tape (Scanpor Surgical Tape, Hollister-Steir). The coverslips were changed at 2, 4, 8 and 24 h postapplication and were mounted cell side up onto glass slides and stained with Wright's stain.

All skin window slides were evaluated without knowledge of the identity of the horse, agent or time of treatments. Differential cell counts were made by counting a total of 500 cells; if this number of cells was not present, as often occurred at the 2 h interval, 100 cells were counted.

Statistical analyses

The count data for both skin windows and biopsies were transformed to the natural logarithm (ln) to achieve normal distributions. Analysis of variance and Duncan's multiple range procedures wre used to detect differences between treatments (Snedecor and Cochran, 1980). Statistical significance, when achieved, was $p<0.05$. To determine if a relationship existed between the leukocyte populations in biopsy and skin windows, a correlation statistic was used (Snedecor and Cochran, 1980).

RESULTS

Skin biopsy (Plates 17–21)

Eosinophils were rapidly recruited following intradermal injection of histamine or tabanid extract (Figs 1, 2). The peak eosinophil response to histamine at 2 h postinjection (PI), was superceded at 4 h by maximal infiltrates produced by LTB_4, tabanid extract and carrageenan (Figs 1, 2). From 2 to 24 h PI, these three agents were equally effective in their ability to recruit and maintain large numbers of eosinophils in inflammatory foci (Table 1). Peripheral eosinophil counts were within normal limits in all horses (results not shown).

Although histamine did not recruit more eosinophils than LTB_4, tabanid extract or carrageenan, it was the only agent that attracted relatively more eosinophils than neutrophils, although this only occurred at 1 h PI (Table 2). Eosinophil and neutrophil infiltrates were quantitatively equivalent for most of the reactions produced by histamine, tabanid extract, for the early and late responses to LTB_4 and for the early responses to carrageenan (Table 2). ZAS,

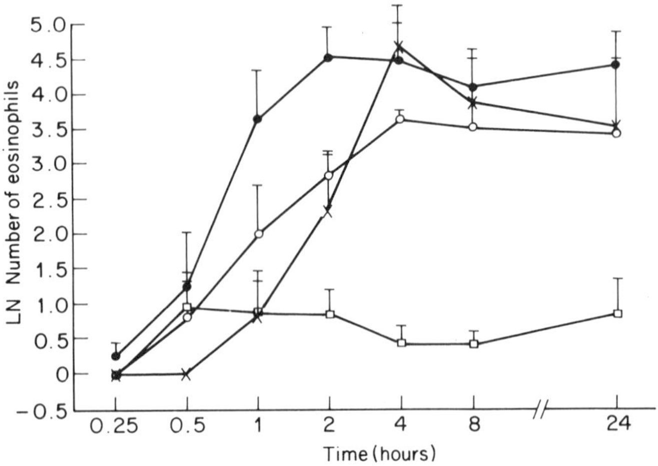

Figure 1 Eosinophil infiltration into equine skin following intradermal injections of carrageenan (o), tabanid extract (•), leukotriene B_4 (X), and ZAS(□). Values are expressed as the mean ± SEM.

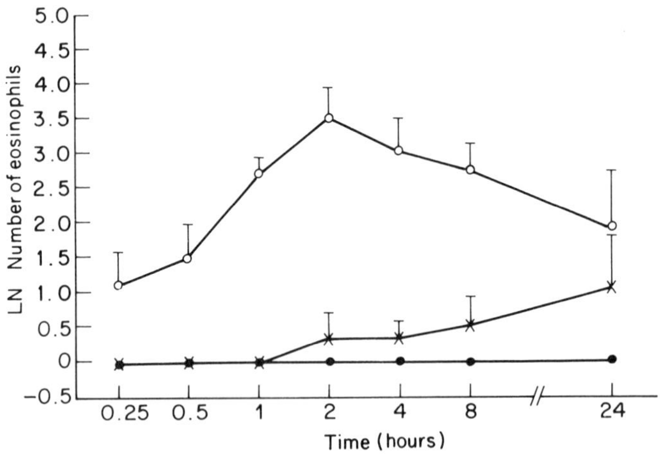

Figure 2 Eosinophil infiltration into equine skin following intradermal injections of histamine (o), leukotriene C_4 (X), and sterile saline (•). Values are expressed as the mean ± SEM.

LTC_4 and sterile saline did not induce a significant eosinophil accumulation (Table 1).

Zymosan activated serum invoked a rapid and marked neutrophil infiltrate that persisted for 24 h PI (Fig. 3). Tabanid extract, LTB_4 and carrageenan also incited an intense, persistent neutrophil response that was equivalent to the

Table 1 Relative effectiveness of the agents that were injected intradermally with respect to dermal eosinophil infiltration

Time (h)	Relative effectiveness
0.25	Histamine* >** TE = Carr = LTB_4 = LTC_4 = Saline = ZAS
0.5	Histamine* = TE > ZAS = Carr = LTB_4 = LTC_4 = Saline
1.0	TE* = Histamine* = Carr* > ZAS = LTB_4 = LTC_4 = Saline
2.0	TE* = Histamine* = Carr* = LTB_4* > ZAS = LTC_4 = Saline
4.0	LTB_4* = TE* = Carr* > Histamine* > ZAS = LTC_4 = Saline
8.0	TE* = LTB_4* = Carr* > Histamine* > LTC_4 = ZAS = Saline
24.0	TE* = LTB_4* = Carr* > Histamine = LTC_4 = ZAS = Saline

* Produced a significantly greater infiltrate than sterile saline, $p < 0.05$ by Duncan's multiple range test.
** >- Produced a significantly greater infiltrate than succeeding agent, $p < 0.05$ by Duncan's multiple range test.
TE: Tabanid extract.
Carr: Carr: Carrageenan.

Table 2 Comparison of relative leukocyte infiltrates produced by intradermal injections of inflammatory mediators, tabanid extract and carrageenan

Relative no. of Leukocytes	Agent/time of occurrence (h) Histamine	LTB_4	LTC_4	ZAS	Tabanid extract	Carr[a]	Saline
Eos[b] >-* PMN[c]	1	NSD[d]	NSD	NSD	NSD	NSD	NSD
Eos = PMN	0.25, 0.5, 2-24	0.25-1, 24	0.25-24	0.25	0.25,1.2, 8,24	0.25-1	0.25-24
PMN > EOS	NSD	2-8	NSD	0.5-24	0.5,4	2-24	NSD
PMN >MN[e]	2	2-8	NSD	2-8	2-8	2-8	NSD
PMN = MN	0.25,1,4,8	0.25,0.5, 24	0.25-24	0.25-1	0.25-1,24	0.25-1, 24	0.25-8
MN > PMN	24	NSD	NSD	24	NSD	NSD	24
MN > EOS	NSD	NSD	NSD	2-24	NSD	NSD	NSD
MN = EOS	0.25,0.5, 2-24	0.25-2 8,24	NSD	0.25-1	0.25,0.5,2, 8,24	0.25-24	0.25-24
EOS > MN	1	4	NSD	NSD	1,4	NSD	NSD

* Produced statistically significant difference at $p < 0.05$ by paired difference *t*-test
[a] Carrageenan.
[b] Eosinophils.
[c] Neutrophils
[d] No significant difference
[e] Mononuclear cells

reaction produced by ZAS from 1. 2 and 4 h PI respectively (Table 3). Small numbers of neutrophils were sporadically recruited by histamine, sterile saline and LTC_4 (Fig. 4. Table 3).

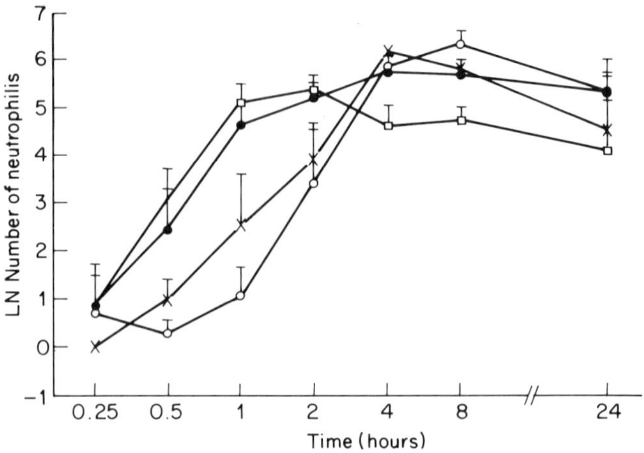

Figure 3 Neutrophil infiltration into equine skin following intradermal injections of carrageenan (o), tabanid extract (•), leukotriene B_4 and ZAS (□). Values are expressed as the mean ± SEM.

Table 3 Relative effectiveness of the agents that were injected intradermally with respect to dermal neutrophil infiltration

Time (h)	Relative effectiveness
0.25	NSA
0.5	ZAS* = TE >** = Histamine = Carr = LTC_4 = Saline
1.0	ZAS* = TE* > LTB_4* > = Histamine* = Carr = LTB_4 = Saline
2.0	ZAS* = TE* = LTB_4* > Carr* > Histamine* > LTC_4 = Saline
4.0	LTB_4* = Carr* = TE* = ZAS* > Histamine = LTC_4 = Saline
8.0	Carr* = LTB_4* = TE* > ZAS* = Histamine* = LTC_4 > Saline
24.0	TE* = Carr* = LTB_4* = ZAS* > Histamine = LTC_4 = Saline

* Produced a significantly greater infiltrate than sterile saline, $p < 0.05$ by Duncan's multiple range test.
** >- Produced a significantly greater infiltrate than succeeding agent, $p < 0.05$ by Duncan's multiple range test.
NSD: No significant difference between potency of agents.
TE: tabanid extract.
Carr: carrageenan.

Neutrophils were the predominant granulocyte in reactions induced by carrageenan and ZAS and were more numerous than mononuclear cells from 2 to 8 h following administration of LTB_4, ZAS, tabanid extract and carrageenan (Table 2).

With the exception of LTC_4 and sterile saline, most agents incited a mononuclear reaction that gradually increased to a maximum inflitrate at 8 h

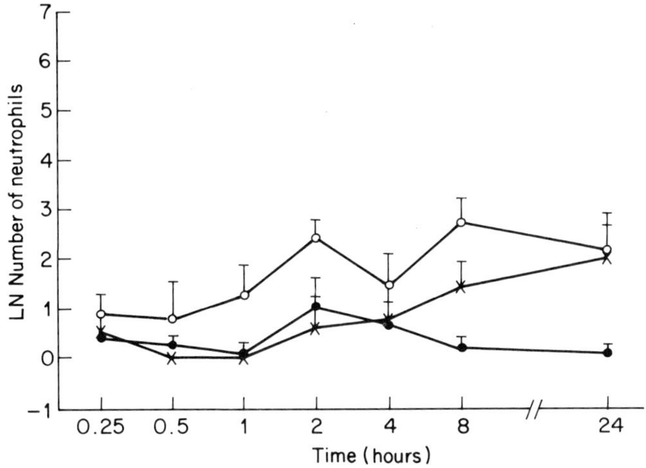

Figure 4 Neutrophil infiltration into equine skin following intradermal injections of histamine (o), leukotriene C_4 (X), and sterile saline (•). Values are expressed as the mean ± SEM.

PI (Figs 5, 6). Mononuclear cells continued to accumulate in sites injected with tabanid extract 24 h previously (Fig. 5). Tabanid extract, ZAS, carrageenan, LTB_4 and histamine were equally effective in recruiting mononuclear cells from 4 to 24 h PI (Table 4).

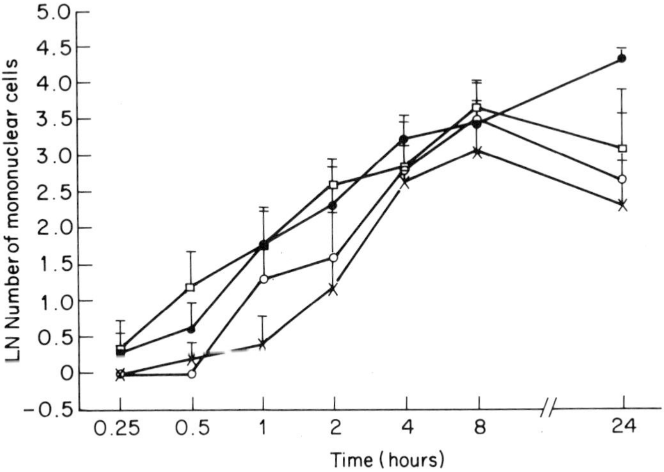

Figure 5 Mononuclear cell infiltration into equine skin following intradermal injections of carrageenan (o), tabanid extract (•), leukotriene B_4 (X), and ZAS (□). Values are expressed as the mean ± .

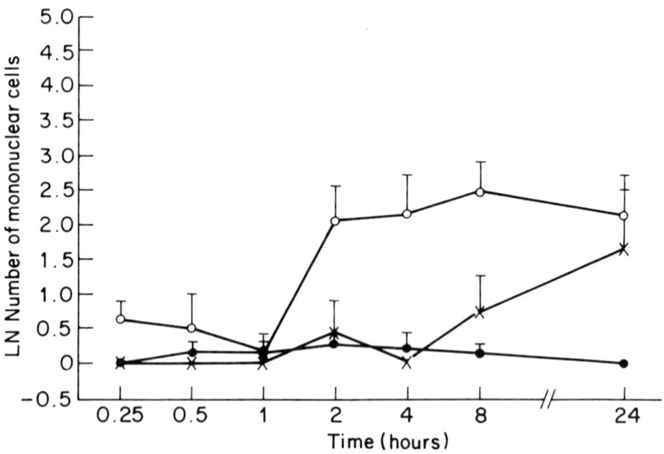

Figure 6 Mononuclear cell infiltration into equine skin following intradermal injections of histamine (o), leukotriene C_4 (X), and sterile saline(•). Values are expressed as the mean ± SEM.

Table 4 Relative effectiveness of the agents that were injected intradermally with respect to dermal mononuclear cell infiltration

Time (h)	Relative effectiveness
0.25	NSD
0.5	NSD
1.0	ZAS* = TE >** Carr = LTB_4 = Histamine = LTC_4 = Saline
2.0	ZAS* = TE* = Histamine* > Carr* > = LTB_4 = LTC_4 = Saline
4.0	TE* = ZAS* = Carr* = LTB_4* = Histamine* > Saline = LTC_4
8.0	ZAS* = Carr* = TE* = LTB_4* = Histamine* > LTC_4 = Saline
24.0	TE* = ZAS* = Carr* = LTB_4* = Histamine* > LTC_4 = Saline

* Produced a significantly greater infiltrate than sterile saline, $p < 0.05$ by Duncan's multiple range test.

** >- Produced a significantly greater infiltrate than succeeding agent, $p < 0.05$ by Duncan's multiple range test.

NSD: No significant difference between potency of agents.

TE: tabanid extract.

Carr: carrageenan.

Skin windows

The relative ability of each agent to recruit leukocytes as measured by the skin window technique is presented in Table 5. There were no significant differences amongst agents regarding their ability to recruit leukocytes, except for the eosinophil accumulation produced by LTB_4 at 4 and 8 h PI, and the saline induced immigration of neutrophils at 2 h PI.

The accumulation of leukocytes by the skin window technique did not frequently correlate with the population of cells infiltrating the dermis as determined by skin biopsy (Table 6). Eosinophil responses to histamine and LTB_4 correlated at 4 h PI. Sporadic positive correlations were also noted for

Table 5 Relative effectiveness of the agents applied topically to recruit leukocytes by the skin window technique

Leukocyte	Time (h)	Relative effectiveness
Eosinophil	2	NSD
	2	LTB_4 = > * LTC_4 = Histamine = Carr = TE = ZAS = Saline
	8	LTB_4* > = Histamine = Carr = TE = ZAS = Saline
	24	NDS
Neutrophil	2	Saline > LTC_4 = Histamine = LTB_4 = Carr = TE = ZAS
	4	NSD
	6	NSD
	8	NSD
	24	NSD
Mononuclear cells	2	NSD
	4	NSD
	6	NSD
	8	NSD
	24	NSD

* Produced a significantly greater infiltrate than sterile saline, $p < 0.05$ by Duncan's multiple range test.
NSD: No significant difference between potency of agents.
Carr: Carrageenan.
TE: Tabanid extract.

Table 6 Correlation of leukocytes accumulations between skin biopsy and skin window

Leukocyte	Agent	Time (h)	Correlation coeffecient*
Eosinophil	Histamine	4	0.979
	LTB_4	3	0.900
Neutrophil	Saline	2	0.956
	Saline	24	0.983
	ZAS	4	0.979
	LTB_4	24	−0.836
	Carrageenan	24	−0.988

$p > 0.05$

neutrophil accumulations to sterile saline and ZAS at 2 and 4 h PI respectively. Negative correlations of neutrophil numbers between biopsy and skin window occurred 24 h following application of sterile saline, carrageenan and LTB_4.

Skin fold thickness

Histamine generated the largest, immediate increase in skin fold thickness, although tabanid extract and ZAS also produced an immediate effect (Figs 7, 8). At 8 h PI, carrageenan, tabanid extract and LTB_4 produced their largest increases in skin fold thickness. From 8 to 24 h PI, carrageenan produced a significantly greater increase in skin fold thickness than all other agents (Table 7).

DISCUSSION

Eosinophils significantly contributed to the acute inflammatory reaction following intradermal injection of histamine, LTB_4, tabanid extract and carrageenan in horses. Histamine was the only agent that recruited relatively more eosinophils than neutrophils, albeit sporadically. The magnitude of the eosinophil response to tabanid extract, LTB_4 and carrageenan, however, significantly surpassed the eosinophil response to histamine. Furthermore, carrageenan, tabanid extract and LTB_4 were equally effective in their ability to

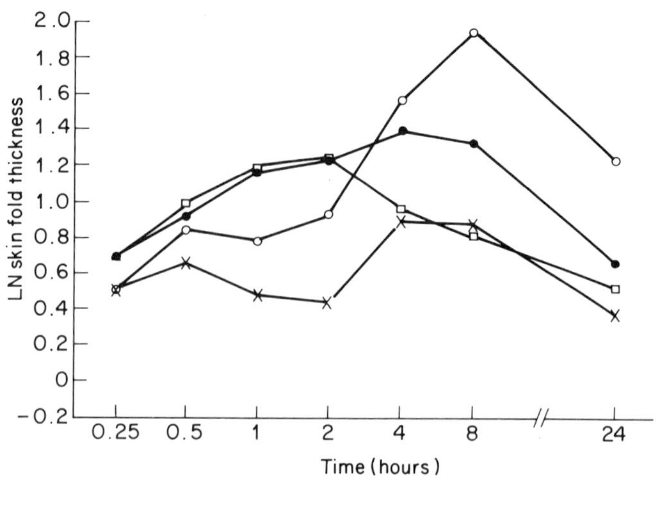

Figure 7 Changes in skin fold thickness following intradermal injections of carrageenan (o), tabanid extract (•), leukotriene B_4 (X), and ZAS (□). Values are expressed as the mean ± SEM.

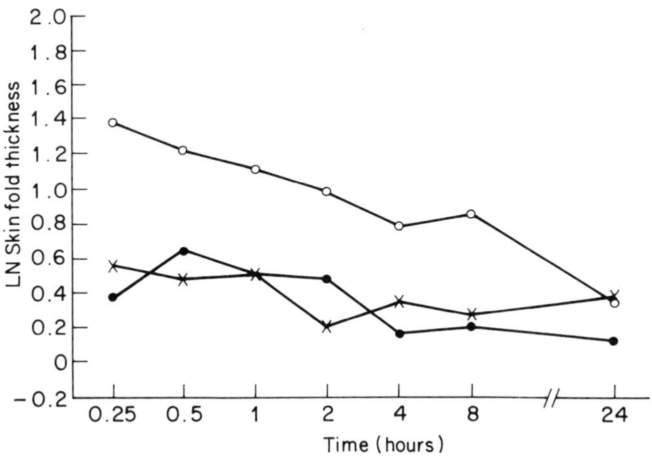

Figure 8 Changes in skin fold thickness following intradermal injections of histamine (o), leukotriene C_4 (X), and sterile saline (•). Values are expressed as the mean + SEM.

Table 7 Relative effectiveness of the agents that were injected intradermally with respect to increase in skin fold thickness

Time (h)	Relative effectiveness
0.25	Histamine* > Tabanid* = ZAS* > LTC_4 = Carr = LTB_4 = NaCl
0.5	Histamine* = ZAS* = Tabanid* = LTB_4 = NaCl = LTC_4
1.0	ZAS* = Tabanid* = Histamine* > Carr = NaCl = LTC_4 = LTB_4
2.0	ZAS* = Tabanid* = Histamine* > Carr* = NaCl = LTC_4 = LTB_4
4.0	Carr* = Tabanid* > ZAS* = LTB_4* = Histamine* > LTC_4 = NaCl
8.0	Carr* > Tabanid* > Histamine* = ZAS* = LTB_4* > LTC_4* = NaCl
24.0	Carr* > Tabanid* > ZAS* = LTB_4 = Histamine* = LTC_4 = NaCl

* Produced a significantly greater infiltrate than sterile saline, $p < 0.05$ by Duncan's multiple range test.

** >- Produced a significantly greater infiltrate than succeeding agent, $p < 0.05$ by Duncan's multiple range test.

Carr: Carrageenan.

invoke a marked, persistent neutrophil infiltrate and also recruit many eosinophils into the equine dermis.

It has been shown that LTB_4 is a potent chemotaxin for equine, human and rabbit eosinophils and neutrophils (Potter *et al.*, 1985; Watson *et al.*, 1987; Czarnetzki and Mertensmeir, 1985; Czarnetzki and Rosenbach, 1986; Camp *et al.*, 1983, 1984; Soter *et al.*, 1983; Carr *et al.*, 1981; Movat *et al.*, 1984; Ford-Hutchinson and Chan, 1985), that *in vitro* preferentially attracts eosinophils over neutrophils (Czarnetzki and Mertensmeir, 1985; Czarnetzki and Rosenbach, 1986). Paradoxically, in humans and rabbits, neutrophils are primarily, if not exclusively, recruited *in vivo* (Camp *et al.*, 1983, 1984; Soter *et al.*, 1983; Carr *et al.*, 1981; Movat *et al.*, 1984; Aked and Foster, 1987). In this study, horses responded to LTB_4 with many neutrophils and fewer (but still numerous) eosinophils. As species differences in the reaction to leukotrienes are documented (Ford-Hutchinson and Chan, 1985; Ueno *et al.*, 1981; Kragballe and Voorhees, 1983), perhaps the conspicuous infiltrate of equine eosinophils in response to LTB_4 reflects an inherent biological variation in this species' reaction to leukotrienes.

Abundant evidence implicates leukotrienes in the genesis of carrageenan-induced inflammation in rats and horses (Higgins and Lees, 1984a, b; Holsapple and Yim, 1984; Simmons *et al.*, 1983). Carrageenan is a phologistin that produces extensive dermal oedema and leukocyte infiltration in a variety of species, including horses (Higgins and Lees, 1984a, b; Sedgwick *et al.*, 1986; DiRosa *et al.*, 1971; Caffesse *et al.*, 1985; Vinegar *et al.*, 1987). The elevated nanogram quantities of LTB_4 recovered from carrageenan-induced inflammatory exudate in rats, rabbits and horses (Higgins and Lees 1984b; Simmons *et al.*, 1983; Aked and Foster, 1987) approximates the concentration of LTB_4 used in our study. Therefore, presumably, the inflammatory reaction of the horses in this study to LTB_4 represents a physiological response rather than a pharmacological phenomenon. Furthermore, inhibition of the lipoxygenase products of arachidonic acid suppresses carrageenan-induced oedema presumably by inhibiting neutrophil infiltration (Holsapple and Yim, 1984), whereas treatment with non-steroidal antiinflammatory drugs does not reduce the leukocyte inflitration in either rats or horses (Higgins *et al.*, 1984; Holsapple and Yim, 1984). This implies that leukotrienes are responsible for mediating some of the effects of carrageenan-induced inflammation in horses (Higgins and Lees, 1984b, Higgins *et al.*, 1984). Our results comply with these findings and further suggest that LTB_4 may have mediated (at least in part), the carrageenan-induced eosinophil infiltration.

If LTB_4 is a putative mediator of carrageenan-induced equine inflammation (Higgins and Lees, 1984a,b) that also recruits substantial numbers of eosinophils, an apparent contradiction exists between our results and those of others (Higgins and Lees, 1984b). The discrepancy between the presence of eosinophils in carrageenan-induced inflammation in our horses and the absence of eosinophils in the preceding studies (Higgins and Lees 1984a,b) may be attributed to differences in methodology. Quantitation of leukocytes from exudates as reported previously (Higgins and Lees, 1984a,b), compared with the histologic sections that we used, are different techniques. The skin window technique, however, traps emigrating leukocytes and accordingly represents an exudate rather than an infiltrate. In agreement with previous reports (Higgins and Lees 1984a,b), we did not consistently see statistically significant numbers of eosinophils in the skin windows even when biopsy sections revealed numerous infiltrating eosinophils, perhaps reflecting a non-linear relationship between the leukocyte emigration in a tissue infitrate and exudate.

Inconsistencies between similar techniques have been noted by others (Ting *et al.*, 1981). Discrepancies between leukocyte numbers, specifically eosinophils, were attributed to the unverified possibility that eosinophils may leave, as well as enter skin lesions (Ting *et al.*, 1981). This concept parallels the idea of selective retention of eosinophils in inflammatory foci (Parish, 1970; Ward, 1969), which requires that neutrophils migrate from the tissue to the circulation. The latter is improbable, as established neutrophil kinetics are not supportive of this hypothesis (Jain, 1986). It may be that the disparity between exudate and infiltrate simply reflects the neutrophil response to the tissue trauma that was part of the leukocyte collection technique, such as epidermal debridement as in the skin windows, or the surgical implantation of foreign objects such as tissue cases or sponges. Therefore, the data obtained from skin windows must be interpreted with the caveat that they do not necessarily reflect only the specific response to the deliberately introduced pholgistin.

Complement fragments are also proposed mediators of carrageenan-induced inflammation in laboratory animals (DiRosa *et al.*, 1971). Addition of zymosan to serum activates the alternate complement cascade, generating the anaphylatoxins C3a and C5a (Fernandez *et al.*, 1977). Serum carboxypeptidase N rapidly converts the latter to C5adesArg, a potent granulocyte chemotaxin devoid of anaphylatoxic properties (Muller-Eberhard, 1988). A C5adesArg analogue produced by incubating zymosan with equine plasma induces adhesion and aggregation of equine neutrophils (Slauson *et al.*, 1987). The large and persistent infiltrate of neutrophils in equine skin observed in our study concurs with the *in vitro* observation by other workers that complement fragments are chemotactic for equine neutrophils (Sedgwick *et al.*, 1986, Zinkl and Brown, 1982). In contrast to rabbits, in which ZAS is 80 times more potent than LTB_4 in attracting neutrophils (Movat *et al.*, 1984; Colditz 1985), ZAS and LTB_4 were equally effective in horses, a finding that emphasizes the inflammatory reaction of horses does differ from other species. ZAS and LTB_4 were also equivalent to carrageenan and tabanid extract in recruiting equine neutrophils *in vivo*. This suggests that ZAS may have contributed to the large neutrophil infiltrate produced by carrageenan and tabanid extract.

An association between neutrophil infiltrates with maximal increases in skin fold thickness, exemplified in this study by the response to LTB_4, ZAS, tabanid extract and carrageenan, has been noted previously (DiRosa *et al.*, 1971); LTB_4 and ZAS increase vasopermeability indirectly by recruiting neutrophils which subsequently damage the vascular endothelium (Wedmore and Williams, 1981; Movat, 1987; Movat *et al.*, 1984). The presumptively neutrophil-associated oedema produced by tabanid extract and carrageenan was possibly initiated in part by LTB_4 and ZAS. The major difference between the reaction to ZAS and LTB_4 was that ZAS did not attract equine eosinophils *in vivo*. Thus, C5adesArg (ZAS) cannot be responsible for the presence of equine eosinophils in the lesions induced by tabanid extract or carrageenan.

As expected, the granulocytic inflammatory response to tabanid extract contained significant numbers of eosinophils as these cells are a hallmark of the response to parasites (Butterworth and David, 1981). The immune status of the horses in this study to tabanids was not determined, but it is unlikely that as mature animals they were immunologically naive to tabanid antigens and consequently hypersensitivity to these parasites may have influenced the inflammatory reaction. Local tissue trauma (Douglas, 1980) and mast cell degranulation following contact with insect derived phospholipases (Cohen and Ottensen, 1983) probably also contributed to the inflammatory reaction. Activated mast cells elaborate a plethora of inflammatory mediators and eosinophil chemotaxins including platelet activating factor, eosinophil chemotactic factor of anaphylaxis, leukotrienes and histamine (Schwartz and Austen, 1984).

Thirty years ago, Archer (1959, 1960) established that histamine recruited eosinophils when injected into the skin of horses. Its effect on other species, however, is controversial and appears to depend on the immune status of the individual (Fechter *et al.*, 1986; Kay, 1985; Parish, 1970; Turnbull and Kay, 1976). Its classification as a direct-acting mediator with short-lived effects (Colditz, 1985; Movat, 1987) agrees with our findings of rapid, but evanescent increases in skin fold thickness and eosinophil infiltration. Histamine, therefore, is unlikely to account for the large and persistent eosinophil accumulations in equine skin as noted in our retrospective survey, or those present in carrageenan-induced lesions. The results of our study agree with previous suggestions that histamine is a relatively insignificant mediator of equine hypersensitivity (Eyre, 1976; Morrow *et al.*, 1986), and that non-amines, such as the leukotrienes, may be more important inflammatory mediators in the horse (Eyre, 1976).

In summary, LTB_4 was equal to tabanid extract and carrageenan in recruiting substantial numbers of eosinophils and neutrophils into the equine dermis. Although ZAS did not attract eosinophils, it produced a neutrophil infiltrate equivalent to LTB_4, tabanid extract and carrageenan. The similarities in the acute inflammatory reactions produced by these compounds in horses suggests that LTB_4 and ZAS (C5adesArg) are plausible mediators of inflammation produced by carrageenan or tabanid extract. Furthermore, there is evidence supporting the role of both LTB_4 and ZAS in carrageenan induced inflammation in horses and other species (Higgins and Lees, 1984b; Higgins *et al.*, 1984; Lees and Higgins, 1984;, 1986; Holsapple and Yim, 1984; Simmons *et al.*, 1983; DiRosa *et al.*, 1971; Vinegar *et al.*, 1987).

The findings of our study also established that the biology of equine inflammation differs from that of other species. The exceptional dermal infiltrate of eosinophils produced by tabanid extract, carrageenan and LTB_4 does not appear to require the induction of a peripheral eosinophilia in horses, in contrast to the dynamics of the eosinophil in acute inflammation in laboratory animals (Bass *et al.*, 1980; Bass, 1975; Runge *et al.*, 1985; Fechter *et al.*, 1986). The presence of eosinophils in the acute inflammatory reaction of horses was first described by Archer (1959, 1960). The precedent of the apparently unique equine response to histamine (Archer, 1959, 1960) can now be extended to include LTB_4. Additional evidence supporting an equine idiosyncratic response to leukotrienes was the failure to induce a significant increase in skin fold thickness following injection of LTC_4. Although humans and guinea pigs develop profound dermal oedema in response to intradermal injections of LTC_4, (Camp *et al.*, 1983; Soter *et al.*, 1983; Ueno *et al.*, 1981) rabbits, pigs and apparently horses, do not (Ford-Hutchinson and Chan, 1985; Ueno *et al.*, 1981). Furthermore, in contrast to the situation in other species (Movat *et al.*, 1984; Colditz, 1985), ZAS and LTB_4 are equally effective in their ability to attract equine neutrophils *in vivo*.

In conclusion, our results suggest that the biology of equine inflammation differs from that of other species, that LTB_4 and complement components (C5adesArg) are important equine inflammatory mediators, and that LTB_4 may be central to eosinophil dominated inflammation in horses. These results have significant implications in the therapy of equine inflammation involving all body systems, since leukotrienes are not inhibited by the frequently used non-steroidal antiinflammatory agents, but are potentiated by this class of drugs (Jorg *et al.*, 1982; Malmsten, 1986; Bottoms *et al.*, 1985). Further clarification of the precise role of LTB_4 as an inflammatory mediator of horses awaits the development of clinically active, selective lipoxygenase inhibitors.

REFERENCES

Aked, D.M. and Foster, S.J. (1987). Leukotriene B_4 and prostaglandin E_2 mediated the inflammatory response of rabbit skin to intradermal arachidonic acid. *British Journal of Pharmacology* **92**: 545-552.

Archer, R.K. (1959). Eosinophil leukocytes and their reactions to histamine and 5-hydroxytryptamine. *Journal of Pathology and Bacteriology* **78**: 95-103.

Archer, R.K. (1960). Eosinophil leukocyte attracting effect of histamine in skin. *Nature* **187**: 155-156.

Bass, D.A. (1975). Behavior of eosinophil leukocyte in acute inflammation II. Eosinophil dynamics during acute inflammation. *Journal of Clinical Investigation* **56**: 870-879.

Bass, D.A., Gonwa, T.A., Sjedja, P., Cousart, M.S., Dechatelet, L.R. *et al.* (1980). Eosinopenia of acute infection. Production of eosinophilia by chemotactic factors of acute inflammation. *Journal of Clinical Investigation* **65**: 1265-1271.

Bjork, J., Hedqvist, P., and Anfors, K.E. (1982). Increase in vascular permeability induced by leukotriene B_4 and the role of polymorphonuclear leukocytes. *Inflammation* **6**: 189-200.

Bottoms, G.D., Johnson, M.A., Lamar, C.H., Fessler, J.F. and Turek, J.J. (1985). Endotoxin-induced eicosanoid production by equine vascular endothelial cells and neutrophils. *Circulatory Shock* **15**: 155-162.

Butterworth, A.E. and David, J.R. (1981). Eosinophil function. *New England Journal of Medicine* **304**: 154-156.

Caffesse, R.G., Nasjleti, C.E. and Kowalski, C.J. (1985). Carrageenan-induced inflammation and its effects on mitotic activity and keratinization of gingival epithelium. *Journal of Periodontology* **56**: 132-138.

Camp, D.J. and Leid, R.W. (1982). Chemotaxis of radiolabelled equine neutrophils. *American Journal of Veterinary Research* **43**: 397-401.

Camp, R.D.R., Coutts, A.A., Greaves, M.W., Kay, A.B. and Walport, M.J. (1983). Responses of human skin to intradermal injection of leukotriene C_4, D_4 and B_4. *British Journal of Pharmacology* **80**:497-502.

Camp, R., Jones, R.R., Brain, S., Woollard, P. and Greaves, M. (1984). Production of intraepidermal microabscesses by topical application of leukotriene B_4. *Journal of Investigative Dermatology* **82**: 202-204.

Carr, S.C., Higgs, G.A., Salmon, J.A. and Spayne, J.A. (1981). The effects of arachidonate lipxygenase products on leukocyte migration in rabbit skin. *British Journal of Pharmacology* **73**: 253P-254P.

Clark, R.A.F., Gallin, J.I. and Kaplan, A.P. (1975). The selective eosinophil chemotactic activity of histamine. *Journal of Experimental Medicine* **142**: 1462-1476.

Cohen, S.G. and Ottensen, E.A. (1983). The eosinophil, eosinophilia and eosinophil-related disorders. *In* E. Middleton, C.E. Reed and E.F. Ellis (eds) *Allergy, Principles and Practice*, pp. 701-769.

Colditz, I.K. (1985). Kinetics of tachyphylaxis to mediators of acute inflammation. *Immunology* **55**: 144-156.

Czarnetzki, B.M. and Mertensmeir, R. (1985). *In vitro* and *in vivo* chemotaxis of guinea pig leukocytes toward leukotriene B_4 and its w-oxidation products. *Prostaglandins* **30**: 5-12.

Czarnetzki, B.M. amd Rosenbach, R. (1986). Chemotaxis of human neutrophils and eosinophils towards leukotriene B_4 and its 20–w-oxidation products *in vitro*. *Prostaglandins* **5**: 851-858.

DiRosa, M., Giroud, J.P. and Willoughby, D.A. (1971). Studies of the mediators of acute inflammatory response induced in rats in different sites by carrageenan and turpentine. *Journal of Pathology* 104: 15-29.

Douglas, W.W. (1980). Autacoids. A.G. Gilman, L.S. Goodman and A. Gilman (eds), *The Pharmacological Basis of Therapeutics*, pp. 608-681. Macmillan, New York.

Duncan, J.R. and Prasse, K.W. (1986). *Veterinary Laboratory Medicine, Clinical Pathology*, Iowa State University Press, Ames.

Eyre, P. (1976). Preliminary studies on pharmacological antagonism of anaphylaxis in the horse. *Canadian Journal of Comparative Medicine* **40**: 149-152.

Fechter, H., Egger, D., Auer, H. and Popper, H. (1986). Experimental eosinophilia and inflammation. The effect of various inflammatory mediators and chemoattractants. *Experimental Pathology* **29**: 153-158.

Fernandez, H.N. Henson, P.M., Otani, A. and Hugli, T.E. (1977). Chemotactic response to human C3a and C5a anaphylatoxins. I. Evaluation of C3a and C5a leukotaxis *in vitro* and under simulated *in vivo* conditions. *Journal of Immunology* **120**: 109-115.

Ford-Hutchinson, A.W. and Chan, C.C. (1985). Pharmacological actions of leukotrienes in the skin. *British Journal of Dermatology* **113S28**: 95-97.

Goetzl, E.J., Wasserman, S.I., and Austen, K.I. (1975). Eosinophil polymorphonuclear leukocyte function in immediate hypersensitivity. *Archives of Pathology* **99**: 1-4.

Higgins, A.J. and Lees, P. (1983). Phenylbutazone inhibition of prostaglandin E_2 production in equine acute inflammatory exudate. *Veterinary Record* **113**: 622-623.

Higgins, A.J. and Lees, P. (1984a). Arachidonic acid metabolites in carrageenin-induced equine inflammatory exudate. *Journal of Veterinary Pharmacology and Therapeutics* **7**: 65-72.

Higgins, A.J. and Lees, P. (1984b). Detection of leukotriene B_4 in equine inflammatory exudate. *Veterinary Record* **115**: 275.

Higgins, A.J., Lees, P., and Taylor, J.B. (1984). Influence of phenylbutazone on eicosanoid levels in equine acute inflammatory exudate. *Cornell Veterinarian* **74**: 198-207.

Holsapple, M.P. and Yim, G.K.W. (1984). Therapeutic reduction of ongoing carrageenin-induced inflammation by lipoxygenase, but not cyclooxygenase inhibitors. *Inflammation* **8**: 223-230.

Jain, N.C. (1986). *Schalm's Veterinary Hematology*. Lea & Febiger, Philadelphia.

Jorg, A., Henderson, W.R., Murphy, R.C. and Klebanoff, S.J. (1982). Leukotriene generation by eosinophils. *Journal of Experimental Medicine* **155**: 390-402.

Kay, A.B. (1985). Eosinophils as effector cells in immunity hypersensitivity disorders. *Clinical and Experimental Immunology* **62**: 1-12.

Kragbelle, K. and Voorhees, J.J. (1983). Arachidonic acid and leukotrienes in dermatology. *Journal of Investigative Dermatology* **81**: 293-296.

Lees, P. and Higgins, A.J. (1984). Flunixin inhibits prostaglandin E_2 production in equine inflammation. *Research in Veterinary Science* **37**: 347-349.

Lees, P. and Higgins, A.J., (1986). Effects of a phenylbutazone paste in ponies: Model of acute non-immune inflammation. *American Journal of Veterinary Research* **47**: 2359-2363.

Malmsten, K.L. (1986). Prostaglandins, thromboxanes and leukotrienes in inflammation. *American Journal of Medicine* **80**: 11-17.

McEwen, B.J., Wilcock, B.P., and Yager, J.A. (1989). Studies of Inflammation of Relevance to Equine Dermatitis. Ph.D. thesis, University of Guelph.

Morrow, A., Quinn, P.J., and Baker, K.P., (1986). Dermal reactivity to histamine, serotonin and bradykinin in relation to allergic skin reactions of the horse. *Journal of Veterinary Pharmacology and Therapeutics* **9**: 40-48.

Movat, H.Z. (1987). The role of histamine and other mediators in microvascular changes in acute inflammation. *Canadian Journal of Physiology and Pharmacology* **65**: 451-457.

Movat, H.Z., Rettl, C., Burrowes, C.E., and Johnston, M.G. (1984). The *in vivo* effect of leukotriene B_4 on polymorphonuclear leukocytes and the microcirculation. Comparison with activated complement (C5adesArg) and enhancement by prostaglandin E2. *American Journal of Pathology* **115**: 233-244.

Muller-Eberhard, H.J. (1988). Complement: chemistry and pathways. *In*: J.I. Gallin, I.M. Goldstein and R. Snyderman (eds), *Inflammation - Basic Principles and Clinical Correlates*, pp. 21-53, Raven Press, New York.

Parish, W.E. (1970). Investigations on eosinophilia. The influence of histamine, antigen-antibody complexes containing 1 or 2 globulins, foreign bodies (phagocytosis) and disrupted mast cells. *British Journal of Dermatology* **82**: 42-64.

Popper, H., Picher, O., and Auer, H. (1982). Reduction of carrageenan-bradykinin- and histamine-induced acute inflammation by experimental eosinophilia in rats. *Immunology* **46**: 589-594.

Potter, K.A., Leid, R.W., Kolattukudy, P.E. and Espelie, K.E. (1985). Stimulation of equine eosinophil migration by hydroxyacid metabolites of arachidonic acid. *American Journal of Pathology* **121**: 361-368.

Rebuck, J.W. and Crowley, J.J. (1955). A method for studying leukocyte function *in vivo*. *Annals of New York Academy of Sciences* **59**: 757-805.

Runge, V.M. Rand, T.H., Clanton, J.A., Jones, J.P., Colley, D.G. *et al.* (1985). ^{111}In-labeled eosinophils. Localization of inflammatory lesions and parasitic infection in mice. *International Journal of Nuclear Medicine and Biology* **12**: 135-144.

Schwartz, L.B. and Austen, K.F. (1984). Structure and function the chemical mediators of mast cells. *In*: K. Ishizaka (ed.) *Mast Cell Activation and Mediator Release. Progress in Allergy* **34**: 271-321.

Sedgwick, A.D., Lees, P. and Higgins, A.J. (1986). Lysosomal enzyme release in equine non-immune acute inflammatory exudate. *Equine Veterinary Journal* **18**: 68-70.

Slauson, D.O., Skrabalak, D.S., Neilsen, N.R. and Zwahlen, R.D. (1987).

Complement-induced equine neutrophil adhesiveness and aggregation. *Veterinary Pathology* **24**: 239-249.
Simmons, P.M. Salmon, J.A. and Moncada, S. (1983). The release of leukotriene B_4 during experimental inflammation. *Biochemical Pharmacology* **32**: 1353-1359.
Smith, J.E. and Cipriano, J.E. (1987). Inflammation-induced changes in serum iron analytes and ceruloplasmin of shetland ponies. *Veterinary Pathology* **24**: 354-356.
Snedecor, G.W. and Cochran, W.G. (1980). *Statistical Methods.* Iowa State University Press, Ames.
Soter, N.A., Lewis, R.A., Corey, E.J. and Austen, K.F. (1983). Local effects of synthetic leukotrienes (LTC_4, LTD_4, LTE_4 and LTB_4) in human skin. *Journal of Investigative Dermatology* **80**: 115-119.
Ting, S., Zwieman, B., Lavker, R.M. and Dunsky, E.H. (1981). In vivo release of eosinophil chemoattractant activity in human allergic skin reactions. *Journal of Immunology* **127**: 557-560.
Turnbull, L.W. and Kay, A.B. (1976). Eosinophils and mediators of anaphylaxis. Histamine and imidazole acetic acid as chemotactic agents for human eosinophil leucocytes. *Immunology* **31**: 797-802.
Ueno, A., Tanaka, K., Katori, M., Hayashi, M. and Arai, Y. (1981). Species differences in increased vascular permeability by synthetic leukotriene C_4 and D_4. *Prostaglandins* **21**: 637-648.
Vinegar, R., Truax, J.F., Selph, J.L., Johnston, P.R., Venable, A.L. *et al*: (1987). Pathway to carrageenan-induced inflammation in the hind limb of the rat. *Federation Proceedings.* **46**: 118-126.
Ward, P.A. (1969). Chemotaxis of human eosinophils. *American Journal of Pathology* **54**: 121-128.
Watson, E.D., Stokes, C.R. and Bourne, F.J. (1987). Influence of arachindonic acid metabolites in vitro and in uterine washings on migration of equine neutrophils under agarose. *Research in Veterinary Science* **43**: 203-207.
Wedmore, C.V. and Williams, T.J. (1981). Control of vascular permeability by polymorphonuclear leukocytes in inflammation. *Nature* **289**: 646-650.
Zinkl, J.G. and Brown, P.D. (1982). Chemotaxis of horse polymorphonuclear to N-formyl-methionyl-L-leucyl-L-phenylalanine. *American Journal of Veterinary Research* **46**: 613-616.

3.3 Feline Psychogenic Alopecia and the Role of the Opioid System

Ton Willemse[1], Berry M. Spruijt[2] and Anita van Osterwyck[2]

[1]Department of Clinical Sciences of Companion Animals, Dermatology Section, and [2] Division of Molecular Neurobiology, Rudolf Magnus Institute and Institute of Molecular Biology and Medical Biotechnology, University of Utrecht, The Netherlands

INTRODUCTION

Since arousing conditions such as novelty and stress stimuli are among the activators of both grooming and the hypothalamo-pituitary-adrenal systems (Dunn *et al.*, 1979; Gispen and Isaacson, 1981) the relationship between pituitary hormones and grooming has been extensively investigated. In an attempt to assess the biological relevance of ACTH-induced grooming detailed frequency and duration analysis of the behavioural elements, collectively constituting grooming behaviour, were made by Gispen and Isaacson (1981). It appeared that ACTH enhances the display of grooming behaviour of rats without changing the frequency distribution of elements.

Although ACTH was the first peptide reported to induce excessive grooming (Ferrari, 1958), it soon became apparent that in rats, other peptides like α-MSH and β-MSH were as active as the sequence ACTH and no qualitative differences in the behavioural responses were observed (Gispen *et al.*, 1975; Spruijt *et al* ., 1985). In addition, experiments of Gispen and Wiegant (1976), Gispen *et al.* (1976) and Zwiers *et al.* (1981) showed that in rats ACTH, MSH, β-endorphin and dinorphin-induced grooming can be blocked by the opioid antagonist naloxone.

An aberrant form of grooming has been seen in cats (Muller *et al.*, 1989). Upon stress these animals develop stereotypic behavioural patterns, characterized by frequent grooming, self-licking and hair pulling. This enhanced grooming behaviour usually results in localized alopecia. In addition, Willemse *et al.* (unpublished data, 1989) showed that α-MSH is one of the important peptides which are involved in stress and stress regulation of cats.

The hypothesis was forwarded that enhanced grooming, resulting from the stress-induced α-MSH, leads to the production of endorphins, which serves to protect the animal against damage from continuous stress. Moreover, by their reinforcing properties, they are thought to maintain the performance of stereotypic behaviour. If the endorphins play a role in the maintenance of this behaviour then a blockade of these reinforcing properties with naloxone should at least temporarily diminish the excessive grooming.

MATERIAL AND METHODS

Animals

Cats entering the study were animals which were referred to the Department of Clinical Sciences of Companion Animals (University of Utrecht) for the presence of a so-called psychogenic alopecia. They were otherwise healthy. The clinical criteria for inclusion were excessive self-licking and hair pulling, resulting in alopecia and the presence of broken hairs in these areas. Other skin diseases were ruled out by skin scrapings, Wood's light examination, dietary tests and extensive flea control programmes.

Five European shorthaired cats (three males and two females) were included in the study. Their age at onset ranged between 6 months and 7 years, with a median of 4 years. The duration of the alopecia varied from 2 weeks to 3¼ years (medium 1 year).

Research protocol

The cats were studied on an in-patient basis. They were housed separately in large stainless steel/glass cages, which allowed videocamera observation. Twice a day at 06.00 and 18.00 h the cats were fed a complete canned food. Water was available during the entire day.

The observation period was between 0.800 and 16.00 h daily for at least a period of 4 consecutive days. At the second day of observation the cats were injected with naloxone at a dose of 1 mg/kg bodyweight subcutaneously at 09.00 h. During that day the video registration was extended to 15 h. A limited period of registration was chosen as no circadian grooming pattern is present in cats (Willense, 1989, unpublished data).

Subsequently to the observation period in the clinic the cat's behaviour was recorded daily by the owner along the lines of a questionnaire for a period of 4 weeks.

Data analysis

The videotapes were analysed for information about the total duration of the grooming, and the duration and sequence of the individual grooming elements. A comparison was made between these data before and after the injection of naloxone. The individual recorded grooming elements were: grooming of the head, the forelimbs, the hindlimbs and the lumbosacral area, the dorsum, the anogenital region, and the tail.

The information from the questionnaire was directed to the same items as mentioned above.

RESULTS

As possible initiating factors of the excessive grooming the following stressors had been detected: move to another home (one) loneliness (one), and a poor relation to other pets in the same household (two). On one occasion the reason for the abnormal behaviour was unknown.

One cat showed no change in grooming behaviour before and after the naloxone injection. The four cats which finally responded to the naloxone, exhibited a decrease after 3–6 h. However, 8–12 h after the injection these animals had a reoccurrence of the excessive grooming, sometimes similar to the situation before the treatment.

Looking at the sequence of the grooming elements, the sequence 'scratching — grooming of the dorsum' seems to be characteristic for the investigated animals before the naloxone injection. After the injection the sequences 'grooming of the hindlimbs — grooming of the tail', and 'grooming anogenital region — grooming of the hindlimbs' have become more typical.

The answers to the questionnaire allowed calculation of the long-term percentage of improvement (decrease in grooming time and/or regrowth of hairs) observed by the owners.

Considering this percentage and the time after which deterioration occurred, the following results were obtained: one cat showed 25% improvement during the first week after the injection, one cat showed 50% improvement from the first week until 3 months later, one cat showed 70% improvement from the second week after the injection for a period of 6 months, and one cat showed 95–100% improvement — gradually over 4 weeks.

DISCUSSION

The cats presenting with clinical manifestations of psychogenic alopecia were all European shorthaired cats. This observation is in contrast to the literature (Muller *et al.*, 1989), where Siamese and Burmese cats are said to be predisposed. As four of the five cats with psychogenic alopecia responded temporarily to the naloxone, it may be concluded that this opioid antagonist has a modulatory effect on stress-induced excessive grooming of cats.

However, the contribution of the change of environment, resulting from the cats' stay at the university clinic, cannot be estimated. Therefore it seems important to perform a double-blind cross-over study to establish the sole effect of opioid antagonists on stereotypic behaviour of cats. Nevertheless the preliminary results of the present study are in agreement with the findings in rats, where naloxone acts as blocking agents for experimentally induced excessive grooming (Gispen and Wiegant, 1976; Zwiers *et al.*, 1981).

REFERENCES

Dunn, A.J., Green, E.J. and Isaacson, R.L. (1979). Intracerebral adrenocorticotropic hormone mediates novelty-induced grooming in the rat *Science* **203**: 281-283.

Ferrari, W. (1958). Behavioural changes in animals after intracisternal injection with adrenocorticotrophic hormone and melanocyte stimulating hormone. *Nature* **181**: 925-926.

Gispen, W.H. and Isaacson, R.L. (1981). ACTH-induced excessive grooming in the rat. *Pharmacological Therapy* **12**: 209-246.

Gispen, W.H. and Wiegant, V.M. (1976). Opiate antagonists suppress $ACTH_{1-24}$-induced excessive grooming in the rat. *Neuroscience Letter* **2**: 159-164.

Gispen, W.H., and Weigant, V.M., Greven, H.M. and De Wied, D. (1975). The induction of excessive grooming in the rat by intraventricular application of peptides derived from ACTH; Structure-activity studies. *Life Sciences* **17**: 645-652.

Gispen, W.H., Wiegant, V.M., Bradbury, A.F. *et al.* (1976). Induction of excessive grooming in the rat by fragments of lipotropin. *Nature* **264**: 794-795.

Muller, G.H., Kirk, R.W. and Scott, D.W. (1989). *Small Animal Dermatology*, 1007 pp. W.B. Saunders Company, Phadelphia.

Spruijt, B.M., De Graan, P.N.E., Eberle, A.N. *et al.* (1985) Comparison of structural requirements of α-MSH and ACTH for inducing excessive grooming and pigment dispersion. *Peptides* **6**: 1185-1189.

Zwiers, H., Aloyo, V.J. and Gispen, W.H. (1981). Behavioural and neurochemical effects of the new opioid peptide $dynorphin_{1-13}$. Comparison with other neuropeptides. *Life Sciences* **28**: 254-255.

3.4 Mononuclear Cell Response of the Rat to Experimental Infection with *Dermatophilus congolensis* and its Effect on Epidermal Cell Kinetics

Julia Woodman

Unité de Recherche Université-INRA d'Immunologie-Parasitaire, Station de Pathologie-Porcine, Centre INRA de Tours, Nouzilly, France

INTRODUCTION

Dermatophilosis is characterized by invasion and partial destruction of the epidermis occurring both as a result of direct damage by *Dermatophilus congolensis* and of the host inflammatory response. The disease is normally confined to the epidermis (Amakiri, 1974) and symptoms range from non-spreading, transient infections, such as those induced experimentally, through to a chronic, generalized exudative dermatitis. Both extremes of the disease spectrum are characterized by regeneration of the epidermis but in the chronic form the newly formed epidermis also becomes infected and the process repeats itself (Roberts, 1967). In transient infections one of the contributing factors to the prevention of further invasion may be a response of the epidermis itself. Amakiri (1974) proposed that the acanthosis and hyperkeratosis observed in *D. congolensis* infections were a means of eliminating the organism. Furthermore, Zlotnik (1955) suggested that epidermal hyperproliferation at *D. congolensis* infection sites was caused by the lymphocytic infiltrate. Indeed, studies of other skin diseases point, not only to an active role for the epidermis in defence against infection, but to involvement of immune mechanisms in its control. Thus, the resolution of experimentally induced *Candida albicans* infections is associated with enhanced desquamation and the onset of a delayed-type hypersensitivity reaction (Sohnle *et al.*, 1976); furthermore, epidermal proliferation at the infection site is greater in immune than in naive animals (Sohnle and

Kirkpatrick, 1978). The epidermal proliferation rate is also increased in *Trichophyton mentagrophytes* infections with the maximum proliferation correlating with the commencement of healing both in primary and subsequent infections, the latter producing faster resolving lesions (Tagami, 1985). *Dermatophilus congolensis* infections are also characterized by accelerated healing on subsequent infections and this has been observed to correlate with the onset of a delayed-type hypersensitivity reaction suggesting that a cell-mediated immune response may be involved in recovery (Roberts, 1966).

Mononuclear cells (MC) become primed following experimentally induced *D. congolensis* infection of rats and will subsequently give a strong and specific *in vitro* proliferative response to inactivated *D.congolensis* cocci. The majority (56%) of the proliferating cells were found to be T-helper lymphocytes and these appeared to be actively secreting lymphokines since the MC culture supernatants contained significant macrophage migration inhibitory activity (Woodman, 1989).

In this study, culture supernatants of *D.congolensis* -stimulated MC isolated from infected rats were tested for their effect on the proliferation rates of cultured rat epidermal cells. Comparisons were made between the effect of supernatants from *D.congolensis* -stimulated MC and control, non-stimulated MC. Similarly produced supernatants from naive rats were also assessed to determine whether the observed effects were specific to *D.congolensis* infection. In the first set of experiments, epidermal cells were grown in low calcium-concentration medium since these cultures are inherently more stable and uniform than those grown at normal calcium concentration (Hennings *et al.*, 1980). However, due to the physiological importance of calcium, the experiments were repeated with epidermal cells cultured in normal calcium concentration medium; problems with culture instability were not encountered due to the relatively short period of the assay. The epidermal cultures were assayed at the stage when they were well-established but were still sub-confluent since cells in the exponential growth phase are most susceptible to growth stimulatory or inhibitory factors (Kappler and Marrack, 1986). The impetus for this work was the hypothesis that the cell-mediated arm of the immune response may induce epidermal hyperproliferation and that this may be an important defence mechanism against some skin pathogens.

MATERIALS AND METHODS

Dermatophilus congolensis isolate

An ovine *D.congolensis* isolate from a confirmed, chronic case of dermatophilosis in Scotland was used throughout. The infectivity of the isolate, when tested on rats and calves, was equal to that of Caribbean isolates from cases of generalized dermatophilosis. The isolate was stored, as pure primary and secondary cultures, at −20°C in 15% glycerol in Colombia broth

(Gibco). For infection of rats or for *in vitro* stimulation of MC, *D.congolensis* cocci were harvested from 48 h blood agar plate secondary cultures by addition of phosphate-buffered saline (PBS) and by gentle rubbing over the colonies with a Pasteur pipette. The bacterial suspension, containing predominantly cocci, was left to stand 1 h at 37°C to allow the filaments to sediment. The cocci-containing supernatant was recovered and aliquots checked for purity and serially diluted for viable counts.

Animals and infection

Epidermal cells were obtained from neonatal, inbred, sibling, Wistar rats which were usually under 24 h and always under 48 h old.

Mononuclear cells were isolated from 3–5 month-old, inbred, male, Wistar rats. Skin sites were prepared for infection by shaving an area of flank, rubbing with ether to remove sebum and then lightly scarifying. Two to twelve million cocci in 25 μl PBS were then spread evenly across the site. Second and third infections were induced at different sites at 10-day intervals. Non-infected, control rats were subjected to the same regimen except that only PBS was applied.

Production of supernatants from *D.congolensis* -stimulated mononuclear cells

Mononuclear cells were isolated from the spleens of rats ten days after the induction of the third infection and from control, non-infected rats 10 days after the third scarification. The spleens were disaggregated and single cell suspensions were separated on Ficoll-paque gradients (density 1.077 g/ml, Pharmacia). The washed MC fraction was resuspended in RPMI-1640 medium containing 8% heat-inactivated fetal calf serum (FCS), 25 mM Hepes, 5×10^{-5} M 2-mercaptoethanol, 2 mM L-glutamine, 100 units ml penicillin and 100 μg/ml streptomycin (complete RPMI). The MC were incubated in 25 cm^2 culture flasks at an initial cell concentration of 5×10^6/ml either in the presence or the absence of inactivated *D.congolensis* cocci. The cocci had been incubated in complete RPMI medium for 1 h at 37°C during which time they were inactivated by the antibiotics in the medium. Non-viability following this treatment was demonstrated by a subsequent inability to grow on blood agar or in broth even after washing. The concentration of cocci in the MC cultures was the same as that which had been previously shown to cause optimal stimulation of the proliferation of presensitized MC in a lymphocyte transformation test (Woodman, 1989).

The cultures were incubated at 37°C under a 5% CO_2, humidified atmosphere for 24 h and were then chilled to 4°C. To allow for any effects of *D.congolensis* products on epidermal growth, complete RPMI medium containing cocci (which had been incubated under the same conditions as the MC cultures) was added to the control, non-stimulated cultures to give an equivalent cocci concentration to that found in the stimulated cultures. The MC were pelleted out (700 **g**, 10 min, 4°C) and the supernatants filtered (low protein-binding, 0.22 μm filters) then half of each was stored at −20°C. The remaining halves were dialysed against incomplete medium (100 volumes, 4°C, 24 h with one change of medium), filter-sterilized and stored at −20°C.

Epidermal cell cultures

The trunk skin was excised from neonatal rats and the underside scraped free of adherent fat. Narrow strips of skin were incubated in 0.2% dispase (grade two, neutral protease, Boehringer Manheim) in minimal essential medium (MEM) containing 100 units/ml penicillin and 100 μg/ml streptomycin at 4°C for 80–90 min. The epidermis was peeled away from the dermis and the former incubated in 0.25% trypsin in 0.02% ethylenediamine tetraacetic acid (EDTA) in PBS for 15 min at 37°C with occasional agitation. An excess of FCS was then added to the strips which were gently agitated for 10 min to allow further release of basal cells. The cell suspension was collected following rinsing of the remaining strips and centrifuged at 400 **g** for 10 min at 15°C. The cells, which consisted of 80% basal cells as assessed by morphology, were resuspended in minimal essential suspension medium (SMEM, Gibco) containing 5% heat-inactivated, Myoclone FCS (Gibco), 0.4 μg/ml hydrocortisone (Sigma), 10 ng/ml cholera toxin (Sigma), 0.75 mg/ml sodium bicarbonate, 20 mM Hepes, 2mM L-glutamine, 50 units/ml penicillin and 50 μg/ml streptomycin (complete SMEM). The calcium concentration of complete SMEM was 0.2 mM (low calcium medium); for some experiments calcium chloride was added to complete SMEM to give a final calcium concentration of 1.4 mM (normal calcium medium).

Epidermal cells, either in low or normal calcium concentration medium, were seeded at an initial cell density of 2×10^5 cells/cm in 96-well, flat-bottomed plates and incubated at 37°C under a 5% CO_2, humidified atmosphere. Ten replicate cultures were set up for each of the treatments tested.

Epidermal cell proliferation assay

After 24 h the medium was removed from the epidermal cell cultures and replaced with the MC culture supernatants. The various supernatants tested for their effect on epidermal proliferation were produced from MC which derived either from *D.congolensis* -infected or non-infected rats, were either from *D.congolensis*- stimulated or non-stimulated MC cultures and were either dialysed or non-dialysed. The supernatants were diluted with complete SMEM, low or normal calcium concentration as appropriate, to give 1/2, 1/10, 1/100 and 1/1000 of the initial strength. The epidermal cultures were then returned to normal incubation conditions.

To determine whether any of the observed effects of the supernatants were due to the presence of *D.congolensis* products, supernatants prepared from cocci incubated in culture medium under identical conditions to those for the MC cultures but for the absence of MC were tested on epidermal cells in the same way as for MC supernatants.

Four hours before the epidermal cell cultures were harvested, 0.5 μCi ^{3}Ci/ml, and the cultures returned to normal incubation conditions. The epidermal cells were harvested 24 or 48 h after the addition of the supernatants as follows: the medium was completely removed from each well and 200 μl 0.25% trypsin in 0.02% EDTA in PBS was added. The plates were incubated for 30 min at 37°C and then the cells were transferred onto glassfibre filter papers using an automated cell harvester. Samples were counted with 1ml scintillation fluid (Opti-scint hi-safe, LKB) in a liqud scintillation analyser.

Analysis of Results

Data were expressed as counts per minute (cpm) and the results treated in two ways. Firstly, epidermal cell proliferation, as assessed by ^{3}H-thymidine incorporation, in the presence of the various supernatants was compared with that in culture medium alone, whereby:

$$SI = \text{md S}/\text{md M} \qquad \text{(Eq. 1)}$$

where SI is the stimulation index, md S is the median cpm of ten replicate cultures incubated with MC supernatant and md M is the median cpm of ten replicate cultures incubated in medium alone.

Secondly, epidermal proliferation in the presence of supernatants from *D.congolensis*-stimulated MC cultures was compared with that in the presence of supernatants of non-stimulated, control MC culture supernatants derived from the same rat, whereby:

$$SI = \text{md SS}/\text{md CS} \qquad \text{(Eq. 2)}$$

where SI is the stimulation index, md SS is the median cpm of ten replicate cultures incubated with *D.congolensis* -stimulated supernatant and md CS is the median cpm of ten replicate cultures incubated with control supernatant.

The Mann-Whitney U test was used to determined statistical significance.

RESULTS

Although the cultures remained subconfluent throughout the assay period the high ^{3}H-thymidine incorporation rates suggested that the cells were growing well. The median incorporation rates reached up to 27 000 cpm/well 24 h after addition of the supernatants and up to 40 000 cpm/well at 48 h and varied with the dilution and type of supernatant. An exception was the poor growth occurring in the presence of dialysed supernatants at the lowest dilution with maximum ^{3}H-thymidine incorporation of 3000 cpm/well.

The predominant effect of the MC culture supernatants, compared with that of medium alone, was stimulation of epidermal cell proliferation as assessed by ^{3}H-thymidine incorporation ($p<0.01$, Table 1). However, at the two lower dilutions of dialysed supernatant the effect was one of significant inhibition of growth compared with that in medium alone ($p<0.01$, Table 1). The same overall pattern was observed for the control, non-stimulated supernatant and also for epidermal cells cultured in normal calcium concentration medium.

Table 1 Effect of *D.congolensis*-stimulated MC supernatants on epidermal proliferation compared with that in medium alone

Dilution of supernatant	Stimulation index			
	24 h		48 h	
	Dialysed	Non-dialysed	Dialysed	Non-dialysed
1/2	0	0.61	0	1.55
1/10	0.32	1.12	0.54	1.61
1/100	1/16	1.08^{NS}	1.10	1.29
1/1000	1.33	1.07^{NS}	1.05^{NS}	1.23

Stimulation indices were calculated as described in the text (eq. 1). All values below 1 indicate significant inhibition of epidermal proliferation. ($p<0.01$) and all values above 1 indicate significant stimulation of epidermal proliferation ($p<0.01$) unless marked (NS). The epidermal cells were cultured in low calcium medium and the supernatants derived from an infected rat.

The contribution of *D. congolensis* products to the observed effects of the MC supernatants was shown to be one of inhibition. The supernatants produced from 'cultures' lacking MC, caused significant inhibition of epidermal growth compared with culture medium alone ($p<0.01$) with corresponding stimulation indices of between 0.46 and 0.78.

A comparison of the effects of supernatants from *D.congolensis* -stimulated MC from infected rats with control supernatants derived from the same animals showed that the former caused significant inhibition of the proliferation of epidermal cells in low calcium concentration medium at the two lower dilutions tested ($p<0.01$ Fig. 1). The inhibition was observed regardless of whether the supernatant was dialysed or not and of the time of assay. In contrast, the two higher dilutions caused significant stimulation of epidermal proliferation ($p<0.01$) and dialysis enhanced this effect (Fig. 1). The same pattern of responses was observed in two further repeat experiments except that significant stimulation occurred with all three of the higher dilutions of dialysed supernatant ($p<0.01$).

When supernatants of *D.congolensis* -stimulated MC derived from infected rats were tested on epidermal cells cultured in normal calcium concentration medium both stimulatory and inhibitory effects, as compared with proliferation in the presence of control supernatants, were again observed.

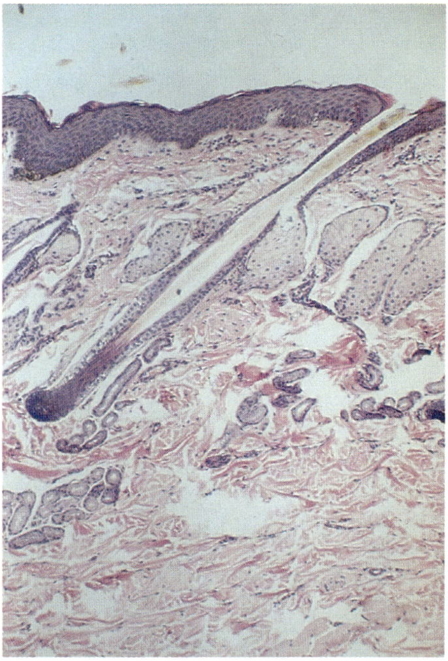

Plate 1A *Normal equine skin. Simple hair follicle (HE-stain × 50). (See p.7.)*

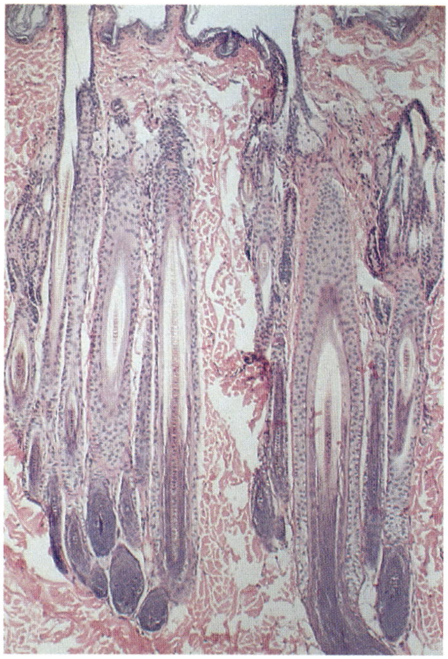

Plate 1B *Normal feline skin. Compound hair follicle (HE-stain × 50). (See p.7.)*

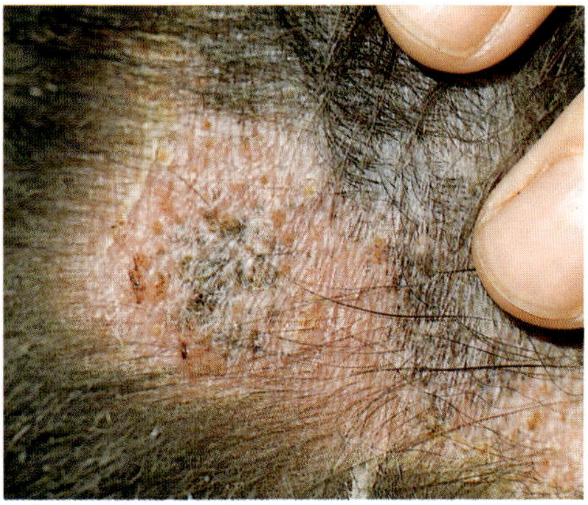

Plate 1C *Canine staphylococcal folliculitis. Annular area of alopecia, erythema and crust with peripheral epidermal collarette and central hyperpigmentation. (See p.16.)*

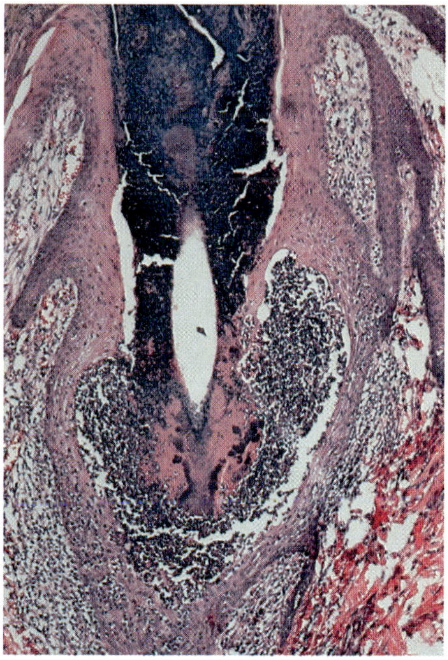

Plate 1D *Porcine staphylococcal folliculitis. Suppurative folliculitis and bacterial colonies (HE-stain × 125). (See p.16.)*

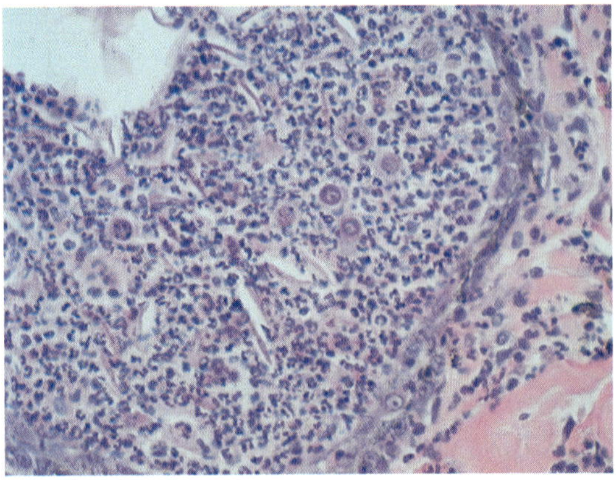

Plate 2A *Canine pemphigus foliaceus. Suppurative folliculitis with numerous acanthocytes (HE-stain × 500). (See p.17.)*

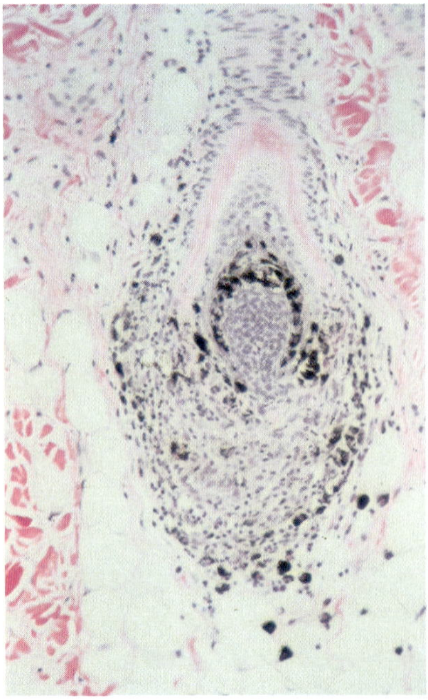

Plate 2B *Canine alopecia areata. Peribulbar lymphohistiocytic infiltrate and pigmentary incontinence (HE-stain × 125). (See p.17.)*

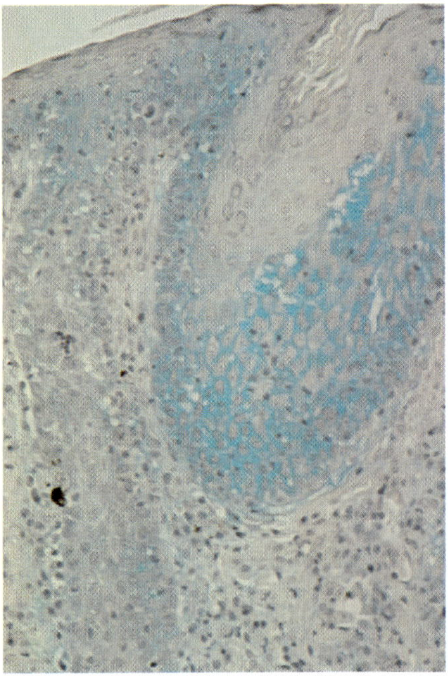

Plate 2C *Feline alopecia mucinosa. Lymphocytic perifolliculitus and marked mucinosis of follicular outer root sheath (Hales stain × 125). (See p.17.)*

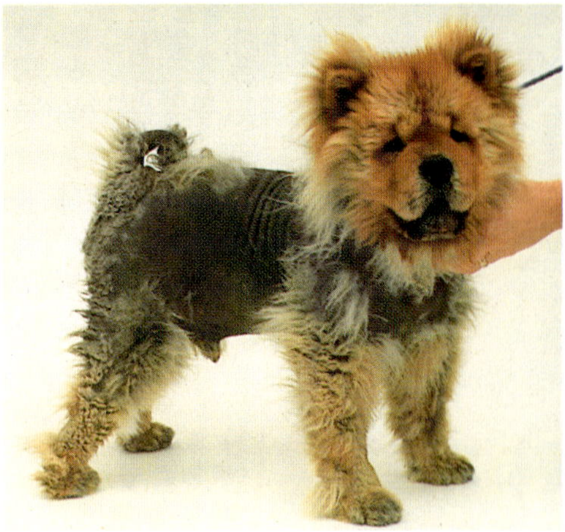

Plate 2D *Canine adult-onset hyposomatotropism. Chow chow with symmetrical truncal/alopecia and hyperpigmentation. (See p.18.)*

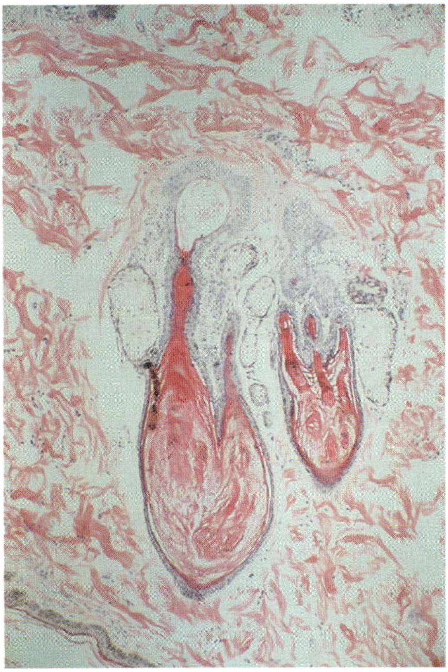

Plate 3A *Canine endocrinopathy. Telogenization and orthokeratotic hyperkeratosis of hair follicles (HE-stain × 50). (See p.18.)*

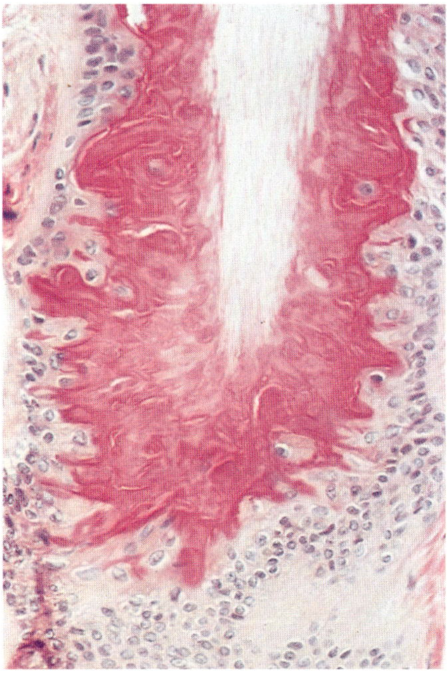

Plate 3B *Canine hypothyroidism. Excessive tricholemmal keratinization (flame follicle) (HE stain × 500). (See p.18.)*

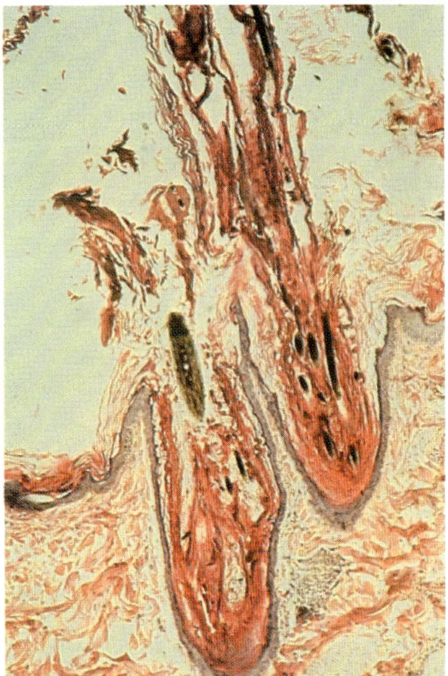

Plate 3C *Canine vitamin A-responsive dermatosis. Disproportionate orthokeratotic hyperkeratosis of hair follicles (HE-stain × 50). (See p.21.)*

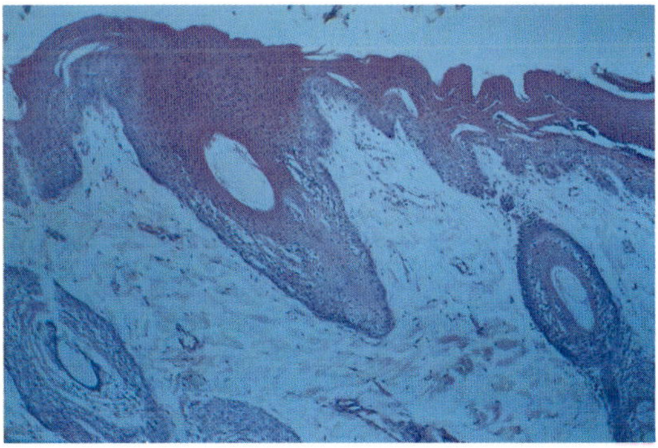

Plate 3D *Canine thallotoxicosis. Parakeratotic hyperkeratosis and neutrophilic microabscesses in outer root sheath of hair follicles (HE-stain × 40). (See p.22.)*

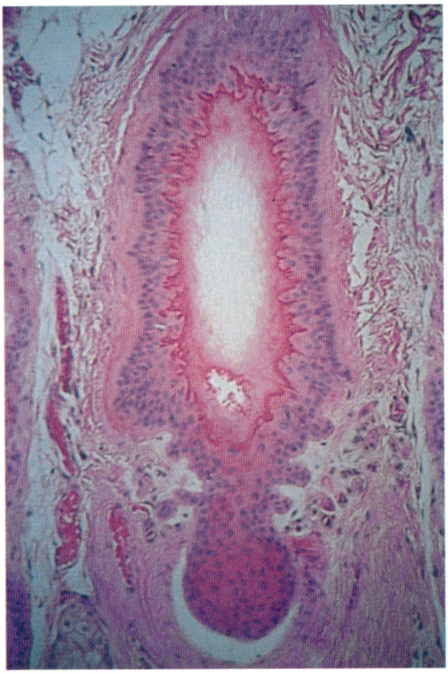

Plate 4 *Histopathology of a skin biopsy demonstrating hypereosinophilic tricholemmal keratinization. Courtesy of Dr R. W. Dunstan, Michigan State University.* *(See p.35.)*

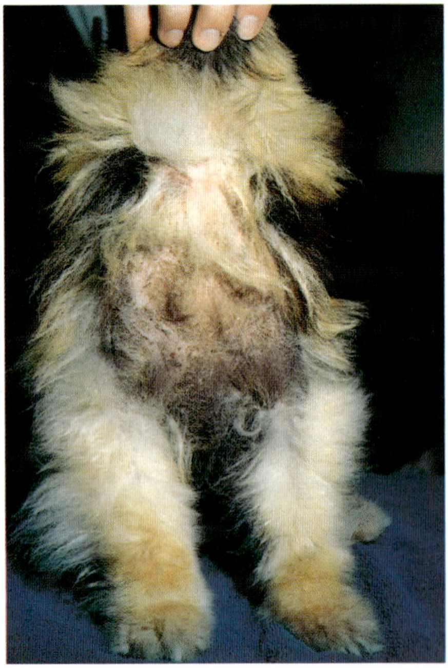

Plate 5 *Alopecia and mild hyperpigmentation around the neck and chest region of a pomeranian.* *(See p.39.)*

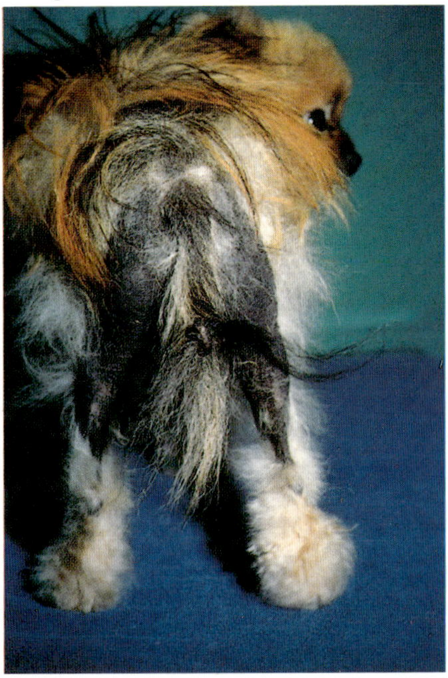

Plate 6 *Alopecia and marked hyperpigmentation of the perineal region and posterior and medial thighs in a pomeranian.* *(See p.40.)*

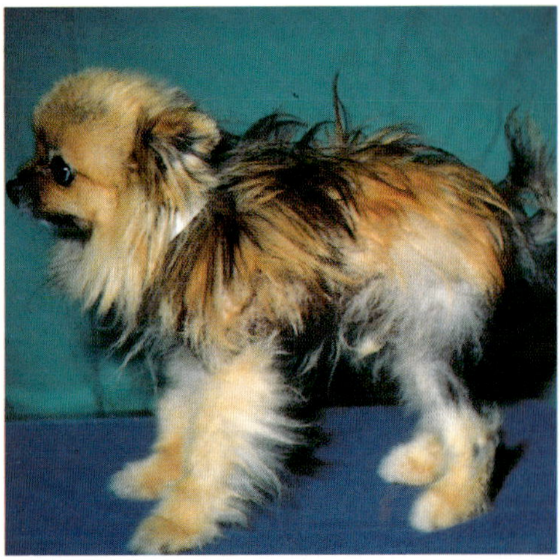

Plate 7 *Rust discolouration and black streaking in the hair coat of a pomeranian.* *(See p.40.)*

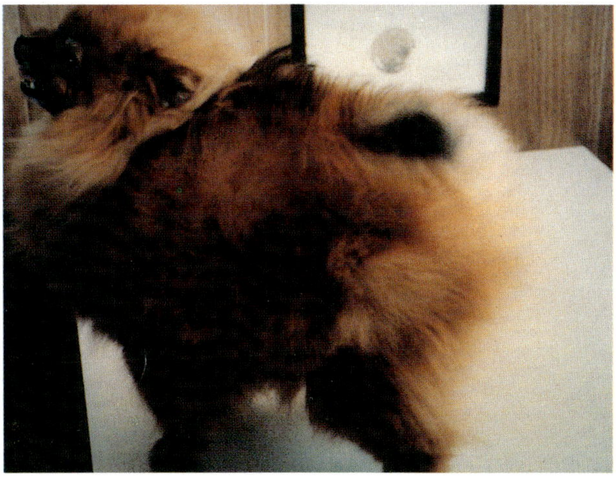

Plate 8 *Pomeranian 3 months after castration. Note complete regrowth of hair and tan coat colour — the original colour before onset of disease.* *(See p.40.)*

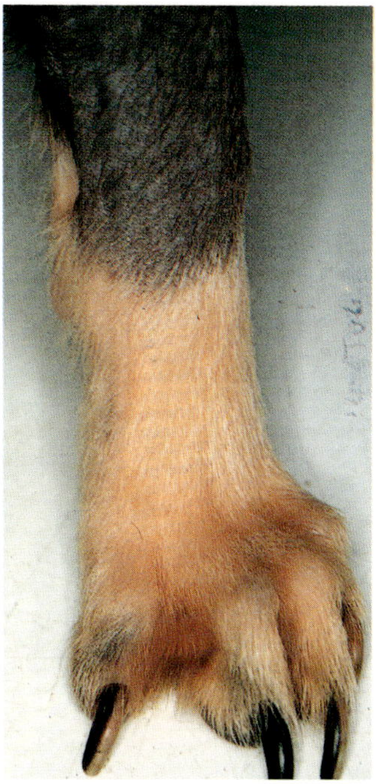

Plate 11 *(Above) Colour mutant alopecia in a blue chihuahua. The blue area is alopectic whereas the tan point is normal.* *(See p.44.)*

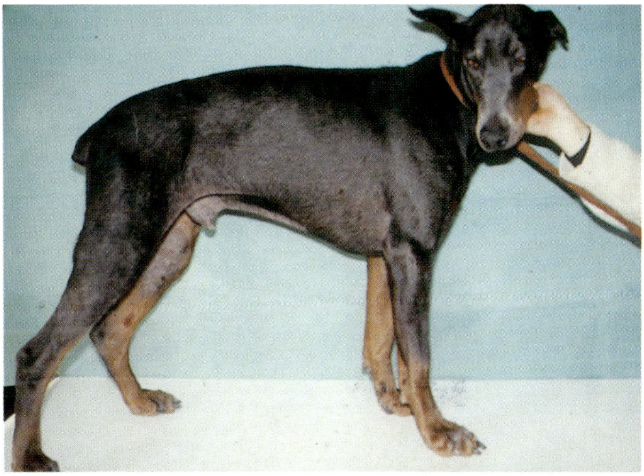

Plate 9 *(Left) Colour mutant alopecia in a blue doberman pinscher. Note that the tan points are almost normal (a biopsy has been taken on the left hock), whereas demodicosis and folliculitis/furunculosis are present in the blue areas.* *(See p.44.)*

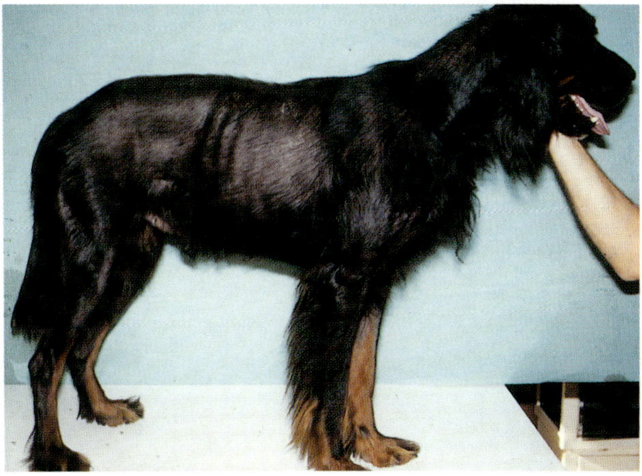

Plate 10 *(Left) Black hair follicular dysplasia in a gordon setter. The points are normal.* *(See p.44.)*

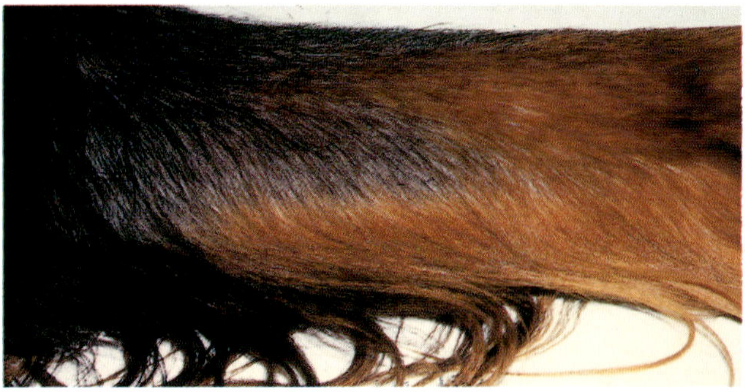

Plate 12 *Black hair follicular dysplasia in a gordon setter (same dog as in Plate 10). The black area is alopectic whereas the tan point is normal. Compare with Plate 11. (See p.44.)*

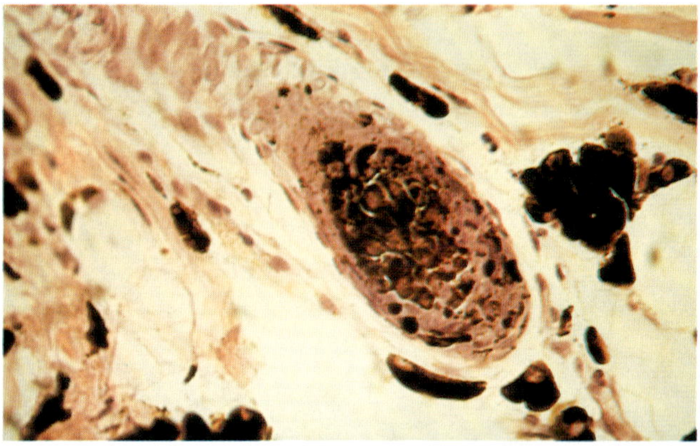

Plate 13 *Histopathology of the skin of a black and white cocker spaniel with black hair follicular dysplasia. Prominent clumping of melanin both around and within hair follicles in a black area of the coat (Photomicrograph by J.P. Magnol, × 300).(See p.44.)*

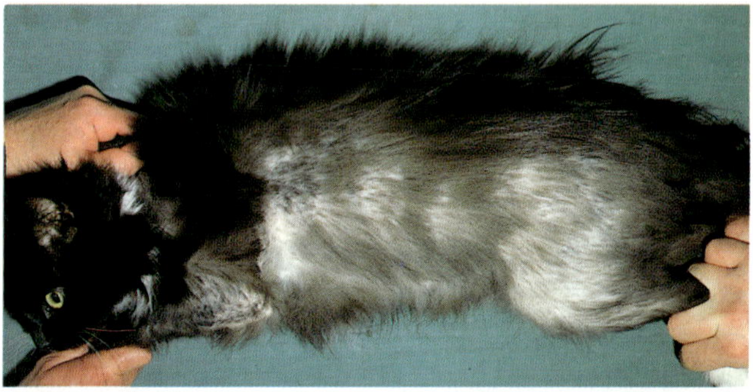

Plate 14A *A 10-year-old, neutered female, domestic short-haired cat with idiopathic feline symmetric alopecia of 11 months' duration (T_3 totally responsive group). (See p.51.)*

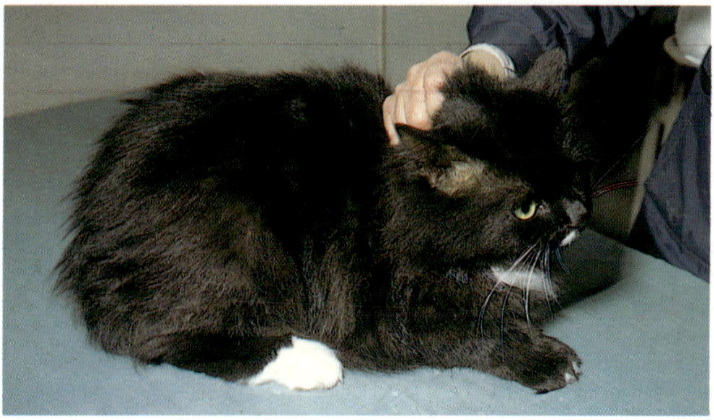

Plate 14B *The same cat 18 weeks after beginning treatment with T_3. (See p.52.)*

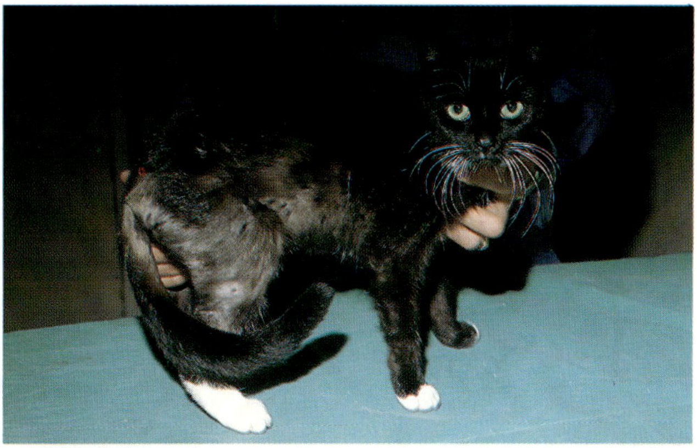

Plate 15A *A 6-year-old, entire female, domestic short-haired cat in which flea infestation was suspected as the cause of the symmetric alopecia. The case responded totally to flea control.* *(See p.59.)*

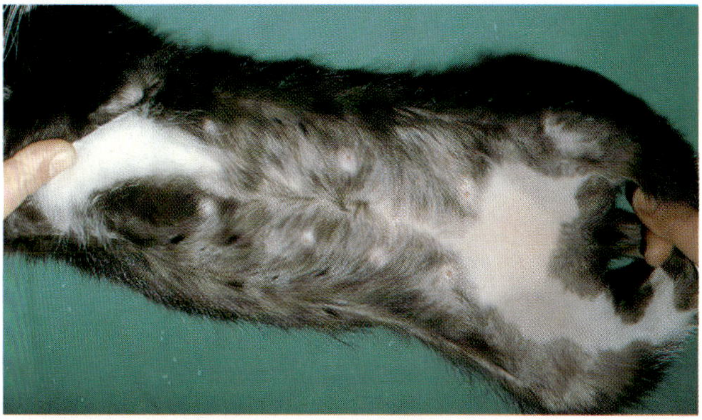

Plate 15B *The ventral surface of the cat in Plate 15A.* *(See p.59.)*

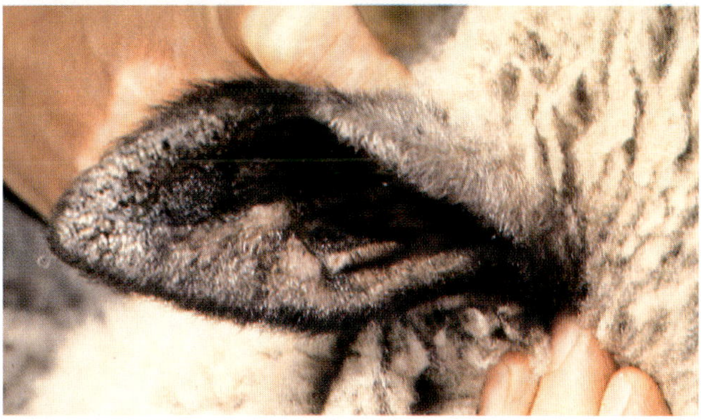

Plate 16A *Crusting lesions on the ears of a sheep suspected of suffering from hypersensitivity to* Culicoides obsoletus. *Reproduced with permission from Connan, RM and Lloyd S., Seasonal allergic dermatitis in sheep.* Veterinary Record **123** *335–337.* *(See p.112.)*

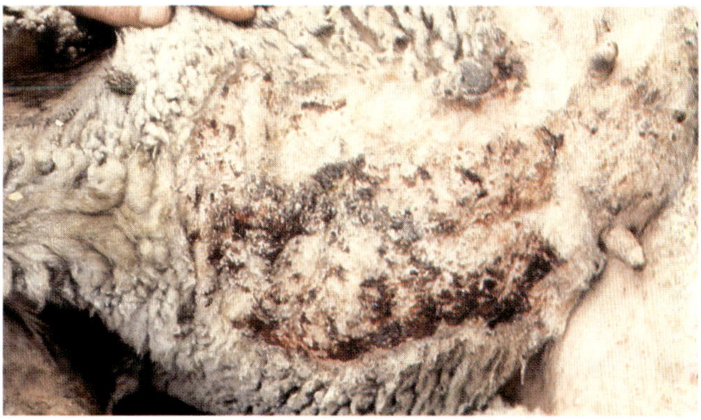

Plate 16B *Crusting lesions on the ventral abdomen of the same sheep as in plate 16A. Reproduced with permission, as Plate 16A.* *(See p.112.)*

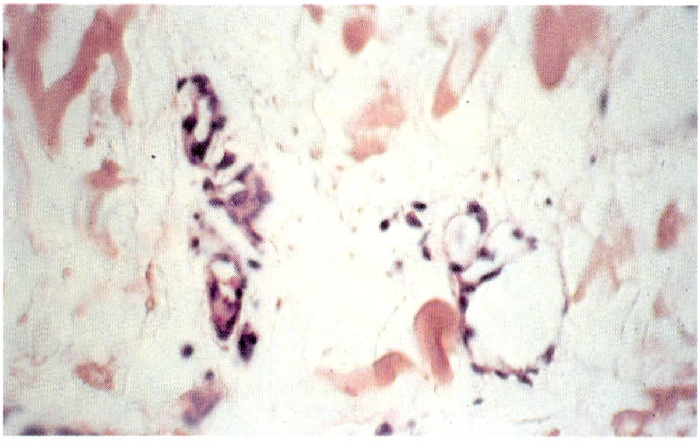

Plate 17 *Response to inflammatory mediators in equine skin. At 4 h postinoculation, sterile saline did not invoke an appreciable leukocytic infiltrate.* *(See p.179.)*

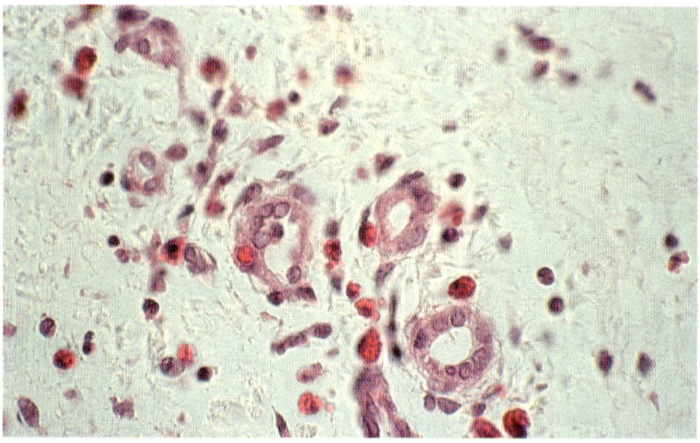

Plate 18 *Response to inflammatory mediators in equine skin. Histamine-induced moderate oedema and a mild eosinophil infiltrate at 4 h postinoculation.* *(See p.179.)*

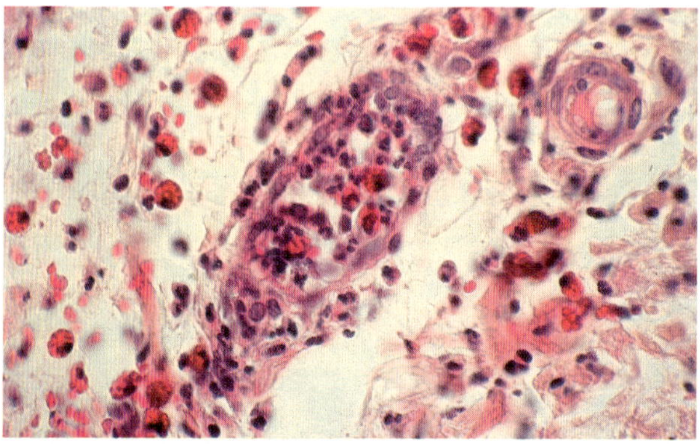

Plate 19 *Response to inflammatory mediators in equine skin. A marked eosinophil and neutrophil infiltrate followed the intradermal injection of leukotriene B_4 at 4 h postinoculation.* *(See p.179.)*

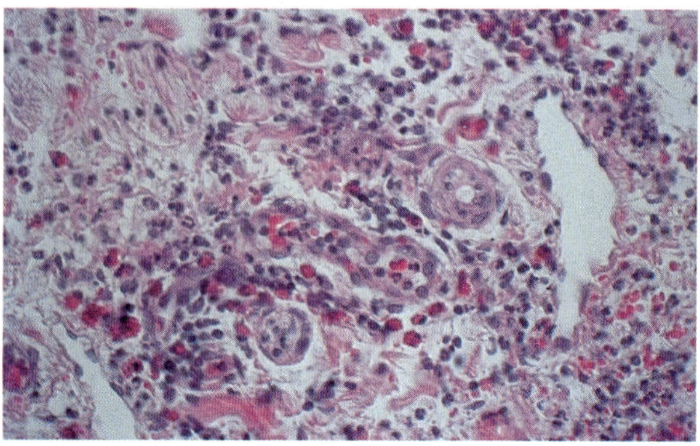

Plate 20 *Response to inflammatory mediators in equine skin. Carrageenin provoked a substantial eosinophil and neutrophil infiltrate 4 h postinoculation. Dermal lymphatics are dilated.* *(See p. 179.)*

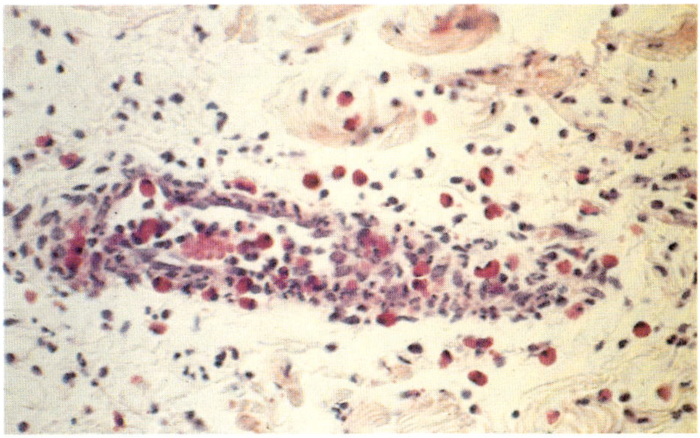

Plate 21 *Response to inflammatory mediators in equine skin. Tabanid extract induced a marked eosinophil and neutrophil infiltrate at 4 h postinoculation. (See p.179.)*

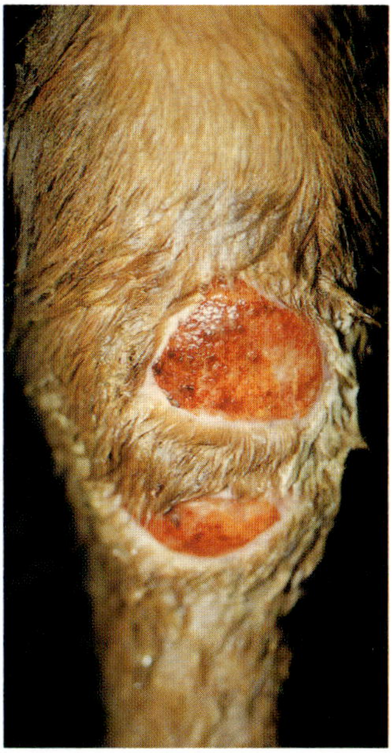

Plate 22 *During ketanserin treatment: fine regular granulation tissue. Dry aspect of lesion. No infection. Large epithelialization zone. (See p.222.)*

Plate 23A *Cervical apocrine glands of the mink. Low-power photomicrograph of the cervical skin from a 1-day-old control kit illustrating the hypertrophic apocrine glands in the subcutaneous tissue. (HE) (See p.294.)*

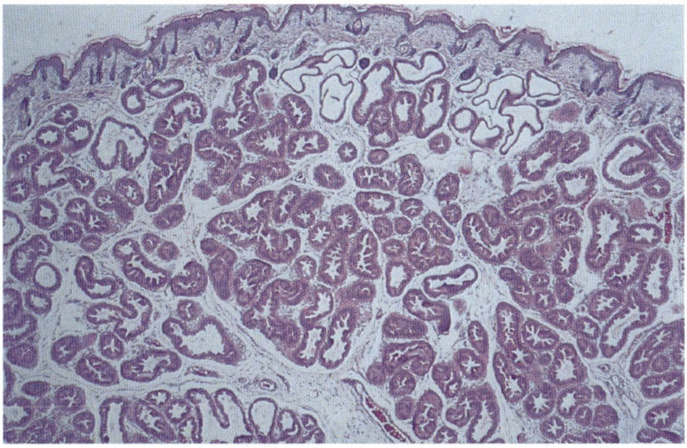

Plate 23B *Higher magnification of the cervical apocine gland from the same kit showing typical apocrine 'secretory vesicles' at the luminal surface. (HE) (See p.294.)*

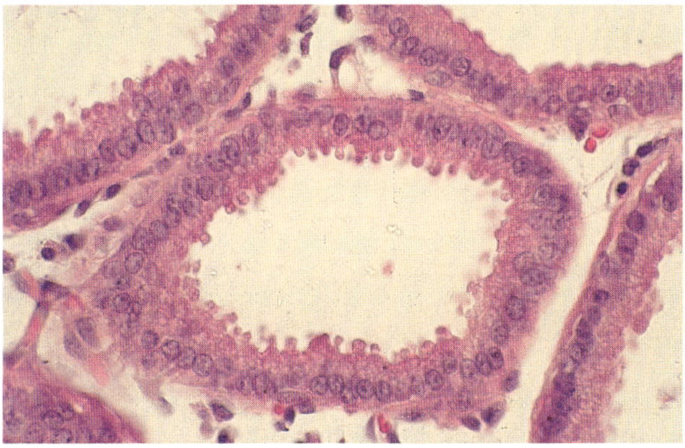

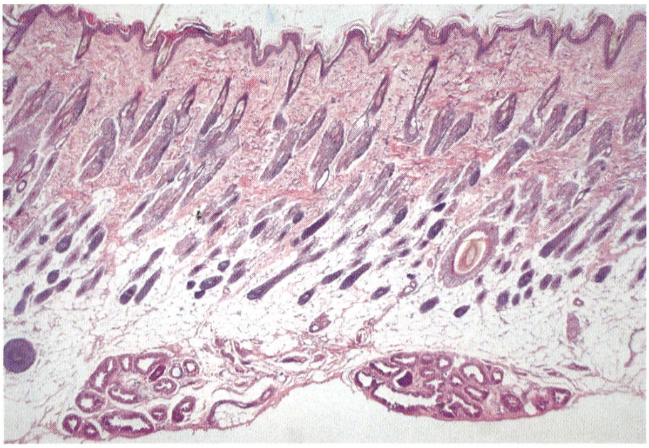

Plate 24A *Low power photomicrograph of the remnants of the cervical apocrine gland in a 5-week-old normal control kit. (HE)* *(See p.294.)*

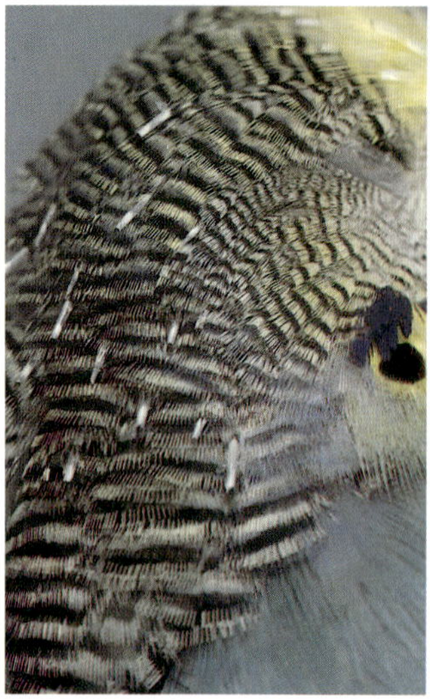

Plate 25 *(Above) Retarded moult: individual feathers persist in the elongated and thickened keratin sheath. A suggested new paramyxovirus infection (budgerigar).* *(See p.388.)*

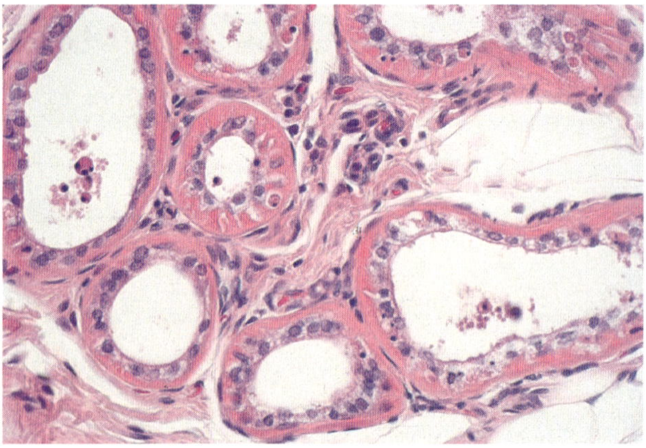

Plate 24B *Higher power photomicrograph of the gland from the same kit showing the markedly thickened basement membrane and degenerating epithelium with several apoptotic cell bodies. (HE)* *(See p.294.)*

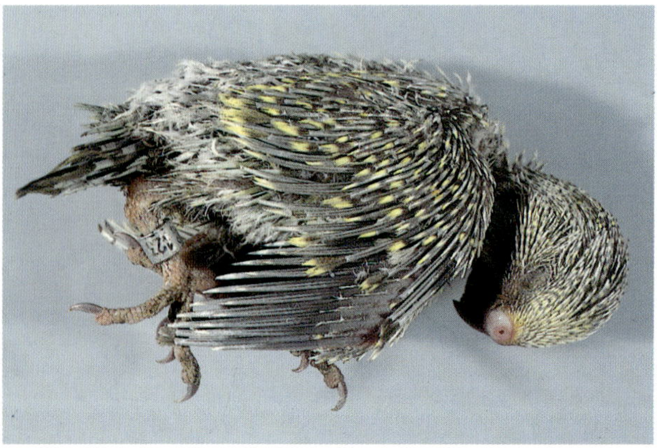

Plate 26 *(Left) French moult disease. A new feature in juvenile budgerigars: all growing feathers of the body have a retained sheath. A poliomavirus infection.* *(See p.387.)*

Plate 27 *Papillomatosis on the feet (bumblefoot-like). Massive fibrosis, hyperkeratosis and ulcerated surface are prominent. A new papillomavirus infection (swan). (See p.387.)*

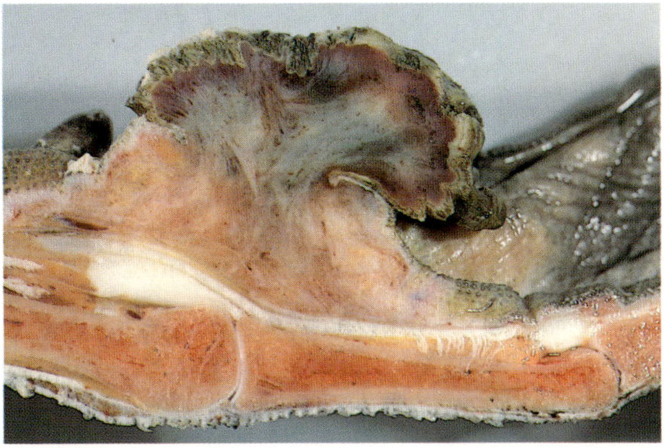

Plate 28 *Lentigo simplex in an orange cat. (See p.395.)*

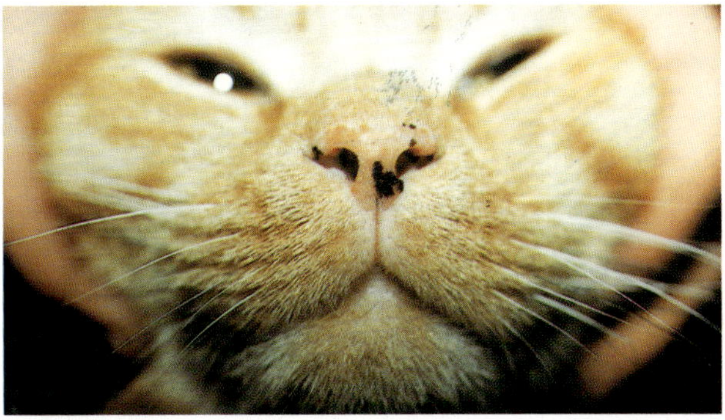

Plate 29 *Colour mutant alopecia in a doberman: (blue doberman syndrome). (See p.395.)*

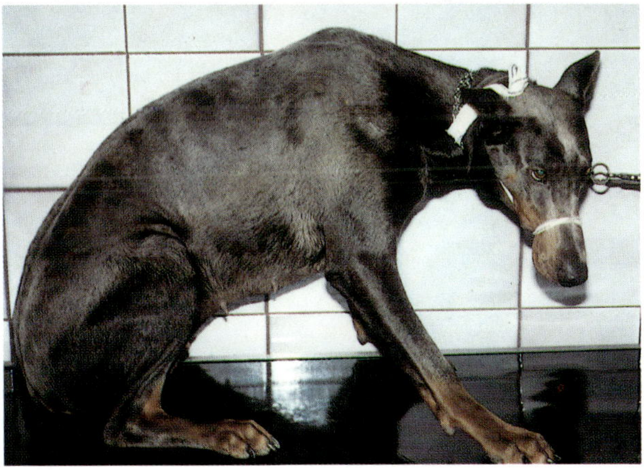

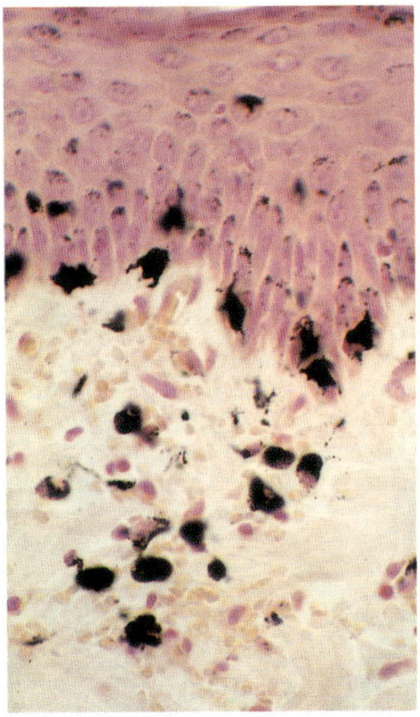

Plate 30 *(Left) Colour mutant alopecia in a doberman: homogeneous distribution of melanocytes, with a melanosomic overload, melanophages, pigmentary incontinence (HE stain × 220). (See p.396.)*

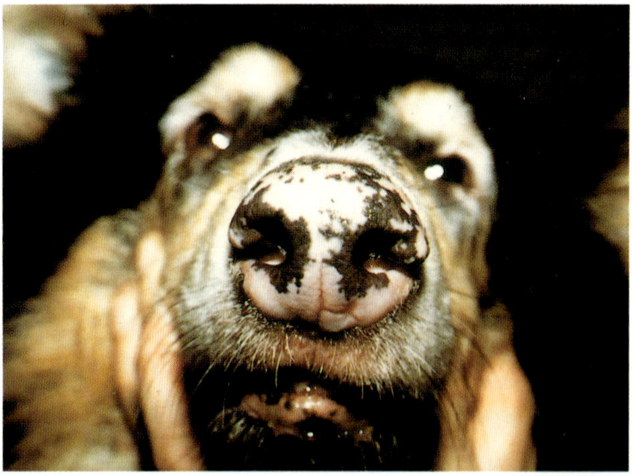

Plate 31 *Vitiligo in a collie: gradual depigmentation of the nose. (See p.398.)*

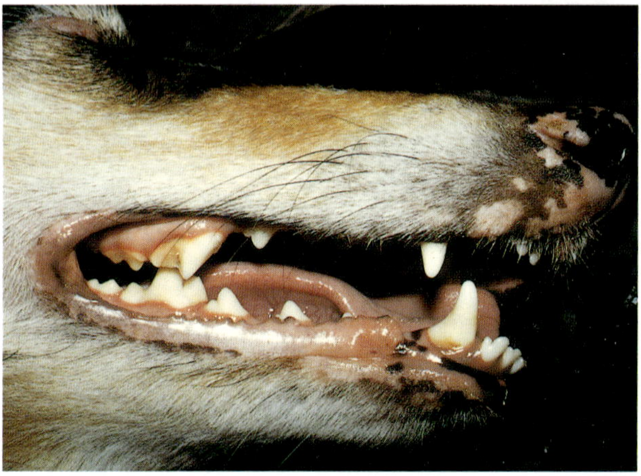

Plate 32 *Vitiligo in a collie: depigmentation of the nose, lips, oral mucosa, eyelids. (See p.398.)*

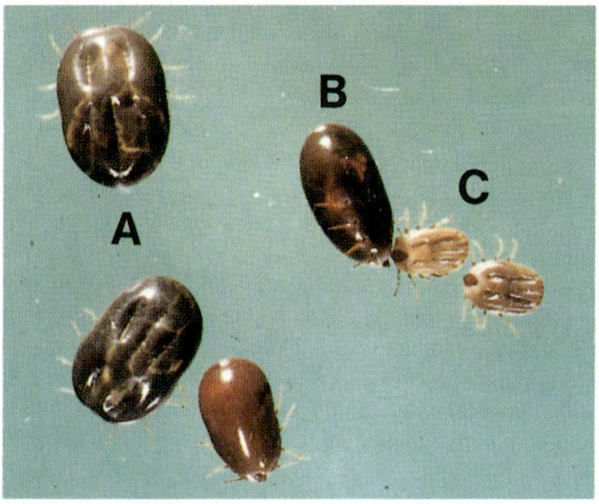

Plate 33 *Examples of types of cattle tick* (Boophilus microplus) *dropped from cattle. A: Fully engorged adult female ticks. B: Damaged adult female ticks. These ticks were damaged by feeding on cattle previously vaccinated with membrane antigens extracted from midguts of ticks. C: Partly fed adult female ticks. (See p.402.)*

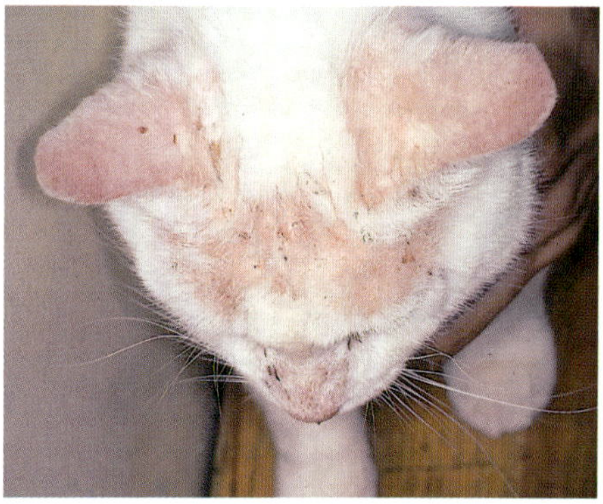

Plate 34 *Castrated male domestic shorthair 2-year-old cat with pruritus, erythema and alopecia of head and ears due to food hypersensitivity. (See p.404.)*

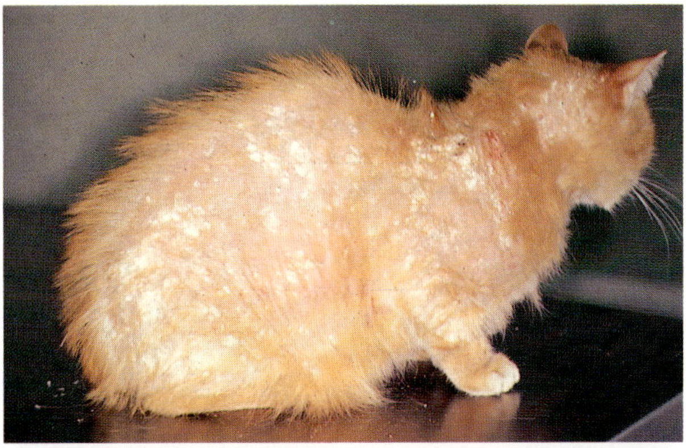

Plate 35 *Castrated male domestic shorthair 12-year-old cat with severe generalized pruritis, alopecia and seborrhoea sicca due to food hypersensitivity. (See p.404.)*

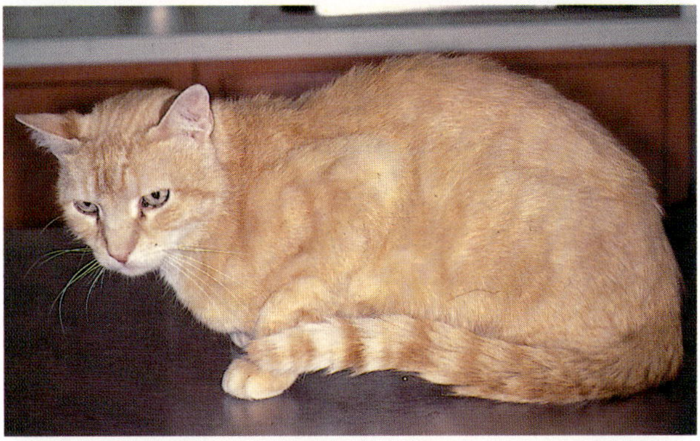

Plate 36 *Same cat as Plate 35, 6 weeks after lamb-based baby food diet. (See p.404.)*

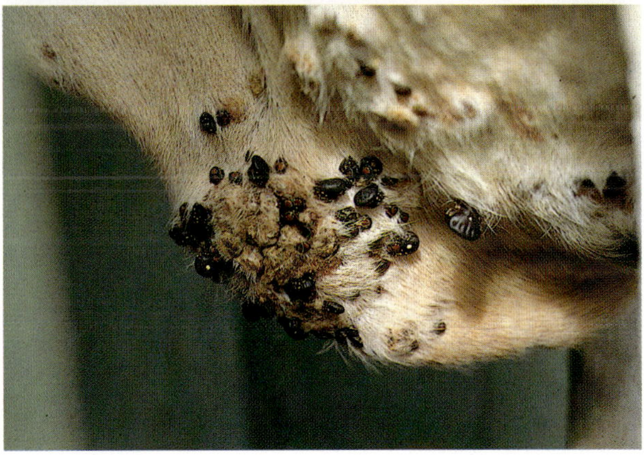

Plate 37 *Chronic skin lesions on the dewlap of a creole cow with* Dermatophilus *infection induced by the mouthparts of ticks. (See p.407.)*

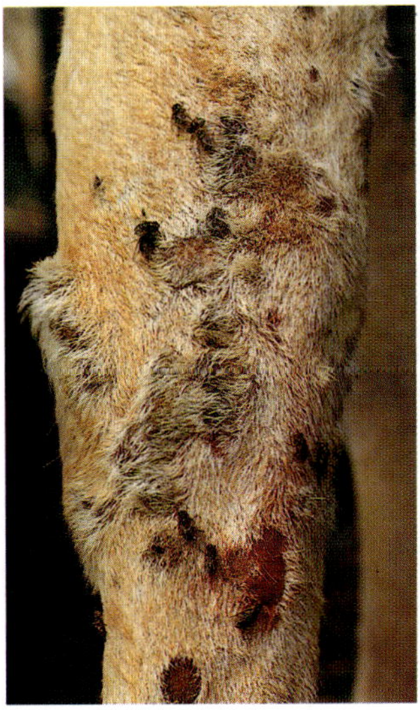

Plate 38 *(Left) Primary lesions of dermatophilosis on the front legs of a brahman heifer at one of the preferential feeding sites of the biting fly* Stomoxys calcitrans. *(See p.407.)*

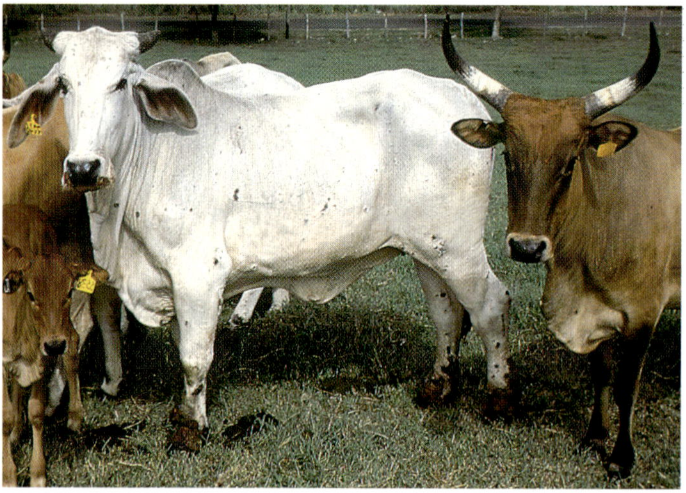

Plate 39 *Brahman herd with skin lesions due to* Dermatophilus congolensis *6 months after import from Martinique; 50% of the animals died. None of the local Zebu cattle had any skin lesions.* *(See p.407.)*

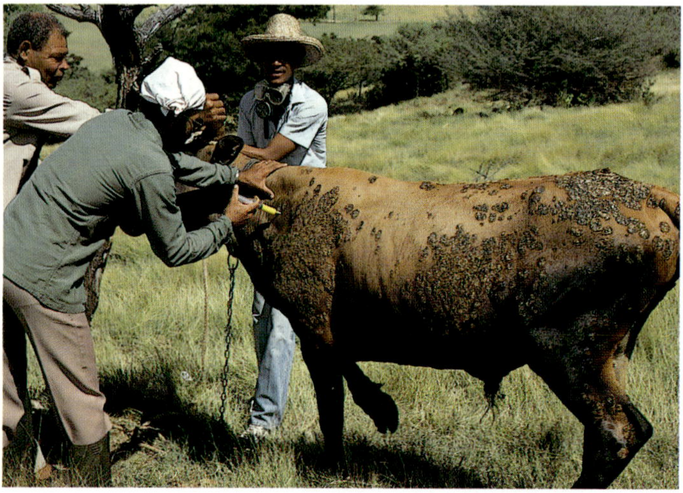

Plate 40 *Bull suffering from* Dermatophilus *infection with severe generalized skin lesions. As experimental infections only induce mild lesions, the factors responsible for severe generalized lesions are unknown.* *(See p.407.)*

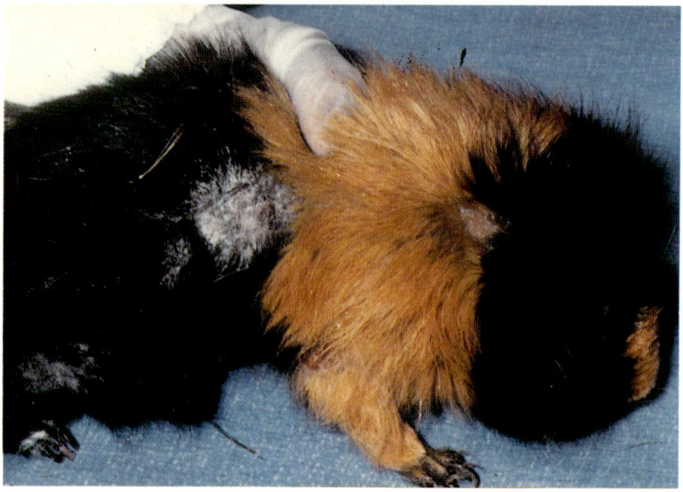

Plate 41 *Patchy alopecia and dermatitis in a guinea pig caused by the mite* Trixacarus caviae. *(See p.424.)*

Plate 42 *Nasal dermatitis in a gerbil associated with lacrimal porphyrin irritation and* Staphylococcus aureus. *(See p.425.)*

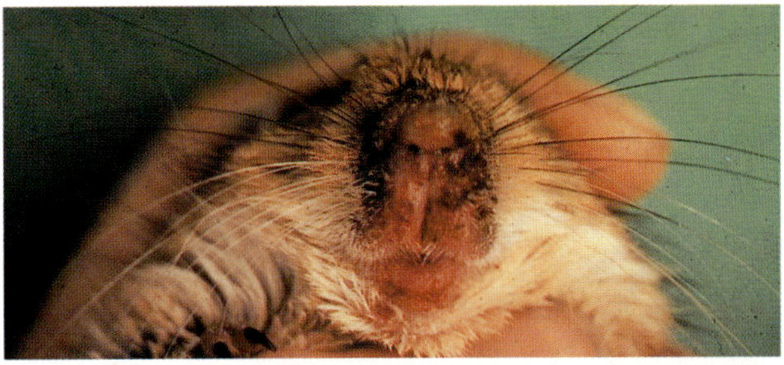

Plate 43 *Ulceration of the ventral scrotum of a German shepherd caused by a fixed-drug eruption due to diethylcarbamazine. (See p.426.)*

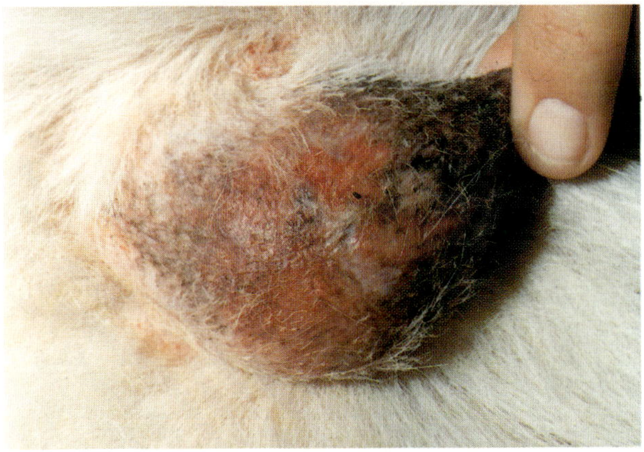

Plate 44 *A Maltese terrier with erythema multiforme manifesting as erythematous macules caused by levamisole. (See p.427.)*

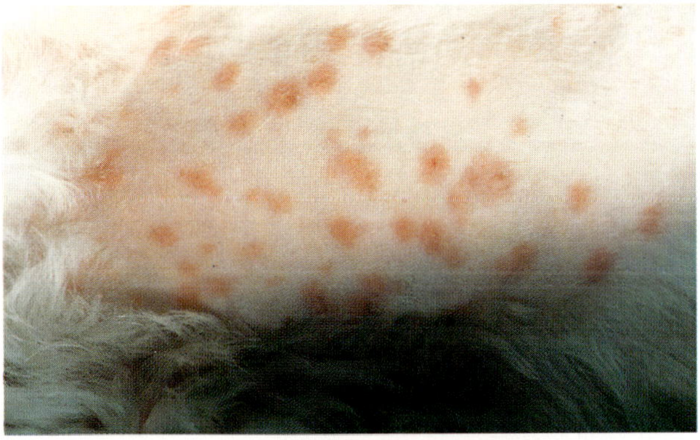

Plate 45 *Adriamycin-caused toxic epidermal necrolysis in a beagle. (See p.428.)*

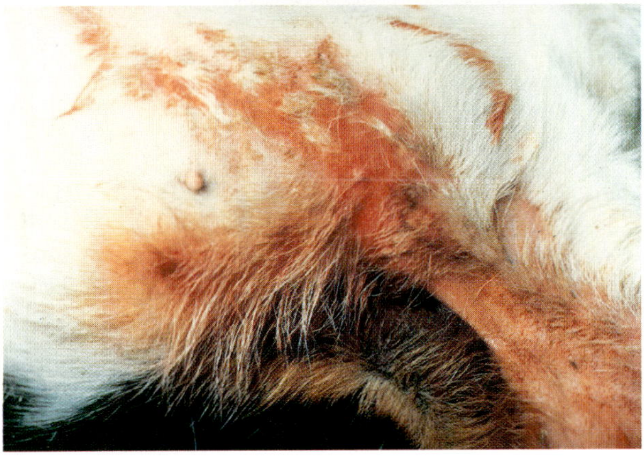

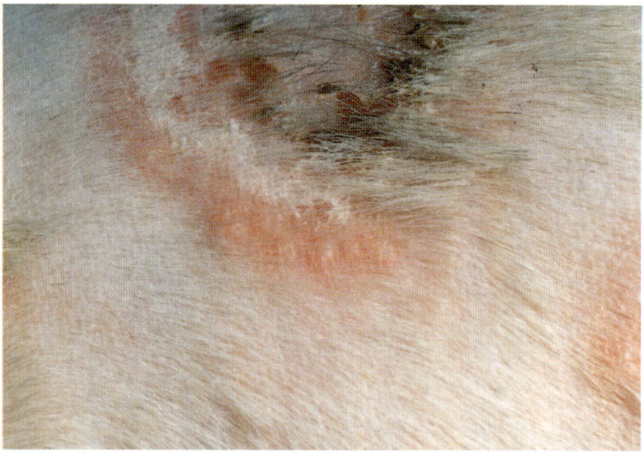

Plate 46 *A pustular eruption resembling pemphigus foliaceus in a cocker spaniel on multiple drug therapy. The eruption resolved on withdrawal of an antibiotic mixture. (See p.429.)*

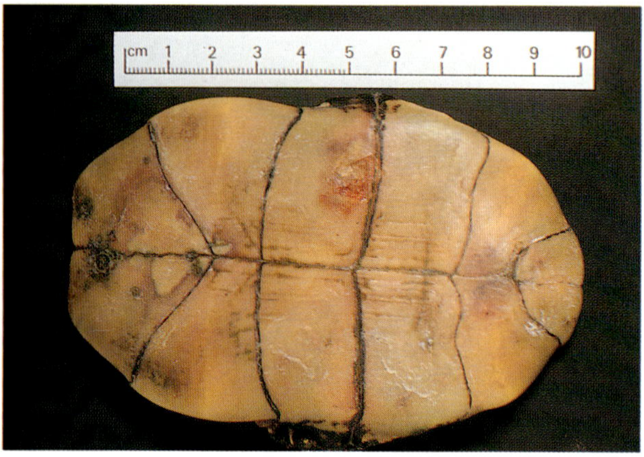

Plate 47 *The 'shell' of a chelonian consists of bone covered by heavily keratinized epithelium. This terrapin* (Emys orbicularis) *shows pitting due to traumatic damage and an area of ulceration and haemorrhage, probably caused by a bacterial infection. (See p.438.)*

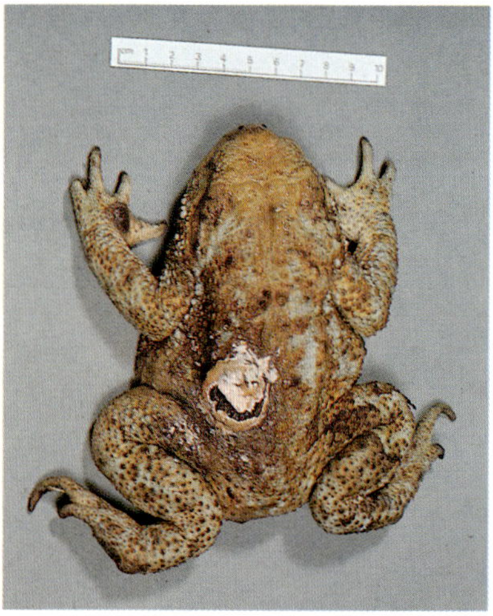

Plate 48 *Fungal lesions are common in amphibians. This toad* (Bufo spinosus) *has a raised fungal granuloma, partly covered with ointment, on its back. The pigmented lesion on the left forefoot is another (early) mycotic focus. (See p.438.)*

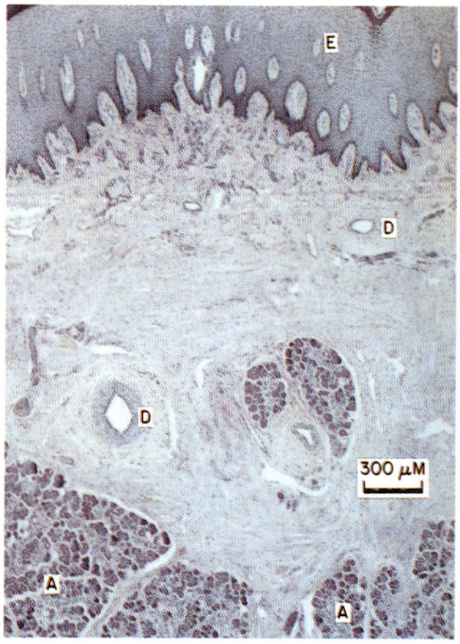

Plate 49 *A section of cow muzzle illustrating mucus-containing dermal acinar glands (A). Sections of the ducts (D) which ultimately penetrate the thick epidermis (E) can be seen (Celestin blue). (See p.229.)*

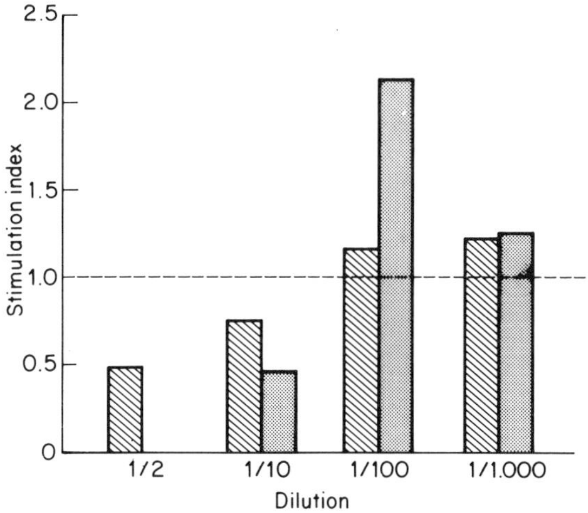

Figure 1 Effect of *D.congolensis*-stimulated MC supernatants derived from infected rats on epidermal proliferation rates in low calcium concentration medium. Stimulation indices were calculated as described in the text (Eq. 2). Striped bars represent non-dialysed and hatched bars dialysed supernatants which were tested at a range of dilutions. All values above 1 indicate significant stimulation and below 1 significant inhibition of proliferation ($p<0.01$). Note that statistical significance refers to the stimulation/inhibition by each supernatant and not to differences between dialysed and non-dialysed supernatants. The results shown were from an assay carried out 24 h after addition of supernatants.

However, the pattern of the response was the reverse of that seen for epidermal cells cultured in low calcium medium. The dialysed supernatants caused significant stimulation of proliferation but at the lower dilutions (the three lower at 24 h and the lowest dilution at 48 h, $p<0.01$) whereas the other dilutions had no effect (48 h results shown in Fig. 2). The non-dialysed supernatants caused significant inhibition at all dilutions although the effect diminished on dilution ($p<0.01$, Fig. 2). A repeat experiment gave similar results.

In contrast, when the MC derived from non-infected rats, *D.congolensis* -stimulated supernatants failed to stimulate epidermal proliferation in low calcium medium, as compared with control supernatants, at any dilution or time with the only significant effect being one of inhibition at the lower dilutions ($p<0.01$, Fig. 3). These results were repeated in a further two experiments, the only exception being very slight but significant stimulation ($SI=1.12$ and $SI=1.10$, $p<0.05$) caused by the two higher dilutions of non-dialysed supernatant in one of the experiments. Likewise, supernatants from non-infected rats caused the same pattern of effects on epidermal cells in normal calcium concentration medium in two identical experiments.

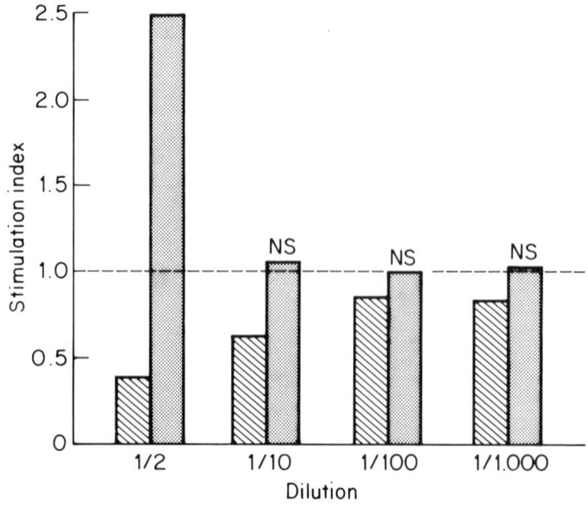

Figure 2 Effect of *D.congolensis*-stimulated MC supernatants derived from infected rats on epidermal proliferation rates in normal calcium concentration medium. For explanation see caption to Fig. 1. NS: not significant. The results shown were from an assay carried out 48 h after addition of supernatants.

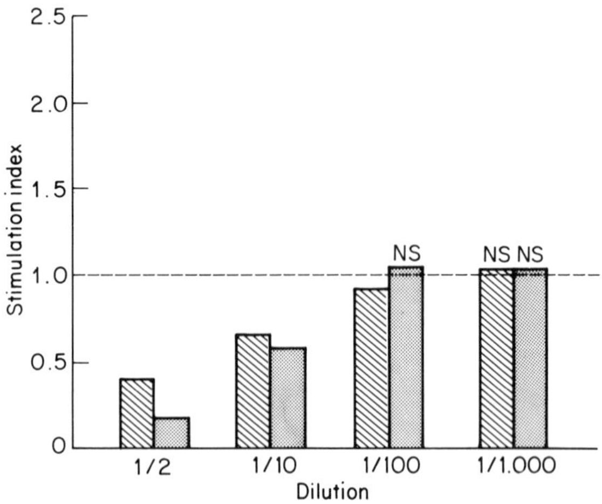

Figure 3 Effect of *D.congolensis*-stimulated MC supernatants derived from non-infected rats on epidermal proliferation rates. For explanation see caption to Fig. 1. NS: not significant. The results shown were from an assay on epidermal cells in low calcium medium carried out 24 h after addition of supernatants.

DISCUSSION

Overall, the results suggest the presence of several factors in the MC supernatants, some of which are stimulatory and others of which are inhibitory to the growth of epidermal cells. Both dialysable and non-dialysable activities were present suggesting molecular weight entities of both below and above 10 000 daltons.

Regardless of their origin, MC supernatants predominantly caused significant stimulation of epidermal proliferation compared with that in medium alone although dialysis removed some of the activity. The stimulation may have been partially due to small molecular weight by-products of MC metabolism creating the well-recognized phenomenon of conditioned-medium growth enhancement (Ling and Kay, 1975). Some of the inhibitory effects observed with the dialysed supernatants at low dilutions may have been caused by larger molecular weight products released from non-viable MC. In addition, the products of *D.congolensis* itself cause inhibition of epidermal cell proliferation as shown by the effect of supernatants produced in the same way as normal but for the absence of MC.

To overcome the problem in interpreting the data caused by such non-specific effects, the results were expressed by comparing the effect of the supernatants deriving from *D.congolensis* -stimulated MC with those deriving from control, non-stimulated MC originating from the same animals. The *D.congolensis* -stimulated supernatants derived from infected rats appeared to contain a preponderance of inhibitory factors for epidermal cells cultured in low calcium concentration medium. Stimulatory factors were also present but only became apparent when the effect of the inhibitory substances had been diluted out. This may reflect different cell surface receptor affinities for the various factors such that the stimulatory factor(s) is recognized by a receptor with a higher affinity than that of the receptor(s) for the inhibitory factor(s). Some of the inhibitory activity was removed by dialysis causing an enhancement of stimulation. Likewise, Krueger and Jederberg (1980) found that MC supernatants were generally inhibitory to HeLa cell proliferation but that dialysis removed some of the inhibition.

Both stimulatory and inhibitory activities were again observed when the same type of supernatants were tested on epidermal cells cultured in normal calcium concentration medium. However, the pattern of response was different from that in low calcium medium with the lower, rather than the higher, dilutions of dialysed supernatants causing stimulation. The epidermal cells may have been responding to different growth-regulating factors in calcium-deficient and in normal calcium level media, or the kinetics of the responses may have been different. Calcium plays a central role in the multitude of growth-related activities; for example, exogenous calcium is essential for the phytohaemagglutinin-induced DNA synthesis by lymphocytes (Whitney and Sutherland, 1972). Since most, if not all, growth factors act via specific cell surface receptors some of the differences in response in low and normal calcium medium may have been caused by the expression of certain receptors being calcium-dependent. Calcium, at a concentration equivalent to that in normal culture medium, can also inhibit the activities of certain factors such as lymphotoxin, a lymphokine which is either growth-inhibitory or cytotoxic depending on its concentration (Okamoto and Mayer, 1978).

Mononuclear cells derived from non-infected rats also produced growth regulatory factors for epidermal cells following *in vitro* stimulation with *D.congolensis*. However, unlike those from infected rats, the predominant effect was one of inhibition of proliferation. That the supernatants of MC from naive rats may affect epidermal cell proliferation might be predicted from the fact that *D.congolensis* cocci do cause a small degree of non-specific stimulation of proliferation of cultured MC; on the other hand, it appears that MC from naive rats may not be stimulated to release lymphokines since their supernatants were found to have no macrophage migration inhibitory activity (Woodman, 1989). One explanation for the strong inhibition of epidermal proliferation by the supernatants of MC from naive rats is that *D.congolensis* cocci have a degree of toxicity for MC (an effect counteracted when the MC derive from infected rats) with the subsequent release of inhibitory breakdown products into the MC culture medium.

The supernatants were not characterized so the growth-regulatory factors remain to be identified by, for example, blocking experiments whereby the effect of the supernatants would be examined following treatment with various antilymphokine monoclonal antibodies. Certain lymphokines are already known to affect *in vitro* epidermal cell growth such as γ interferon which, at high concentrations, causes inhibition (Nickoloff *et al.*, 1984). Interleukin 1 (IL-1), produced by monocytes, may also have been present in the supernatants although the effect it is likely to have had is controversial. Ristow (1987) found that IL-1 caused a three-fold increase in ^{3}H-thymidine uptake by cultured mouse epidermal cells, whereas Morhenn (1988) observed no stimulation. A possible reason for this anomaly could have been interference through the secretion of IL-1 by the epidermal cells themselves since epidermal cell-derived thymocyte activating factor, which acts as an autocrine growth factor (Gilchrest and Sauder, 1984), is identical to IL-1 (Sauder, 1985).

Thus, MC derived from experimentally infected rats stimulated *in vitro* with *D.congolensis* produced both growth-enhancing and growth-inhibitory factors for epidermal cells, the predominant effect being concentration dependent and presumably determined by competition between factors with opposite effects. One can predict that some of these factors would be produced at infection sites and that the net effect of stimulation or inhibition would be a function of the size of the MC infiltrate, the degree of MC activation and the distance of the activated cells from the proliferative cells of the epidermis. Although it is not possible to relate the *in vitro* concentration of growth regulatory factors to that *in vivo*, it is interesting to note that during the course of an experimental infection W3/25 (T-helper) cells were observed immediately underneath and within the epidermis; moreover, the cells were expressing interleukin 2 receptor and Class II molecules (Woodman, 1989). The proximity of these activated cells to the epidermal basal cells suggests that the concentration of any released factors would be relatively high in the locality of the proliferative epidermal cells and furthermore the overriding effect of the MC supernatants, when at the highest concentration, was stimulation of epidermal proliferation at normal calcium levels.

Further work is required to characterize the supernatants and to try and relate the finding to the *in vivo* situation. However, primed and stimulated MC do appear to be able to regulate epidermal growth and may contribute to the transience of *D.congolensis* infections if an activated MC infiltrate did indeed bring about hyperproliferation since the subsequent increased desquamation rate may hinder further invasion. In contrast, one can predict that chronic, generalized infections may result if the MC response is suppressed. This may occur in the presence of the numerous external factors such as high biting arthropod burdens which are associated with the chronic type of infection.

ACKNOWLEDGEMENTS

This work was funded by Edinburgh University and the Overseas Development Administration. The automated cell harvester and liquid scintillation counter were provided by the Wellcome Trust.

REFERENCES

Amakiri, S.F. (1974). Extent of skin penetration by *Dermatophilus congolensis* in bovine streptothricosis. *Tropical Animal Health and Production* **6**: 99–105.

Gilchrest, B.A. and Sauder, D.N. (1984). Autocrine growth stimulation of human keratinocytes by epidermal cell-derived thymocyte activating factor (ETAF). *Journal of Investigative Dermatology* **82**: 439 (abstract).

Hennings, H., Michael D., Cheng, C *et al.* (1980). Calcium regulation of growth and differentiation of mouse epidermal cells in culture. *Cell* **19**: 245–254.

Kappler, J. and Marrack, P. (1986). Lymphokines. In: Weir DM, Herzenberg LA, Blackwell, C. and Herzenberg, L.A. (eds) *Handbook of Experimental Immunology* Volume II: *Cellular Immunology* 4th edn, pp. 59; 1–59; 10. Blackwell Scientific Publications, Oxford.

Krueger, G.G. and Jederberg, W.W. (1980). Alteration of HeLa cell growth equilibrium by supernatants of peripheral blood mononuclear cells from normal and psoriatic subjects. *Journal of Investigative Dermatology* **74**: 148–153.

Ling, N.R. and Kay, J.E. (1975) *Lymphocyte Stimulation*. North Holland Publishing Company, Amsterdam.

Morhenn, V.B. (1988). Keratinocyte proliferation in wound healing and skin diseases. *Immunology Today* **9**: 104–107.

Nickoloff, B.J. Basham, T.Y., Merigan, T.C. and Morhenn, V.B. (1984). Anti-proliferative effects of recombinant and interferons on cultured human keratinocytes. *Laboratory Investigation* **51**: 697–701.

Okamoto, M. and Mayer, M.M. (1978). Studies on the mechanism of action of guinea-pig lymphotoxin II. Increase of calcium uptake rate in lymphotoxin-damaged target cells. *Journal of Immunology* **120**: 279–285.

Ristow, H.J. (1987). A major factor contributing to epidermal proliferation in inflammatory skin diseases appears to be interleukin-1 or a related protein *Proceedings of the National Academy of Science of the USA* **84**: 1940–1944.

Roberts, D.S. (1966). The influence of delayed hypersensitivity on the course of infection with *Dermatophilus congolensis*. *British Journal of Experimental Pathology* **47**: 9–16.

Roberts, D.S. (1967). *Dermatophilus* infection. *Veterinary Bulletin* **37**: 513–521.

Sauder, D.N. (1985). Biologic properties of epidermal cell thymocyte activating factor (ETAF). *Journal of Investigative Dermatology* **85** (suppl. 1): 176–182.

Sohnle, P.G. and Kirkpatrick, C.H. (1978). Epidermal proliferation in the defence against experimental cutaneous candidiasis. *Journal of Investigative Dermatology* **70**: 130–133.

Sohnle, P.G., Frank, M.M. and Kirkpatrick, C.H. (1976). Mechanisms involved in elimination of organisms from experimental cutaneous *Candida albicans* infections in guinea-pigs. *Journal of Immunology* **117**: 523–530.

Tagami, H. (1985). Epidermal cell proliferation in guinea-pigs with experimental dermatophytosis. *Journal of Investigative Dermatology* **85**: 153–155.

Whitney, R.B. and Sutherland, R.M. (1972). Requirement for calcium ions in lymphocyte transformation stimulation by phytohaemagglutinin. *Journal of Cell Physiology* **80**: 329–337.

Woodman, J.P. (1989). The cell-mediated immune response in epidermal defence against *Dermatophilus congolensis*. PhD thesis, University of Edinburgh.

Zlotnik, I. (1955). Cutaneous streptothricosis in cattle. *Veterinary Record* **67**: 613–614.

3.5 Eicosanoid Levels in Canine Inflammatory Skin Diseases

Manfred Kietzmann

Department of Pharmacology, Toxicology and Pharmacy
School of Veterinary Medicine
Hannover, FRG

INTRODUCTION

The past years have witnessed major advances in the knowledge of eicosanoids. Prostaglandins and leukotrienes play a major role in inflammatory mechanisms. Like other mediators, eicosanoids are involved in reactions like vasodilatation, vasoconstriction, platelet aggregation, chemotaxis and pyrexia (Greaves *et al.*, 1971; Ruzicka and Printz, 1982; Duell and Vorhees, 1983; Vorhees, 1983; Camp *et al.*, 1984; Kragballe and Vorhees, 1984; Ruzicka *et al.*, 1986). Interactions between different mediators are complicating the understanding of the pathophysiology of inflammatory reactions. Increasing effort to elucidate molecular mechanisms in skin disorders, i.e. the pathophysiology of inflammatory diseases, is leading to therapeutic consequences.

Skin irritation induces the release of arachidonic acid from biomembranes. The reaction is catalysed by phospholipase A_2. While biomembrane bound arachidonic acid cannot be metabolized, the free acid is rapidly converted by cyclooxygenase or lipoxygenases (Brain and Williams, 1989). Products of the cyclooxygenase pathway are prostaglandins, prostacyclin and thromboxanes. Hydroperoxyeicosatetraenoic acids, hydroxyeicosatetraenoic acids and leukotrienes are products of the lipoxygenase pathway. Leukotriene B_4 (LTB_4) and the peptidoleukotrienes leukotriene $C_4/D_4/E_4$ ($LTC_4/D_4/E_4$) are 5-lipoxygenase products. Prostaglandins and leukotrienes are involved in the regulation of keratinocyte proliferation; LTB_4 is known as a stimulator of epidermal cell growth (Kragballe *et al.*, 1985). Measured in human beings, eicosanoid concentrations are altered in various skin disorders (Greaves, 1987). Cyclooxygenase and lipoxygenase products found in inflamed human skin are listed in Table 1. Information about eicosanoid levels in canine skin is lacking. The present study was performed to measure the concentration of prostaglandin E_2 (PGE_2) as well as of LTB_4 and $LTC_4/D_4/E_4$ in canine skin. Additionally, ornithine decarboxylase activity was measured and thymidine triphosphate, histidine and leucine incorporation into the epidermis determined.

Table 1 Lipoxygenase and cyclooxygenase products increased in inflamed human skin (Greaves, 1987)

Disease	Lipoxygenase products
Psoriasis	LTB_4, 12-HETE, PGE_2
Allergic contact dermatitis	LTB_4, PGE_2, $PGF_{4\alpha}$
Eosinophilic cellulitis	LTB_4, LTC_4/D_4
Urticaria	PGD_2
UVA-erythema	12-HETE, PGE_2, PGD_2, 6-keto-$PGF_{1\alpha}$
UVC-erythema	PGE_2, PGD_2, $PGF_{2\alpha}$, 6-keto-$PGF_{1\alpha}$
UVC-erythema	PGE_2, $PGF_{2\alpha}$

MATERIALS AND METHODS

Skin samples (biopsies) were taken from various body regions in female and male dogs (different breeds) after clinical examination. The controls were 18 healthy dogs. The study included 22 cases of pyoderma, 15 cases of seborrhoea, five cases of atopic dermatitis, three cases of flea allergy dermatitis and four cases of skin disease caused by hypothyroidism. The diagnosis based on clinical, histopathological and laboratory examinations.

Samples were immediately frozen (−196°C) in an EDTA buffer with addition of indomethacin. Using the EDTA buffer, epidermis was dissected from the dermis according to Lubach and Kietzmann (1988). Thereafter the epidermis was homogenized (Ultra Turrax) and centrifuged (2000 ***g***, 15 min, 4°C). The eicosanoids were extracted from the supernatant by solid phase extraction with octadecyl reversed-phase columns. The extract was dried in a stream of nitrogen. Using specific antibodies, PGE_2, LTB_4 and $LTC_4/D_4/E_4$ were measured by radioimmunoassay with appropriate RIA kits (Amersham, Braunschweig, FRG). For measurement of the ornithine decarboxylase activity (ODC), the determination of $^{14}CO_2$-release from ^{14}C-ornithine hydrochloride was used. The incorporation rate of thymidine triphosphate into DNA as well as that of leucine and histidine into protein was determined using labelled precursors. The thymidine triphosphate incorporation was used as a parameter for the DNA polymerase activity. Leucine, incorporated predominantly into basal epidermal layer proteins, represents the metabolism of proliferating cells. Histidine, which is incorporated into upper epidermal layer proteins, is used as a parameter of keratinocyte differentiation.

RESULTS

Table 2 shows the results (mean ± SD) measured in controls. Figures 1 and 2 represents the parameter ranges in dogs with pyoderma and seborrhoea. The first and the third quartile are shown. The range of the first to the third quartile includes 50% of the measured data. The second quartile is identical with the median value. Because of the limited number of cases, in Figs 3 and 4 the minimal, median and maximal values found in dogs with atopic dermatitis and hypothyreoidism are shown. Table 3 summarizes the results.

Compared with controls, changes in skin from dogs with pyoderma (n = 22) are presented in Fig. 1. An enhanced concentration of PGE_2 and LTB_4 was detected. A slight increase of the thymidine triphosphate and histidine incorporation rate was found in a few animals.

In seborrhoeic dogs (n = 15) an enhanced LTB_4 concentration was observed; $LTC_4/D_4/E_4$ concentration was diminished (Fig. 2).

Dogs with atopic dermatitis (n = 5) showed a diminished leukotriene concentration (Fig. 3); however, some of these may have been pretreated with glucocorticoids. Therefore an additional controlled study will be started to examine changes of eicosanoids in dogs with atopic dermatitis as well as effects of glucocorticoid treatment in these dogs. A slightly enhanced incorporation rate of thymidine triphosphate into DNA and of histidine into protein was found in some animals.

In three dogs with flea allergy dermatitis there were no obvious changes.

Table 2 Concentration of PGE_2, LTB_4 and $LTC_4/D_4/E_4$, thymidine triphosphate incorporation rate into DNA, ornithine decarboxylase activity as well as leucine and histidine incorporation into protein in epidermal specimens of healthy dogs.

PGE_2	203 ± 64	pg/mg DNA
LTB_4	3.1 ± 2.0	pg/mg DNA
$LTC_4/D_4/E_4$	48.5 ± 18.2	pg/mg DNA
Thymidine triphosphate incorporation rate	215 ± 70	CPM/mg DNA
Ornithine decarboxylase activity	520 ± 107	CPM/mg DNA protein
Leucine incorporation rate	1193 ± 215	CPM/mg DNA protein
Histidine incorporation rate	1206 ± 314	CPM/mg DNA protein

Data are given as mean ± SD of 18 animals.

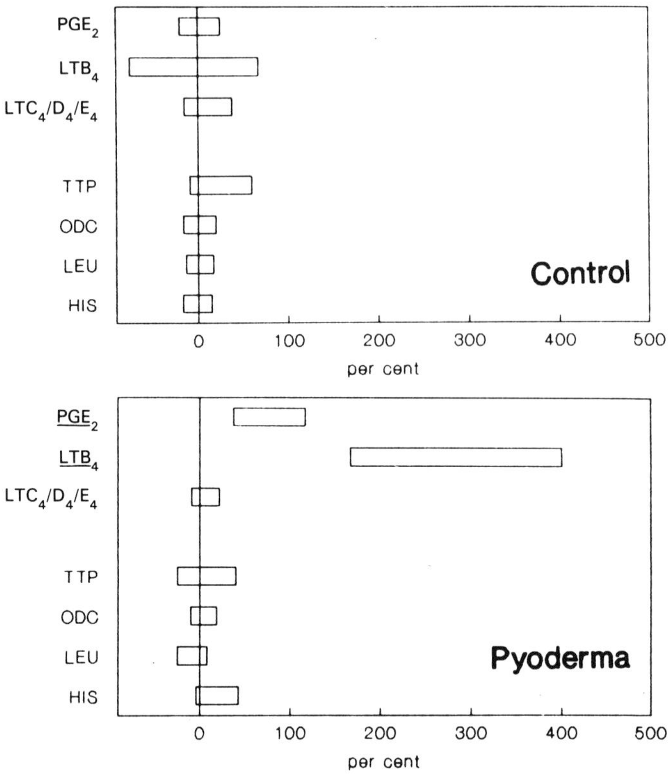

Figure 1 PGE_2, LTB_4 and $LTC_4/D_4/E_4$ concentration, thymidine triphosphate incorporation rate into DNA, ornithine decarboxylase activity as well as leucine and histidine incorporation into protein, measured in skin specimens of dogs with pyoderma (n = 22). Differences are presented in %, compared with controls median (n = 18). The left and the right side of the rectangles present the first and the third quartile.

Hypothyroidism (n = 4) was accompanied by an enhanced LTB_4 concentration, while the $LTC_4/D_4/E_4$ concentration was slightly diminished (Fig. 4). The changes found do not permit any conclusion regarding the involvement of eicosanoids in hypothyreoidism.

The enhanced LTB_4 concentration might be caused by secondary bacterial infection. Additional examinations including also histopathologic evaluations are necessary.

Correlating the measured results and clinical signs, i.e. pruritus, erythema, hyperproliferation (enhanced thymidine triphosphate incorporation), atrophy or hyperpigmentation, the following changes were observed. The PGE_2 concentration was enhanced in erythematous and atrophic skin. Pruritus was associated with an increased concentration of LTB_4, while the $LTC_4/D_4/E_4$ concentration was diminished. An enhanced LTB_4 concentration was mostly

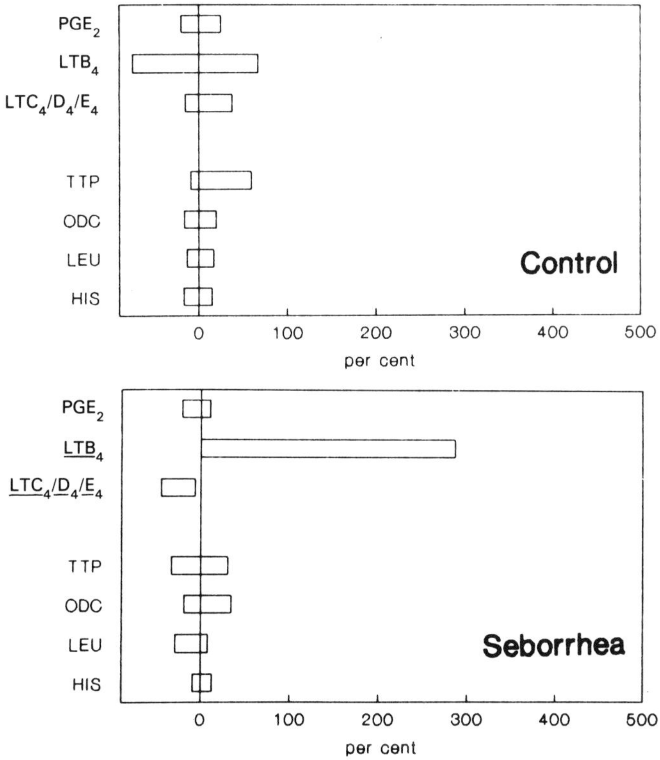

Figure 2 PGE_2, LTB_4 and $LTC_4/D_4/E_4$ concentration, thymidine triphosphate incorporation rate into DNA, ornithine decarboxylase activity as well as leucine and histidine incorporation into protein, measured in skin specimens of dogs with seborrhoea (n = 15). Differences are presented in %, compared with controls median (n = 18). The left and the right side of the rectangles present the first and the third quartile.

accompanied by a slight decrease of the $LTC_4/D_4/E_4$ concentration. An increase of the LTB_4 concentration was also found, when the skin was erythematous, hypertrophic, scaling and hyperpigmented. The ODC activity as well as the thymidine triphosphate incorporation rate were enhanced in hyperkeratotic skin. The leucine incorporation was diminished in hyperpigmentated skin specimens. The incorporation of histidine was increased, when pruritus and/or erythema were obvious.

DISCUSSION

The knowledge about the regulation of epidermal and dermal metabolic reactions by different mediators is essential for a causal treatment of skin

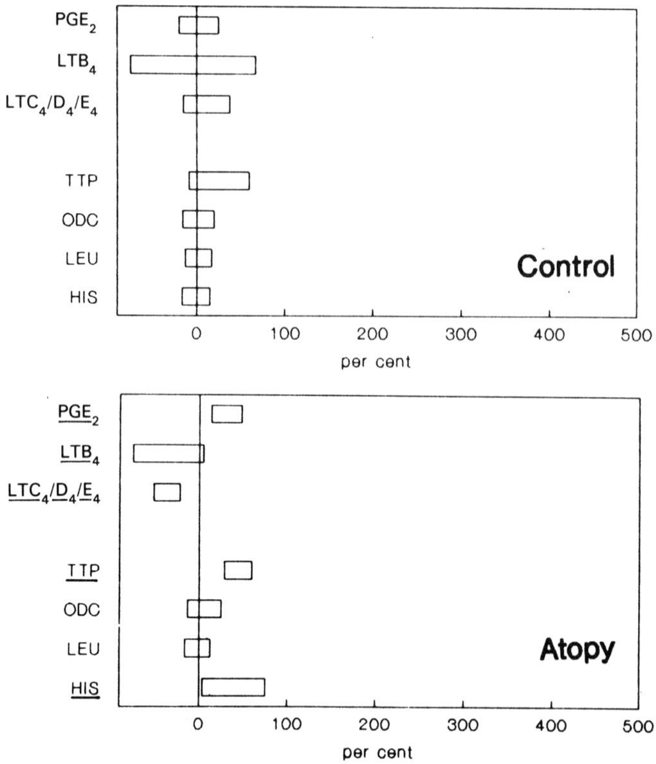

Figure 3 PGE_2, LTB_4 and $LTC_4/D_4/E_4$ concentration, thymidine triphosphate incorporation rate into DNA, ornithine decarboxylase activity as well as leucine and histidine incorporation into protein, measured in skin specimens of dogs with atopic dermatitis (n = 5). Differences are presented in %, compared with controls median (n = 18). The left and the right side of the rectangles present the minimal and the maximal value.

diseases. Eicosanoids seem to be important mediators in the regulation of epidermal proliferation and differentiation (Ziboh and Lord, 1979; Ziboh *et al.*, 1984a,b; Kietzmann *et al.*, 1988; Kietzmann and Lubach, 1989). The study described was performed to investigate changes in eicosanoid concentrations in canine skin with dermatological disease.

The preliminary results presented show that changes in cutaneous levels of LTB_4 seem to be associated with various skin disorders (like atopic dermatitis or seborrhoea). Because 5-lipoxygenase products are most likely secreted by leukocytes, the increase of LTB_4 measured in the epidermis of dogs with hypothyroidism might be caused by secondary bacterial infection with leukocyte infiltration. Additional studies including histopathologic evaluation are necessary to compare the eicosanoid concentration in hypothyroidism with and without secondary bacterial infection. The LTB_4 concentration was

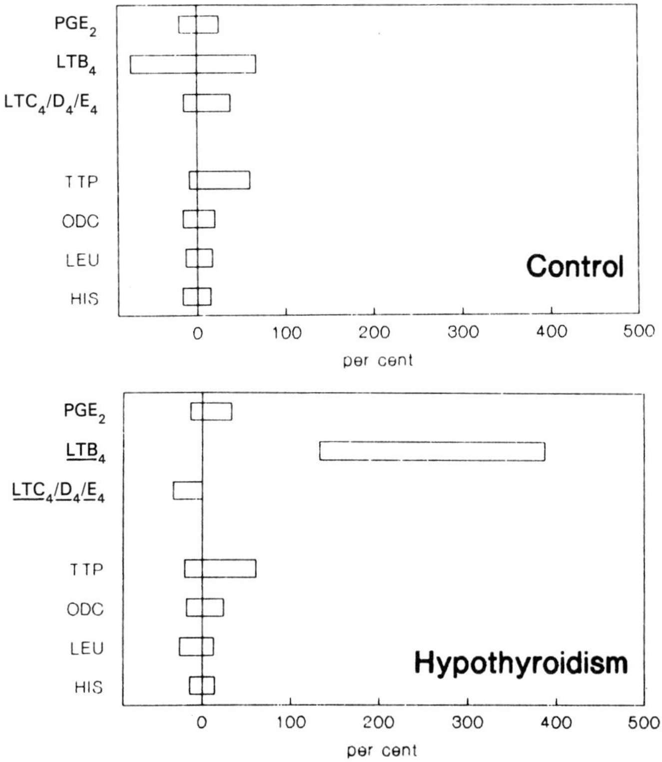

Figure 4 PGE_2, LTB_4 and $LTC_4/D_4/E_4$ concentration, thymidine triphosphate incorporation rate into DNA, ornithine decarboxylase activity as well as leucine and histidine incorporation into protein, measured in skin specimens of dogs with hypothyroidism (n = 4). Differences are presented in %, compared with controls median (n = 18). The left and the right side of the rectangles present the minimal and the maximal value.

Table 3 Summary of changes found in skin disorders in comparison to controls

	PGE_2	LTB_4	$LTC_4/D_4/E_4$	TTP	ODC	LEU	HIS
Pruritus		+	−				+
Erythema	+	+					+
Hyperproliferation		+		+	+		
Atrophy	+						
Hyperpigmentation		+				−	
Pyoderma	+	+					
Seborroea		+	−				
Atopic dermatitis		−	−	+			+
Hypothyroidism		+	−				

(+: increase, −: decrease)

enhanced in pruritic, erythematous and hyperproliferative skin. The concentration of peptidoleukotrienes was decreased in pruritic skin. The concentration of PGE_2 was enhanced in clinically atrophic skin. From these findings it is simple to conclude that a hyperproliferation is accompanied by an enhanced LTB_4 concentration. Calculating a ratio LTB_4/PGE_2, a ten-fold increase was registered in hyperproliferation. Further studies are necessary to investigate the hypothesis that this ratio can be a suitable parameter to characterize the proliferative epidermal state. From studies in cultured human keratinocytes it is known that LTB_4 enhances keratinocyte proliferation (Kragballe *et al.*, 1985). In psoriatic skin of human beings an increase of lipoxygenase products is measurable (Brain and Williams, 1989). Therefore it is simple to conclude that lipoxygenase products may play a role in hyperproliferative skin diseases. It is to confine that other mediators, like cytokines, are yet involved in regulatory processes of keratinocyte proliferation and differentiation.

The incorporation of thymidine triphosphate into DNA, measured simultaneously, was increased in the hypertrophic and scaling canine skin confirming results of Baker and Maibach (1987). A decrease of the thymidine incorporation rate was found in clinically obvious atrophic skin. The measured changes confirm results of studies in laboratory animals (Lubach and Kietzmann, 1988; Kietzmann and Lubach, 1989). Based on experimental studies, it was therefore concluded that the thymidine triphosphate incorporation rate is a suitable parameter to elucidate the proliferative state of the epidermis. Additionally to histometric studies the thymidine triphosphate incorporation rate is used to characterize the postmitotic lifespan of keratinocytes. This enables a distinction between hyperplasia caused by hyperproliferation or hyperplasia caused by retention of keratinocytes. An enhanced cell turnover is found in hyperproliferative epidermis, resulting in so-called proliferation hyperplasia (Lubach and Kietzmann, 1988). For example, proliferation hyperplasia is found in experimentally irritated skin (Kietzmann and Lubach, 1989). In contrast, a prolonged postmitotic keratinocyte lifespan causes an hyperplasia, when the cell proliferation remains unchanged. This so-called retention hyperplasia is induced by different agents like benzoyl peroxide, sulphur or minoxidil (Kietzmann *et al.*, 1990).

The ODC activity is enhanced in various proliferative states. The enzyme is involved in the ornithine metabolism. Reaction products are the polyamines putrescine, spermidine and spermine (Lowe, 1980). ODC activity and polyamine concentration are correlated with the continuous growth of cells. Skin irritation induces an increase of epidermal ODC activity and polyamine concentration, resulting in enhanced mitotic activity (Kietzmman *et al.*, 1988; Kietzmann and Lubach, 1989). Confirming this, an enhanced ODC activity was measurable in hyperproliferative dog skin.

From histoautoradiographic studies it is known (Fukuyama and Epstein, 1968; Kietzmann *et al.*, 1990) that leucine is incorporated predominantly in basal epidermal cells, while histidine incorporation is localized in upper epidermal layers (granular layer). Therefore Freinkel and Wier (1975) used the incorporation rates of these amino acids to characterize epidermal proliferation (leucine) and differentiation (histidine). In skin specimens of atopic dogs (atopic dermatitis, pruritus and erythema) an enhanced histidine incorporation rate was found. A decrease of the leucine incorporation was demonstrated in clinically obvious hyperpigmentation.

In conclusion, eicosanoids are involved in various canine skin diseases. This demonstrates also the efficacy of glucocorticoids in dermatological therapy (Greaves, 1987). Glucocorticoids, inhibiting phospholipase A_2 and causing a diminished epidermal eicosanoid concentration, are the most frequently used and prescribed drugs for dermatological therapy. Studies have been started to elucidate the efficacy of 5-lipoxygenase inhibitors or leukotriene antagonists in the treatment of skin disorders, which are accompanied by an increase in the concentration of lipoxygenase products. Investigations, concerning the role of eicosanoids in skin pathophysiology and pharmacology, include also the non-steroidal antiinflammatory drugs (inhibitors of cyclooxygenase) as well as the search for dermatocorticoids with a minimum of side-effects.

REFERENCES

Baker, B.B. and Maibach, H.J. (1987). Epidermal cell renewal in seborrhoic skin of dogs. *American Journal of Veterinary Research* **48**: 726–728.

Brain, S.D and Williams, T.J. (1989). Prostaglandins, leukotrienes, related compounds and their inhibitors. In: Greaves, M.W., and Shuster, S. (eds) *Pharmacology of the Skin I: Handbook of Experimental Pharmacology*, Vol. 87/I, pp. 347-366. Springer Verlag, Berlin.

Camp, R., Jones, R.R., Brain, S., Woollard, P. and Greaves, M.W. (1984). Production of intraepidermal microabscesses by topical application of leukotriene B_4. *Journal of Investigative Dermatology* **82**: 202–204.

Duell, E.A. and Vorhees, J.J. (1983). Control of epidermal growth. In: Goldsmith, L.A. (ed) *Biochemistry and Physiology of the Skin*, pp. 241-268. Oxford University Press, Oxford.

Freinkel, R.K. and Wier, K.A. (1975). Changing patterns of incorporation of ^{14}C-histidine and ^{3}H-leucine into epidermal proteins during differentiation of fetal rat skin. *Journal of Investigative Dermatology* **65**: 482–487.

Fukuyama, K. and Epstein, W.L. (1968). Epidermal keratinisation: Localisation of isotopically labelled amino acids. *Journal of Investigative Dermatology* **47**: 551-560.

Greaves, M.W., Sondergaard, J. and McDonald-Gibson, W. (1971). Recovery of PGs in human cutaneous inflammation. *British Medical Journal* **2**: 258–260.

Greaves, M.W. (1987). Pharmacology and significance of nonsteroidal anti-inflammatory drugs in the treatment of skin diseases. *Journal of the American Academy of Dermatology* **16**: 751-764.

Kietzmann, M. and Lubach, D. (1989). Epidermal effects of etretinate, diflorasone and cyclosporin A after different skin irritations. *Naunyn Schmiedeberg's Archives of Pharmacology* **339** (Suppl): R9.

Kietzmann, M., Lubach, D. and Heynck, L. (1988). Prostaglandins, leukotrienes and polyamines in mechanically irritated skin. In: Simon, F. (ed) *Veterinary*

Pharmacology, Toxicology and Therapy in Food Producing Animals Vol. I, p. 24. (Abstracts of the 4th EAVPT Congress, Budapest).

Kietzmann, M., Bigler, B., von Tscharner, C., Heitmann, H. and Müther, T. (1990). Untersuchungen zur Verträglichkeit, Wirkung im epidermalen Stoffwechsel und Metabolisierung von Benzoylperoxid beim Hund. *Kleintierpraxis* **35**: 31-34.

Kragballe, K. and Vorhees, J.J. (1984). Modulation of epidermal cell division and growth by oxygenation products of arachidonic acid. *Journal of Allergy and Clinical Immunology* **74**: 426-429.

Kragballe, K. Desjarlais, L. and Vorhees, J.J. (1985). Leukotrienes B_4, C_4 and D_4 stimulate DNA synthesis in cultured human epidermal keratinocytes. *British Journal of Dermatology* **113**: 43-52.

Lowe, N.J. (1980). Epidermal ornithine decarboxylase, polyamines cell proliferation and tumour promotion. *Archives of Dermatology* **116**: 822-825.

Lubach, D., Kietzmann, M. (1988). Effects of etretinate in epidermal metabolism and histology after abrasion of superficial layers (mouse tail assay). *Arzneimittelforschung (Drug Research)* **38**: 54-59.

Ruzicka, T. and Printz, M.P. (1982). Arachidonic acid metabolism in skin: A review. *Reviews of Physiology, Biochemistry and Pharmcacology* **100**: 121-160.

Ruzicka, T., Simmer, T., Peskar, B.A. and Ring, J. (1986). Skin levels of arachidonic acid-derived inflammatory mediators and histamine in atopic Dermatitis. *Journal of Investigative Dermatology* **86**: 105-108.

Vorhees, J.J. (1983). Leukotrienes and other lipoxygenase products in the pathogenesis and therapy of psoriasis and other dermatoses. *Archives of Dermatology* **119**: 541-547.

Ziboh, V.A. and Lord, J.T. (1979). Phospholipase A activity in the skin — modulators of arachidonic acid release from phosphatidylcholine. *Biochemical Journal* **184**: 283-290.

Ziboh, V.A., Casebolt, T.L., Marcelo, C.L. and Vorhees, J.J. (1984a). Lipoxygenation of arachidonic acid by subcellular preparations from murine keratinocytes. *Journal of Investigative Dermatology* **83**: 248-251.

Ziboh, V.A., Casebolt, T.L., Marcelo, C.L. and Vorhees, J.J. (1984b). Biosynthesis of lipoxygenase products by enzyme preparations from normal and psoriatic skin. *Journal of Investigative Dermatology* **83**: 426-430.

3.6 Effects of the S_2-Antagonist Ketanserin on Wound Repair in Horses

K. Vlaminck

Janssen Pharmaceutica NV, Beerse, Belgium

INTRODUCTION

Wound healing is a biological event, part of the general repair processes necessary for the survival of the individual. Although the wound healing process has a basically similar pattern in all mammals, there are some species peculiarities. Specific for horses is the easy formation of exuberant granulation tissue (Silver, 1982). The aim of this study was to evaluate the effect of ketanserin on the wound healing process in horses, especially on the incidence of formation of exuberant granulation tissue.

PROFILE OF THE COMPOUND

Ketanserin, a quinazolinedione derivative, is a potent and selective serotonin$_2$-antagonist. It has also weak α_1-adrenergic and histamine-$_1$ antagonistic properties (Van Nueten *et al* 1987). It has no antibacterial activity *in vitro* (Van Cutsem, 1985). On the basis of acute, subacute and chronic toxicity studies, ketanserin may be considered a safe drug. It is also devoid of teratogenic, mutagenic or carcinogenic effects. No dermal irritation or skin sensitization has been observed after topical application. Ketanserin is primarily a serotonin$_2$-antagonist and influences wound healing by its effect on microcirculation, fibroblasts and probably also interferon-γ. Ketanserin antagonizes serotonin-induced vasoconstriction of the blood vessels, inhibits platelet activation and aggregation as well as the release of platelet derived mediators and it decreases the vascular permeability and the accumulation of fibrinogen in the interstital fluid (Van Neuten *et al.*, 1987). As a result of this effect on microcirculation, the oxygen and nutrient supply to the lesion increases.

An *in vitro* study with human dermal fibroblasts revealed a stimulatory effect of ketanserin on the m-RNA steady state level of collagen type I and III (Kellens *et al.*, 1988). In a sponge granuloma model a biphasic effect was observed. First a stimulation of the cellular infiltration and the collagen content of the sponges was noted, and after 8 days the collagen content was stabilized. Due to its effects on dermal collagen, ketanserin can contribute to the rapid formation of healthy, non-exuberant granulation tissue (Plate 22).

A study in murine bone marrow macrophages revealed that ketanserin increases the capability of these macrophages to participate in the immune response as antigen presenting cells by inhibition of the negative modulation induced by interferon-γ (Sternberg *et al.*, 1986).

A pharmacokinetic study in two wounded horses demonstrated that the plasma levels of ketanserin remained mostly below the HPLC-detection limit (1 ng/ml) after topical application of a 0.25% gel twice daily during 3 weeks. One lesion was located on the elbow and had a surface of 19 cm^2. The other was located dorsally on the tarsal joint and had a surface of 62 cm^2 (Vlaminck *et al.*, 1988b).

MATERIALS AND METHODS

The therapeutic trials in wounded horses were open studies. They included hospitalized horses as well as horses treated under field conditions. In the hospitalized horses usual wound management was kept unchanged, except for the fact that a 0.25% ketanserin gel was applied as topical therapy. Under field conditions ketanserin 0.25% gel was applied twice daily, mostly on open wounds. Fresh as well as old lesions were included. Most lesions were located on the legs of the horses, as the tendency of proud flesh formation is the strongest in these lesions.

RESULTS

The trials in hospitalized horses are summarized in Table 1. All lesions were located distally on the legs, from the carpal and tarsal joints onwards.

From these trials it appeared (Keller, 1987; Stornetta and Diehl, 1987):

1. that the 0.25% ketanserin gel seemed to influence the aspect of the granulation tissue: it became red, regular and finely granular;
2. that based on the clinical experience of the investigation at the veterinary faculty there was no obvious effect on the rate of epithelization;
3. the most prominent effects were noted when the gel was applied daily, without wound dressing.

Table 1 Efficacy of 0.25% gel in wound management in hospitalized horses

	University of Berlin Prof. H. Keller	University of Bern Dr M. Diehl
Number of horses	7	18
Type of lesions	old natural (4) surgical (3)	old natural
Location of lesions	distal on legs	distal on legs
Application of 0.25% gel	daily, 3 x/week (2) 3 x/week (5)	1-2 x/day
Duration of treatment (days)	natural wounds: 15-103	natural wounds: 9-78
Wound dressings	yes	no
Observations	healthy, fine, regular granulation tissue, when daily application no effect on epithelization rate	intensive red colour less exudation inhibition of formation of excessive granulation tissue no effect on epithelization rate no infection

In view of these results the participants in the field trials were advised to treat the lesions, whenever possible and advisable, as open wounds and to apply the gel twice daily after rinsing the lesions. The results of these trials (Table 2) confirmed the effect of ketanserin 0.25% gel on granulation tissue: it had a red, regular and finely granular aspect with a very low incidence of formation of exuberant granulation tissue. No topical or systemic adverse reactions due to ketanserin 0.25% gel were observed. No incompatibility with commonly used disinfectants, penicillin and sulphonamide preparations was noted (Vlaminck and Dony, 1987; Vlaminck *et al.*, 1988a,b).

DISCUSSION

Wound healing proceeds essentially in three phases. First there is the initial lag phase during which the organism reacts with vasoconstriction and blood clotting, followed by an inflammatory reaction, and the start of formation of granulation tissue and epithelization.

This phase is followed by the phase of wound contraction and remodelling. In the horse, the formation of excessive granulation tissue is a major problem. Finally the phase of epithelialization results in closure of the lesion (Jacobs, 1986).

Table 2 Efficacy of 0.25% gel in wound management in horses under field conditions

	Belgium	Multicentre
Number of horses	91	62
Type of lesions	13 days old (< 1–1460) natural	fresh, old, natural
Location of lesions	legs (77%)	legs (74%)
Application of 0.25% gel	2 x/day	2 x/day at renewal of wound dressing
Wound dressings	no	no (71%) yes (29%)
Concomitant treatment	no	no (62%) yes (38%)
Duration of treatment (days)	42	15
Median extremes	5–247	8–39
Evaluation excellent/good	87.8%	90%
Observations	uneventful wound healing short initial period of exudation, later dry aspect and marked red color low incidence of excessive granulation tissue (5.5%)	uneventful wound healing low incidence of excessive granulation tissue (4%) aspect of scar esthetically good (86%)

Thanks to its pharmacological properties ketanserin can influence the wound healing process during the intitial lag phase by reactivating the microcirculation and decreasing the vascular permeability. In addition, ketanserin increases the oxygen and nutrient supply to the lesion. During the phase of wound contraction ketanserin can promote the formation of healthy non-exuberant granulation tissue through its effect on fibroblasts and dermal collagen. During the epithelialization phase no direct effect of ketanserin can be expected.

From the therapeutic trials it appeared that the most prominent feature of the application of the 0.25% ketanserin gel was its effect on granulation tissue. As the formation of excessive granulation tissue is a major problem in wound healing in horses, this property of ketanserin constitutes a major advantage. No adverse effects due to the application of ketanserin 0.25% gel were observed during the therapeutic trials. Nor was there any incompatibility with commonly used disinfectants, antibiotics or chemotherapeutics.

It can be concluded that the ketanserin 0.25% gel is a safe, well-tolerated product which can bring a major advantage in wound management in horses.

REFERENCES

Jacobs, K.A. (1986). Skin wound management techniques. Part I: Unsutured wounds. *Proc. 8th Bain-Fallon Memorial Lectures Equine Medicine, Australia, 1986*, pp. 92–97.

Kellens, P., Lambert, CH., Paye, M., Nusgens, B. and Laptere, CH.M. (1988). Effects of ketanserin, a serotonin-antagonist, on human dermal fibroblasts. *Abstract 18th Annual Meeting of the European Society of Dermatological Research, Munich, 1988.*

Keller, H. (1987) *Klinischer Einsatz von Ketanserin-Gel 0, 25% bei der Wundbehandlung von Pferden.* Report, Freie Universität Berlin.

Silver, I.A. (1982). Basic physiology of wound healing in the horse. *Equine Veterinary Journal* **14** (1): 7–15.

Sternberg, E.M., Trial, J. and Parker, CH.W. (1986). Effect of serotonin on murine macrophages: suppression of Ia expression by serotonin and its reversal by 5-HT_2 serotonergic receptor antagonists. *Journal of Immunology* **137** (1): 276–282.

Stornetta, D. and Diehl, M. (1987). Essai d'application du gel ketanserin Janssen dans le traitement des plaies chez le cheval. Report, Université de Berne.

Van Cutsem, J. (1985). *The Antimicrobial Activity of Ketanserin.* Preclinical Research Report N 49065, Janssen Pharmaceutica, Beerse.

Van Nueten, J.M., Janssen, P.A.J., Symoens J., Janssens W.J., Heykants, J. *et al.* (1987). *New Cardiovascular Drugs — Ketanserin*, pp. 1–56 Raven Press, New York.

Vlaminck, K. and Dony, J. (1987). *The Efficacy of Ketanserin 0.25% gel in Wound Care in Horses: A Field Trial.* Report V 6544, Janssen Pharmaceutica, Beerse.

Vlaminck, K., Van den bergh, J. and Van der Westhuizen, B. (1988a) Multicentre evaluation of the efficacy of ketanserin 0.25% gel in wound care in horses. Report V 6952, Janssen Pharmaceutica, Beerse.

Vlaminck, K., Dony, J., Monbaliu, J. & Woestenborghs, R. (1988b) *Absorption and Plasma Levels of Ketanserin after Topical Application of 0.25% Ketanserin Gel on Wounded Horses.* Preclinical Research Report V 6910, Janssen Pharmaceutica, Beerse.

PART 4

EPIDERMAL METABOLISM

4.1 Sweat and Sebaceous Glands and their Function in Domestic Animals

D. McEwan Jenkinson

Moredun Research Institute, Edinburgh

THE SKIN GLANDS

Sweat and sebaceous glands are exocrine skin glands, the former, tubular and the latter, alveolar. Both are widely dispersed throughout the general body surface skin of mammals including the glabrous regions, although they are not present in all species or in all body areas. The tubular glands in specialized cutaneous glands, e.g. the ear (Fernando, 1965) and the eyelids (Moll's glands), are therefore, by definition, sweat glands; similarly, specialized alveolar structures such as the Meibomian and preputial glands are sebaceous glands. The mammary gland is classed as a specialized sweat gland, although it has been suggested that it may originate from the sebaceous gland (Carlisle, 1954).

In contrast, the third type of exocrine skin gland, the acinar gland, (Plate 49), which has a structure similar to that of salivary glands and is presumed to function in an analogous manner (Majeed *et al.*, 1970), has been located only in specialized body regions such as the bovine muzzle (Mackie and Nisbet, 1959). The hippopotamus has developed subdermal acinar glands which produce a red fluid (Allbrook, 1962). However, since these are neither tubular nor in the skin, the secretion is not, by definition, sweat although it has for convenience been so described (Luck and Wright, 1964).

THE SEBACEOUS AND SWEAT GLANDS

Location

In haired species the sebaceous and sweat glands are located in association with the hair follicles as part of the basic hair follicle unit (Fig. 1a). Embryologically, the glands both develop from the epidermis via the hair follicle bud (Hardy and Lyne, 1956; Yasuda *et al.*, 1957; Lyne and Heideman, 1959) and because of this and their anatomical disposition beside the hair, the former has been classed as *pilosebaceous* (Thody and Shuster, 1989) and the latter as *epitrichial* (Bligh, 1967). In haired skin therefore, the ducts of both the sweat and sebaceous glands generally open into the pilosebaceous canal.

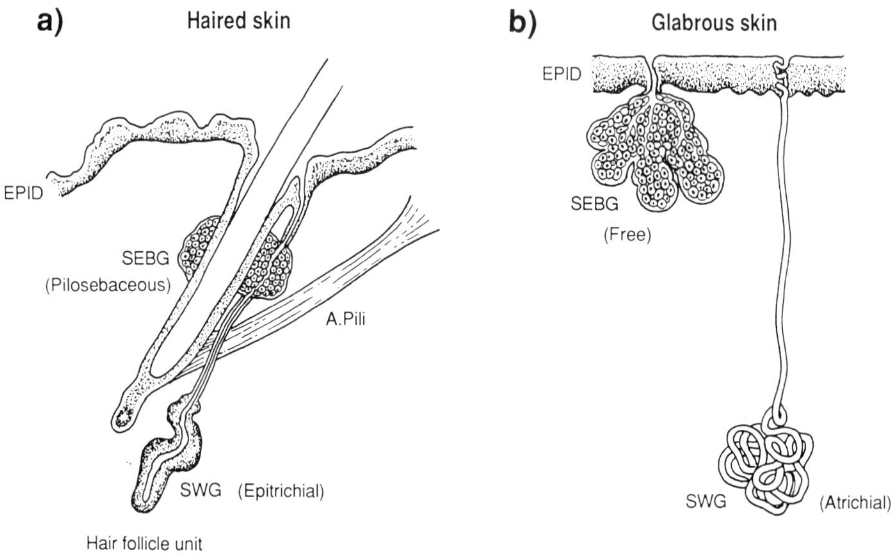

Figure 1 A diagram illustrating the locations of sweat (SWG) and sebaceous (SEBG) glands. (a) In haired skin both are generally found in association with the hair follicle and arrector pili muscle (APili) as part of what is termed the hair follicle unit and they open into the follicular canal (EPID: epidermis). b) In glabrous skin the sebaceous and sweat glands emerge directly through the epidermis.

Variations from this general pattern occur in some species; for example, in the sheep and dog which exhibit hair follicle grouping (Webb and Calhoun, 1954; Carter, 1955; Lovell and Getty, 1957), there are no sweat glands (or arrectores pilorum muscles) and sometimes no sebaceous glands associated with the secondary hairs. In the mole (Giacometti and Machida, 1965) and some of the higher primates (including man), the sebaceous gland still forms part of the hair follicle unit but the sweat gland is no longer associated with the hair follicle; it now opens through the epidermis and in man at least, develops directly from it. Such sweat glands have been called *atrichial* (Bligh, 1967). Atrichial sweat glands have also been located in the axilla of man (Sato *et al.*, 1987) and they are occasionally present in the skin of the dog and cow among the hair follicle units (Aoki, personal communication; Jenkinson personal observations).

In skin where the hair is no longer present, the sweat and sebaceous glands both develop directly from the epidermis and open through it. Thus the sweat glands in glabrous regions such as the footpads of the dog, cat and rat, and the human hands and feet, are also *atrichial*. The sebaceous glands in such regions have been designated as *free* (Fig. 1b).

Structure

Sebaceous gland

The sebaceous gland is a composite of basic lobes. In the haired skin of many species the gland is bilobular while in glabrous regions it is often multilobular and much larger, with the several lobes separated by trabeculae giving an outward appearance of a bunch of grapes. Each lobe consists of cells at varying degrees of development surrounded by a peripheral zone composed of low cuboidal cells (Fig. 2). The duct is short and linked with a keratinizing epithelium which becomes contiguous with the lining of the follicular canal or epidermis.

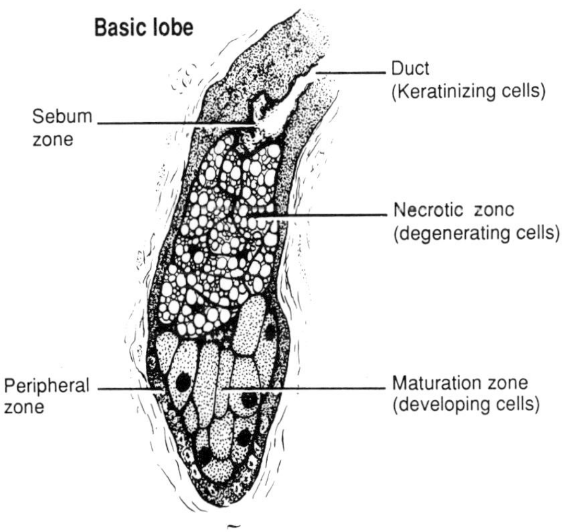

Figure 2 A diagram showing the general structure of the lobe of the sebaceous gland which consists of cells at various stages of development surrounded by a zone of peripheral cells. Zones where the cells are maturing, degenerating and coalescing can be distinguished. The duct is short and lined with keratinized cells.

Sweat gland

The structure of the epitrichial and atrichial glands is basically the same and consists of a duct and a fundus (Fig. 3). The intrafollicular region of the duct in the former equates with that of the intraepidermal region in the latter and hence the general ductal structure is similar in most species (Jenkinson, 1986). A notable exception is the duct of the human sweat gland which has a specialized region, the coiled duct, within the glandular coil.

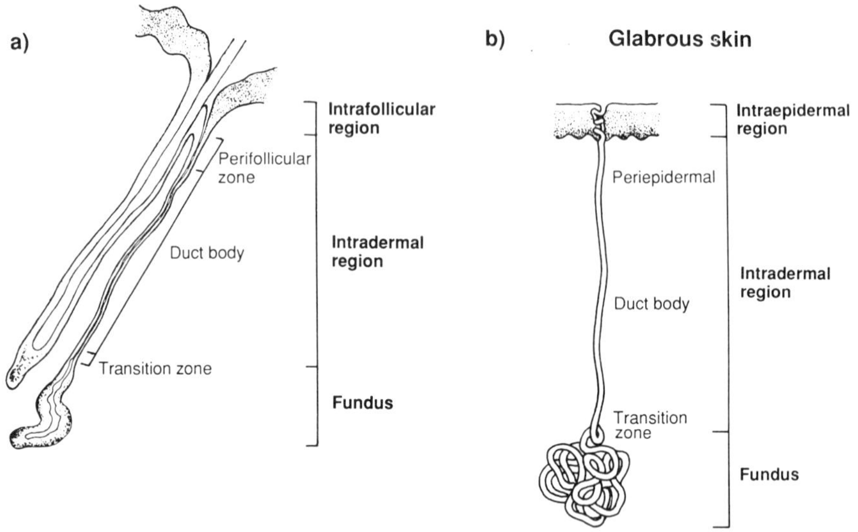

Figure 3 Diagrams illustrating that the general structure of a) the epitrichial and b) the atrichial sweat gland is essentially the same. The ductal intrafollicular and perifollicular regions of the former are histologically similar to the intraepidermal and periepidermal regions respectively, in the latter.

Although the fundus can vary outwardly in shape from a tight coil to a simple sac, in all species it consists of two layers of epithelium, an inner secretory and outer myoepithelium, surrounded by a sheath of fibrocytes (Fig. 4). The appearance of the secretory cells is, however, variable between species; they are for example, low cuboidal in the cow with few secretory vesicles whereas in the horse they are low columnar and packed with large secretory vesicles (Fig. 5a,b). The only major difference from the basic fundus structure is again found in man where two types of secretory cells have been identified indicating diversification of secretory function; cannaliculi, which extend almost from the basal lamina, thereby greatly increasing surface area, are also prominent. The myoepithelium in the sheep and cow forms a complete layer around the secretory cells, but in the horse, man and rat footpad glands it is a loose network through which the secretory cells extend to the basal lamina.

PURPOSE OF SEBUM AND SWEAT

Both the sebaceous and sweat glands are involved in body protection.

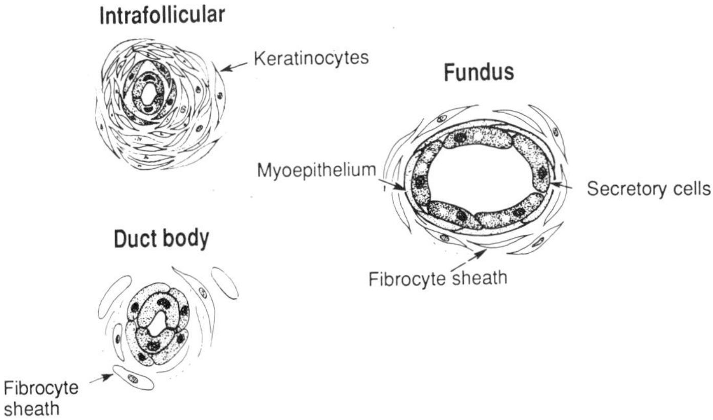

Figure 4 Histology of a sweat gland. The fundus of all sweat glands consists of an inner secretory epithelium surrounded by a layer of myoepithelial cells and an outer fenestrated fibrocyte sheath. The duct body is generally composed of two cell layers and in the intrafollicular/intraepidermal region there is, in the vicinity of the skin surface, an inner ring of keratinized cells.

Sebum

Sebum is important in the protection against microbial invasion. It forms a mixture, probably an emulsion, with sweat within the stratum corneum of the epidermis (Lloyd, *et al.*, 1979) and provides a 'cement' (Fig. 6) at the surface and around the hair pores, which if disrupted can lead to bacterial invasion of the epidermis (Lloyd *et al.*, 1980). Its constituent fatty acids, as both nutrients and inhibitors of microbial growth, provide the basis for physical, chemical and biological defence mechanisms (Jenkinson, 1980) which limit the variety of microbial species capable of surviving at the skin surface. Sebum also protects against excessive water loss through the skin and modification of surface texture. Third, sebum protects against extinction of species; sebaceous glands, particularly in specialized body regions such as the legs (Quay and Muller-Schwarze, 1970, 1971) and forehead (Jenkinson *et al.*, 1967; Johnson and Leask, 1977) provide pheromones which attract the opposite sex and aid species survival.

Topically applied pyrethroids are capable of travelling across the skin within the emulsion (Jenkinson *et al.*, 1986) which is therefore, apparently capable of mobility. A need to maintain a mobile surface emulsion for overall protection would provide an explanation for the wide variation in sebum and sweat compositions between species (Nicolaides *et al.*, 1968; Jenkinson *et al.*, 1974; Lindholm *et al.*, 1981). If complimentary sweat and sebum compositions are required to produce a mobile surface mixture, then variations in composition would be expected, especially in species which lack sweat glands or which have a low density of sebaceous glands.

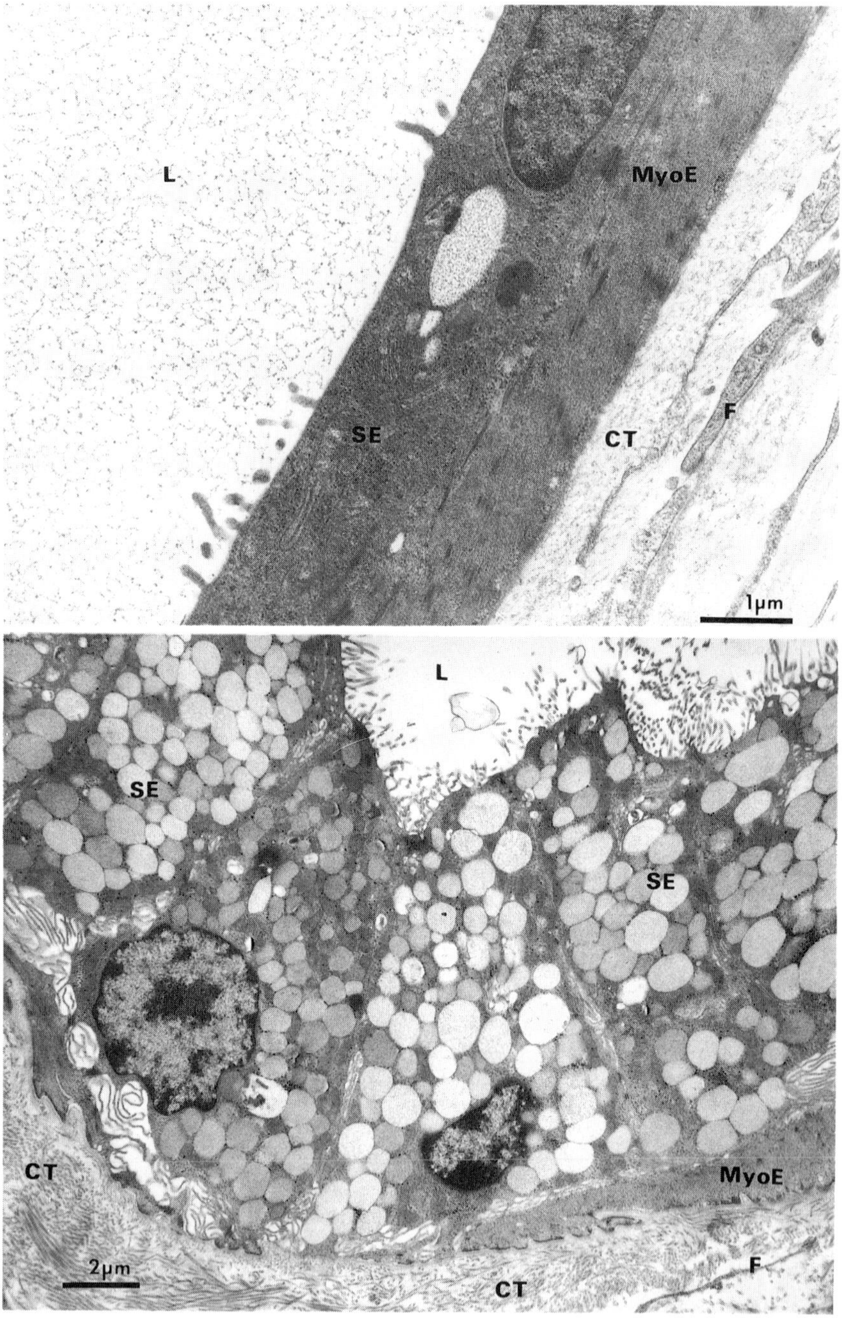

Figure 5 An electron micrograph of the wall of a sweat gland fundus from a cow. Note the low cuboidal secretory epithelium (SE) and the well-developed outer myoepithlium (MyoE). The surrounding fibrocyte sheath (F) encloses a layer of connective tissue (CT). (L-lumen.)

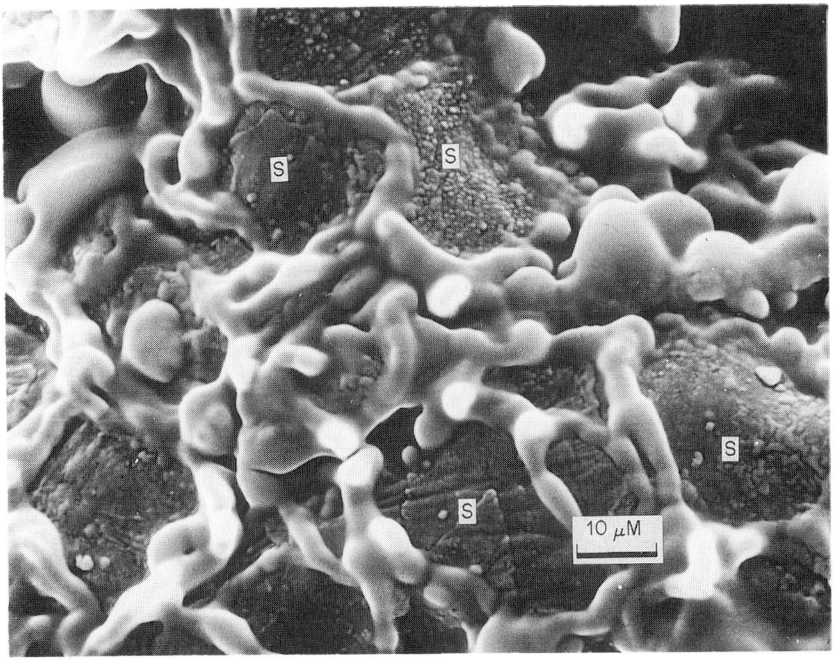

Figure 6 Scanning electron micrograph of the surface of freeze-dried bovine skin. The squames (S) are surrounded by lipid apparently derived from the underlying layers.

Sweat

The traditional view, based on the responses of man and the horse to heat and exercise, that sweat glands are primarily thermoregulatory organs, does not hold for mammals in general. Only those of equidae, some primates and some bovidae are of importance to body temperature regulation (Jenkinson, 1986). It is now considered that sweat has a number of protective roles, one or more of which may be present in many given species or body region. It has been suggested that sweat can help to protect against, 1) microorganisms as part of the surface emulsion; 2) frictional damage in regions such as the footpads and eyelids; 3) accumulation of waste products in the blood; 4) excessive increase in body temperature; and 5) extinction of the species (Jenkinson, 1986). The role of the mammary gland in this last context is obvious but pheromone substances produced by specialized sweat glands in species such as the deer (Quay and Muller-Schwarze, 1970, 1971; Johnson and Leask, 1977), by attracting the opposite sex, may have an important role in reproduction.

It is now evident that, with the exception of the few species where the glands have a role in thermoregulation, profuse secretion is not a prerequisite for efficiency of function. This concept is supported by the fact that Moll's glands contribute to the highly efficient protection of the eyes where a high output would be detrimental to sight.

MODE OF PRODUCTION OF SEBUM AND SWEAT

Historical concept of secretory mechanisms

Both free and pilosebaceous alveolar glands, according to traditional theory, exhibit holocrine secretion, by which cells increase their size and lipid content as they develop, then ultimately die to form the secretory product (Bell, 1986; Wheatley, 1986; Ross *et al.*, 1989). By this definition therefore, sebum is simply an aggregation of the contents and membranes of dead glandular cells. In contrast, it is believed that the artrichial and epitrichial sweat glands exhibit eccrine and apocrine secretion respectively. Eccrine glands are considered to transport their secretory products through the luminal membrane without disrupting it, while apocrine glands are, in addition, believed to exhibit necrobiotic discharge involving cell enlargement and loss of the apical portion of the cell by blebbing (Schiefferdecker, 1917).

Mode of sebum formation

It is widely considered that sebum is ultimately derived from progenitor cells in the peripheral layer around the lobe (Fig. 2) which develop as they grow inwards towards the centre of the gland and subsequently disintegrate to form the secretion (Rhodin, 1974; Ross *et al.*, 1989). Recently, this theory has been challenged following the discovery that the lateral peripheral cells bordering the lumen, some of which are keratinized, are unlikely to be able to develop into sebocytes (Jenkinson *et al.*, 1985). It is now considered that progenitor cells at the base of the lobe give rise to a column of cells which develop and die as they approach the duct of the gland (Fig. 7). The inwardly-growing lateral peripheral cells of the lobe almost certainly contribute keratin to this cell mass. Keratin would seem therefore to be a constituent of sebum and not simply a product acquired during the outward passage of the secretion through the short duct, which is a stratified squamous epithelium, and the hair follicle canal.

The source of the progenitor cells at the base of the lobe is still unknown; they may, as in the embryo, be derived from the hair follicle by lateral cell movement along the outer lining layer to the base of the lobe. Bloom and Fawcett (1966) state, although without supporting evidence, that mitoses are numerous close to the walls of the excretory ducts where the new cells move into the secretory regions. Alternatively, the progenitor cells may be resident at the base of the lobe and divide there to produce two cell populations, one for sebocyte development and the other to provide outer peripheral cells in a manner akin to inner root sheath formation in the hair follicle (Fig. 7). The

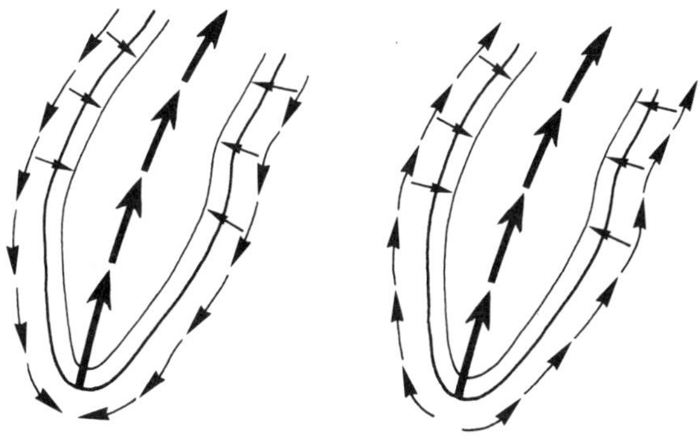

Figure 7 Putative method of sebum formation. It is conceived that cells derived from peripheral cells at the base of the lobe develop and disintegrate in a column. Keratin is added from inward-growing lateral peripheral cells. It is not known if the progenitor cells a) originate at the margins of the hair follicle and progress downwards or b) are situated at the base of the lobe and give rise to the peripheral layer as well as the developing column.

sebaceous gland could well be a hair follicle analogue which produces a secretory product rather than a solid structure. Kinetic studies are now required to test this hypothesis.

The mechanism of sebum formation, however, appears to be more than simple holocrine secretion. Lanthanum can pass from the dermis to the ductal lumen, between the developing cells (Jackson *et al.*, 1986), confirming the absence of tight junctions between sebocytes (Kitson and Van Lennep, 1984). Consequently, it is almost certain that, at the very least, the ionic composition of sebum is influenced by paracellular transport; it still has to be established whether or not larger molecules can be transported to the lumen by this route. Moreover, it is also not known if intact sebocytes secrete while maturing and to what extent any such secretory products contribute to sebum formation. In cattle, after stimulation of the gland, mitotic activity is unaffected and the number of cells necessary to produce sebum purely by a holocrine mechanism greatly exceeds the estimated level of cell production (Smith and Jenkinson, 1975). Active secretion may well occur within sebaceous glands and this possibility should not be dismissed lightly, as it has been in the past, without serious consideration and careful scrutiny.

Therefore, from current evidence, it can be postulated that sebum is formed from the products of *cell death* and possibly *secretion* including paracellular transport (Fig. 8).

Rate of sebum output

Sebum appears to be stored in the hair follicle canal and hence has a slow rate of excretion. After intradermal injection of ^{14}C-acetate in the sheep and man

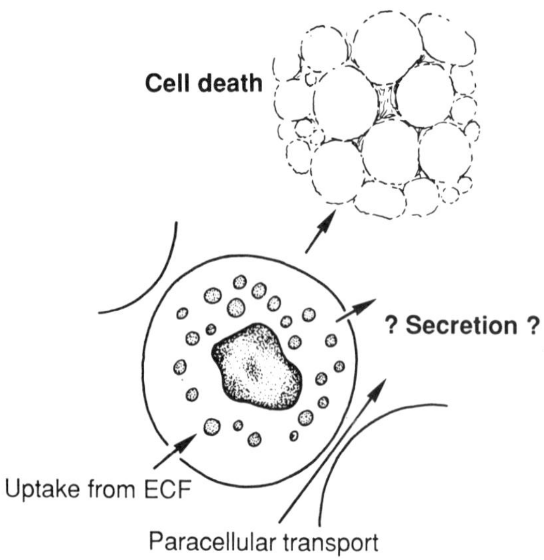

Figure 8 Sebum seems to be produced from the products of cell death and probably also those of secretion including paracellular transport. (ECF: extracellular fluid.)

(Downing *et al.*, 1975) and the horse (Colton and Downing, 1985), radioactivity was not detected in the surface lipids for 3–4 days. The delay between injection and maximum output of radioactivity averaged 6 days in the sheep, 4 in man and 16–25 in the horse. In cattle, ^{14}C-linoleic acid was incorporated into the glandular triglyceride fraction within 3 h of intradermal injection and radiolabelled triglycerides were detected on the skin within a day (MacMaster *et al*, 1986). Maximum labelling of the triglycerides, however, occurred at about 9 days and the duration of storage in the follicular canal was estimated to be about 6.5 days. Elevation of the ambient temperature reduced the time taken for maximum output from 9 to about 4 days.

Mode of sweat formation

The concepts of eccrine and apocrine secretion are based on light and ultrastructural studies of unstimulated sweat glands (Schiefferdecker, 1917; Charles, 1959; Kurosumi and Kawabata, 1976; Inoue, 1979; Meyer and Neurand, 1987) and the existence of apocrine secretion in sweat glands has been disputed (Weiner and Hellman, 1960; Biempica and Montes, 1965; Jenkinson, 1967; Montgomery *et al.*, 1984), although the nomenclature has been retained to the extent that 'apoeccrine' glands have been described (Sato *et al.*, 1987). In the last decade however, the ultrastructural changes in the gland have been studied following *in vivo* activation by thermal or pharmacological stimulation and these provide a different picture.

In species where the glands respond to heat, three different patterns of sweat output have been described (Fig. 9). The first, which is exhibited by the cow, shows a stepwise increase in evaporative loss to a plateau level which can be sustained for more than 5 h. The second, found in sheep and goats, is characterized by discrete decremental discharges to a state of fatigue and the third, seen in the horse and man, shows a smooth onset to a plateau level which is sustained, although after about 4 h there is often a decline in activity. Bligh (1967) attributed the first pattern to the effect of a rapidly rising secretory rate superimposed upon myoepithelial contractions. The second, he considered to be due to phasic myoepithelial contractions expelling a secretion produced in a slow uncontrolled manner. The third, he believed resulted from secretory activity with little or no myoepithelial action.

The role of the myoepithelium in the expulsion of sweat is, however, still uncertain. Tucker (1968), from study of the highly developed contractile system in the palm glands of the koala, considered that the myoepithelial cells regulate the fluids within the gland. Repetitive, though sporadic myoepithelial contractions have been reported following stimulation of the glands of the bat

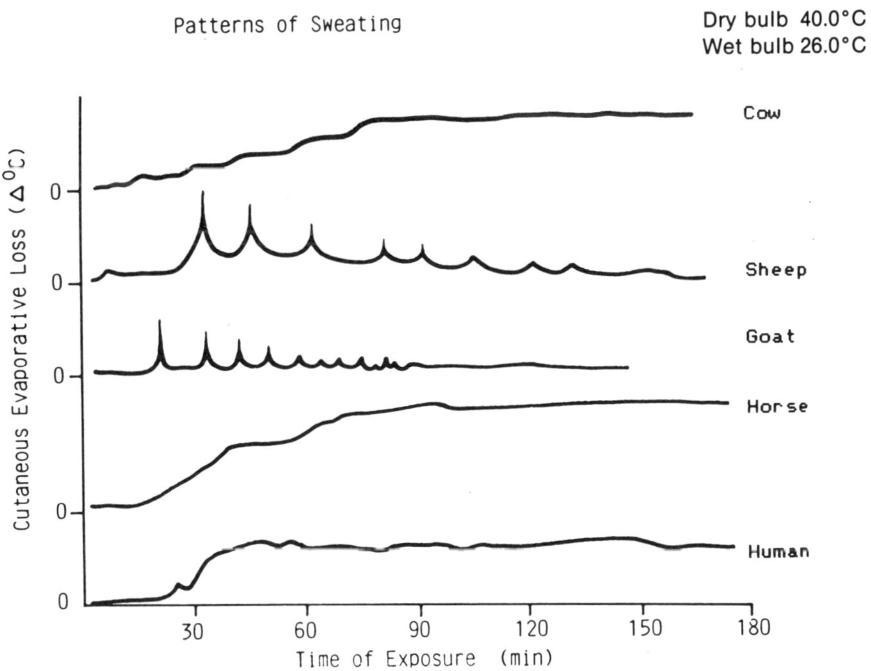

Figure 9 A diagram incorporating the work of a number of authors showing the three different patterns of mammalian cutaneous evaporative loss. Data for cow from Jenkinson (1969); for sheep from Robertshaw (1968); for goat from Jenkinson and Robertshaw (1971); and for the human from Montgomery *et al.* (1984).

wing (Murphy, 1960; Cortese and Nicholl, 1970) and Nicolaidis and Sivadjian (1972) observed pulsatile sweat output on the human forehead which they attributed to rhythmical myoepithelial contractions. Tubular contraction, attributed to myoepithelial activity, was also observed in isolated atrichial glands from the monkey and epitrichial glands from man in response to pharmacological stimuli, although these studies demonstrated that initial contraction did not expel significant amounts of preformed sweat and led to the conclusion that the major function of the myoepithelium is the provision of structural support to the secretory epithelium. (Sato, 1977, 1980; Sato *et al.*, 1979). This view is endorsed by the fact that the myoepithelium of the active cow, sheep, goat and horse gland was always seen contracted when examined by electron microscopy (Jenkinson *et al.*, 1979; Montgomery *et al.*, 1982a). There is thus a need for more detailed information on the contribution, if any, of the myoepithelial cells to sweat output in different species.

The ultrastructural evidence on the mode of sweat formation (Jenkinson *et al.*, 1979; Montgomery *et al.*, 1982a,b, 1984, 1985; McWilliams *et al.*, 1988) obtained from glands sampled by biopsy at known times during activity from species exhibiting different patterns of output is summarized in Table 1. These data illustrate that the flat secretory cells in the 'apocrine' gland of the cow do not alter in height nor do they exhibit apical blebbing during activity. There is, however, circumstantial evidence of cell death. In contrast microapocrine blebbing is found in the 'eccrine' human gland where complete secretory cell disruption is evident (Wilborn and Montes, 1978). In the human coiled duct and the 'eccrine gland' of the rat footpad, blebbing of the apical microvilli in a

Table 1 Secretory cell ultrastructure upon activity

Species	Before activation	After activation		
	Cell shape	Cell shape	Evidence of secretion	Evidence of cell death
Sheep/ goat	Cubical	Columnar	Vesicle exocytosis	Secretory cell debris in duct
Horse	Low columnar	Low cubical	Exocytosis Microapocrine	Secretory cell debris in duct
Cow	Low cubical	Low cubical	Exocytosis	Increased surface DNA
Man	Cubical	Columnar	Exocytosis Microapocrine	Gaps in secretory epithelium
Rat footpads	Cubical	Columnar	Exocytosis Microapocrine Blebbing of apical microvilli	Moribund cells in epithelium

manner reminicent of apocrine secretion occurs. It is apparent therefore that the apocrine/eccrine classification is no longer tenable.

One feature common to all sweat glands, following activity, is cell death and in most instances moribund secretory cells can be detected in the duct lumina. It follows therefore that the contents of dead cells are an integral component of sweat. Although lanthanum does not appear to pass the tight junctions of some species during activity (Jenkinson *et al.*, 1983) the possibility of paracellular ionic transport cannot be eliminated and in man, transport must occur through the gaps in the secretory epithelium. It seems therefore that sweat is produced by two processes *cell death* and *secretion* including a possible paracellular pathway (Fig. 10). The secretory processes are mainly ion and water transport and vesicle exocytosis. However, in some species, microapocrine secretion and in others, blebbing of the microvilli, may also occur.

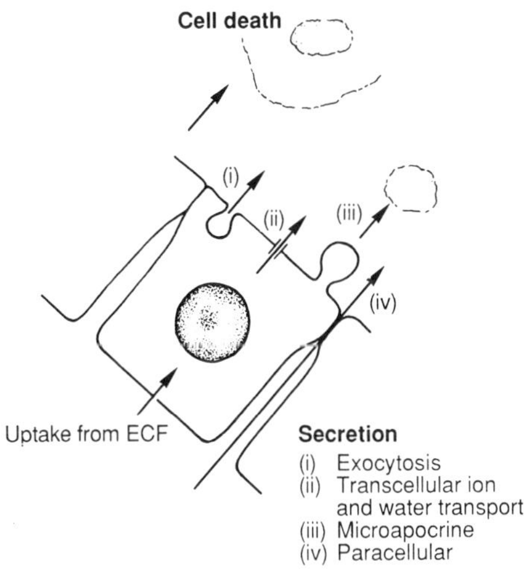

Figure 10 Putative method of sweat formation. Sweat, like sebum, appears to be formed from the products of cell death and those of secretion. In this instance, however, several secretory processes have been identified. ECF: Extracellular fluid

The source of cell replacement in the sweat gland is still unknown. Possible sources include differentiating duct cells and the fundus itself. The first seems a distinct possibility as different cells have been detected in the transitional zone between the duct and fundus (Montgomery *et al.*, 1982b). Evidence from injured glands (Lobitz and Dobson, 1957) supports the latter possibility, although it remains to be determined how far recovery from injury reflects the physiological situation. As for the sebaceous gland, there is a need for kinetic studies of cell turnover in the sweat gland.

There is also little or no information on the mechanisms underlying the exocytotic and microapocrine processes in the sweat gland. However, information is now emerging on the systems governing water and ion transport. The current paradigm, the essential elements of which are given in Fig. 11, is largely based upon data from the shark rectal gland and mammalian salivary and lacrimal glands (Silva *et al.*, 1977; Epstein *et al.*, 1983; Hannafin *et al.*, 1983; Petersen and Maruyama, 1984; Morris *et al.*, 1987; Petersen and Gallacher, 1988; Singh, 1988). Recent work on the human and primate sweat glands suggests that the basic similarity is close (Quinton and Tormey, 1976; Sato, 1977; Bijman, 1987; Quinton, 1987; Saga *et al.*, 1988; Sato and Sato, 1988; Wilson *et al.*, 1988a; Bovell *et al.*, 1989) and translation of the paradigm to the sweat gland is justified.

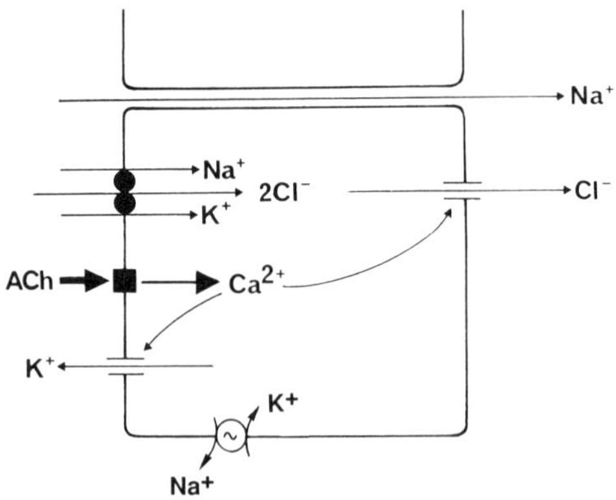

Figure 11 A simplified picture of the current theory of ion and water transport through the secretory cell of the sweat gland. The active expulsion of Na ions by a Na^+/K^+ pump on the basolateral membrane lowers the internal concentration of Na^+ and creates an inward gradient for this ion; Na ions enter the cell via an electroneutral co-transport system which consequently causes a rise in intracellular Cl^-. Secretagogues such as acetylcholine (Ach) induce a rise in the concentration of intracellular Ca ions which promotes the opening of Cl^- channels on the luminal membrane. Cl and hence Na, ions flow out of the cell and draw water into the lumen by osmosis. The secretary drive is maintained by the loss of K ions through calcium-sensitive, voltage-dependent channels on the basolateral membrane.

It is envisaged that, in common with other cell types, the basic driving force is provided by a Na^+/K^+ pump on the basolateral membrane (Fig. 11) powered by ATP breakdown. By driving Na ions out and K ions in, this pump maintains a low Na^+ concentration inside the cell and hence produces a large sodium gradient from outside to in. Na ions therefore move into the cell taking with them K and Cl ions probably via a $Na^+/K^+/2Cl^-$ electro-neutral co-transporter situated on the basolateral membrane. The Cl ions accumulate within the cell above the concentration defined by the chloride equilibrium potential. Cell activation by secretagogues such as acetylcholine (Ach) initiates a cascade of second messenger mechanisms which result in a rise in intracellular Ca ions. These in turn open calcium-sensitive chloride channels on the luminal membrane and chloride ions flow out down their electrochemical gradient. The lumen thus becomes more negative and this lumen-negative transepithelial potential draws cations principally Na^+ with it (shown as paracellular although it may be transcellular) and hence water by osmosis. The loss of Cl ions also makes the cell less negative, i.e. it tends to depolarize and this would reduce the driving force for secretion. However, secretion is maintained by the loss of K ions through calcium-sensitive and voltage-dependent channels on the basal membrane. α-Adrenergic agonists appear to stimulate secretion in a similar manner but with β-adrenergic agonists it seems that cyclic-AMP is the second messenger and calcium is not involved (Sato and Sato, 1981a).

It remains to be seen if the paradigm also applies to the glands of domestic animals. Electron microprobe studies have revealed a K^+ efflux from the horse gland (Wilson *et al.*, 1988b) but not from those of the sheep and goat subjected to thermal stimulation (Bovell *et al.*, 1988). If a K^+ efflux is absent from the latter, this could explain the early glandular fatigue which occurs in these species.

Concept of a common mechanism of sweat and sebum formation

It can therefore now be postulated that the mechanisms of sweat and sebum formation are basically similar and that in sebaceous glands and atrichial and epitrichial sweat glands there are two main components, *cell death* and *secretion* (Figs 8, 10).

The proportional contribution of these two processes is likely to vary between the two gland types and also between sweat glands in different body regions and in various mammals. The contribution from cell death for example is almost certainly greater in the sweat glands of the sheep than in those of the cow and is likely to be the major component in the formation of sebum. Some variation in the mode of secretion e.g. differences in ionic transport mechanisms, would also be expected between sweat glands which exhibit different patterns of output in response to heat and those in specialized areas which are not thermally responsive. The importance of the underlying processes of mitosis and cell development to the necrobiotic component and of vesicle production, protein synthesis and lipogenisis to secretion, require more detailed investigation.

It is not at all unreasonable to suppose that the glandular cells in both glands, as modified epidermal cells, provide products of importance to surface defence in a manner analagous to the cells of the epidermis which transport materials during life and ultimately die to provide a defensive layer.

CONTROL OF GLANDULAR ACTIVITY

Sebaceous gland

Sebaceous output is influenced by endocrine factors (Shuster and Thody, 1974) which, since they have been recently reviewed by Thody and Shuster (1989), are merely summarized in Fig. 12. These hormones can act synergistically and on different aspects of glandular function e.g. androgens increase both mitotic rate and sebum output whereas oestrogens reduce output but appear to have no action on glandular mitotic activity. Most of this evidence has been obtained from studies on man and laboratory animals which mature later in life; changes occur in the human sebaceous glands at puberty which are associated with acne.

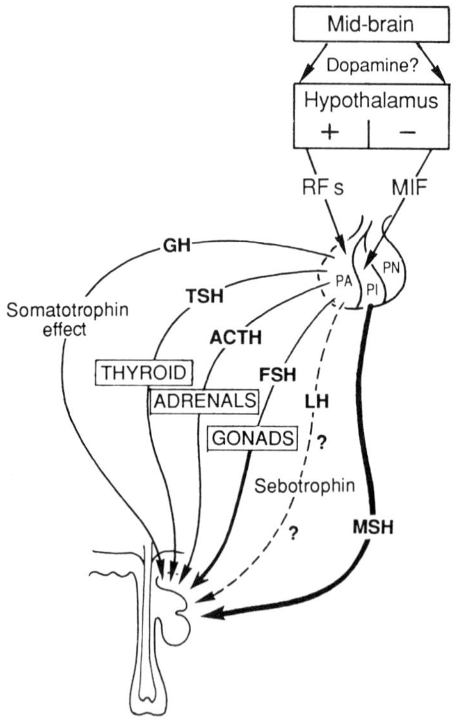

Figure 12 A diagram illustrating the importance of the endocrine system in the control of sebum output. From Shuster and Thody (1974).

It remains to be determined how far this evidence on endocrine control can be translated to domestic animals, such as the cow, where the glands have an adult output and composition within a few weeks of birth (Mabon *et al.*,

1983). Blasquez *et al.* (1987) found that oestradiol reduced the volume of the sebaceous glands in the neck of the cow but enlarged the specialized alveolar glands in the perineal region of the same animal. This suggests the possibility that the hormonal action is influenced by local receptors or that the effects of the hormone were nullified in the specialized glands by other overriding, possibly even non-endocrine, control mechanisms. There is good evidence for the participation of non-endocrine factors in the control of the rat sebaceous gland, where hypophysectomy does not reduce sebum output to below one-third of normal and where repeated removal of sebum stimulates a sustained increase in surface lipid (Thody and Shuster, 1989). Non-endocrine factors may be of prime importance in some specialized glands such as the rat Meibomian gland, which may not be under an endocrine control (Thody and Shuster, 1989). There is little information on the action of the nervous system on sebaceous gland activity other than the fact that cholinergic blocking agents have no effect on output (Cartlidge *et al.*, 1972) and there is need for more detailed investigation of the non-endocrine mechanisms involved in the control of sebum output.

Sweat gland

In contrast to the sebaceous glands, there is limited information on the actions of hormones, other than the catecholamines, on sweat output although there is some evidence on the effects of antidiuretic hormone and aldosterone on sweating in man (MacKinnon and Harrison, 1961; Furman and Beer, 1963; Fasciolo *et al.*, 1969; Allen and Roddie, 1974; Robertshaw, 1977).

Sweat output in response to heat is dependent on an intact sympathetic nervous system and circulating catecholamines supplement neural stimulation during exercise (Robertshaw and Taylor, 1969; Robertshaw, 1977). Adrenaline and noradrenaline induce a sweat response in all species so far studied and in the sweat glands of specialized body areas but acetylcholine is effective in only some species such as man and the horse. Acetylcholine has no stimulatory effect on the sweat glands of the cow, sheep, goat and pig (Kimura and Aoki, 1962; Findlay and Robertshaw, 1965; Ingram, 1967; Hayashi, 1968) although it does elicit a response in the dog (Aoki, 1955) and in the footpad glands of the cat and rat.

The picture is further complicated by the fact that the sweat glands in species such as the cow, the sheep and the goat do not seem to be innervated. The nerves are located around the cutaneous blood vessels and there appears to be a peripheral non-neural component in the control mechanism (Jenkinson *et al.*, 1978). The glands of the horse and man have a closely associated nerve supply but it has still to be established whether or not this is primarily to the gland or to blood vessels within the fibrocyte sheath.

A unified theory of sudomotor control (Fig. 13) was proposed by Jenkinson *et al.*, (1978) to explain these findings. It is conceived that in species where the nerves are over 10μm from the gland, the sympathetic adrenergic and

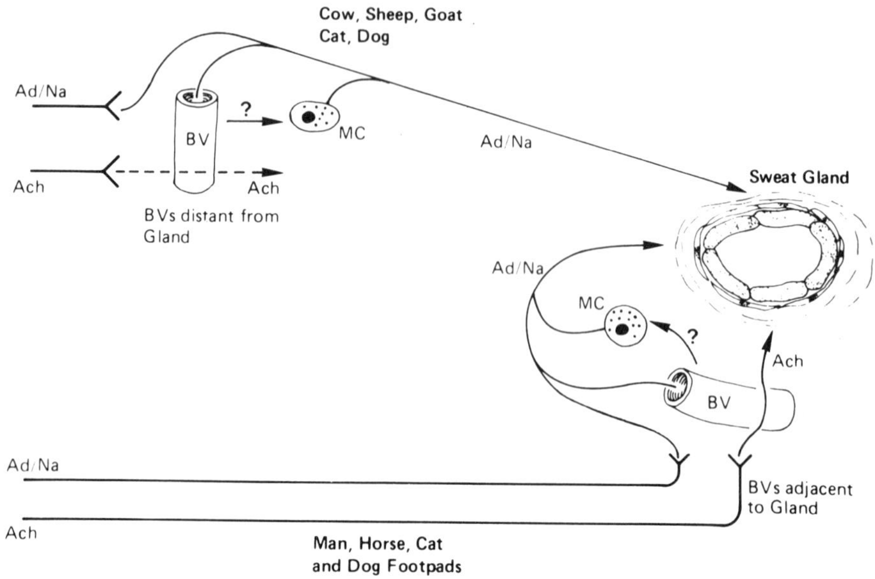

Figure 13 Concept of a unified sudomotor mechanism. It is postulated that as shown for the cow, sheep, goat, cat and dog, the action of sympathetic adrenergic and cholinergic nerves on cutaneous blood vessels (BV) elicits a local transfer to the gland of threshold quantities of a local transmitter possibly adrenaline (Ad) or noradrenaline (Na) from the circulation or from dopamine stores in mast cells (MC) in close opposition to capillaries. In species such as man and the horse it is suggested that the glands may also be controlled directly by transmitters (catecholamines and acetylcholine (Ach)) released at the sympathetic endings, especially from nerves located adjacent to blood vessels within the fibrocyte sheath. (From Jenkinson *et al.*, 1978 with permission from Cambridge University Press.)

cholinergic nerves to the blood vessels when stimulated, elicit a local transfer to the gland of threshold quantities of a transmitter or transmitters which have still to be identified. The most likely candidates are the catecholamines, universal stimulators of sweating, which could possibly emanate from the circulation or be produced locally from cellular stores of dopamine in mast cells in the vicinity of the blood vessels. Acetylcholine released at the nerve endings to the blood vessels would be inactivated and would thus have no stimulatory action on remote glands. In species where the blood vessels are in close proximity to the glands (Fig. 13), the transmitters produced at the nerve endings to the vessels are likely to have in addition, a direct action on the glands. Indeed, in some instances, the cholinergic component has become more dominant. In primates including man, for example, receptors for both acetylcholine and adrenaline have been identified on the secretory cell membranes (Sato and Sato, 1981b; Bovell *et al.*, 1989). It will be interesting to see if, as would be predicted from the unified theory (Fig. 13), cholinergic receptors are absent from the secretory cells in the cow, sheep and goat.

In the past, sweat and sebaceous gland function have been studied within a very limited sample of mammals with a tendency to concentrate on the differences found. It is hoped that in the future a much wider mammalian population will be examined and greater emphasis given to the similarities. When the theme has been grasped, the variations will be better appreciated.

REFERENCES

Allbrook, D. (1962). The morphology of the subdermal glands of Hippopotamus amphibius. *Proceedings of the Zoological Society, London* **139**: 67–73.

Allen, J.A. and Roddie, I.C. (1974). The effect of antidiuretic hormone on human sweating. *Journal of Physiology* **236**: 403–412.

Aoki, T. (1955). Stimulation of the sweat glands in the hairy skin of the dog by adrenaline, noradrenaline, acetylcholine, mecholyl and pilocarpine. *Journal of Investigative Dermatology* **24**: 545–556.

Bell, M. (1986). Sebaceous glands. In: Bereiter Hahn, J., Matoltsy, A.G., Richards, K.S. (eds) *Biology of the Integument* Vol. 2, pp. 318–338. Springer-Verlag, Berlin.

Biempica, I. and Montes, L.F. (1965). Secretory epithelium of the large axillary sweat glands. A cytochemical and electron microscopic study. *American Journal of Anatomy* **117**: 47–72.

Bijman, J. (1987). Transport processes in the eccrine sweat gland. *Kidney International* **32** (Suppl 21): S109–S112.

Blazquez, N.B., Long, S.E., Perry, G.C. and Watson, E.D. (1987). Effect of oestradiol 17β on perineal and neck skin glands in heifer calves. *Journal of Endocrinology* **115**: 43–46.

Bligh, J. (1967). A thesis concerning the process of secretion and discharge of sweat. *Environmental Research* **189**: 28–45.

Bloom, W. and Fawcett, D.W. (1966). *A Textbook of Histology* 8th edn, p. 386. W.B. Saunders Company, Philadelphia.

Bovell, D.L., Jenkinson, D. McEwan, Elder, H.Y. and Wilson, S.M. (1988). Effects of thermal stimulation on intracellular sodium, potassium and chlorine in the sweat glands of the cow, sheep and goat. *Research in Veterinary Science* **44**: 388–390.

Bovell, D.L., Elder, H.Y., Jenkinson, D. McEwan and Wilson, S.M. (1989). The control of potassium ($^{86}Rb^{+}$) efflux in the isolated human sweat gland. *Quarterly Journal of Experimental Physiology* **74**: 267–276.

Carlisle, D.B. (1954). On the relationship between mammary, sweat and sebaceous glands. *Quarterly Journal of Microscopical Science* **95**: 79–83.

Carter, H.B. (1955). The hair follicle group in sheep. *Animal Breeding Abstracts* **23**: 101–116.

Cartlidge, M., Burton, J.L. and Shuster, S. (1972). The effect of prolonged application of an anticholinergic agent on the sebaceous glands. *British Journal of Dermatology* **86**: 61–63.

Charles, A. (1959). An electron microscopic study of the human axillary apocrine gland. *Journal of Anatomy* **93**: 226–232.

Colton, S.W. and Downing, D.T. (1985). Measurement of the time between biosynthesis and surface excretion of sebaceous lipids in the horse. *Biochimica et Biophysica Acta* **635**: 98–103.

Cortese, T.A. and Nicholl, P.A. (1970). *In vivo* observations of skin appendages in the bat. *Journal of Investigative Dermatology* **54**: 1–10.

Downing, D.T., Strauss, J.S., Ramasastry, P., Abel, M., Lees, C.W. *et al.* (1975). Measurement of the time between synthesis and surface excretion of sebaceous lipids in sheep and man. *Journal of Investigative Dermatology* **64**: 215–219.

Epstein, F.H., Stoff, J.S. and Silva, P. (1983). Mechanism and control of hyperosmotic NaCl-rich secretion by the rectal gland of *Squalus acanthias*. *Journal of Experimental Biology* **106**: 25–41.
Fasciolo, J.C., Totel, G.L. and Johnson, R.E. (1969). Antidiuretic hormone and human eccrine sweating. *Journal of Applied Physiology* **27**: 303–307.
Fernando, S.D.A. (1965). A histological and histochemical study of the glands of the external auditory meatus of the ox. *British Veterinary Journal* **121**: 223–227.
Findlay, J.D. and Robertshaw, D. (1965). The role of the sympatho-adrenal system in the control of sweating in the ox (*Bos taurus*). *Journal of Physiology* **179**: 285–297.
Furman, K.I. and Beer, G. (1963). Dynamic changes in sweat electrolyte composition induced by heat stress as an indication of acclimatization and aldesterone activity. *Clinical Science* **24**: 7–12.
Giacometti, L. and Machida, H. (1965). The skin of the mole (*Scapanus townsendii*). *Anatomical Record* **153**: 31–40.
Hannafin, J., Kinne-Saffran, E., Friedman, D. and Kinne, R. (1983). Presence of a sodium-potassium chloride cotransport system in the rectal gland of *Squalus acanthias*. *Journal of Membrane Biology* **75**: 73–83.
Hardy, M.H. and Lyne, A.G. (1956). The pre-natal development of wool follicles in merino sheep. *Australian Journal of Biological Sciences* **9**: 423–441.
Hayashi, H. (1968). Functional activity of the sweat glands in the hairy skin of the sheep. *Tohoku Journal of Experimental Medicine* **94**: 361–375.
Ingram, D.L. (1967). Stimulation of cutaneous glands in the pig. *Journal of Comparative Pathology* **77**: 93–98.
Inoue, T. (1979). Scanning electron microscopic study of the human axillary apocrine glands. *The Journal of Dermatology* **6**: 299–308.
Jackson, D., McQueen, L., Jenkinson, D. McEwan, Nimmo, M.C. *et al.* (1986). Passage of lanthanum through the intercellular spaces of the sebaceous gland. *Research in Veterinary Science* **40**: 48–53.
Jenkinson, D. McEwan (1967). On the classification of sweat glands and the question of an apocrine secretory process. *British Veterinary Journal* **123**: 311–316.
Jenkinson, D. McEwan (1969). Sweat gland function in domestic animals. In: Botelho, S.Y., Brooks, F. and Shelley, W.B. (eds) *The Exocrine Glands*, pp. 201–221. University of Pennsylvania Press, Philadelphia.
Jenkinson, D. McEwan (1980). The topography, climate and chemical nature of the mammalian skin surface. *Proceedings of the Royal Society of Edinburgh* **79B**: 3–22.
Jenkinson, D. McEwan (1986). Thermoregulatory function. In: Thody, A.J. and Friedman, P.S. (eds) *Scientific Basis of Dermatology*, pp. 89–112. Churchill Livingstone, Edinburgh.
Jenkinson, D. McEwan and Robertshaw, D. (1971). Studies on the nature of sweat gland 'fatigue' in the goat. *Journal of Physiology* **212**: 455–465.
Jenkinson, D. McEwan, Mabon, R.M. and Manson, W. (1974). Sweat proteins. *British Journal of Dermatology* **90**: 175–181.
Jenkinson, D. McEwan, Montgomery, I. and Elder, H.Y. (1978). Studies on the nature of the peripheral sudomotor control mechanism. *Journal of Anatomy* **125**: 625–639.
Jenkinson, D. McEwan, Montgomery, I. and Elder, H.Y. (1979). The ultrastructure of the sweat glands of the ox, sheep and goat during sweating and recovery. *Journal of Anatomy* **129**: 117–140.
Jenkinson, D. McEwan, Nimmo, M.C., Jackson, D. McQueen, L., Elder, H.Y. *et al.* (1983). Comparative studies of the effect of thermal stimulation on the permeability of the luminal cell junctions of the sweat gland to lanthanum. *Tissue and Cell* **15**: 573–581.

Jenkinson, D. McEwan, Blackburn, P.S. and Proudfoot, R. (1967). Seasonal changes in the skin glands of the goat. *British Veterinary Journal* **123**: 541-549.

Jenkinson, D. McEwan, Elder, H.Y., Montgomery, I. and Moss, V.A. (1985). Comparative studies of the ultrastructure of the sebaceous gland. *Tissue and Cell* **17**: 683-698.

Jenkinson, D. McEwan, Hutchison, G., Jackson, D. and MacQueen, L. (1986). Route of passage of cypermethrin across the surface of sheep skin. *Research in Veterinary Science* **41**: 237-241.

Johnson, E. and Leask, J.T.S. (1977). Metabolism of testosterone by forehead skin of the roebuck (Capreolus capreolus). *Journal of Endocrinology* **75**: 363-372.

Kimura, A. and Aoki, T. (1962). Functional activity of the apocrine sweat gland in the goat. *Tohoku Journal of Experimental Medicine* **76**: 8-82.

Kitson, N. and Van Lennep, E.W. (1984). Intercellular junctions and the permeability barrier in human sebaceous glands. *British Journal of Dermatology* **110**: 601-606.

Kurosumi, K. and Kawabata, I. (1976). Transmission and scanning electron microscopy of the human ceruminous apocrine gland. 1. Secretory glandular cells. *Archivum Histologicum Japonicum* **39**: 207-229.

Lindholm, J.S., McCormick, J.M., Colton, S.W.V.I. and Downing, D.T. (1981). Variation of skin lipid composition among mammals. *Comparative Biochemistry and Physiology* **69B**: 75-78.

Lloyd, D. H., Dick, W.D.B. and Jenkinson, D. McEwan (1979). Structure of the epidermis in Ayrshire bullocks. *Research in Veterinary Science* **26**: 172-179.

Lloyd, D.H. and Jenkinson, D. McEwan (1980). The effect of climate on experimental infection of bovine skin with *Dermatophilus congolensis. British Veterinary Journal* **136**: 122-134.

Lobitz, W.C. and Dobson, R.L. (1957). Responses of the secretory coil of the human eccrine sweat gland to controlled injury. *Journal of Investigative Dermatology* **28**: 105-120.

Lovell, J.E. and Getty, R. (1957). The hair follicle, epidermis, dermis and skin glands of the dog. *American Journal of Veterinary Research* **18**: 873-885.

Luck, C.P. and Wright, P.G. (1964). Aspects of the anatomy and physiology of the skin of the hippopotimus (H. amphibius). *Quarterly Journal of Experimental Physiology* **49**: 1-14.

Lyne, A.G. and Heideman, M.J. (1959). The pre-natal development of skin and hair in cattle (*Bos Taurus* L). *Australian Journal of Biological Sciences* **12**: 72-95.

Mabon, R.M., Noble, R.C. and Jenkinson, D. McEwan (1983). Bovine sebum composition during the first 6 weeks post partum. *Journal of Agricultural Science Cambridge* **101**: 503-505.

Mackie, A.M. and Nisbet, A.M. (1959). The histology of the bovine muzzle. *Journal of Agricultural Science* **52**: 376-379.

McKinnon, P.C.B. and Harrison, J. (1961). The influence of hormones associated with pituitary-adrenal and sexual-cycle activity in palmar sweating. *Journal of Endocrinology* **23**: 217-225.

MacMaster, J.D., Jenkinson, D. McEwan, Noble, R.C. and Elder, H.Y. (1986). Output of triglyceride from the sebaceous gland and to the skin of cattle. *Research in Veterinary Science* **41**: 242-246.

McWilliams, S.A., Montgomery, I., Elder, H.Y., Jenkinson, D. McEwan, Wilson, S.M. (1988). Effects of stimulation on the ultrastructure and Na, K, Cl composition of the fundus of the rat plantar sweat gland. *Tissue and Cell* **20**: 109-118.

Majeed, M.A., Zaidi, I.H. and Ilahi, A. (1970). The nature of nasolabial gland secretion (NLGS) in large domestic ruminants. *Research in Veterinary Science* **11**: 407-410.

Meyer, W. and Neurand, K. (1987). A comparative scanning electron microscopic view of the integument of domestic animals. *Scanning Microscopy* **1**: 169–180.

Montgomery, I., Jenkinson, D. McEwan, and Elder, H.Y. (1982a). The effects of thermal stimulation on the ultrastructure of the fundus and duct of the equine sweat gland. *Journal of Anatomy* **135**: 13–28.

Montgomery, I., Jenkinson, D. McEwan, and Elder, H.Y. (1982b). The ultrastructure of the sweat gland duct of the ox, sheep and goat before and during sweating. *Journal of Anatomy* **134**: 741–755.

Montgomery, I., Jenkinson, D. McEwan, Elder, H.Y., Czarnecki, D. and MacKie, R.M. (1984). The effects of thermal stimulation on the ultrastructure of the human atrichial sweat gland. 1. The fundus. *British Journal of Dermatology* **110**: 385–397.

Montgomery, I., Jenkinson, D. McEwan, Elder, H.Y., Czarnecki, D. and MacKie, R.M. (1985). The effects of thermal stimulation on the ultrastructure of the human atrichial sweat gland. 2. The duct. *British Journal of Dermatology* **112**: 165–177.

Morris, A.P., Gallacher, D.V., Irvine, R.F. and Petersen, O.H. (1987). Synergism of inositol trisphosphate and tetrakisphosphate in activating Ca^{2+}-dependent K^+ channels. *Nature* **330**: 653–655.

Murphy, R.C. (1960). Fluoresence studies in the wing of the living bat. *Anatomical Record* **136**: 127–135.

Nicolaidis, S. and Sivadjian, J. (1972). High-frequency pulsatile discharge of human sweat glands: Myoepithelial mechanism. *Journal of Applied Physiology* **32**: 86–90.

Nicolaides, N., Fu, H.C. and Rice, G.R. (1968). The skin surface lipids of man compared with those of eighteen species of animals. *Journal of Investigative Dermatology* **51**: 83–89.

Petersen, O.H. and Gallacher, D.V. (1988). Electrophysiology of pancreatic and salivary acinar cells. *Annual Review of Physiology* **50**: 65–80.

Petersen, O.H. and Maruyama, Y. (1984). Calcium-activated potassium channels and their role in secretion. *Nature* **307**: 693–696.

Quay, W.B. and Muller-Schwarze, D. (1970). Functional histology of integumentary glandular regions in black-tailed deer (*Odocoileus hemionus columbianus*). *Journal of Mammalogy* **51**: 675–694.

Quay, W.B. and Muller-Schwarze, D. (1971). Relations of age and sex to integumentary glandular regions in rocky mountain mule deer (*Odocoileus hemionus hemionus*). *Journal of Mammalogy* **52**: 670–685.

Quinton, P.M. (1987). Physiology of sweat secretion. *Kidney International* **32** (Suppl. 21): 5102–5108.

Quinton, P.M. and Tormey, J.M. (1976). Localisation of Na/K-ATPase sites in the secretory and reabsorptive epithelia of perfused eccrine sweat glands; a question to the role of the enzyme in secretion. *Journal of Membrane Biology* **29**: 383–399.

Rhodin, J.A.G. (1974). *Histology A Text and Atlas*. London: Academic Press.

Robershaw, D. (1968). The pattern and control of sweating in the sheep and goat. *Journal of Physiology* **198**: 531–539.

Robertshaw, D. (1977). Neuroendocrine control of sweat glands. *Journal of Investigative Dermatology* **69**: 121–129.

Robershaw, D. and Taylor, C.R. (1969). Sweat gland function of the donkey (Equus asinus). *Journal of Physiology* **205**: 79–87.

Ross, M.H., Reith, E.J. and Romrell, L.G. (1989). *Histology: A Text and Atlas* 2nd edn. Williams & Wilkins, Baltimore.

Saga, K., Sato, F. and Sato, K. (1988). K^+ efflux from the monkey eccrine secretory coil during the transient of stimulation with agonists. *Journal of Physiology* **405**: 205–217.

Sato, K. (1977). The physiology, pharmacology and biochemistry of the eccrine sweat gland. *Review of Physiology, Biochemistry and Pharmacology* **79**: 51–131.

Sato, K. (1980). Pharmacological responsiveness of the myoepithelium of the isolated human axillary apocrine sweat gland. *Clinical and Laboratory Investigations* **103**: 235–243.

Sato, K. and Sato, F. (1981a). Clyclic AMP accumulation in the β-adrenergic mechanism of eccrine sweat secretion. *Pflungers Archives* **390**: 49–53.

Sato, K. and Sato, F. (1981b). Pharmacological responsiveness of isolated single eccrine sweat glands. *American Journal of Physiology* **240**: R44–R51.

Sato, K. and Sato, F. (1988). Relationship between quin2-determined cytosolic [Ca^{2+}] and sweat secretion. *American Journal of Physiology* **254**: C310–C317.

Sato, K., Nishiyama, A. and Kobayashi, M. (1979). Mechanical properties and functions of the myoepithelium in the eccrine sweat gland. *American Journal of Physiology* **237**: C177–C184.

Sato, K., Leidal, R. and Sato, F. (1987). Morphology and development of an apocrine sweat gland in human axillae. *American Journal of Physiology* **252**: R166–R180.

Schiefferdecker, P. (1917). Die Hautdrusen des Menschen und der Saugetiere; ihre biologische und rassenanatomische Bedeitung sowie die Muscularis sexualis. *Biologisches Zentralblatt* **37**: 534–562.

Shuster, S. and Thody, A.J. (1974). The control and measurement of sebum secretion. *Journal of Investigative Dermatology* **62**: 172–190.

Silva, P., Stoff, J., Field, M., Fine, L. and Forrest, J.N. *et al.* (1977). Mechanism of active chloride secretion by shark rectal gland; role of Na-K-ATPase in chloride transport. *American Journal of Physiology* **233**: F298–F306.

Singh, J. (1988). Acetylcholine-evoked potassium and sodium transport in rat lacrimal segments: evidence for a sodium-chloride co-transport system. *Quarterly Journal of Experimental Physiology* **73**: 767–775.

Smith, M.E., Jenkinson, D. McEwan (1975). The mode of secretion of the sebaceous glands of cattle. *British Veterinary Journal* **131**: 610–618.

Thody, A.J. and Shuster, S. (1989). Control and function of sebaceous glands. *Physiological Reviews* **69**: 383–416.

Tucker, R. (1968). The organisation of a contractile system in glands. 1. The contractile system in the palmar apocrine glands of the Koala Phascolarctos cinereus. *Research in Veterinary Science* **9**: 29–34.

Webb, A.J. and Calhoun, M.L. (1954). The microscopic anatomy of the skin of mongrel dogs. *American Journal of Veterinary Research* **15**: 274–280.

Weiner, J.S. and Hellman, H. (1960). The sweat glands. *Biological Reviews* **35**: 141–186.

Wheatley, V.R. (1986). *The Physiology and Pathophysiology of the Skin* Vol. 9. *The Sebaceous Glands*, pp. 2763–2796. Academic Press, London.

Wilborn, W.H. and Montes, L.F. (1978). Scanning electron microscopy of axillary apocrine sweat glands. *Scanning Electron Microscopy* **2**: 131–138.

Wilson, S.M., Elder, H.Y., Sutton, A.M., Jenkinson, D. McEwan, Cockburn, F. *et al.* (1988a). The effects of thermally-induced activity *in vivo* upon the ultrastructure and Na, K and Cl composition of the epithelial cells of sweat glands from patients with cystic fibrosis. *Tissue and Cell* **20**: 691–700.

Wilson, S.M., Elder, H.Y., Jenkinson, D. McEwan, McWilliams, S.A. (1988b). The effects of thermally induced activity in vivo upon the levels of sodium, chlorine and potassium in the epithelia of the equine sweat gland. *Journal of Experimental Biology* **136**: 489–494.

Yasuda, K., Kaga, T., Goto, T., Kashimura, T., Furusawa, H. *et al* (1957). A study of the development of the sweat glands of the cattle embryos. *Keio Journal of Medicine* **6**: 159–209.

4.2 Keratinocyte Differentiation in the Dog

Maja M. Suter, Dana M. Pantano, Hellmut G. Augustin-Voss, Mark Varvayanis, Flavio M. Crameri and John E. Wilkinson

Department of Pathology, New York State College of Veterinary Medicine, Cornell University, Ithaca, NY, USA

INTRODUCTION

Stratified squamous epithelium consists of well organized layers of keratinocytes, resulting in a complete multilayered sheet well equipped for a multitude of functions. After the keratinocytes leave the basal layer, they undergo an orderly and progressive differentiation during their migration to the stratum corneum. Recent immunohistochemical studies on mouse, human, and canine stratified squamous epithelium demonstrated a marked heterogeneity of cells involved in the process of differentiation. Various cytoplasmic components such as involucrin, filaggrin, and some keratins are present only in differentiated keratinocytes. In addition to cytoplasmic changes during the process of differentiation, the expression of cell surface molecules has been shown to be differentiation dependent. Changes in the expression of some of these differentiation markers have been proposed to be involved in the pathogenesis of some skin diseases, e.g. the different forms of pemphigus.

The recent establishment of undifferentiated and differentiated cultures of normal neoplastic keratinocytes has provided the basis for *in vitro* studies on the pathogenesis of diseases involving canine stratified squamous epithelium. The assessment of the degree of differentiation of cells grown in these *in vitro* systems is crucial to such experiments. The purpose of this study is to demonstrate differentiation-dependent expression of cell surface markers in canine keratinocytes *in vivo* and *in vitro*.

MATERIAL AND METHODS

Keratinocyte cultures

Submerged keratinocyte cultures

Cultures of normal keratinocytes were established from canine oral mucosa as described recently (Wilkinson *et al.*, 1987). Established cell cultures were grown in complete William's Medium E (WME; GIBCO Laboratories, Grand Island, NY) containing 10% fetal bovine serum (FBS; Hyclone Co., Logan, UT), 10^{-10} M cholera toxin (CT; INC Biomedicals, Irvine, CA), and 10 ng/ml epidermal growth factor (EGF; Collaborative Research Inc., Bedford, MA). Neoplastic keratinocytes were established from biopsies from dogs with spontaneous oral squamous cell carcinoma. Briefly, single cell suspension was obtained by incubation of multiple tissue pieces in 0.5% trypsin/0.25% EDTA (Gibco Co., Grand Island, NY) for 60 min at 34°C. The cells were plated at $1-2\times10^5/cm^2$, grown to confluency, and passaged at a 1:5 dilution. Established cultures were grown in complete WME.

Keratinocyte cultures grown at the air–liquid interface

Differentiated stratified squamous epithelium was established *in vitro* from normal and neoplastic keratinocytes by growth of keratinocytes at the air–liquid interface as described recently (Wilkinson *et al.*, 1989a). Briefly, keratinocytes were cultured on cellulose acetate membranes (Millicell-HA^R, 13 mm; Millipore Co., Bedford, MA) coated with or without collagen. Cells on a confluent monolayer at passage 3–8 were trypsinized, resuspended, and plated at 3:1 ($3-6\times10^5$ cells/cm^2) onto the artificial membranes placed in 24-well tissue culture plates. They were grown submerged for 5 days (normal cells) and 3 days (neoplastic cells) in complete WME to achieve confluency. Upon confluency culture medium was added to be in basal cell contact only, exposing the suprabasilar layers to air. Cells were then cultured for 14 days (normal cells) or 10 days (neoplastic cells).

Production of monoclonal antibodies

Antikeratinocyte surface monoclonal antibodies were produced as described recently (Suter *et al.*, 1987; 1990). Briefly, paraformaldehyde-induced plasma membrane vesicles from cultured canine keratinocytes were used as the antigen source for the immunization of Balb/c mice. Sp2/O hybridoma cells were fused 1:1 with 1×10^8 spleen cells using polyethylene glycol of MW 1300-1600 (Kodak, Rochester, NY) as the fusogen. Hybridomas were grown in Dulbecco's minimum essential medium (DMEM) supplemented with 20% FBS. Using an indirect peroxidase method, hybridoma supernatants were evaluated for antikeratinocyte cell surface antibody on cryostat sections of canine oesophagus. Hybridomas which produced cell surface-specific antibodies were cultured, cloned by limiting dilution, and reevaluated for antibody production. Five monoclonal antibodies (D9, E10, 1F, 2D and 13E) which showed three different staining patterns on canine oesophagus were used for this study. These patterns have been described elsewhere (Suter *et al.*, 1987).

Immunohistochemistry

An indirect immunoperoxidase method was used to screen monoclonal antibodies for their reactivity with cultured keratinocytes as described recently (Suter *et al.*, 1987). Briefly, undiluted supernatants were incubated on frozen sections of canine oesophagus or lifted cultures for 30 min at 21°C. Peroxidase-conjugated goat antimouse immunoglobulin (Cappel, Malvern, PA) at a dilution of 1:150 was applied for 30 min. Finally, 3-amino 9-ethylcarbazole (AEC; Sigma Chemical Co., St Louis, MO) was used as the chromogen. A peroxidase antiperoxidase (PAP) method was used to test the reactivity of the monoclonal antibodies on submerged keratinocyte cultures as previously described (Suter *et al.*, 1984). Briefly, antimouse immunoglobulin (Sternberger-Meyer, Jarretsville, MD) was used as the linking antibody (diluted 1:40), followed by incubation with mouse PAP complex (Sternberger-Meyer, Jarretsville, MD) at a 1:100 dilution. AEC was used as the chromogen. The following negative controls were included: Complete DMEM and supernatant of a hybridoma cell line producing non-keratinocyte related monoclonal antibodies of the immunoglobulin G1 isotype (Antibody 79). Additionally, oesophagus sections were incubated with diluted samples of each monoclonal antibody which were preabsorbed with the plasma membrane vesicles obtained from cultured keratinocytes.

Lectin histochemistry

To determine the differentiation-associated expression of lectin binding sites of canine keratinocytes, formalin-fixed and paraffin-embedded sections of normal skin (one to three cell layers), moderately hyperplastic skin (up to six cell layers) and markedly hyperplastic skin (more than six cell layers) were evaluated. Additionally, formalin-fixed and paraffin-embedded sections of neoplastic keratinocytes grown at the air–liquid interface for 3, 6, 9, and 12 days were examined. Lectin binding patterns were determined with an indirect immunoperoxidase technique. The following three lectins were used: Soybean agglutinin (SBA), *Ulex europaeus* agglutinin I (UEA-I), and peanut agglutinin (PNA). Briefly, endogenous peroxidase was quenched in deparaffinized and rehydrated tissue sections. Unspecific staining was blocked with diluted non-immune rabbit serum. Sections were incubated with unconjugated lectins (SBA 5μg/ml, UEA-I 40μg/ml, PNA 5μg/ml; Vector Lab., Burlingame, CA) for 60 min at 37°C, followed by incubation with the corresponding goat antilectin antibody (5μg/ml, 30 min, 37°C; Vector Lab., Burlingame, CA). A biotinilated rabbit antigoat antibody was used as secondary antibody (10 min, 21°C) after which the sections were incubated with the streptavidin-biotin-peroxidase complex (1:20, 5 min, 21°C; Zymed Lab., South San Francisco, CA). The resulting immune complex was visualized using 3,3 diaminobenzidine (DAB). To determine specificity of lectin binding, a hapten inhibition test was carried out by incubation of negative control sections with lectins which were preabsorbed with the appropriate inhibiting sugar.

Reactivity of hyperplastic epidermal and mucosal keratinocytes with antikeratinocyte monoclonal antibodies

Twelve epidermis and two nasal planum biopsies taken for diagnostic purposes from canine patients with a history of inflammatory dermatitides were tested for reactivity with three antikeratinocyte monoclonal antibodies using the indirect peroxidase method as described above. The antibodies used were D9, E10, and 1F.

Retinoic acid studies

Cultures of neoplastic keratinocytes grown at the air-liquid interface were incubated with 10^{-6}M retinoic acid for 2 or 8 days respectively before harvesting. Non-retinoic acid treated cultures served as control. Half of the cultures were formalin-fixed, paraffin-embedded, and stained with haematoxylin/eosin (HE). Morphologic changes were assessed by light microscopy. Using the indirect peroxidase assay, 4μm frozen sections of the second half of the cultures were tested for reactivity with four monoclonal antibodies (D9, 1F, 13, 2D).

RESULTS

Expression of differentiation antigens and lectin binding sites by keratinocytes *in vivo*

The three monoclonal antibodies used bound to normal, fully differentiated oral stratified squamous epithelium in three distinct distribution patterns as described recently (Suter *et al.*, 1987). D9 reacts with all cell layers, E10 binds to all layers but spares the basal cells, and 1F stains only the superficial, differentiated cell layers. Normal canine skin only expresses the D9 antigen while the antigens of differentiated cells (E10 and 1F) are absent. The reactivity of 12 epidermis and two nasal planum biopsies of dogs with inflammatory lesions with the three antibodies is detailed in Table 1. The hyperplastic epidermis of all dermatitides newly expressed the 1F differentiation antigen (Fig. 1) independent of the type of dermatosis.

Table 1 Expression of cell surface antigens by hyperplastic epidermal keratinocytes

Diagnosis	No. of layers	Monoclonal antibodies			
		D9	E10	1F	79
Skin					
superf. perivascular dermatitis ($n=2$)	>9	+	–	+	–
superf. perivascular dermatitis ($n=2$)	5	+	–	+[a]	–
superf. periv. derm./demodex foll.	5	+	–	+[a]	–
lupus erythematosus ($n=2$)	>9	+	–	+	–
lupus erythematosus	>12	+	–	–	
pemphigus foliaceus	>12	+	–	+	–
pemphigus foliaceus ($n=2$)	5–8	+	–	+[a]	–
dermatomyositis	5	+	–	+[a]	
Nose					
lupus	8	+	+	+	–
subcorneal pust. dermatosis	>10	+	+	+	–
Controls					
normal skin	1–3	+	–	–	—
normal lip	8	+	+	+	—

Antibody patterns: D9 – all layers, E10 – suprabasal, 1F – superficial, 79 – negative control; [a] = patchy distribution.

However, the antigen was only expressed in a patchy pattern in moderately hyperplastic skin with four to six keratinocyte layers. In contrast, the suprabasilar antigen E10 which is present in normal nasal and oral mucosa, is absent in hyperplastic skin.

Table 2 summarizes the expression of lectin binding sites on normal and hyperplastic canine skin. SBA binding sites are increasingly expressed from the basal to the suprabasilar layers and decrease in the superficial layers. UEA-1 reacted exclusively with superficial, differentiated cells of hyperplastic skin. In contrast, PNA binding sites are expressed in basal and suprabasal cells and are absent in superficial cells. Lectin staining of PNA and SBA are similar between normal and hyperplastic skin.

Expression of differentiation antigens and lectin binding sites on canine keratinocytes *in vitro*

Normal keratinocytes cultured submerged in medium form only four to five flat cell layers and lack the morphology of a well differentiated stratified squamous epithelium (Wilkinson *et al.*, 1987). These cells reacted with monoclonal antibodies D9 and E10. Antigen 1F is not expressed by these cells. If these same normal keratinocytes are grown at the air–liquid interface, they

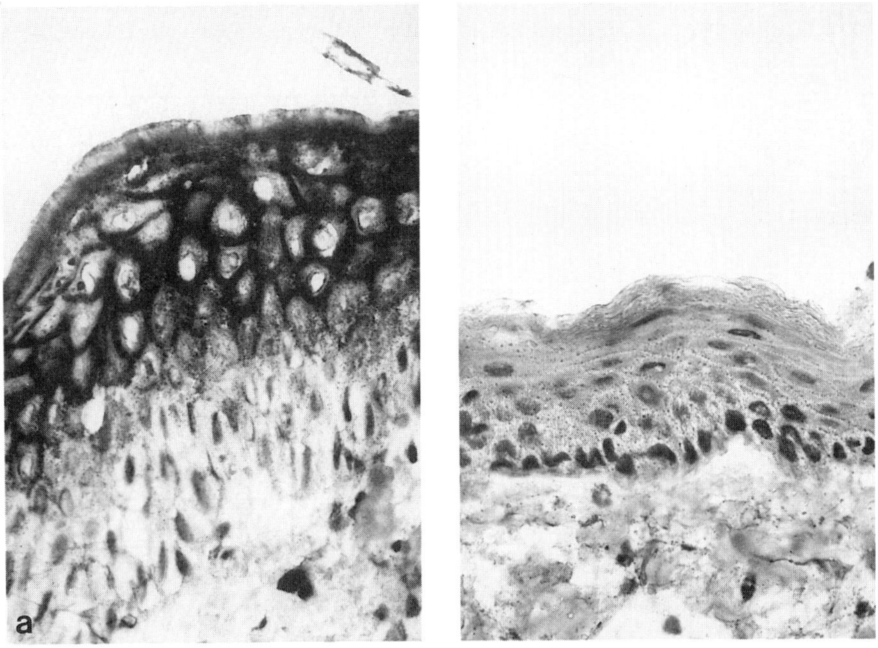

Figure 1 Immunohistochemical staining of mildly and severely hyperplastic epidermis with monoclonal antibody 1F. (a) Severe hyperplasia. Note the distinct staining of the cell surface of the superficial keratinocyte layers. (b) Mild hyperplasia. No antibody binding to the cell surface of keratinocytes is present.

Table 2 Lectin binding patterns of normal and hyperplastic canine epidermis

Lectins	Normal skin		Hyperplastic skin					
	1–3 layers		4–6 layers		>6 layers			
	B	S	B	S	U	B	S	G
SBA	–/+	++	–	++	+	–	++	–/+
UEA-I	–	–	–	–	–/+	–	–	–/+
PNA	+	++	+	++	–	+/++	++	–

B: basal cell layer; S: suprabasal cell layers; U: upper, superficial cell layers.

change their morphology to a full thickness stratified squamous epithelium as seen *in vivo*, in e.g. oral epithelium. However, these cells did not express the differentiation antigen 1F, unless grown on collagen-coated membranes (Table 3).

Neoplastic keratinocytes grown at the air–liquid interface also show increased differentiation and form a stratified squamous epithelium comparable to that of normal cells. However, multifocally they form clusters

Table 3 Reactivity of monoclonal antibodies with normal canine keratinocytes grown at the air–liquid interface

Antibody	Lip	Culture		
		Submerged	Lifted	Lift/Coll
Monoclonal antibodies				
mAb D9	+	+	+	+
mAb E10	+	+	+	+
mAb 1F	+	–	–	+

Lifted: culture at the air–liquid interface; Coll: collagen.

Table 4 Lectin binding patterns of neoplastic canine keratinocyte cultures grown at the air–liquid interface

Lectin	Grown at the air–liquid interface				
	3 days		9 days		
	B	S	B	S	U
SBA	–	+ +	+	+ +	–
UEA-1	–	+	–	+	–/+
PNA	+/+ +	–	+ +	+	–

B: basal cell layer; S: suprabasal layers; U: upper, superficial layers.

of unorganized cells with basal cell morphology or whorls with a few central cells resembling suprabasilar cells. Lectin binding patterns of these cultures is similar to that of native stratified squamous epithelium (Table 4). Soybean agglutinin binding sites are strongly expressed in suprabasal cell layers and decrease in the superficial cell layers; UEA-1 binds to some suprabasal cells but mainly to the superficial cell layers, while PNA staining is seen on the surface of basal cells while decreasing intensity towards the surface of the culture (Fig. 2).

Effect of retinoic acid on the differentiation of canine keratinocytes *in vitro*

In lifted cultures grown in the presence of retinoic acid the basal cells and one to two suprabasal cell layers show disorganization of cells and an increased number of cells with basal cell morphology. There was a distinct difference in the staining patterns of all superficially binding monoclonal antibodies (Table 5). The three antibodies tested (1F, 2D, and 13) strongly reacted with all suprabasal keratinocyte layers in the control culture. After 2 days of incubation with retinoic acid, binding of these superficial antibodies was present only from the fourth layer up. In cultures treated for 10 days, the three antibodies reacted only with clusters of superficial cells.

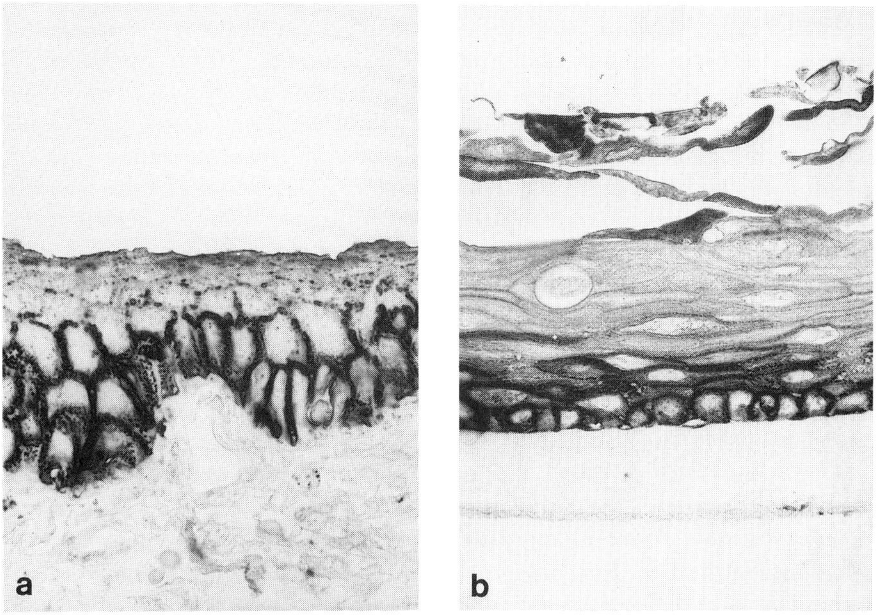

Figure 2 Lectin immunohistochemistry demonstrating binding of PNA to hyperplastic epidermis (a) and keratinocyte culture grown at the air–liquid interface (b). Strong lectin binding is present within the basal cell layer of both epithelia. The spinous cells of the epidermis have a higher expression of the lectin binding site than the lifted culture.

Table 5 Effect of retinoic acid on the expression of cell surface antigens of neoplastic keratinocytes at the air–liquid interface

mAb	Staining pattern	Control	Retinoic acid	
			2 days	9 days
D9	Entire epithelium	+ +	+ +	+ +
1F	Superficial layers	+ +	nd	−/+
13	Superficial layers	+ +	+	−
2D	Superficial layers	+ +	+	−/+

mAb: monoclonal antibody.

DISCUSSION

Stratified squamous epithelium is a well organized tissue with clearly defined layers of epithelium. These layers show variability in morphology and function. The cells of the basal layer are the proliferating cell population as has been demonstrated in healthy skin of beagles and cocker spaniels (Kwochka and Rademakers, 1989). After leaving the basal cell layer, the cells gradually move upward in an orderly manner and undergo a process of differentiation. In human and murine keratinocytes distinct heterogeneity between these cell layers has been demonstrated (Staiano-Coico *et al.*, 1986; Buidin *et al.*, 1988; Skerrow *et al.*, 1989). While keratins 5 and 15 are mainly expressed in basal cells of the human epidermis, keratins 1 and 10 are present in terminally differentiated cells (Fuchs, 1988). Additionally, keratins 6 and 16 which are not normally expressed in the epidermis, are present in keratinocytes during wound-healing and in hyperproliferative stages (Kopan and Fuchs, 1989). Some keratins are specific to cetain body sites, e.g. keratin 9 (Knapp *et al.*, 1986; Moll *et al.*, 1987). In addition to differentiation-dependent changes in cytoplasmic components such as various keratins (Fuchs, 1988; Kopan and Fuchs, 1989), involucrin (Watt, 1987; Walts *et al.*, 1985; Banks-Schlegel and Green, 1981; Etoh *et al.*, 1986; Murphy *et al.*, 1984), transglutaminase (Thacher, 1989; Thacher and Rice, 1985), and some lesser defined proteins (e.g. protein 195lD or Gp37) (Zambruno *et al.*, 1986; Ma and Sun, 1986; Simon and Green, 1984), the expression of certain cell surface markers changes during differentiation. In the dog, monoclonal antibodies directed against cell surface antigens have been used to define distinct subpopulations of keratinocytes in different layers of the stratified squamous epithelium and in stratified squamous epithelia of different tissue origin (Suter *et al.*, 1987; 1990). Some of these antibodies have been used in this study to demonstrate the alteration of cell surface antigen expression in hyperplastic epidermis. The differentiation-specific molecule reacting with monoclonal antibody 1F, which is not expressed by normal epidermal cells, appears on hyperplastic keratinocytes. The expression of new cell surface antigens in hyperplastic skin of chronic dermatitides may play a role in the pathogenesis of immune-mediated dermatoses. Autoimmune diseases, e.g., can develop subsequent to chronic dermatitis. Interestingly, we have demonstrated the presence of pemphigus foliaceus antigen only on highly differentiated lifted keratinocyte cultures and not on undifferentiated submerged cultures (Wilkinson *et al.*, 1989b). The antigen of antibody E10, present on differentiated lip epithelium could not be demonstrated on hyperplastic skin and seems to be specific for epithelia which normally show a higher degree of differentiation than the epidermis such as nasal, oral and oesophageal mucosa (Suter *et al.*, 1990). Canine keratinocytes derived from normal epithelium have been established and characterized in culture (Wilkinson *et al.*, 1987). In submerged cultures these cells show only a minor degree of differentiation and fail to express the differentiation markers shown by monoclonal antibody binding. In contrast, keratinocytes develop into a well differentiated stratified squamous epithelium when grown at the air–liquid interface. An even further degree of differentiation is seen when the cells are plated on a collagen matrix. These 'lifted cultures' express most of the antigens demonstrated on well differentiated native stratified squamous epithelium. Therefore, these cultures of fully differentiated stratified squamous epithelium represent a close imitation of the *in vivo* tissue and can be used for the study of the pathogenesis of a variety of canine skin diseases including autoimmune dermatoses and keratinization defects.

These differentiation markers are useful tools to define the degree of differentiation of such keratinocyte cultures. In tissue culture experiments it is important to be able to ascertain the extent of the degree of differentiation of a stratified squamous epithelium, because submerged monolayer cultures are not terminally differentiated and are not fully representative of *in vivo* stratified squamous epithelium (Wilkinson *et al.*, 1987). The differentiation-dependent antigen recognized by antibody 1F was only expressed on cultures plated on collagen-coated membranes and grown at the air–liquid interface, not on submerged cultures. The determination of the degree of differentiation is critical for the use of these cultures in pathogenicity studies of certain dermatoses. Pemphigus foliaceus antibody, e.g., only reacts with keratinocytes of lifted, collagen-coated cultures similar to antibody 1F (Wilkinson *et al.*, 1989b). Cultured epithelial cell sheets are used as skin grafts for severely burned patients or those with other extensive epidermal defects. The survival rate of such grafted cell sheets is dependent on an advanced degree of differentiation of the cultured keratinocytes (Staiano-Coico *et al.*, 1986; Faure *et al.*, 1987). Adequate markers for differentiation are therefore vital to the success of this procedure. It has been shown, by studies on the embryogenesis of stratified squamous epithelium that expression of differentiation markers such as high molecular weight keratins occur before morphologic evidence of keratinization (Fisher and Holbrook, 1987).

The synthesis of cell surface glycoproteins is clearly regulated and appears to be important in many intercellular interactions (Dennis and Laferte, 1987). Lectin binding surface glycoproteins have been proposed to be involved in the control of cell growth during fetal development (Mann *et al.*, 1988), in cell–cell interactions during differentiation (Morrison *et al.*, 1988), in endocytosis (Monsigny *et al.*, 1988) and in the metastatic potential of tumour cells (Dennis and Laferte, 1987). The expression of *Helix pomatia* (HPA) binding sites on adult human keratinocytes is restricted to differentiated cells (Mansbridge and Knapp, 1984) and UEA-I binding is confined to suprabasilar cells in neonatal rat keratinocytes (Brown *et al.*, 1987; Ku and Bernstein, 1989). Expression of lectin binding sites on the cytoplasmic membrane of canine keratinocytes is also dependent on the state of differentiation; PNA binding sites are heavily expressed on basal keratinocytes and its expression decreases as the cells migrate upwards. In contrast, UEA-I binds only to highly differentiated superficial keratinocytes and SBA is preferentially present on spinous cells.

Neoplastic keratinocytes obtained from spontaneous squamous cell carcinomas have been established in culture. These neoplastic cells can also be grown at the air–liquid interface, under which conditions the degree of differentiation is increased. They form a well differentiated stratified squamous epithelium with a mild irregularity and hyperplasia of the basal cell layer. Human keratinocytes seeded on deepidermized dermis and grown at the air–liquid interface recover the specific morphology of the tissue of origin (tumour versus normal epithelium) (Regnier *et al.*, 1988). The expression of lectin binding sites was analogous to that of the epidermis *in vivo*. SBA and UEA-I being differentiation-dependent, are increasingly expressed on differentiated keratinocytes, while PNA binding site expression decreases towards the superficial layers.

The expression of differentiation markers by keratinocytes is influenced by a variety of factors. The differentiation of murine and human keratinocyte cultures is dependent on the calcium concentration in the culture medium (Morrison *et al.*, 1988; Brown *et al.*, 1987; Dale *et al.*, 1983; Stanley and Yuspa, 1983). In neonatal rat keratinocyte cultures, the binding of basal cells to *Griffonia simplicifolia* (GS-I) was decreased and UEA-I binding of suprabasilar cells was increased as the cells underwent differentiation under the influence of calcium (Brown *et al.*, 1987; Ku and Bernstein, 1989). Retinoic acid inhibits final differentiation of keratinocytes (Ponec *et al.*, 1988; Eichner, 1986) which has to be demonstrated by their altered keratin expression. Human keratinocytes, in cultures treated with retinoic acid (Kopan and Fuchs, 1989). Canine keratinocytes show decreased organization in the lower layers of stratified squamous epithelium and loosening of cell–cell contacts in the spinous layers, changes similar to those described in human keratinocytes (Eichner, 1986). A marked decrease in the expression of the superficially located antigens recognized by monoclonal antibodies was seen in these cultures.

In summary, specific antikeratinocyte monoclonal antibodies and certain lectins are excellent markers to assess the degree of differentiation of canine keratinocytes *in vivo* and *in vitro*. Furthermore, the characterization of the differentiation of canine keratinocytes in these *in vitro* systems has established a powerful and elegant research tool for the study of both pathogenetic mechanisms and therapeutic modulation of inflammatory and neoplastic diseases.

REFERENCES

Banks-Schlegel, S.P. and Green, H. (1981). Involucrin synthesis and tissue assembly by keratinocytes in natural and cultured human epithelia. *Journal of Cell Biology* **90**: 732–737.

Brown, R., Ku, W.W. and Bernstein, I.A. (1987). Changes in lectin binding by differentiating cutaneous keratinocytes from the newborn rat. *Journal of Investigative Dermatology* **88**: 719–726.

Buidin, B., Goldstein, J., Parent, D. *et al.* (1988). Detection of a heterogeneity of basal keratinocytes in human hyperpapillomatous epidermimis: a monoclonal antibody study. *Archives of Dermatologic Research* **280**: 64–66.

Dale, B.A., Schofield, J.A., Hennings, H. *et al.* (1983). Identification of filaggrin in cultured mouse keratinocytes and its regulation by calcium. *Journal of Investigative Dermatology* **81** (Suppl 1): 90s–95s.

Dennis, J.W. and Laferte, S. (1987). Tumor cell surface carbohydrate and the metastatic phenotype. *Cancer and Metastasis Reviews* **5**: 185-204.

Eichner, R. (1986). Epidermal effects of retinoids: *In vitro* studies. *Journal of the American Academy of Dermatology* **15**: 789-796.

Etoh, Y., Simon, M. and Green, H. (1986). Involucrin acts as a transglutaminase substrate at multiple sites. *Biochemical and Biophysical Research Communications* **136**: 51-56.

Faure, M., Mauduit, G., Schmitt, D. *et al.* (1987). Growth and differentiation of human epidermal cultures used as auto- and allografts in humans. *British Journal of Dermatology* **116**: 161-170.

Fisher, C. and Holbrook, H.A. (1987). Cell surface and cytoskeleton associated with epidermal stratification and differentiation in organ cultures of embryonic human skin. *Developmental Biology* **119**: 231-241.

Fuchs, E. (1988). Keratins as biochemical markers of epithelial differentiation. *TIG* **4**: 277-281.

Knapp, A.C., Franke, W.W., Heid, H. *et al.* (1986). Cytokeratin No. 9, an epidermal type I keratin characteristic of a special program of keratinocyte differentiation displaying body site specificity. *Journal of Cell Biology* **103**: 657-667.

Kopan, R. and Fuchs, E. (1989). The use of retinoic acid to probe the relation between hyperproliferation-associated keratins and cell proliferation in normal and malignant cells. *Journal of Cell Biology* **109**: 295-307.

Ku, W.W. and Bernstein, I.A. (1989). Lectin binding as a probe of proliferative and differentiative phases in primary monolayer cultures of cutaneous keratinocytes. *Experimental Cell Research* **175**: 298-316.

Kwochka, K.W. and Rademakers, A.M. (1989). Cell proliferation of epidermis, hair follicles, and sebaceous glands of Beagles and Cocker Spaniels with healthy skin. *American Journal of Veterinary Research* **50**: 587-591.

Ma, A.S. and Sun, T.-T. (1986). Differentiation-dependent changes in the solubility of a 195kD protein in human epidermal keratinocytes. *Journal of Cell Biology* **36**: 827-834.

Mann, P.L., Swartz, C.M. and Holmes, D.T. (1988). Purification of keratinocyte transglutaminase and its expression during squamous differentiation. *Mechanisms of Ageing and Development* **44**: 17-33.

Mansbridge, J.N. and Knapp, A.M. (1984). The binding of helix promatia and ulex europeus agglutinins to normal and psoriatic skin. *Journal of Investigative Dermatology* **82**: 170-175.

Moll, I., Heid, H., Franke, W.W. *et al.* (1987). Distribution of a special subset of keratinocytes characterized by the expression of cytokeratin 9 in adult and fetal human epidermis of various body sites. *Differentiation* **33**: 254-265.

Monsigny, M., Roche, A.-C., Kieda, C. *et al.* (1988). Characterization and biological implications of membrane lectins in tumor, lymphoid and myeloid cells. *Biochimie* **70**: 1633-1649.

Morrison, A.I., Keeble, S. and Watt, F.M. (1988). The peanut lectin-binding glycoprotein of human epidermal keratinocytes. *Experimental Cell Research* **177**: 247-256.

Murphy, G.F., Flynn, T.C., Rice, R.H. *et al.* (1984). Involucrin expression in normal and neoplastic human skin: A marker for keratinocyte differentiation. *Journal of Investigative Dermatology* **82**: 453-457.

Ponec, M., Weerheim, A., Kempenaar, J. *et al.* (1988). Proliferation and differentiation of human squamous carcinoma cell lines and normal keratinocytes: Effects of epidermal growth factor, retinoids, and hydrocortisone. *In vitro Cellular Development and Biology* **24**: 764-770.

Regnier, M., Desbas, C., Bailly, C. *et al.* (1988). Differentiation of normal and tumoral human keratinocytes cultured on dermis: Reconstruction of either normal or tumoral architecture. *In vitro Cellular Development and Biology* **24**: 625-632.

Simon, M. and Green, H. (1984). Participation of membrane-associated proteins in the formation of the cross-linked envelope of the keratinocyte. *Cell* **36**: 827–834.

Skerrow, C.J., Clelland, D.G. and Skerrow, D. (1989). Changes to desmosomal antigens and lectin-binding sites during differentiation in normal human epidermis: A quantitative ultrastructural study. *Journal of Cell Science* **92**: 667–677.

Staiano-Coico, L., Higgins, P.J., Darzynkiewicz, Z. *et al.* (1986). Human keratinocyte culture: Identification and staging of epidermal cell subpopulations. *Journal of Clinical Investigation* **77**: 396–404.

Stanley, J.R. and Yuspa, S.H. (1983). Specific epidermal protein markers are modulated during calcium-induced terminal differentiation. *Journal of Cell Biology* **24**: 764–770.

Suter, M.M., Palmer, D.G., Zindel, S. *et al.* (1984). Pemphigus in the dog: comparison of immunofluorescence and immunoperoxidase method to demonstrate intercellular immunoglobulins in the epidermis. *American Journal of Veterinary Research* **45**: 367–369.

Suter, M.M., Wilkinson, J.E., Greenberger, L.J. *et al.* (1987). Monoclonal antibodies: Cell surface markers for canine keratinocytes. *American Journal of Veterinary Research* **48**: 1367–1371.

Suter, M.M., Greenberger, L.J., Wilkinson, J.E. *et al.* (1990). Differential expression of cell surface antigens on canine keratinocytes defined by monoclonal antibodies. *Journal of Histochemistry and Cytochemistry* **38**: 541–549.

Thacher, S.M. (1989). Purification of keratinocyte transglutaminase and its expression during squamous differentiation. *Journal of Investigative Dermatology* **92**: 578–584.

Thacher, S.M. and Rice, R.H. (1985). Keratinocyte-specific transglutaminase of cultured human epidermal cells: Relation to cross-linked envelope formation and terminal differentiation. *Cell* **40**: 685–695.

Walts, A.E., Said, J.W., Siegel, M.B. *et al.* (1985). Involucrin, a marker of squamous and urothelial differentiation. An immunohistochemical study on its distribution in normal and neoplastic tissues. *Journal of Pathology* **145**: 329–340.

Watt, F.M. (1987). Influence of cell shape and adhesiveness of stratification and terminal differentiation of human keratinocytes in culture. *Journal of Cell Science* (Suppl.) **8**: 313–326.

Wilkinson, J.E., Smith, C.A., Suter, M.M. *et al.* (1987). Long term cultivation of canine keratinocytes. *Journal of Investigative Dermatology* **88**: 202–206.

Wilkinson, J.E., Smith, C.A., Suter, M.M. *et al.* (1989a). Role of plasminogen activator in pemphigus vulgaris. *American Journal of Pathology* **134**: 561–569.

Wilkinson, J.E., Smith, C.A., Suter, M.M. *et al.* (1989b). Characterization of canine keratinocyte cultures grown at the air-liquid interface. Manuscript in preparation.

Zambruno, G., Reano, A., Meissner, K. *et al.* (1986). GP37 expression in normal and diseased human epidermis: a marker for keratinocyte differentiation. *Acta Dermtolo-Venereologica (Stockh)* **66**: 185–192.

4.3 The Cellular Defect in Idiopathic Seborrhoea of Cocker Spaniels

Kenneth W. Kwochka and Daniel D. Smeak

College of Veterinary Medicine, The Ohio State University, Columbus, Ohio, USA

INTRODUCTION

Primary idiopathic seborrhoea is a chronic, exfoliative skin disease found in several breeds of dogs including cocker spaniels (Horwitz and Ihrke, 1977; Dunstan and Rosser, 1987; Muller *et al.*, 1989). The disease is characterized by varying degrees of scaling and crusting, dryness or oiliness, keratinaceous plaques, comedones, alopecia, inflammation, and odour. In addition to cocker spaniels, this condition may be seen in springer spaniels, bassett hounds, Irish setters, German shepherd dogs, doberman pinschers, West Highland white terriers, dachshunds, Chinese Shar Peis, labrador retrievers, and poodles (Muller *et al.*, 1989). The dermatitis usually becomes clinically apparent at 1–3 years of age. Idiopathic seborrhoea persists for the life of the dog and is at best controllable with continual topical therapy (Dunstan and Rosser, 1987; Muller *et al.*, 1989).

Histologically, idiopathic seborrhoea in the cocker spaniel is characterized by excessive basketweave to laminated orthokeratotic hyperkeratosis occasionally alternating with layers of parakeratosis, cystic keratin plugging of follicular infundibula, and parakeratotic mounds over the lips of the follicular ostia (Dunstan and Rosser, 1987). Focal spongiosis and a mild-to-moderate superficial perivascular dermatitis composed predominantly of small mononuclear cells are generally present.

Although the complete pathogenesis of the condition is unknown, accelerated epidermopoiesis plays some role in the disease. By labelling keratinocytes in DNA synthesis (S phase) with ^{3}H-thymidine, Baker and Maibach (1987) demonstrated that epidermopoiesis is accelerated in the skin of seborrhoeic cocker spaniels and Irish setters. Kwochka and Rademakers (in press) showed that in cocker spaniels there is basal cell hyperproliferation not only of the interfollicular epidermis but also of the hair follicle infundibulum. Additionally, keratinocytes without dermal components from seborrhoeic canine epidermis have been grown in primary cell culture. These cells show significantly greater proliferation than keratinocytes from dogs with normal skin at the same stage of growth (Kwochka *et al.*, 1987).

These findings suggest the possibility of a primary epidermal cell defect accounting for the accelerated epidermopoiesis. However, the potential role of host factors and dermal–epidermal interactions on expression or non-expression of the hyperproliferation and the clinical signs of the disease must be considered. The keratinocytes may be inherently abnormal, or they may be normal cells responding to abnormal stimuli, or a combination of both may exist as has been defined for psoriasis in man (Krueger *et al.*, 1981; Fraki *et al.*, 1982).

The overall objective of this study was to establish if the epidermal cell hyperproliferation in idiopathic seborrhoea of cocker spaniels is a primary cellular defect or one controlled by host factors from dermal–epidermal interactions. Specifically, we first wished to ascertain if epidermal cells grown *in vitro* would retain their distinctive morphologic and kinetic characteristics when autografts were prepared. Secondly, we proposed to determine the role of dermal–epidermal interactions in expression of the disease by recombinant grafting, autografts and allografts, followed by assessment of structure and proliferation of the grafted epidermis.

MATERIALS AND METHODS

Dogs

Three adult beagle dogs with healthy skin and three adult cocker spaniels with primary idiopathic seborrhoea were used. Determination of healthy skin and coats was made by physical examination, CBC, serum biochemistry evaluation, urinalysis, faecal examination for parasites, and results of cutaneous biopsy examination of the lateral thoracic skin stained with haematoxylin and eosin (HE) and examined by routine light microscopy. None of these dogs had a known prior history of skin disease.

In the cocker spaniels with primary idiopathic seborrhoea, the skin disease had started within the first 3 years of life and had gradually progressed since that time. The cutaneous abnormalities consisted of a greasy skin surface and hair coat, follicular plugging (comedones), generalized excessive scaling, hair loss, mild erythema, ceruminous otitis externa, and variable numbers of focal keratinous plaques composed of a thick layer of tightly adherent yellow scales and crusts. The diagnosis was further confirmed by histologic examination of cutaneous biopsies with findings as described in the previous section.

Other potential causes for the dermatitis were eliminated by negative or normal skin scrapings, fungal culture, bacterial culture or lack of response to antibiotics, intradermal allergy testing, food elimination diet, CBC, serum biochemistry evaluation, urinalysis, faecal examination for parasites, and base-line serum thyroxine or postthyrotropin stimulation thyroxine levels.

All dogs were housed individually in inside runs kept at a temperature of 22°C with a 12-h light cycle. They were acclimated to this environment for at least 1 week before the study. Dog food and water were available at all times. No topical or systemic treatment had been administered for at least 4 weeks prior to the study.

Preparation of cultures

Dogs were maintained under general anaesthesia throughout the skin harvesting procedure. Hair was shaved from the dorsal lumbar area using a No. 40 clipper blade followed by a safety razor. The area was washed three times with chlorhexidine scrub and 70% alcohol. A thin layer of sterile lubricant was applied to the skin surface. Split thickness strips of skin were harvested aseptically using a Brown air dermatome at a thickness adjustment of 0.038 cm. Split thickness skin was immediately immersed in minimal essential medium (MEM) with 1000 units/ml of penicillin, 1 mg/ml of streptomycin, 2.5 μg/ml of Amphotericin B, and 10% fetal calf serum at 4°C. Within 10 h, skin sheets were cut into 0.25 cm^2 sections, immersed in 0.02% EDTA for 15 min, and then transferred to 0.25% trypsin at 4°C for 15–18 h. Epidermis was separated from dermis using watchmaker's forceps. In separate procedures, epidermis and dermis were scissored into smaller pieces. Keratinocytes and fibroblasts were dispersed by gentle pipeting in a trypsin-EDTA solution. Hair and other debris were removed by passage through a 100 μ nylon mesh and cells were concentrated by centrifugation at $180 \times g$ for 10 min at 4°C. Cells were resuspended in culture media and pipeting, filtering, and centrifugation were repeated a second time. Cell counts were performed using a haemocytometer and cell viability was determined by trypan blue exclusion.

Keratinocytes and fibrolasts were seeded separately into plastic dishes at a density of 2.5×10^5 cells/cm^2. Culture media consisted of MEM plus non-essential amino acids, 2mM L-glutamine, 0.4 μg/ml of hydrocortisone, 10% fetal bovine serum, and penicillin, streptomycin, and Amphotericin B at the concentrations listed above. The pH was adjusted to 7.4. Cells were incubated at 36°C in water-saturated air containing 5% CO_2. Cells were fed every 48 h.

Keratinocyte and fibroblast cultures were observed daily by phase contrast microscopy for the 21-day period prior to grafting. Direct cell counts and cell viability were determined weekly from selected samples. Immediately prior to grafting, a representative epidermal cell culture sample was fixed and processed for routine light microscopy to confirm the presence of a fully stratified epithelium.

Epidermal grafts

The fibroblast cultures were dispersed into single cell suspensions by trypsinization 24 h prior to grafting. Fibroblasts were then replated at the same concentration and in the same media in tissue culture dishes to which a Type-I collagen film (Collagen Film F1310, American Biomaterials) had been added to the bottom of the dish. Fibroblasts impregnated the fibrillar matrix of the film over the 24 h prior to grafting.

Immediately before grafting, the media was aspirated from the epidermal cultures followed by one wash in calcium and magnesium-free phosphate buffered saline. The epidermis was then released in a large sheet from each dish by incubation at 36°C in 4 ml of serum-free MEM containing 1.2 units/ml of Dispase II® (Boehringer-Mannheim). The sheets of epidermis were placed over the fibroblast impregnated Type-I collagen films with the basal cell layer in contact with the film. The epidermal sheets were then covered with a Type-I collagen sponge (Helistat®, American Biomaterials). This three-layered collagen-epidermis-collagen 'sandwich' was used for grafting.

The six dogs were divided into three pairs with one beagle and one cocker spaniel per pair. A dermatome was used to prepare a large graft bed on the dorsal and lateral thorax of each dog. Full-thickness skin was removed down to well vascularized connective tissue to insure that no adnexal structures remained to reepithelialize the surface in the grafted areas. Additionally, wide, non-grafted areas (control sites) were prepared around each graft to counter wound contraction over the 6-week course of the study.

Each dog received autografts consisting of autologous epidermis and allografts consisting of epidermis from the other dog in the pair. Regardless of the source of the epidermis, the grafted fibroblasts impregnated into the collagen film were autologous. Each graft was sutured to the connective tissue of the graft bed at four places along its edge with non-absorbable suture material. After all grafts were attached on each dog, the graft beds were covered with a vaseline gauze and a padded bandage held in place with stent sutures. A total of eleven autografts and ten allografts were prepared on the three pairs of dogs. Bandages were changed twice per week until the graft sites were covered by a viable epithelium.

Biopsies

Once per week for 6 weeks, 6 mm punch biopsies were taken of graft sites for HE staining and histologic examination.

Cell labelling

All graft sites and adjacent non-grafted skin were radiolabelled 6 weeks after grafting to assess epidermal cell proliferation. Epidermal cell labelling was accomplished by the intradermal injection of ^{3}H-thymidine (specific activity

> 20 Ci/mM) at a dosage of 10 μCi in 0.1 ml sterile saline per site using a 27-gauge, 1.27 cm needle. All injections were performed between 08.00 and 10.00 h. Biopsies were performed 1 h after labelling by clipping the hair (only necessary in the non-grafted areas) with a No. 40 clipper blade, infusion of 1 ml of 2% lidocaine SC, and sample collection with a 6 mm disposable biopsy punch.

Skin samples were flattened on nitrocellulose filters, placed in Bouin solution for 2 h, and then fixed in 10% neutral formalin for at least 48 h before processing. Samples were dehydrated, embedded in glycol methacrylate, sectioned at 3 μm, and mounted on glass slides. Autoradiographs were prepared, exposed, developed, and stained according to past reports (Messier and Leblond, 1957; Kopriwa and Leblond, 1962; Kwochka and Rademakers, 1989).

Cell counts were performed from areas in which there was uniform labelling of the epidermis. Basal cells with more than five silver grains present in the nucleus were considered adequately labelled. As a measure of epidermal proliferation, an epidermal basal cell labelling index was established by counting a total of 2000 labelled and non-labelled basal cells from each biopsy site on each dog. The labelling index was expressed as a percentage: Epidermal basal cell labelling index (%) = (labelled epidermal basal cells/total epidermal basal cells) × 100.

Statistical analysis

The data were expressed as single datum (mean ± SD). Epidermal basal cell labelling indices were compared between the normal and seborrhoeic dogs and between allografts and autografts on the same dogs using the Mann-Whitney U test. Differences were considered significant at $p < 0.05$.

RESULTS

Gross and histologic observations

The non-grafted control sites surrounding the epidermal grafts appeared to be pink, glistening, healthy granulation tissue which bled easily when traumatized. During the 6 weeks of the study, these areas did not demonstrate epithelial covering. However, in some areas wound contraction and epithelial migration from the edge of the intact skin necessitated removing an additional strip of skin with the dermatome to help insure the purity of the grafted epidermis. Skin biopsies of control sites (Fig. 1) on all animals revealed no evidence of epithelialization or cutaneous adnexal structures. A healthy bed of granulation tissue was observed with oedematous collagenous tissue, fibroblasts, capillaries, and a mild mononuclear cell infiltrate.

During the first 1–2 weeks after grafting, the epidermis appeared as a fine,

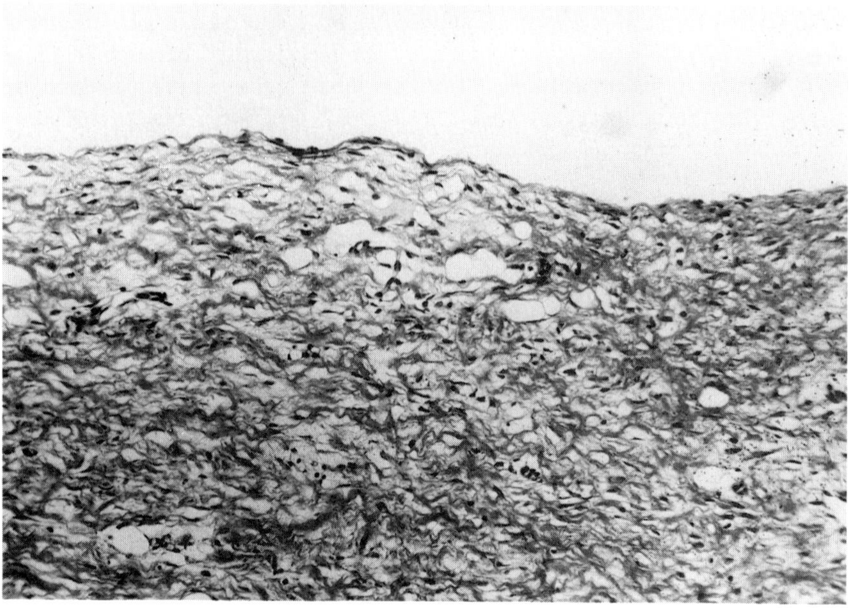

Figure 1 Photomicrograph of a non-grafted control site. A healthy granulation tissue bed is present without epidermis or adnexal structures. HE stain, ×122.5.

glistening whitish covering and was three to 15 layers thick and completely covered the surface of the graft site (Fig. 2). The collagen films and sponges had been absorbed and were not detected on histologic examination. In the newly forming epidermis, there was no apparent stratum corneum or stratum granulosum and the epithelioid cells adjacent to the dermal tissue had not yet organized into a columnar basal layer with a basement membrane. Some cells appeared vacuolated and anuclear. The granulation tissue showed moderate numbers of mononuclear and polymorphonuclear cells.

After the initial 2 weeks, the grafted epidermis matured quickly showing all of the characteristics of non-grafted epidermis *in vivo* but without the adnexal structures. Nine of the eleven autografts and nine of the ten allografts were successful at 6 weeks after grafting. All graft sites appeared to have fully matured into healthy, tough epithelium forming a viable covering of the graft beds. There were no gross or microscopic signs of graft rejection. Those that failed were infected. Grossly, autografts and allografts (onto seborrhoeic dermis) from the beagles with normal skin were essentially normal except for the lack of hair. Histologically, the autografts showed mild epidermal hyperplasia and some intracellular oedema (Fig. 3). Small numbers of mononuclear cells were observed in the dermis. The allografts were essentially the same, showing mild epidermal hyperplasia without intracellular oedema (Fig. 4).

Autografts and allografts (onto normal dermis) from the seborrhoeic cocker

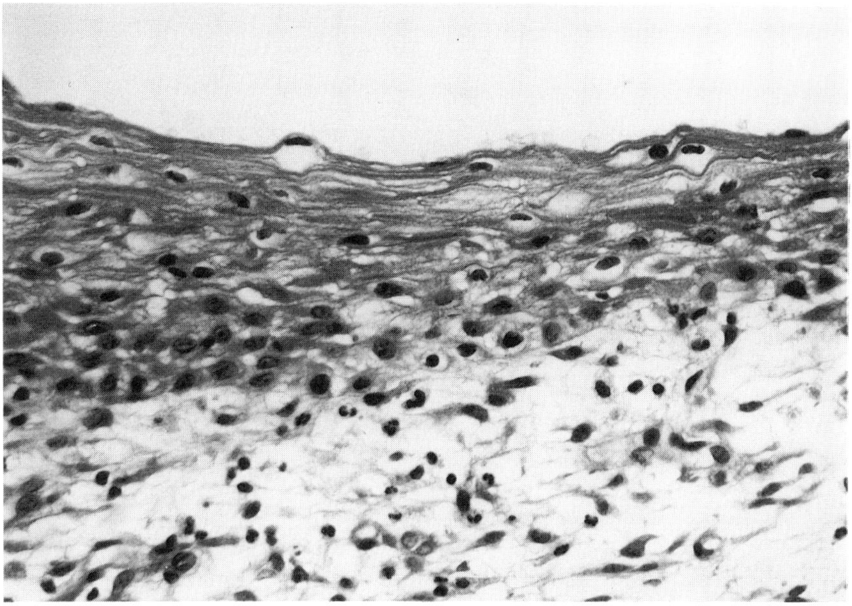

Figure 2 Photomicrograph of a cocker spaniel autograft 7 days after grafting. The epidermis is several cell layers thick but neither stratum corneum nor a stratum granulosum is present. Some of the cells are anuclear and vacuolated. Epithelioid cells adjacent to the dermis have not formed a columnar basal cell layer with a demonstrable basement membrane. HE stain, ×31.5.

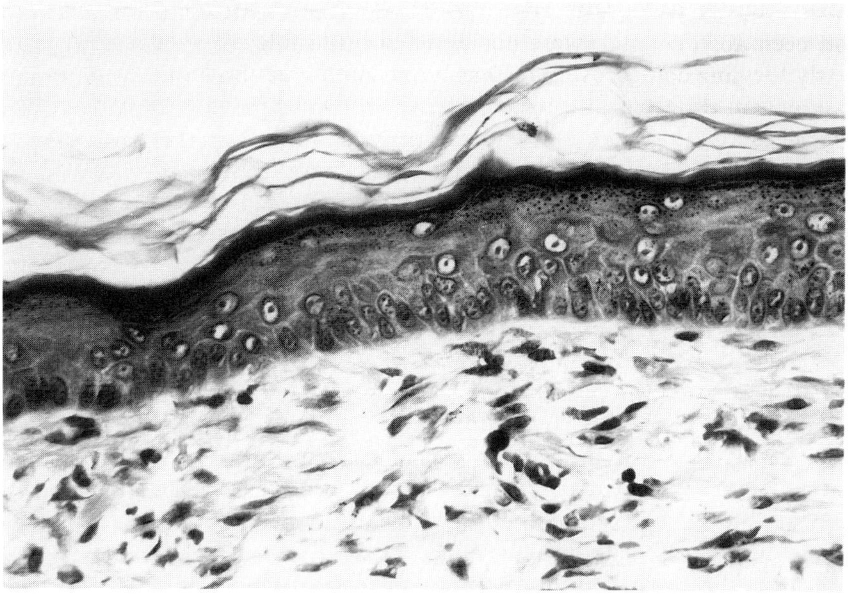

Figure 3 Photomicrograph of a beagle autograft 6 weeks after grafting. There is mild epidermal hyperplasia with some intracellular oedema. HE stain, ×305.

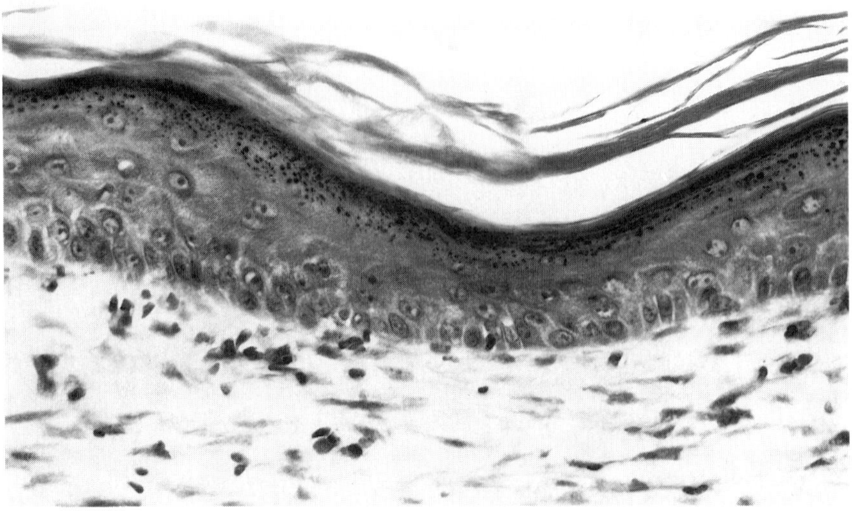

Figure 4 Photomicrograph of a beagle allograft 6 weeks after grafting. There is mild epidermal hyperplasia. HE stain, ×305.

spaniels showed visible exfoliation of large sheets of dry scale and on occasion brown crusts. Autografts appeared histologically to have severe epidermal hyperplasia, intracellular oedema, and disorganization of basal and migrating keratinocytes (Fig. 5). Allografts cultured onto graft beds of normal beagles showed two different histologic patterns. In two of the dogs, mild epidermal hyperplasia with severe basketweave orthokeratotic hyperkeratosis (Fig. 6) was present. The third dog's allografts were characterized by severe parakeratotic hyperkeratosis, hypergranulosis, and irregular epidermal hyperplasia with rete ridge formation along with hypercellularity of the papillary dermis (Fig. 7).

Labelling indices

All basal keratinocyte cell labelling indices are found in Table 1. The labelling index of the epidermis from the skin adjacent to the graft sites was significantly greater in the seborrhoeic cocker spaniels than in the beagles with normal skin. Beagle autografts had a virtually identical labelling index when compared to the adjacent non-grafted skin. The same was true for the cocker spaniel autografts. The labelling index of the cocker spaniel autografts was significantly greater than that from the beagles with normal skin.

Beagle allografts cultured onto the graft beds of seborrhoeic cocker spaniels had an increased but not significantly greater labelling index than the beagle

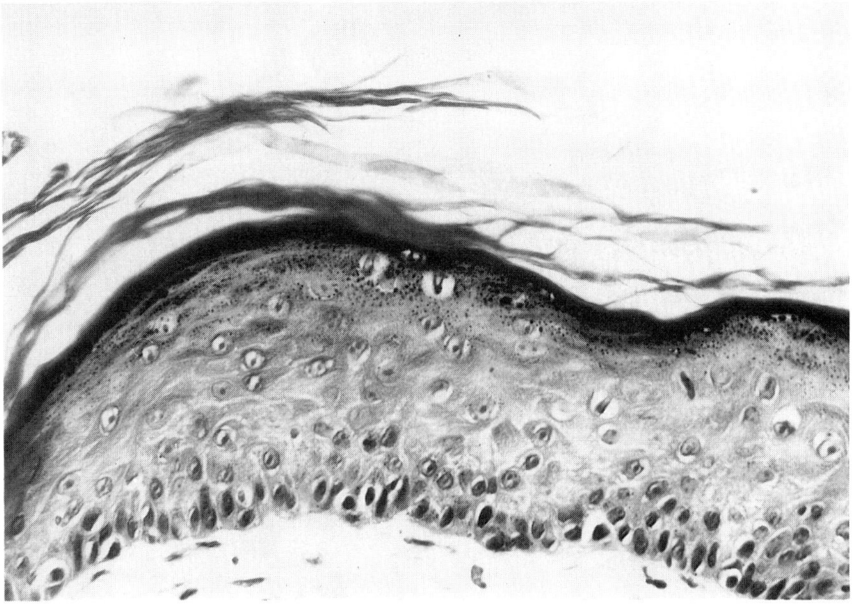

Figure 5 Photomicrograph of a cocker spaniel autograft 6 weeks after grafting. There is severe epidermal hyperplasia, intracellular oedema, and disorganization of basal and migrating keratinocytes. HE stain, ×305.

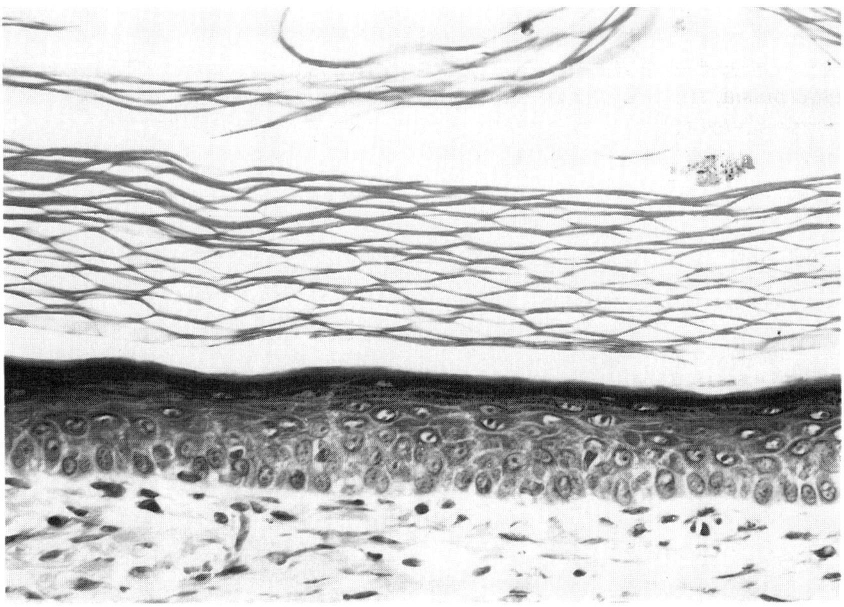

Figure 6 Photomicrograph of a cocker spaniel allograft 6 weeks after grafting. There is mild epidermal hyperplasia with severe basketweave orthokeratotic hyperkeratosis. HE stain, ×305.

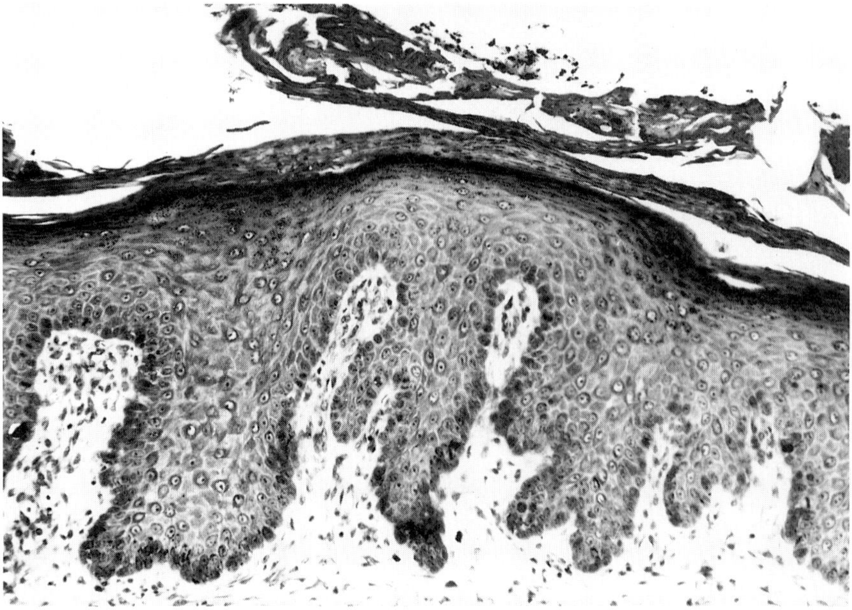

Figure 7 Photomicrograph of a cocker spaniel allograft 6 weeks after grafting. There is parakeratotic hyperkeratosis, hypergranulosis, and irregular epidermal hyperplasia. HE stain, × 122.5.

Table 1 Labelling indices of basal keratinocytes in skin grafts cultured from beagles with normal skin and cocker spaniels with primary idiopathic seborrhoea

Dogs	Basal keratinocyte labelling index (%)		
Breeds/Condition	Skin adjacent to graft site	Autograft	Allograft
Beagles/ Normal skin	1.82	1.79	2.98
	2.16	1.95	3.06
	2.55	2.56	3.75
	2.64	3.19	4.11
	2.77	3.25	
	3.14		
Mean ± SD	2.51 ± 0.47	2.55 ± 0.68	3.48 ± 0.55
Cocker spaniels/ Primary ideopathic seborrhoea	4.19	3.68	7.68
	4.63	4.51	7.95
	4.65	5.63	9.06
	5.49	6.37	9.90
	5.68		10.03
	6.38		
Mean ± SD	5.17 ± 0.82[a]	5.05 ± 1.19[a]	8.92 ± 1.08[a,b]

[a] Significantly different ($p<0.05$) from the corresponding value from the beagles with normal skin.

[b] Significantly different ($p<0.05$) from the labelling index of beagle autografts and cocker spaniel autografts.

autografts. Conversely, seborrhoeic cocker spaniel allografts cultured onto the graft beds of normal beagles showed a significantly increased labelling index over cocker spaniel autografts. Additionally, the cocker spaniel allograft labelling index was significantly greater than beagle autografts and allografts.

DISCUSSION

The success of the autografts (nine of eleven) and allografts (nine of ten) in producing a grossly and histologically viable epidermis 6 weeks after grafting confirms the results of a previous study which used dogs to investigate the potential usefulness of cultured epidermal grafts for wound coverage (Eisinger *et al.*, 1980). Similar studies have also been successful in man in which burned skin was replaced with cryopreserved allogeneic dermis and autologous cultured keratinocytes (Langdon *et al.*, 1988). Although the cultured epidermis appears to become fully integrated with the dermis, we have not yet performed electron microscopic studies to determine whether a complete basement membrane is formed at the dermal–epidermal junction.

When performing epidermal grafting studies, it is important to be sure that the epithelialization is truly from the grafted epidermis and not from the healing wound edge or from mitotically active basal epithelial cells in hair follicles. Deep graft beds were prepared with the dermatome to insure that all adnexal structures had been removed from graft sites. To be certain that dermal components would still be present in these deep graft beds, the Type-I collagen film impregnated with autologous fibroblasts was used under the cultured epidermis. Histologic evaluation of biopsies from non-grafted control sites revealed no epithelialization and no adnexal structures after 6 weeks. In some cases, additional strips of skin were removed from wound edges to interfere with contraction and reepithelialization. Biopsies from the grafted sites (autografts and allografts) also failed to demonstrate adnexal structures, thus negating their potential role in contributing to epithelialization in grafted sites. From this study, we cannot comment on whether epidermal growth and contraction from the wound edge would eventually replace the grafted epidermis over a longer period of time.

Not only do the grafts have a high percentage of success, but the cultivated epidermal cells grown *in vitro* for 21 days have the ability to resume normal functioning *in vivo* with a well-organized epidermis formed on the graft bed. Epidermal autografts from both beagles and cocker spaniels retained their essential morphological characteristics and proliferation indices 6 weeks after transplantation.

The allograft basal cell labelling indices give further support to the cutaneous defect in primary idiopathic seborrhoea of cocker spaniels being primarily epidermal cell in origin. When normal beagle epidermis was grafted onto the dermis of seborrhoeic cocker spaniels, the labelling index was slightly but not significantly elevated. This indicates no significant increase in cell proliferation and correlates well with the histologic observation of only mild epidermal hyperplasia. These findings indicate that there is no apparent influence of host factors or dermal-epidermal interactions from the seborrhoeic cocker spaniels which stimulate the normal epidermis to significant hyperproliferation.

Seborrhoeic cocker spaniel epidermis grafted onto the dermis of normal beagles retained its increased proliferation based on the elevated basal cell labelling index. In fact, the labelling index of these allografts was significantly increased over cocker spaniel autografts and beagle allografts indicating very severe hyperproliferation. These data demonstrate that the epidermal cells themselves are inherently abnormal resulting in aberrant epidermal proliferation in the skin of cocker spaniels with primary idiopathic seborrhoea. However, since the seborrhoeic epidermis becomes significantly more proliferative when grafted onto normal dermis, it appears that some host factors or dermal-epidermal interactions must also play a role in the full expression of the disease. It is possible that the beagle provides host factors not present in the cocker spaniel which stimulate an already hyperproliferative epidermis to greater proliferation. It is also possible that the cocker spaniel produces factors which partially inhibit proliferation of the abnormal epidermis.

Similar recombinant grafting studies have been performed on epidermal hyperproliferative diseases of man including psoriasis (Fraki *et al.*, 1982). Clinically involved psoriatic epidermis maintains its histological appearance and increased labelling index after being grafted onto athymic nude mice, while uninvolved psoriatic epidermis develops an increased labelling index after grafting. Both indices are significantly increased over control skin. These results also suggest a primary epidermal cell defect and that skin can display markers of psoriasis independent of the host.

In conclusion, our data support the hypothesis that primary idiopathic seborrhoea in cocker spaniels is due to a primary epidermal cell defect resulting in aberrant epidermal proliferation. However, host factors or dermal-epidermal interactions also play a role in the full expression of the disease. Further work is needed to elucidate factors in the canine epidermis and dermis which control epidermal cell proliferation. Additionally, studies of keratin expression of the normal and seborrhoeic epidermis *in vivo* and *in vitro* will provide information on the keratinization process. Finally, further cell kinetic studies to evaluate epidermal basal cell growth fraction and full cell cycle characteristics will help to define the cell abnormality and possibly means to control the epidermal hyperproliferation associated with the disease.

REFERENCES

Baker, B.B. and Maibach, H.I. (1987). Epidermal cell renewal in seborrheic skin of dogs. *American Journal of Veterinary Research* **48**: 726–728.

Dunstan, R.W. and Rosser, E.J. (1987). Newly recognized and emerging genodermatoses in domestic animals. *Current Problems in Dermatology* **17**: 216-235.

Eisinger, M., Monden, M., Raaf, J.H. and Fortner, J.G. (1980). Wound coverage by a sheet of epidermal cells grown *in vitro* from dispersed single cell preparations. *Surgery* **88**: 287-293.

Fraki, J.E., Briggaman, R.A. and Lazarus, G.S. (1982). Uninvolved skin from psoriatic patients develops signs of involved psoriatic skin after being grafted onto nude mice. *Science* **215**: 685-687.

Horwitz, L.N. and Ihrke, P.J. (1977). Canine seborrhea. In: Kirk, R.W. (ed.) *Current Veterinary Therapy* Vol. VI, pp. 519-524. W.B. Saunders Company, Philadelphia.

Kopriwa, B.M. and Leblond, C.P. (1962). Improvements in the coating technique of radioautography. *Journal of Histochemistry and Cytochemistry* **10**: 269-284.

Krueger, G.G., Chambers, D.A. and Shelby, J. (1981). Involved and uninvolved skin from psoriatic subjects: are they equally diseased? *Journal of Clinical Investigation* **68**: 1548-1557.

Kwochka, K.W. and Rademakers, A.M. (1989). Cell proliferation of epidermis, hair follicles, and sebaceous glands of Beagles and Cocker Spaniels with healthy skin. *American Journal of Veterinary Research* **50**: 587-591.

Kwochka, K.W. and Rademakers, A.M. (in press). Cell proliferation kinetics of epidermis, hair follicles, and sebaceous glands of Cocker Spaniels with idiopathic seborrhea. *American Journal of Veterinary Research.*

Kwochka, K.W., Rademakers, A.M. and Schultz, K.T. (1987). Development and characterization of an *in vitro* cell culture system for the canine epidermis. *Proceedings of the Annual Members' Meeting of the American Academy and American College of Veterinary Dermatology, Phoenix, 1987*, p. 9.

Langdon, R.C., Cuono, C.B., Birchall, N. *et al* (1988). Reconstitution of structure and cell function in human skin grafts derived from cryopreserved allogeneic dermis and autologous cultured keratinocytes. *Journal of Investigative Dermatology* **91**: 478-485.

Messier, B. and Leblond, C.P. (1957). Preparation of coated radioautographs by dipping sections in fluid emulsion. *Proceedings of the Society for Experimental Biology and Medicine* **96**: 7-10.

Muller, G.H., Kirk, R.W. and Scott, D.W. (1989). *Small Animal Dermatology* pp. 25-33. W.B. Saunders Company, Philadelphia.

4.4 Human Skin Reconstructed *in vitro* as a Model for Studying Epidermal Permeability: Effect of Retinoic Acid

M. Regnier, M. Darmon and H. Schaefer

Centre International de Recherches Dermatologiques (CIRD), Valbonne, France

INTRODUCTION

It is presently possible to 'reconstruct' human skin *in vitro* by growing epidermal keratinocytes on various dermal substrates, such as de-epidermized human dermis (Régnier *et al.*, 1981) or collagen gels (Fusenig *et al.*, 1978; Lillie *et al.*, 1980) which may contain viable cells (Bell *et al.*, 1981; Pruniéras *et al.*, 1983). Human keratinocytes can be obtained after dissociation of interfollicular epidermis (Medawar, 1941; Régnier *et al.*, 1981) or derived from outgrowth of the hair follicle outer root sheath (Lenoir *et al.*, 1988). Under these conditions, the cultured epidermis seems equivalent to normal epidermis with respect to morphological and biochemical criteria.

In the present work, epidermis was reconstructed *in vitro* by growing human keratinocytes on acellular de-epidermized dermis and maintaining the culture at the air–liquid interface. The architecture and differentiation of the cultured epidermis were very similar to those of epidermis *in vivo*. All the differentiation markers studied were localized to the appropriate epidermal layers. Suprabasal cells were distributed in several layers including granular layers and the compact stratum corneum (Régnier *et al.*, 1988). Using ultramicroscopy, it was possible to demonstrate the presence and normal location of structures such as hemidesmosomes and membrane coating granules. Biochemical studies showed that markers of epidermal differentiation such as high molecular weight keratins were also present. The cultured epidermis described here is responsive to hormones and pharmacological agents (Asselineau *et al.*, 1989; Régnier and Darmon, 1989b; Régnier *et al.*,

1989). In order to investigate the permeability barrier function of this reconstructed tissue, we measured the fluxes of tritiated water across the reconstructed epidermis as a function of various culture conditions.

MATERIAL AND METHODS

Tissue culture

Preparation of the substrate

De-epidermized dermis (DED) was prepared according to the technique already described (Pruniéras *et al.*, 1979; Régnier *et al.*, 1984). Briefly, split human cadaver skin was submerged in magnesium and calcium-free phosphate buffered saline at 37°C for 10 days. Epidermis was then separated from the dermis. Dermal cells were killed by successive freezings and thawings and stored at −70°C until use. After separation of epidermis from dermis, the resulting de-epidermized dermis (DED) is still covered with its lamina densa as shown by electron microscopy. Laminin, collagen IV and proteoglycan antigens can also be detected by immunofluorescence (Woodley *et al.*, 1982).

Preparation of reconstructed epidermis on DED

Adult human skin was obtained after skin excision in plastic surgery. Dermatomized skin (0.4 mm thick), was floated on a trypsin solution (0.25%) overnight at 4°C. Epidermis was separated from dermis and further dissociated in a trypsin-EDTA solution as previously described (Régnier *et al.*, 1981). Epidermal suspensions were harvested on mitomycin-blocked 3T3 feeder cells (Rheinwald and Green, 1975; Kubilus *et al.*, 1981). When subconfluent, cells were trypsinized and kept in liquid nitrogen to constitute a stock of frozen cells. Second passage epidermal cells ($5 \times 10^5/cm^2$) were seeded into a steel ring put on the epidermal side of the acellular de-epidermized dermis (Fig. 1). After one day of culture, necessary for the attachment of keratinocytes, the dermis bearing the epidermal cells was lifted up on a grid to maintain the cultured epithelium at the air–liquid interface (Pruniéras *et al.*, 1983).

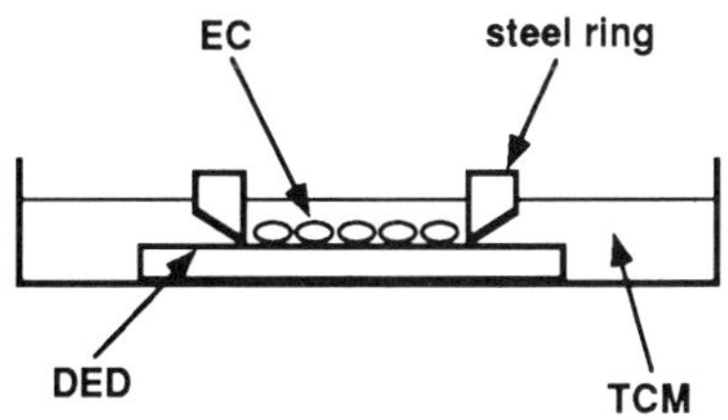

Figure 1 Seeding keratinocytes on DED.

Media

Various culture media were compared: a) mixture of Dulbecco modified minimum essential medium (DMEM) and Ham F12 (3:1), supplemented with either 10% total or delipidized (Rothblat *et al.*, 1976) fetal calf serum (TFCS, DFCS respectively); b) a defined medium MCDB 153 (Boyce and Ham, 1986) without bovine pituitary extract, supplemented with 1.2 mMCa+ + (MCDB).

Relative humidity

TFCS cultures were maintained under an atmosphere of controlled relative humidity (100%, 60% or 25%) in the presence of 5% CO_2 at 37°C.

Variation of time in culture

TFCS cultures were observed after 14, 21, 28 and 35 days; DFCS cultures were taken for permeability assay after 21 and 28 days. Incubation was at 37°C and under 100% relative humidity.

Modulation of epidermal differentiation

TFCS cultures were left in DMEM/F12 medium without serum and growth factors for 6 days. TFCS cultures were also treated for 6 days with 10^{-6} M 1,25 $(OH)_2$ vitamin D_3 to stimulate differentiation and increase the thickness of the stratum corneum (Régnier and Darmon, 1989a). DFCS cultures were treated throughout the culture period with 10^{-6} M retinoic acid which is known to induce parakeratosis (Asselineau *et al.*, 1989; Régnier and Darmon, 1989c). All the culture conditions used are summarized in Table 1.

Table 1 Summary of the culture conditions used for water flux measurements

Culture conditions			
Medium	Relative humidity (%)	Duration of the culture (days)	Modulators of differentiation
TFCS	100, 60, 25	14, 21, 28, 35	
DFCS	100	21, 28	RA
MCDB	100	28	
TFCS/0%FCS	100	22/6	
TFCS/0%FCS	100	22/6	D_3

TFCS: total fetal calf serum; DFCS: delipidized fetal calf serum; MCDB: defined medium; FCS: fetal calf serum; RA: retinoic acid; D_3: 1.25 dihydroxyvitamin D_3.

Characterization of the cultures

Histology

Samples were fixed either in 10% formaldehyde for histological studies or in

Karnovski's fixative for electron microscope observations. Semi-thin sections were stained with toluidine blue.

Indirect immunofluorescence

Samples were embedded in OCT compound (Tissue-Tek, Miles Laboratories, Naperville, Il) and frozen in liquid nitrogen. Cryostat sections were reacted with bullous pemphigoid serum diluted 1:100, (Prof. Saurat, Geneva, Switzerland); suprabasal cells were identified after reaction with anti-K1/K10 keratin (dilution 1:50, Bioyeda, Israel) and antimembrane-bound transglutaminase (Dr S.M. Thacher, Texas, USA) monoclonal antibodies; anti-involucrin polyclonal and antifilaggrin monoclonal (BIT, Cambridge, Ma) antibodies recognized granular cells. Appropriate fluorescein conjugates were used as second antibodies. Fluorescent stainings were examined with a Zeiss epifluorescence microscope.

Biochemical studies

Keratinocytes of the reconstructed epidermis were labelled for 1 h with ^{35}S methionine (300 μCi/ml, Amersham, 1000 Ci/mmol). The epidermis was then gently detached from the dermis. The soluble proteins were extracted in high salt butter (Winter *et al.*, 1980), the keratins were solubilized in 5% SDS, 5% β-mercaptoethanol, 10 mM tris-HC1 ph8 at 65°C for 1 h and migrated on polyacrylamide gel. After electrophoresis, gels were dried and exposed to hyper MP film (Amersham) for 4 days. Keratinocytes of the reconstructed epidermis were detached from dermis by scraping. The samples were boiled for 30 min in a reaction mixture consisting of 2% sodium dodecylsulphate and 2% β-mercaptoethanol. The envelopes were centrifuged and resuspended in a small volume of the same mixture. Morphological observations were made under Nomarski contrast microscopy according to Michel *et al.* (1988).

Water flux

After 1 h at room temperature and a relative humidity of 54%, reconstructed skin specimens were mounted in diffusion cells (Franz, 1978) (Fig. 2); 3 ml of 0.9% sodium chloride were introduced into the lower chamber. Tritiated water (Amersham 5 Ci/ml) was diluted with water to a volumetric activity of 0.025 μCi/μl. A volume of 40 μl (1 μCi) was applied onto the epidermis. Every 2 h during a 6-h period, fluid in the lower chamber was withdrawn and replaced with fresh sodium chloride solution; 500 μl samples were counted for ^3H by liquid scintillation counting. Eight separate determinations were performed for each type of sample. The mean rate of HTO flux was determined and expressed in $\mu g/cm^2/h$.

Control samples

Normal human skin (NHS) was obtained from plastic surgery; de-epidermized dermis (DED) was maintained air-exposed with TFCS at 37°C in 100% relative humidity for 28 days.

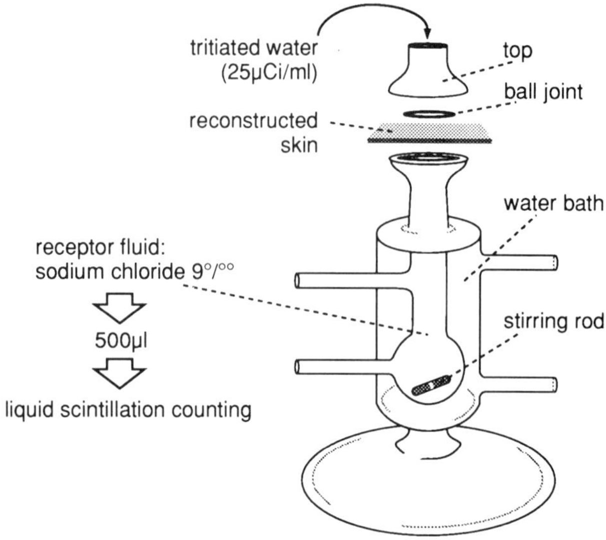

Figure 2 Franz diffusion cell for *in vitro* percutaneous absorption.

RESULTS

Architecture of the epidermis reconstructed on de-epidermized dermis

After 7 days of culture of keratinocytes on de-epidermized dermis (DED), a stratified and fully differentiated epidermis is obtained (Fig. 3). All classical ultrastructural markers of differentiation are present: normal hemidesmosomes present at the dermal–epidermal junction, desmosomes, tonofilaments, intra- and extracellular membrane coating granules, homogeneous and heterogeneous keratohyaline granules, and thickening of the cell wall of anucleated corneocytes (Régnier *et al.* 1981) (Table 2). Immunofluorescence studies revealed the presence of bullous pemphigoid antigen at the basal side of basal cells, suprabasal keratins K1/K10 in all suprabasal layers, and filaggrin in the granular cells. Moreover, a compact stratum corneum was formed (Régnier and Darmon, 1989c) (Table 3).

Biochemical markers

Keratin synthesis
All normal epidermal keratins, including K1 and K10 which are specific for suprabasal cells, were observed. In addition, K6 and K16/17 (the so-called 'hyperproliferative' keratins) were also present as in all types of cultures of keratinocytes.

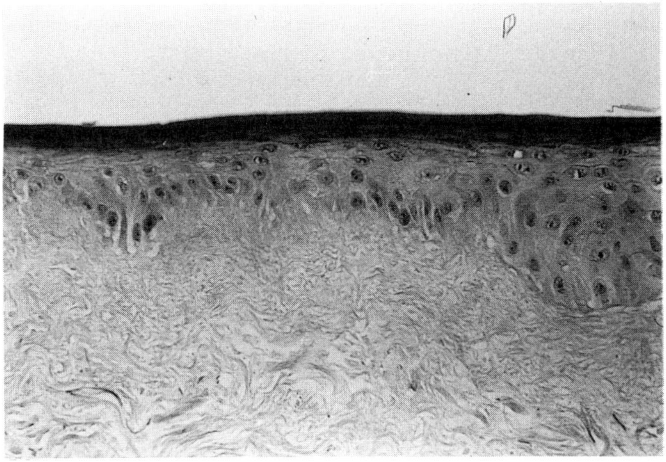

Figure 3 Histological section of the epidermis reconstructed on DED. A stratified and well keratinized epidermis is formed after 7 days of culture.

Table 2 Ultrastructural markers of differentiation

Epidermis *in vivo*	Epidermis cultured on DED
Hemidesmosomes	+
Desmosomes	+
Tonofilaments	+
Homogeneous keratohyalin granules	+
Heterogeneous keratohyalin granules	+
Intra/extracellular membrane coating granules	+
Membrane thickening	+
Keratin pattern	0

Table 3 Markers of differentiation detected by immunofluorescence

Immunological markers	Epidermis *in vivo*	Epidermis cultured on DED
Bullous pemphigoid	Basal cells	Basal cells
Keratins 1/10	Suprabasal cells	Suprabasal cells
Membrane-bound transglutaminase	Suprabasal cells	Suprabasal cells
Involucrin	Granular cells	Suprabasal cells
Filaggrin	Granular cells	Granular cells

Envelope formation

Nomarski contrast microscopy revealed the two morphological types of envelopes already described in human epidermis (Michel *et al.*, 1988). One has a polygonal 'rigid' type, the other has an irregular, withered and 'fragile' appearance. These results are summarized in Table 4.

Table 4 Markers of differentiation studied at the biochemical level

Keratin synthesis	Epidermis *in vivo*	Epidermis cultured on DED
K1/K10	+	+
K5/K14	+	+
K6/K16–17	0	+
Envelope formation		
Rigid	+	+
Fragile	+	+

Water flux

Effect of the composition of the culture media

Cultures were maintained for 28 days in three different media: a classical one, DMEM/F12 containing total fetal calf serum (TFCS cultures); the same base-medium supplemented with delipidized serum (DFCS cultures) and a defined medium enriched in growth factors in which Ca+ + level was elevated to 1.2 mM (MCDB cultures). The flux of tritiated water through DFCS cultures was 10 times faster than across normal dermatomized skin (NHS), although it was 30 times faster through TFCS cultures maintained at 100% relative humidity than through NHS. Penetration across MCDB cultures showed a water flux equivalent to that found through DED devoid of epidermis (Fig. 4).

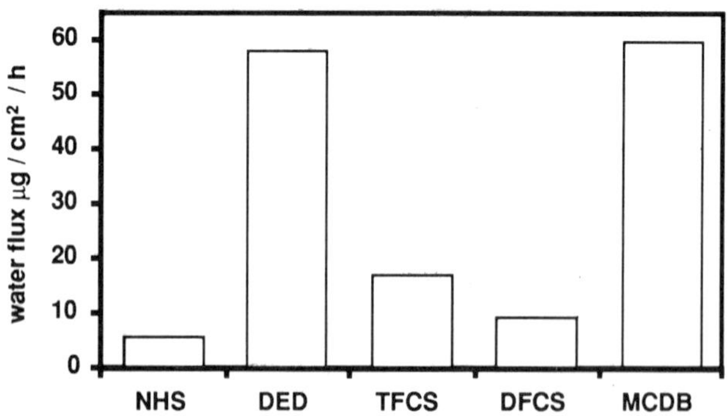

Figure 4 Water fluxes through normal human skin (NHS), de-epidermized dermis (DED) and reconstructed epidermis on DED cultured in DMEM/F12 medium containing total (TFCS) or delipized (DFCS) fetal calf serum and in defined medium (MCDB).

Effect of relative humidity

TFCS cultures were observed after 28 days at 100%, 60% or 25% relative humidity (RH). The water fluxes were found to decrease in correlation with the decrease of relative humidity. However, the flux was still 10 times higher through epidermis reconstructed at 25% humidity than through NHS (Fig. 5).

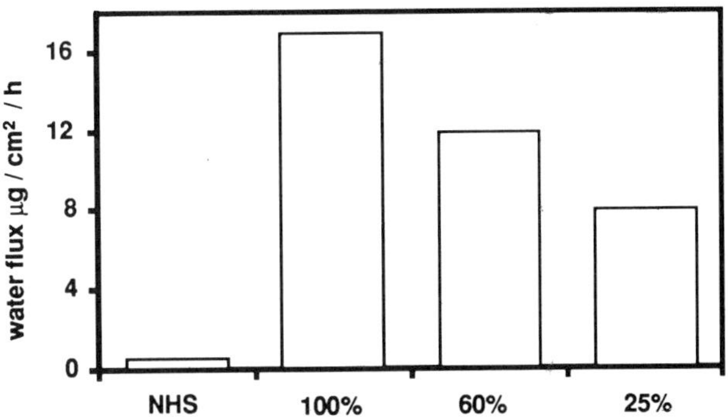

Figure 5 Water fluxes through normal human skin (NHS) and reconstructed epidermis on DED cultured in TFCS for 28 days under 100%, 60%, 25% relative humidity.

Effect of the duration on the cultures

TFCS cultures were maintained at 100% RH for 14, 21, 28 or 35 days. DFCS cultures were observed after 28 and 35 days. Differences in water flux between older and younger cultures were minimal. All values were about 20–30 times higher than the flux through NHS. However, a slight decrease of permeability of the cultured epithelium was observed after 35 days in DFCS cultures (Fig. 6).

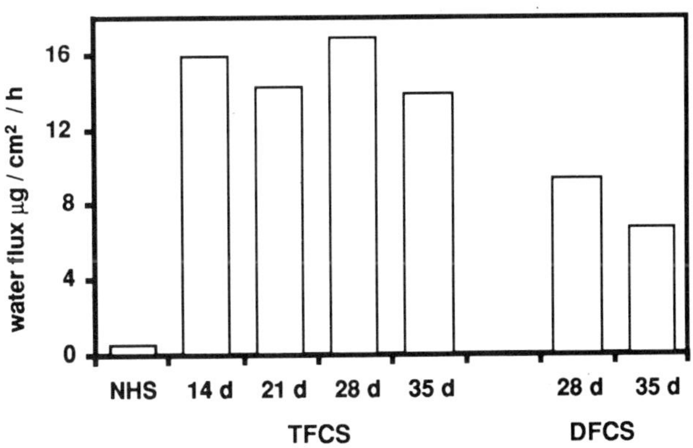

Figure 6 Water fluxes through normal human skin (NHS) and reconstructed epidermis on DED cultured in TFCS for 14, 21, 28, 35 days or in DFCS for 28 and 35 days.

Effect of modulators of epidermal differentiation

Steady state cultures were maintained in serum-free DMEM/F12 medium in the presence and absence of dihydroxyvitamin D_3 for 6 days. After 24 h, DFCS cultures were treated with retinoic acid for 28 days.

A normal viable epidermis was still present in serum-depleted cultures (Fig. 7c). However, the stratum corneum was thicker than in normal cultures. The vitamin D_3-treated epidermis contained only one or two layers of nucleated

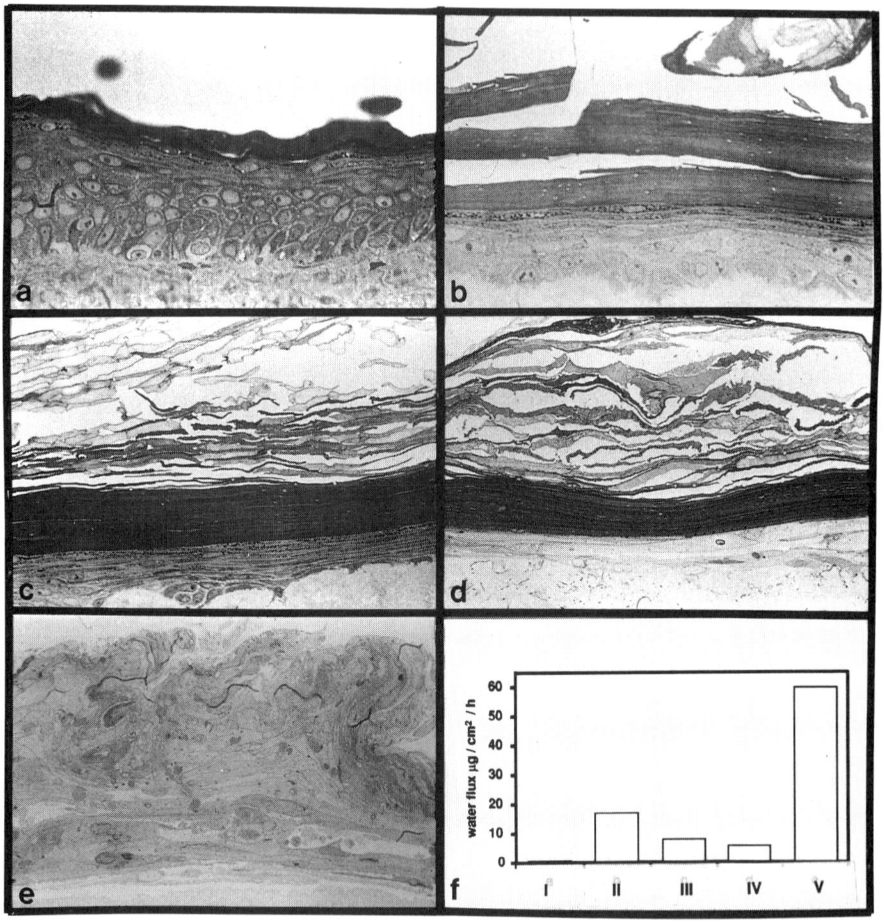

Figure 7 (a)–(e): Semi-thin sections of normal human skin (orthokeratosis) (a) and reconstructed epidermis on DED cultured for 28 days in TFCS (orthokeratosis) (b), for 22 days in TFCS followed by 6 days without serum (orthokeratosis) (c), for 22 days in TFCS followed by 6 days without serum and in presence of 10^{-6} M vitamin D_3 (orthokeratosis, but with diminished nucleated compartment) (d) and for 28 days in presence of 10^{-6} M retinoic acid (parakeratosis and agranulosis) (e). (f) Water fluxes through: (I) normal human skin; reconstructed epidermis on DED in the culture conditions described above: (II) TFCS, (III) without serum, (IV) 10^{-6} M vitamin D_3 retinoic acid.

cells (Régnier and Darmon, 1989a), but the stratum corneum was much thicker than in untreated reconstructed epidermis; at least 10 additional layers of corneocytes were observed in the presence of the vitamin (Fig. 7d). In cultures treated with retinoic acid, the stratum corneum was disorganized and parakeratotic (Fig. 7e). Water fluxes were 10 times higher through epidermis reconstructed in the presence of serum-free medium (Fig. 7f) supplemented with or without vitamin D (Fig. 7f III,IV) than through normal skin. When cultures were treated with retinoic acid, the flux was 20 times higher (Fig. 7f V).

DISCUSSION AND CONCLUSIONS

This work was undertaken to determine whether human epidermis reconstructed *in vitro* retains its barrier function. Our results show that epidermis reconstructed on de-epidermized dermis is equivalent to normal epidermis with regards to its morphology and architecture. All biochemical markers of differentiation are also present. However, we found that the reconstructed epidermis is much more permeable than normal epidermis. Our results correlate well with those reported by Cumpstone *et al.* (1989), who measured water fluxes through mouse keratinocyte cultures performed on collagen-coated filters maintained at the air–liquid interface. In their experiments, permeability of water through the cultures was much higher than through fresh skin. But, instead of using fresh skin as a control if the comparison is made with skin cultured for a short time under the same conditions, the permeability of the reconstructed epidermis is only five times higher. This probably means that the structure of stratum corneum is not completely differentiated and/or functional *in vitro*. Culture conditions seem to play an important role in the barrier function of the cultured epidermis since modulators of differentiation such as retinoic acid and vitamin D_3 significantly modified the permeability of the reconstructed epidermis to water. Thus, improved culture conditions must be elaborated in order to restore an efficient permeability barrier *in vitro*.

ACKNOWLEDGEMENTS

We thank Dr Ph. Sabatier for providing us with skin biopsies. We are grateful to Dr P. Buchan and Dr D. Caron for helpful discussions. We also acknowledge F. Bernerd for preparation of electron microscopy, P. Rossio for histological sections and C. Miquel for her great experience in cell cultures.

REFERENCES

Asselineau, D., Bernard, B.A., Bailly, C. and Darmon, M. (1989). Retinoic acid improves the morphogenesis of human epidermis *in vitro*. *Developmental Biology* **133**: 322–335.

Bell, E., Ehrlich, H.P., Buttle, D. and Nakatsuji, T. (1981). Living tissue formed *in vitro* and accepted as a skin-equivalent tissue of full thickness. *Science* **211**: 1052-1054.

Boyce, S.T. and Ham, R.G. (1986). Normal human epidermal keratinocytes. In: Webber, M.M. and Sekely, L.I. (eds) *In vitro Models for Cancer Research* Vol III, pp. 245-274. CRC Press, Boca Raton, USA.

Cumpstone, M.B., Kennedy, A.H., Harmon, C.S., Phil, D. and Potts, R.O. (1989). The water permeability of primary mouse keratinocyte cultures grown at the air-liquid interface. *Journal of Investigative Dermatology* **92**: 598-600.

Franz, T.J. (1978). The finite dose technique as valid *in vitro* model for the study of percutaneous absorption in man. *Current Problems in Dermatology* **7**: 58-68.

Fusenig, N.E., Amer, S.M., Boukamp, P. and Worst, P.K.M. (1978). Characteristics of chemically transformed mouse epidermal cells *in vitro* and *in vivo*. *Bulletin of Cancer* **65**: 271-280.

Kubilus, J., Rand, R. and Baden, H.P. (1981). Effects of retinoic acid and other retinoids on the growth and differentiation of 3T3 supported human keratinocytes. *In Vitro* **17**: 786-795.

Lenoir, M.C., Bernard, B.A., Pautrat, G., Darmon, M., Shroot, B. (1988). Outer root sheath cells of human hair follicle are able to regenerate a fully differentiated epidermis *in vitro*. *Developmental Biology* **130**: 610-620.

Lillie, J.H., MacCallum, D.K. and Jepsen, A. (1980). Fine structure of subcultivated stratified squamous epithelium grown on collagen rafts. *Experimental Cell Research* **125**: 153-165.

Medawar, P.B. (1941). Sheets of pure epidermal epithelium from human skin. *Nature* **148**: 783.

Michel, S., Schmidt, R., Shroot, B. and Reichart, U. (1988). Morphological and biochemical characterization of the cornified envelopes from human epidermal keratinocytes of different origin. *Journal of Investigative Dermatology* **91**: 11-15.

Pruniéras, M., Régnier, M. and Schlotterer, M. (1979). Nouveau procédé de culture des cellules épidermiques humaines sur derme homologue ou hétérologue: préparation de greffons recombinés. *Annales de Chirurgie Plastique* **24**: 357-362.

Pruniéras, M., Régnier, M. and Woodley, D. (1983). Methods of cultivation of keratinocytes with an air-liquid interface. *Journal of Investigative Dermatology* **81**: 28s-33s.

Régnier, M. and Darmon, M. (1989a). Dihydroxyvitamin D3 provokes a dramatic acceleration of epidermal differentiation. *Journal of Investigative Dermatology* **90**: 600A.

Régnier, M. and Darmon, M. (1989b). Effect of retinoic acid on epidermal differentiation studied in the reconstructed skin model. In: Reichert, U. and Shroot, B. (eds) *Pharmacology of the Skin* Vol. 3, pp. 84-85. Karger, Basel.

Régnier, M. and Darmon, M. (1989c). Human epidermis reconstructed *in vitro*: a model to study keratinocyte differentiation and its modulation by retinoic acid. *In Vitro Cellular and Developmental Biology* **25**: 1000-1008.

Régnier, M., Pruniéras, M. and Woodley, D. (1981). Growth and differentiation of adult human epidermal cells on dermal substrates. *Frontiers of Matrix Biology* **9**: 223-224.

Régnier, M., Desbas, C., Bailly, C., Darmon, Y.M. (1988). Differentiation of normal and tumoral human keratinocytes cultured on dermis: reconstruction of either normal or tumoral architecture. *In Vitro Cellular and Developmental Biology* **24**: 625-631.

Régnier, M., Eustache, J., Shroot, B. and Darmon, M. (1989). Bioassays for retinoic acid-like substances using cultured human keratinocytes. *Skin Pharmacology Journal* **2**: 1-9.

Rheinwald, J.G. and Green, H. (1975). Serial cultivation of strains of human keratinocytes: the formation of keratinizing colonies from single cells. *Cell* **6**: 331-343.

Rothblat, G.H., Arrogast, L.Y., Ouelette, L. and Howard, B.V. (1976). Preparation of delipidized serum protein for use in cell culture systems. *In Vitro* **12**: 557-557.

Winter, H., Schweizer, J. and Goerttler, K. (1980). Keratins as markers of malignancy in mouse epidermal tumors. *Carcinogenesis* **1**: 392-397.

Woodley, D.T., Saurat, J.H., Pruniéras, M. and Régnier, M. (1982). Pemphigoid pemphigus and Pr antigens in adult human keratinocytes grown on non viable substrates. *Journal of Investigative Dermatology* **79**: 23-29.

4.5 The Cervical Apocrine Gland of Neonatal Mink: the Effects of *in utero* Exposure to Polychlorinated Biphenyls on Glandular Development

Julie A. Yager, J.L. Caswell, D. Bruce Hunter and M.A. Hayes

Department of Pathology, Ontario Veterinary College, University of Guelph, Guelph, Ontario, Canada

INTRODUCTION

The importance of chemical communication in determining mammalian behaviour is well recognized (Albone, 1984; Doty, 1986). The secretions of cutaneous glands are a major source of these chemicals, which are often referred to as pheromones but which are more properly termed semiochemicals (Adams, 1980; Albone, 1984; Mykytowycz, 1970). Semiochemicals have been shown to be important in mediating many aspects of reproductive function, including the interaction of mother and young (Albone, 1984; Leon, 1983; Mykytowycz, 1970). While certain glands have been associated with particular behavioural functions, for example the ventral scent marking gland of the gerbil, little is known of the exact source of semiochemicals involved in mediating the interaction of mother and offspring (Harper, 1981; Leon, 1983). Recently, hypertrophic apocrine sweat glands have been described in neonatal mink, *Mustela vison* (Dolnick, 1959; Petskoi and Kolpovsky, 1970; Yager *et al.*, 1988). These glands are not present in the adult and are maximal in size at 2–3 weeks of age. Preliminary behavioural experiments indicate that the glandular secretion may influence maternal recognition of the young (Yager *et al.*, 1988).

There is much public concern about the potential environmental hazard posed by polychlorinated biphenyls (PCBs) to human and animal health (Nath, 1987). Mink are extremely sensitive to the effects of PCBs, and as such may act as a sentinel species for environmental contamination (Roberts *et al.*, 1978). One effect of PCB toxicity in the mink is neonatal mortality (Blevins, 1980). The mechanism of the neonatal mortality is not known but the kits fail to thrive and die from a wasting disease. Passage of PCBs through the milk has been postulated as the route of transfer to the young (Wren *et al.*, 1987).

The effect of PCBs on human health, particularly carcinogenic potential, remains a topic of controversy (Hayes, 1987). Documented adverse effects of human exposure to PCBs include dermatological lesions called chloracne, hepatic dysfunction and decreased pulmonary function (Safe, 1987). Chloracne is characterized clinically by the presence of comedones and histologically by follicular hyperkeratosis and sebaceous gland atrophy (Ebling *et al.*, 1986; Urabe and Asahi, 1985). Dermatological lesions have also been identified after experimental exposure to PCBs in other primates, rabbits and 'hairless' mice (McConnell, 1985) and PCBs have been shown to accumulate in human milk (Hara, 1985), causing concern for the health of the nursing child (Nath, 1987).

In view of the documented pathological effects of PCBs on the mammalian integument, we decided to investigate their effect on the development of the cervical apocrine gland in neonatal mink. We postulated that mink kits exposed *in utero* to PCBs may develop cutaneous lesions which could interfere with secretion and/or production of the putative semiochemicals which assist in maternal recognition. Failure to nurse would readily explain the wasting disease observed in litters from mink fed PCB-contained feed. We found that PCBs affected both body weight and glandular development. The reduction in gland size in the first two weeks of life was greater than could be attributed to the effects on body size alone.

MATERIALS AND METHODS

Ten 1-year-old, pastel colour phase, female mink were housed on a commercial mink farm in wire mink cages. The mink were randomly divided into two equal groups. The five PCB-treated mink were fed a commercial wet mink feed containing 1.0 ppm Aroclor 1254 (originally manufactured by Monsanto Chemical Co., St Louis, Mo, USA) from 2 weeks postbreeding until whelping, a period of approximately 45 days. The five control mink were fed the same diet, without Aroclor.

One live kit was randomly selected from each litter at 1, 7, 14, 21, and 35 days of age and euthanized with pentobarbital. Each kit was weighed, and the length from occiput to tailhead was measured (crown-rump length). After removing the skin the cervical gland was examined from the cutaneous and subcutaneous aspects. The length and width of the gland was recorded. The excised gland was mounted on cardboard and fixed in 10% buffered formalin. After fixation, the cervical gland was sectioned through the widest part, processed for routine histological examination, and stained with haematoxylin and eosin (HE). Morphometric histologic assessment was made using a Zeiss Videoplan. Measurements included total area of all adenomeres beneath a standard length of epidermis, total perimeter of these adenomeres, and average area and perimeter of each adenomere. In addition, total area and the luminal area were measured in 25 adenomeres. From this, the area of glandular cytoplasm of the 25 adenomeres was calculated. This glandular area was expressed as a percentage of total area of the 25 adenomeres.

These data were statistically analysed using a three-way ANOVA procedure to examine the effect of PCB treatment, age of the kit, and interaction between treatment and age on the above measurements and ratios formed by them. Student's t tests were applied to means from each group to evaluate the effect of PCB treatment.

RESULTS

Figure 1(a) compares the body weight of the offspring of PCB treated and control females. The body weights of the offspring of PCB treated mink were significantly lower than those of the controls ($p = 0.05$). These differences increased as the kits aged. A similar trend was noted in the crown to rump length data. Significantly shorter crown to rump lengths ($p = 0.04$) were found in the offspring of PCB treated females.

The macroscopic area off the cervical gland was markedly reduced in the PCB treatment group ($p = 0.0002$) (Fig. 1b). The difference was most apparent in the 1- and 2-week-old kits ($p < 0.05$).

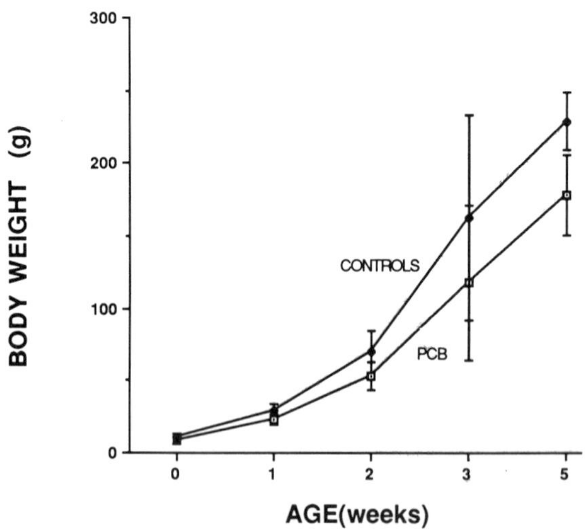

Figure 1a Comparison of the body weight (g) of PCB treated and control mink kits during the first 5 weeks of life. Each datum point represents the mean. The bar represents the standard deviation.

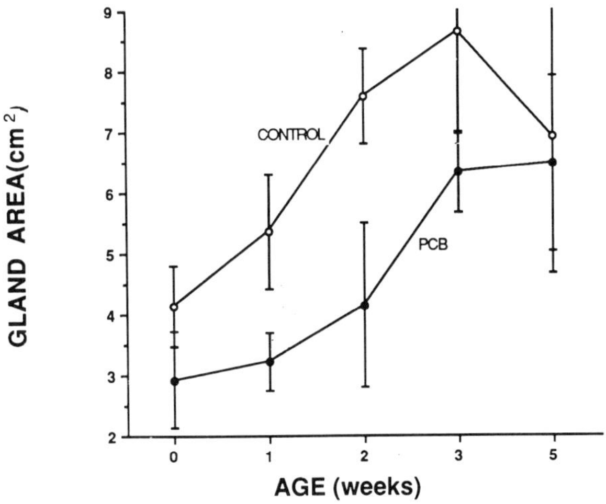

Figure 1b Comparison of the area (cm^2) of the cervical apocrine gland in the offspring of PCB treated and control mink. Each datum point represents the mean; the bar represents the standard elevation.

Ratios of gland area to body weight and body length were calculated to control for the effect of treatment on body size. Both these ratios were smaller in the offspring of the PCB treated group (Figs 2a,b). Differences between the PCB and control groups were highly significantly different when gland area:crown length ratios were compared ($p = 0.0006$). The comparison

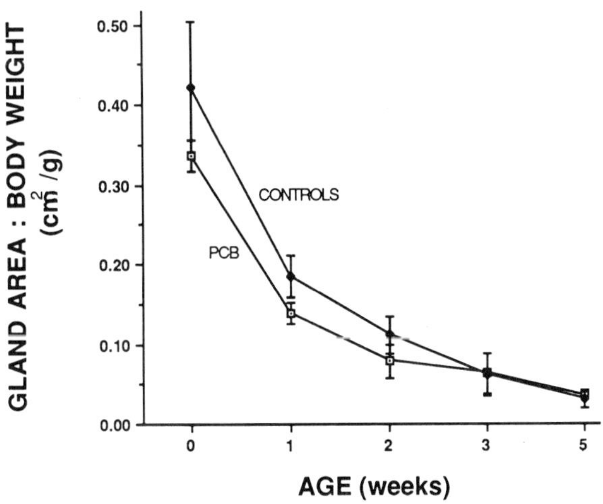

Figure 2a Comparison of the gland area:body weight ratio in the offspring of PCB treated and control mink. Each datum point represents the mean; the bar represents the standard deviation.

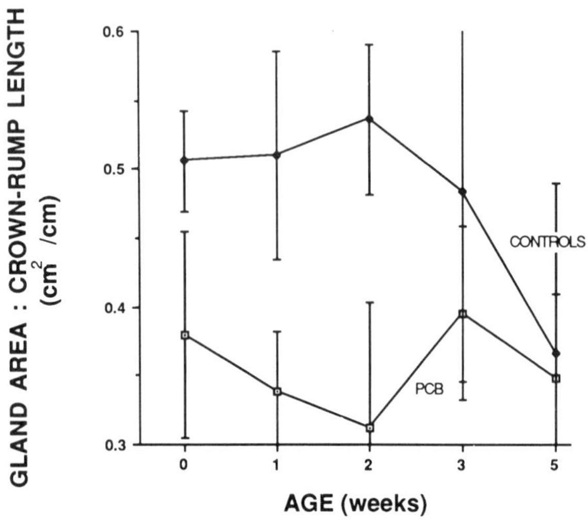

Figure 2b Comparison of the gland area:crown rump length ratio in the offspring of PCB treated and control mink. Each datum point represents the mean; the bar represents the standard deviation.

between the gland area:body weight ratios approached but did not reach statistical significance. The ratios in the treated and control groups in the 3-week and 5-week-old kits were not significantly different.

Morphometric histology of the cervical glands assessed the total area and perimeter of all adenomeres beneath a standard length of epidermis. Offspring of PCB-treated mink had significantly reduced adenomere area ($p = 0.02$) and perimeter ($p = 0.025$) compared to controls (Fig. 3a). These differences were maximal in the 1-week-old kits. The area of glandular cytoplasm was also reduced in the treated mink ($p = 0.04$). This area increased sharply in control mink to reach a maximum at 2-weeks of age. Conversely, glandular cytoplasmic area of treated mink did not increase as rapidly, or reach as large a total area (Fig. 3b). The percentage of each adenomere occupied by epithelial cell cytoplasm as opposed to gland lumen was significantly diminished in the PCB group ($p = 0.05$).

The histological appearance of the cervical apocrine glands in the offspring of the PCB females did not differ qualitatively from those of the controls. In the neonatal period the glands showed typical hypertrophic adenomeres (Plate 23A) lined by actively secreting epithelial cells (Plate 23B). By 5 weeks of age the glands were atrophic (Plate 24A), characterized by thickening of the basement membrane, a lack of secretion and the presence of many apoptotic cells in the degenerating epithelium (Plate 24B). The stratum corneum of the surface epidermis and the follicular infundibula were normal in both groups. There was no indication of follicular hyperkeratosis or comedone formation.

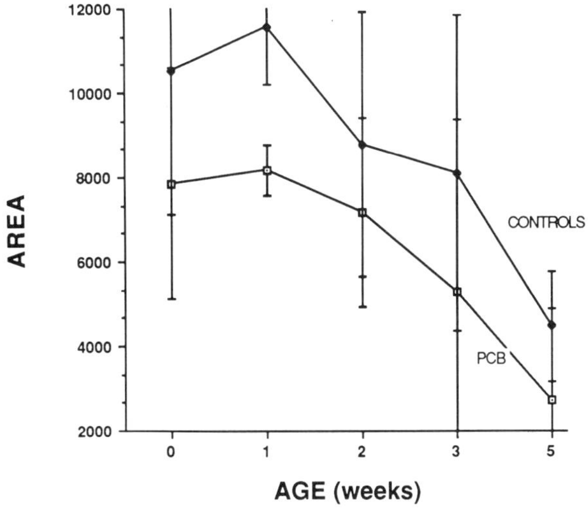

Figure 3a Comparison of the area of the adenomeres subjacent to a standard length of epidermis (1.32 mm) in the cervical apocrine gland of PCB exposed and control mink kits. Each datum point represents the mean expressed in units where 1 unit = 100 μm^2. The bar represents the standard deviation.

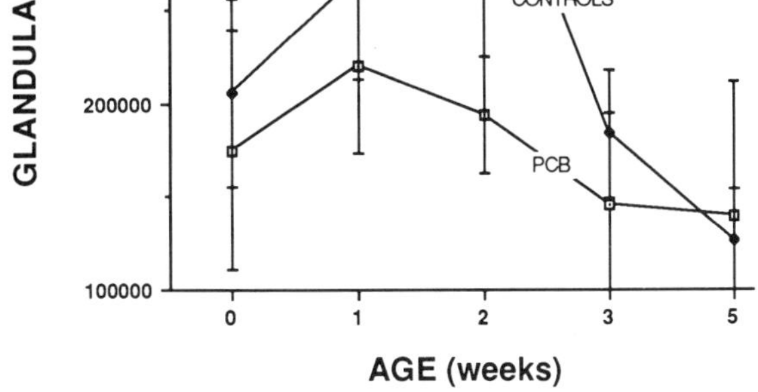

Figure 3b Comparison of the cytoplasmic area in adenomeres of the cervical apocrine glands of mink kits exposed to PCBs and controls. Each datum point represents the mean expressed in units where 1 unit = μm^2. The bar represents the standard deviation.

DISCUSSION

The hypertrophic cervical apocrine glands appear to be unique to members of the Mustelidae (Petskoi and Kolpovsky, 1970; Yager *et al.*, 1988). In the newborn mink kit, the gland is visible as an area of thickened skin on the dorsal neck, extending from the occiput to the thorax. The secretory product is abundant and may be seen macroscopically as dried honey-coloured crusts on the skin surface (Yager *et al.*, 1988). Histologically, the gland is composed of hypertrophic apocrine sweat glands. Morphometric histological assessment showed that the gland enlarges during the first 2 weeks of life and then regresses, so that by the time of weaning at 6 weeks, the gland is composed of a few degenerate glandular acini (Yager *et al.*, 1988). Regression is by the process of apoptosis, otherwise known as programmed cell death.

The timing of the glandular regression to coincide with weaning is a phenomenon which has only been noted in members of the Mustelidae. The transitory presence of the cervical gland during the neonatal period argues for a role in maternal interaction with the kits. Such a role was supported by data from preliminary behavioural studies, in which several parameters of maternal reaction were monitored following exposure of the lactating females to secretions collected from the cervical glands (Yager *et al.*, 1988).

Polychlorinated biphenyls have been widely used in industry as transformer coolants, plasticizers, fire retardants and hydraulic fluids (Safe *et al.*, 1987). The extraordinary stability of these chemicals provided the basis for much of their use, yet this same stability is a major factor in their environmental persistence (Safe *et al.*, 1987). Since PCBs bioaccumulate in body fat, carnivores at the top of the food chain are well-placed to receive higher exposure. Fish-eating species like mink are especially vulnerable because of the bioconcentration and biomagnification of PCBs in ocean and lake sediments (Safe *et al.*, 1987).

Exposure to PCBs affected both the development of the cervical apocrine gland and the growth rate of mink kits born to females receiving the chemical in the diet. The effect on the glandular development was greatest in the first 2 weeks of life, the time when in the normal kit the gland is maximally active (Yager *et al.*, 1988). Morphometric analysis of the histological sections showed that not only were the glandular units reduced in size but the area of epithelial cell cytoplasm was significantly reduced. The mechanism underlying this effect on gland development was not apparent. However, follicular hyperkeratosis, the lesion of chloracne in man, could be ruled out on histological grounds.

Mink are very sensitive to the effects of PCB ingestion. Mortality rates of 50% have been reported in adult mink ingesting 0.05 ppm of the toxic congener 3,4,5,3',4',5'-hexachlorobiphenyl (3,4,5,-HCB) over 135 days (Aulerich *et al.*, 1987). Exposure to a lower dose of 3,4,5-HCB, 0.01 ppm, resulted in a significant loss of body weight in the principals. Feeding Arochlor 1254, a complex mixture of PCBs, to pregnant females at 1 ppm led to reduced growth rate in the kits (Wren *et al.*, 1987). The results of our study confirm that maternal ingestion of PCBs is associated with significant reduction of growth rate in the offspring as well as a significant effect on the development of the cervical apocrine gland. We were not able to determine whether there is a cause and effect relationship between the diminution of the gland and the reduction in body weight. Further studies are needed to determine if these morphological changes are associated with a reduction in the amount and quality of the glandular product. Behavioural studies are also needed to ascertain whether any reduction in gland secretion is associated with diminished mothering activity.

Because PCBs have been identified in the milk of women exposed to these chemicals (Hara, 1985), doubts have been expressed about the safety of breast feeding in certain circumstances (Nath, 1987). The adverse effects of PCB exposure on the growth and development of mink kits may have given some credence to this view. However, the extrapolation of results from toxicity studies in one species to another may be inappropriate because the pathophysiological basis for the toxicity may depend on structures and functions unique to that species, structures such as the cervical apocrine glands of the neonatal mink.

REFERENCES

Adams, M.G. (1980). Odour-producing organs of mammals. *Symposium of the Zoological Society of London* No. 45 pp. 57–86.

Albone, E.S. (1984). The skin and scent glands. In: Albone, E.S. (ed.) *Mammalian Semiochemistry. The Investigation of Chemical Signals between Mammals*, pp. 40–134. John Wiley, New York.

Aulerich, R.J., Bursian, S.J., Evans, M.G. *et al.* (1987). Toxicity of 3,4,5,3',4',5'-hexachlorobiphenyl to mink. *Archives of Environmental Contamination and Toxicology* **16**: 53–60.

Blevins, M.R. (1980). Polychlorinated biphenyls (Arochlors 1016 and 1242): Effects on survival and reproduction in mink and ferrets. *Archives of Environmental Contamination and Toxicology* **9**: 627–635.

Dolnick, E.H. (1959). Histogenesis of hair in the mink and its relationship to dermal fat cells. *Journal of Morphology* **105**: 1–31.

Doty, R.L. (1986). Odor-guided behavior in mammals. *Experientia* **42**: 257–271.

Ebling, F.J.G. *et al.* (1986). The sebaceous glands. In: Rook, A., Wilkinson, D.S. and Ebling, J.G. (eds) *Textbook of Dermatology*, pp. 1931–1932. Blackwell, Oxford.

Hara, I. (1985). Health status and PCBs in blood of workers exposed to PCBs and of their children. *Environmental Health Perspectives* **59**: 85–90.

Harper, L.V. (1981). In: Gubernick, D.J. and Klopfer, P.H. (eds) *Parental Care in Mammals*, pp. 117–177. Plenum Press, New York.

Hayes, M.A. (1987), Carcinogenic and mutagenic effects of PCBs. In: Safe, S. and Hutzinger, O. (eds) *Environmental Toxin* Series 1, pp. 77–93. Springer-Verlag, Berlin.

Leon, M. (1983). Chemical contamination in mother-young interactions. In: Vandenbergh, J.G. (ed.) *Pheromones and Reproduction in Mammals*, pp. 39–77, Academic Press, New York.

McConnell, E.E. (1985). Comparative toxicity of PCBs and related compounds in various species of animals. *Environmental Health Perspectives* **60**: 29–33.

Mykytowycz, R. (1970). The role of skin glands in mammalian communication. In: Johnson, J.W., Moulton, D.G. and Turk, A. (eds) *Communication by Chemical Signals*, pp. 327–360. Appleton Century Crofts, New York.

Nath, U.M. (1987). WHO sounds the alarm over chemicals in breast milk. *New Scientist* 25 June 1987 :30.

Petskoi, P.G. and Kolpovsky, V.M. (1970). Neck glandular structures in animals of the family Mustelidae. *Zoologicheskii Zhurnal (Moscow)* **49**: 1208–1219. (in Russian)

Roberts, J.R., Rodgers, D.W., Bailey, J.R. and Rourke, M.A. (1978). Polychlorinated biphenyls. Biological criteria for an assessment of their effects on environmental quality. *National Research Council of Canada Report 16077.* NRCC/CNRC Publications, Ottawa.

Safe, S. (1987). PCBs and human health. In: Safe, S. and Hutzinger, O. (eds) *Environmental Toxin* Series 1, pp. 133–145. Springer-Verlag, Berlin.

Safe, S., Safe, L. and Mullin, M. (1987). Polychlorinated biphenyls: Environmental occurrence and analysis. In: Safe, S. and Hutzinger, O. (eds) *Environmental Toxin* Series 1, pp. 1–13. Springer-Verlag, Berlin.

Urabe, H. and Asahi, M. (1985). Past and current dermatological status of Yusho patients. *Environmental Health Perspectives* **59**: 11–15.

Wren, C.D., Hunter, D.B., Leatherland, J.F. and Stokes, P.M. (1987). The effects of polychlorinated biphenyls and methylmercury, singly and in combination, on mink. II Reproduction and kit development. *Archives of Environmental Contamination and Toxicology* **16**: 449–454.

Yager, J.A., Hunter, D.B., Wilson, M.R., Allen, O.B. (1988). A source of cutaneous maternal semiochemicals in the mink? *Experientia* **44**: 79–81.

4.6 Percutaneous Absorption of Pesticides in the Isolated Perfused Porcine Skin Flap (IPPSF)

J. Edmond Riviere and Nancy A. Monteiro-Riviere

Director and Professor of Pharmacology and Toxicology; and Assistant Professor of Anatomy and Toxicology, Cutaneous Pharmacology and Toxicology Center, College of Veterinary Medicine, North Carolina State University, Raleigh, North Carolina, USA

INTRODUCTION

Skin is acknowledged as a primary route of systemic exposure of pesticides in man and domesticated animals. Their widespread use as agricultural chemicals, in home gardening and as topical parasiticides in veterinary medicine has generated a great deal of interest in quantitating their percutaneous penetration and absorption after topical exposure. As a direct result of concern for human health, numerous *in vitro* and *in vivo* animal models have been developed to predict pesticide percutaneous absorption in man. The result of this effort has been the development of an extensive database in the literature comparing the absorption of chemicals in numerous species and man. Of most animal species studied including human xenograft rodent models the pig consistently shows the best corrclation to human penetration for the widest variety of chemicals (Bartek *et al.*, 1972; Wester and Maibach, 1977; Reifenrath *et al.*, 1984; Reifenrath and Hawkins, 1986). Porcine skin is structurally, biochemically and functionally similar to that of man (Monteiro-Riviere, 1990). However, *in vivo* techniques for quantitating percutaneous absorption are laborious and time consuming, the results of which are often confounded by systemic metabolism of the compound. Studies with very toxic pesticides often cannot be conducted in a humane manner.

In vitro strategies using full thickness or dermatomed skin slices in static and flow through diffusion cell systems suffer from a lack of anatomical integrity and the absence of a functional cutaneous microvasculature. Epidermal viability is often not optimal in these systems for realistic cutaneous metabolism investigations. Finally, cutaneous metabolism can often be detected only when the skin has been pretreated with enzyme-inducing compounds, a manoeuvre which may affect the validity of extrapolating to the natural *in vitro* setting. Pharmacokinetic studies have revealed that percutaneous absorption is a complicated process, whose final outcome is a delicate balance between the physiochemical process of diffusion, the biochemical pathways of epidermal metabolism, and the physiological function of the cutaneous microcirculation. The integration of these processes can only be studied *in vitro* in an anatomically intact and fully functional skin preparation. The isolated perfusion of fully vascularized skin flaps is one such applicable *in vitro* model system.

The purpose of this paper is to briefly overview the development of the isolated perfused porcine skin flap (IPPSF) developed in our laboratory to assess percutaneous absorption and cutaneous toxicity in a realistic and controllable *in vitro* setting (Monteiro-Riviere *et al.*, 1987; Monteiro-Riviere and King, 1989; Riviere *et al.*, 1986, 1987a,b, 1989; Williams and Riviere, 1989; Williams *et al.*, 1990). A full description of this methodology is beyond the scope of this presentation and the cited utility will be illustrated with percutaneous absorption studies conducted using the organophosphate pesticides parathion and malathion.

METHODS

Female weanling Yorkshire pigs were used in these studies. The skin of the caudal inguinal region of the pig is supplied by direct cutaneous vasculature; the superficial epigastric artery and paired *venae comitantes*. A two-stage surgical procedure is used to create a pair of single-pedicle island tubed skin flaps (Fig. 1) one on each side of the pig, which are then cannulated and transferred to an isolated organ perfusion chamber (Riviere Skin Flap Perfusion Chamber, Diamond Research, Raleigh, NC) (Fig. 2) (Bowman *et al.*, 1990, Riviere *et al.*, 1986). An interval of 2 days between creation and harvest of these flaps was judged optimal for this preparation (Monteiro-Riviere *et al.*, 1987). Skin is perfused with an albumin-based Krebs-Ringer bicarbonate buffered media gassed with 95% O_2/5% CO_2. Glucose is provided as an energy source. Chamber temperature and humidity are controlled and monitored. Viability is assessed by monitoring arterial and venous glucose, lactate and LDH activity as well as perfusate flow and pressure. At the termination of an experiment, skin samples may be collected for both light and transmission electron microscopy. Based on extensive correlative studies, an individual IPPSF has been judged to be viable when cumulative glucose

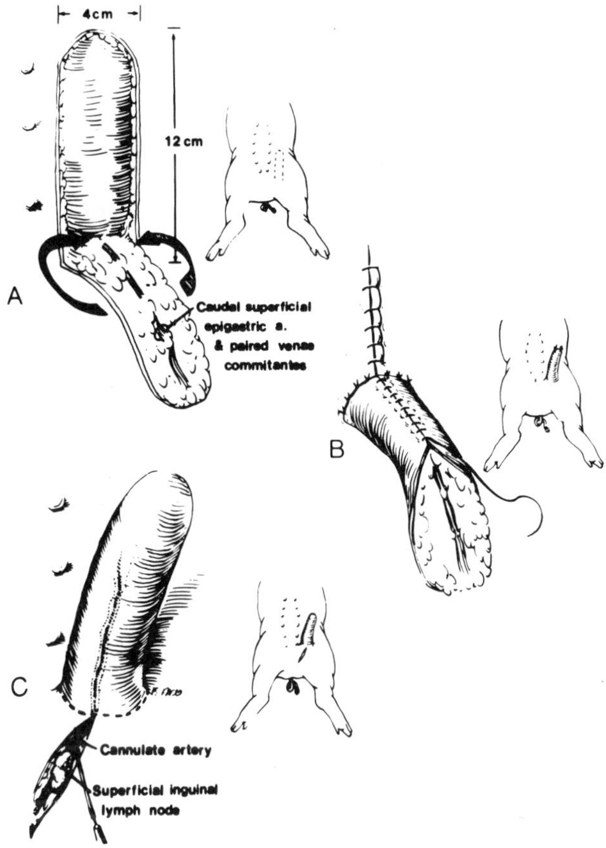

Figure 1 Two-stage surgical procedure used to create (A&B) and harvest (C) skin flaps for isolated perfusion.

utilization is greater than 10 mg/h and perfusate flow is at least 1 ml/min (Riviere *et al.*, 1986, 1987a; Monteiro-Riviere *et al.*, 1987). Figure 3 is a light micrograph taken from a typical viable IPPSF demonstrating essentially normal histology.

For percutaneous absorption studies (Carver and Riviere, 1989; Williams *et al.*, 1990), compound was applied to the surface of an IPPSF which has been perfused for 1–2 h so that equilibration within the *in vitro* chamber could occur. A 5 cm^2 exposure area was demarcated with a flexible plastic template (Stomahesive, ConvaTec, Princeton, NJ) and 40 μg/cm^2 of compound (ethanol vehicle) was applied with a microsyringe (^{14}C-labelled parathion (n = 4) and malathion (n = 5), Amersham, Arlington Heights, IL; 10 μCi total radiolabel dose). Venous efflux samples were then collected every 30 min for the first 4 h and hourly thereafter for a total exposure period of 8 h. At the termination of an experiment, the patch, dosed and surrounding skin and flap

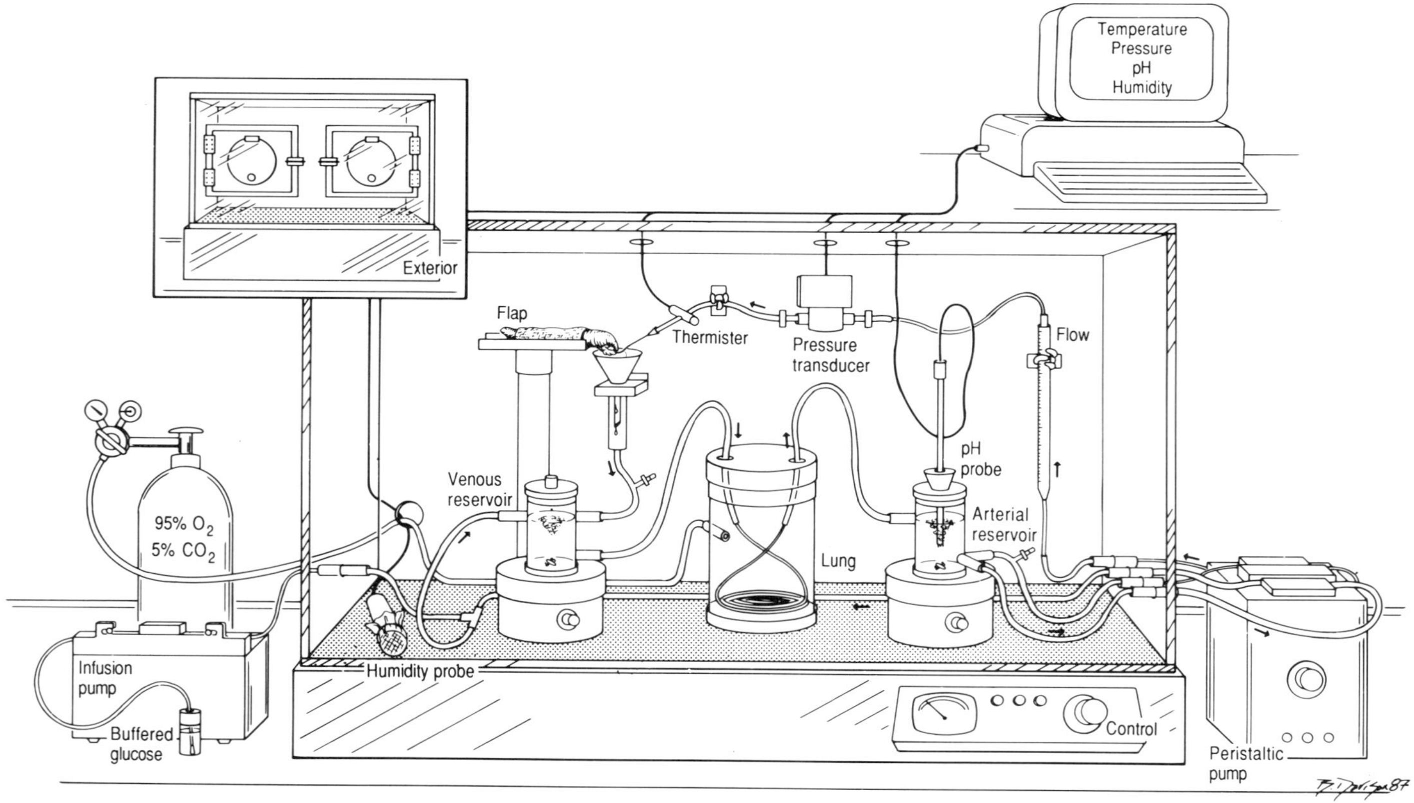

Figure 2 Schematic diagram of the isolated skin perfusion chamber utilized in IPPSF studies.

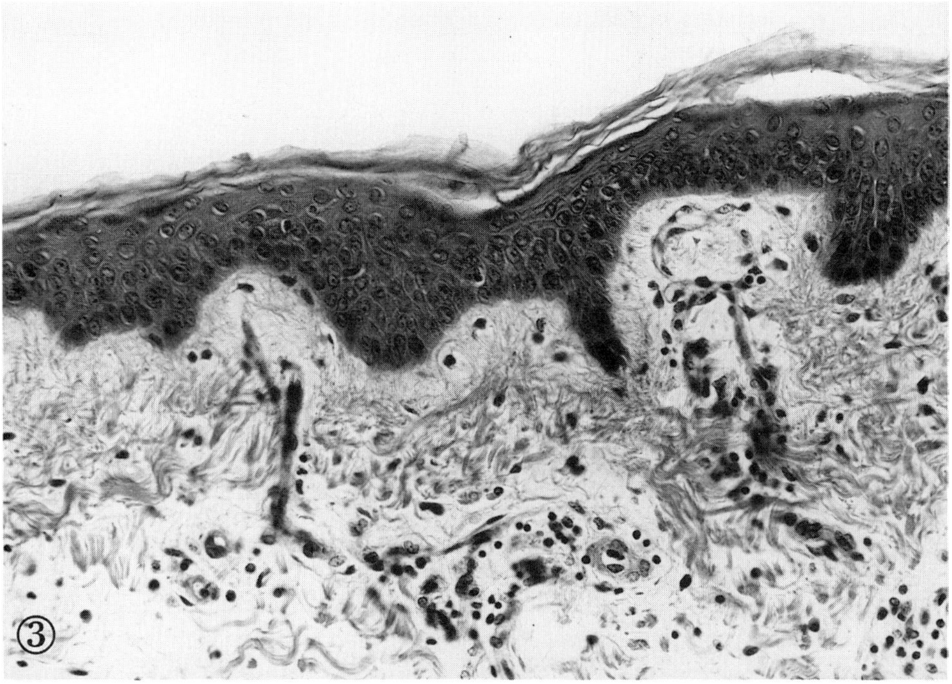

Figure 3 Light micrograph of a typical isolated perfused porcine skin flap after 10 h of stable perfusion. HE × 330.

were collected. All samples were oxidized and counted using scintillation spectroscopy. The resulting venous efflux profiles were fitted to a hybrid physiologically compartmental pharmacokinetic model using a digital computer to provide an estimate of total percutaneous absorption at an infinite time (Williams and Riviere, 1989; Williams *et al.*, 1990). This model was judged superior to an earlier compartmental analysis of the data. The details of this method are beyond the scope of the present article and the reader is urged to consult these references for further details. For parathion, metabolism was also assessed using TLC methodology (Riviere *et al.*, 1987b). Additional flaps were pretreated with the cytochrome P-450 inhibitor ABT to confirm epidermal biotransformation.

Identical exposure conditions were also conducted *in vivo* using intravenous dosing to correct for systemic disposition ($n = 4$ per compound per route) (Carver and Riviere, 1989). In these studies, urine and faeces were collected for 6 days and the excreta and the remaining carcass are counted for radioactivity. The percent absorption is then calculated as:

$$\frac{(\text{topical excretion})}{(\text{i.v. excretion})} \times 100\%$$

This *in vivo* estimate was calculated separately using urine and urine + faeces (total excrement) data.

RESULTS

Table 1 presents the percutaneous absorption estimates and total radiolabel recoveries for the *in vivo* and IPPSF studies. In both model systems, percent radiolabel recoveries were excellent. When urine data alone is used to estimate absorption *in vivo*, there is a slight underestimation of total absorption compared to when total excrement is collected (urine and faeces). As can be appreciated from examining these data, the IPPSF estimates are in excellent agreement with the *in vivo* study. Figure 4 plots the venous efflux profiles for parathion and malathion in IPPSF experiments. These data are compared to *in vivo* literature values in Table 2.

Table 1 Percutaneous absorption of malathion and parathion *in vivo* and *in vitro* through porcine skin

	Malathion	Parathion
In vivo		
% absorption with i.v. urine correction factor	5.4 ± 0.8	5.4 ± 1.1
% absorption with i.v. urine and faeces correction factor	5.2 ± 0.5	6.7 ± 1.3
% total radiolabel recovery	92.2 ± 8.6	83.6 ± 1.2
In vitro IPPSF		
calculated % absorption[a]	5.9	6.6
absorption rate constant (1/min)	0.00164 ± 0.00003	0.00096 ± 0.00003
% total radiolabel recovery	93.4 ± 6.4	94.6 ± 5.9

Mean ± SE.

[a] IPPSF absorptions are not shown with SE because they result from a group simulation for each compound.

The metabolism studies ($n = 4$) in these recirculating flaps indicated that 67.8 ± 2.3% of the absorbed parathion was present as paraoxon and 14.5 + 5.21% as *p*-nitrophenol. When flaps were pretreated with ABT, only 6.6% was converted to paraoxon and 11.9% to *p*-nitrophenol.

DISCUSSION

These experiments confirm previous studies (Bartek *et al.*, 1972; Reifenrath *et al.*, 1984) that the pig is an excellent animal model for estimating human

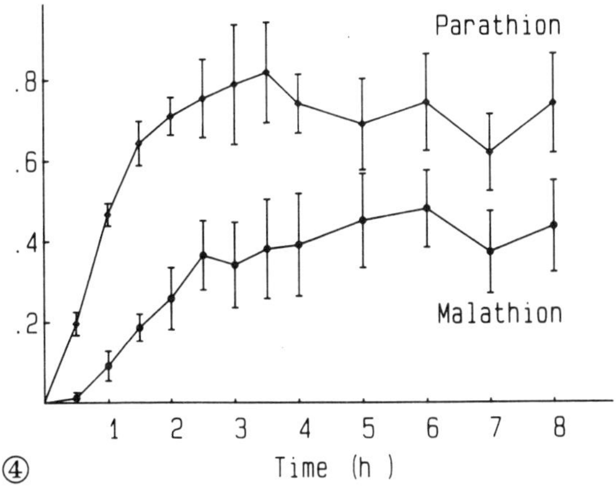

④

Figure 4 IPPSF venous efflux profiles (mean ± SE) for parathion (n = 4) and malathion (n = 5) showing absorption rate (% dose/h) versus time.

Table 2 Comparative percutaneous absorption of malathion and parathion (4μg/cm²)

	Malathion	Parathion
Humans[a]		
forearm	6.8	8.6
abdomen	9.4	18.5
Pigs (back)[b]	4.4	19.0
Rabbits[c]	64.6	97.5
Monkey[c]	19.3	30.3

In vivo absorptions were corrected using parenteral data as described in the text except for the monkey.
[a] Maibach and Feldman (1975).
[b] Reifenrath and Hawkins (1986).
[c] Wester and Maibach (1977).

percutaneous absorption. Penetration in rabbits and rodents for most chemicals is accepted as being much greater than that seen in humans, pigs or monkeys (Wester and Maibach, 1977; Bartek *et al.*, 1972; Shat *et al.*, 1981). Examination of Table 2 confirms this concept for the organophosphate pesticides malathion and parathion.

The IPPSF predicted absorptions were very well correlated to the *in vivo* data. When the extent of IPPSF and *in vivo* percutaneous absorption is compared across an additional five compounds (benzoic acid, caffeine, DFP, testosterone and progesterone), this correlation holds. Using the original compartmental pharmacokinetic model, the correlation coefficient was R = 0.94 while it was 0.97 when the physiological model was employed (Williams *et al.*, 1990). These data support the use of the IPPSF to predict percutaneous absorption in pigs. When the data in both tables are compared, there is an excellent agreement between IPPSF and *in vivo* human absorption values.

The advantages of using an *in vitro* isolated system such as the IPPSF are numerous. First, the presence of cutaneous metabolism can be easily quantitated. For parathion, a significant amount of biotransformation of topically applied parathion to the active metabolite paraoxon occurs. The blocking of this reaction with the cytochrome P-450 inhibitor ABT supports the enzymatic specificity of this process. Since these experiments were conducted in a recirculating system, the fraction metabolized overestimates the true extent of 'first pass' cutaneous metabolism. Careful analysis of this data, in conjunction with arterial perfusion and non-recirculating topical studies, would suggest that 20–30% of the absorbed dose of parathion is metabolized while penetrating the skin. The environmental and physiological determinants of this toxicologically significant first-pass cutaneous metabolism deserves further study. The IPPSF is ideally suited to studying the percutaneous absorption of systemically toxic chemicals since the absorptive phase can be modelled independently. With *in vivo* models, the toxicosis which results after compound absorption often prohibits long-term studies from being conducted. A similar advantage is seen when the IPPSF has been used to study cutaneous vesicant toxicity (Monteiro-Riviere and King, 1989).

The use of a pharmacokinetic model to analyse IPPSF venous efflux profiles allow for the data collected in an 8-h experiment to predict percutaneous absorption totals requiring 6-day *in vivo* studies. These advantages, coupled with the ability to directly assess cutaneous metabolism independent of systemic biotransformation and to pharmacologically modulate the cutaneous microcirculation (Riviere *et al.*, 1990), make the IPPSF a useful humane alternative animal model system. The results can be correlated to human exposure or are directly applicable to assessing pesticide absorption in pigs. Studies are currently being conducted with carbaryl, paraquat and lindane to expand our understanding of this field.

ACKNOWLEDGEMENTS

The research in this manuscript was supported by USAMRDC contract DAMD17-84C-4103 and NIEHS grants ES00044 and ES07046.

REFERENCES

Bartek, M.J., LaBudde, J.A. and Maibach, H.I. (1972). Skin permeability *in vivo*: comparison in rat, rabbit, pig and man. *Journal of Investigative Dermatology* **58**: 114–123.

Bowman, K.F., Monteiro-Riviere, N.A. and Riviere, J.E. (1990). Development of surgical techniques for preparation of *in vitro* isolated perfused porcine skin flaps for percutaneous absorption studies. *American Journal of Veterinary Research* (in press).

Carver, M.P. and Riviere, J.E. (1989). Percutaneous absorption and excretion of xenobiotics after topical and intravenous administration to pigs. *Fundamental and Applied Toxicology* **13**: 714–722.

Maibach, H.I. and Feldman, R. (1975). *Systemic Absorption of Pesticides through the Skin of Man*. Report to the Federal Working Group on Pest Management from the Task Group on Occupational Exposure to Pesticides, Appendix B, pp. 120–127. US Government Printing Office, 0-551-026, Washington DC.

Monteiro-Riviere, N.A. (1990). Comparative anatomy, physiology and biochemistry of mammalian skin. In: Hobson, D.W. (ed.) *Fundamentals and Methods of Dermal and Ocular Toxicology*. The Telford Press, Caldwell, NJ (in press).

Monteiro-Riviere, N.A. and King, J.R. (1989). The dermatoxicity of 2-chloroethyl methyl sulfide and solvent vehicles in isolated perfused porcine skin. In: *Proceedings of the 1989 Medical Defense Bioscience Review*, pp. 53–56, Columbia, Md.

Monteiro-Riviere, N.A., Bowman, K.F., Scheidt, V.J. and Riviere, J.E. (1987). The isolated perfused porcine skin flap (IPPSF) II. Ultrastructural and histological characterization of epidermal viability. *In Vitro Toxicology* **1**: 241–252.

Reifenrath, W.G. and Hawkins, G.S. (1986). The weanling Yorkshire pig as an animal model for measuring percutaneous penetration. In: Tumbleson, M.E. (ed.) *Swine in Biomedical Research* Vol. 1, pp. 673–680. Plenum Press, New York.

Reifenrath, W.G., Chellquist, E.M., Shipwash, E.A., Jederberg, W.W. and Krueger, G.G. (1984). Percutaneous penetration in the hairless dog, weanling pig and grafted athymic nude mouse: evaluation of models for predicting skin penetration in man. *British Journal of Dermatology* **3** (Suppl. 27): 123–135.

Riviere, J.E., Bowman, K.F., Monteiro-Riviere, N.A., Dix, L.P. and Carver, M.P. (1986). The isolated perfused porcine skin flap (IPPSF) I. A novel *in vitro* animal model for percutaneous absorption and cutaneous toxicology studies. *Fundamental and Applied Toxicology* **7**: 444–453.

Riviere, J.E., Bowman, K.F. and Monteiro-Riviere, N.A. (1987a). On the definition of viability in isolated perfused skin preparations. *British Journal of Dermatology* **116**: 739–741.

Riviere, J.E., Carver, M.P., Monteiro-Riviere, N.A. and Bowman, K.F. (1987b). Percutaneous absorption of organophosphates, steroids, caffeine and benzoic acid *in vivo* and *in vitro* using the isolated perfused porcine skin flap (IPPSF). In: *Proceedings of the Sixth Medical Chemical Defense Bioscience Review*, pp. 763–766, Columbia, Md.

Riviere, J.E., Sage, B.H. and Monteiro, N.A. (1990). Transdermal lidocaine iontophoresis in isolated perfused porcine skin. *Journal of Toxicology: Cutaneous & Ocular* **9**: 493–504.

Shah, P.V., Monroe, R.J. and Guthrie, F.E. (1981). Comparative rates of dermal penetration of insecticides in mice. *Toxicology and Applied Pharmacology* **59**: 414–423.

Wester, R.C. and Maibach, H.I. (1977). Percutaneous absorption in man and animals: a perspective. In: Drill, V.A. and Lazar, P. (eds) *Cutaneous Toxicity*, pp. 111–126. Academic Press, New York.

Williams, P.L. and Riviere, J.E. (1989). Definition of a physiologic pharmacokinetic model of cutaneous drug distribution using the isolated perfused porcine skin flap. *Journal of Pharmaceutical Science* **78**: 550–555.

Williams, P.L., Carver, M.P. and Riviere, J.E. (1990). A physiologically relevant pharmacokinetic model of xenobiotic percutaneous absorption utilizing the isolated perfused porcine skin flap (IPPSF). *Journal of Pharmaceutical Science* **79**: 305–311.

PART 5

BACTERIAL SKIN DISEASE

5.1 Bacterial Skin Infections in Domestic Animals and Man

W.C. Noble

Professor of Microbiology, Department of Microbial Diseases, Institute of Dermatology, United Medical & Dental Schools, St Thomas' Hospital, London

INTRODUCTION

The two principal groups of organisms colonizing human skin are the coryneforms and the staphylococci; skin infection is caused mostly by these organisms, by streptococci, and more rarely by a wide variety of other microorganisms (Noble, 1981). Relatively little attention has been paid to coryneforms from animal skin and this is partly the result of poor taxonomy since, with few exceptions, we cannot easily classify coryneforms even to the species level. In contrast, the taxonomy of the staphylococci is well worked out (Schleifer *et al.*, 1979) though new species continue to be recognized from human and animal sources (Freney *et al.*, 1988; Varaldo *et al.*, 1988). Both staphylococci and coryneforms colonize skin and specialized sites such as the nares, and potential pathogens spread from these localized habitats to cause infection or superinfection elsewhere. This paper will briefly review carriage of coryneforms and staphylococci, will consider infection due to these organisms, to streptococci and to some exotica such as the mycobacteria, and will speculate on the role of plasmid DNA in infective processes and on therapy.

SKIN COLONIZATION

It has become customary in human skin microbiology to allot organisms to one of two major categories, 'transients' and 'residents' with the term 'nomads' for those organisms which stay for a short while only. There have been few entirely successful studies of this, even in man, but it is evident that some organisms may be recovered only occasionally from the skin whilst others are permanent inhabitants, at least over periods of a few months

(Somerville-Millar and Noble, 1974). Individual humans differ in the composition of their skin flora though some generalizations may be made. Studies of this type seem not to have been carried out in animals, partly because of the difficulty inherent in sampling a hairy skin surface and partly because of the logistic problems of handling large numbers of diverse organisms. It seems probable, however, that animals also have a resident and transient flora. Lists of genera found on the skin of man and animals are similar (Table 1) as might be expected from warm blooded creatures inhabiting a similar environment.

Table 1 Genera of bacteria recovered from the skin

Genera/species *n* =	Man	Cats 10	Dogs 10
Staphylococcus aureus	±	+	+ +
Staphylococcus 'albus'	+ +	+	+ +
Micrococcus	+ +	+ +	+ +
Alpha streptococci	±	+ +	+ +
Coliforms	±	±	±
Bacillus	±	±	±
Coryneforms	+ +	−	±
Acinetobacter	+ +	+ +	+ +

Based on Noble (1981), Krogh and Kristensen (1976).
+ + very commonly found; + commonly found; ± found in substantial minority; − not reported.
Staphylococcus 'albus' encompasses all the coagulase negative species.
Staphylococcus aureus encompasses all the coagulase positive species.

THE CORYNEFORMS

In man at least three genera of coryneforms are regularly present on the skin, *Brevibacterium*, *Corynebacterium* and *Propionibacterium*. *Brevibacterium* spp. have a limited distribution appearing most frequently in the toewebs and similar niches, various *Corynebacterium* spp. are found on most body areas whilst *Propionibacterium* are abundant on the highly sebaceous areas such as the face and shoulders and are the most numerous organisms on human skin. *Propionibacterium* spp. and to a lesser extent *Corynebacterium* spp. are lipophilic, that is they grow very much better *in vitro* in the presence of lipid, especially oleates. Resident carriage of *P. acnes* in man does not occur until about puberty when lipid secretion increases in quantity and changes its composition (Nordstrom and Noble, 1985). In man the skin surface fatty acids are derived by microbial hydrolysis of sebaceous triglycerides. Studies of the skin lipid composition in a number of animals including laboratory and domestic species (Nicolaides *et al.*, 1968; Nikkari, 1974) show that abundant sebaceous triglycerides and their breakdown products are unique to man. As a result, extensive colonization with *P. acnes* is confined to man. The most common skin disease of young human adults, acne vulgaris, does not occur in the same form in animals. In man acne is characterized by comedones, pustules and inflammatory lesions, appears at about puberty and persists into young adulthood and is associated with *P. acnes*. Canine acne is more often characterized by deep folliculitis and furunculosis and disappears at puberty. Bedford and Young (1981) reported studies of skin lipid in hairless dogs showing clinical signs of acne and concluded that the fatty acids found in the comedones, pustules and abscesses were epidermal rather than sebaceous in origin corresponding in a rather general way to those found in man though with a longer mean chain length. In unaffected areas of skin in these dogs the lipid was approximately 80% sterols and sterol esters as has been reported by others. There do not seem to be reports of the involvement of *Propionibacterium* in canine acne though this organism is reported as a rare cause of abscesses in dogs and cats (Berg *et al.*, 1979).

Many species of *Corynebacterium* are resident on human skin (Pitcher and Noble, 1978); data on animals are scarce but *C. bovis* is reportedly present on cattle skin. Overgrowth of *Corynebacterium* species on normal skin of man results in skin infections or affections. Erythrasma is a scaling disease which occurs in interriginous areas such as the toewebs and groins and is due to an overgrowth of *C. minutissimum* which increase 20-fold over its normal resident level. There is apparently no veterinary equivalent of this disease. In man overgrowth of axillary coryneforms results in trichomycosis axillaris in which nodular microbial colonies grow on the axillary hair shafts. This is, in itself, trivial but is often associated with pungent axillary odour. The coryneforms are able to form malodorous compounds from steroids secreted by the apocrine glands. There are suggestions that these compounds are involved in maternal/neonate recognition in humans and that they may act as human pheromones. It may be of veterinary interest that amongst the compounds formed in the human axilla is the boar pheromone 5 α androstenone, which causes a sow in oestrus to adopt the mating stance and which, like the presence of a boar in a breeding unit, accelerates puberty in piglets (see Gower *et al.*, 1988 for a wide ranging review). A physically similar nodular growth on the hair of a single beagle dog has been reported (Muller *et al.*, 1989). Although man may suffer skin lesions due to *C. diphtheriae* (Ayyagari *et al.*, 1979; Harnish *et al.*, 1989) infections of skin do not seem common in animals infected with *C. pseudotuberculosis* (*C. ovis*) or *C. ulcerans* which express the same toxins as *C. diphtheriae* when lysogenized by the same phages. Abscesses caused by infection with *C. pseudotuberculosis* (*C. ovis*) are only very rarely seen in man (Richards and Hurse, 1985) but are well described in horses (Miers and Ley, 1980; Heffner *et al.*, 1988). Abscess formation is also associated with pitting oedema, dermatitis and lameness and it may be that either the diphtheria toxin which is produced by lysogenized strains (Wong and Groman, 1984) or the toxin specific to *C.*

pseudotuberculosis and *C. ulcerans* (Onon, 1979) is responsible. Abscess formation in horses has a pronounced seasonal and locational occurrence, peaking sharply in October/November in California, USA. 'Contagious acne' of horses, a rare disease, is also caused by this organism (Scott and Manning, 1980) as are more deep seated lesions in sheep and goats. Skin infections with such well known pathogens as *Rhodococcus equi* seem as rare in animals as they are in humans, where they are most frequent in the immunosuppressed (Barton and Hughes, 1980; Higgins and Paradis, 1980; Ellis-Pegler *et al.*, 1983).

Brevibacterium, in common with a number of other coryneforms or near relatives, is probably underreported in human infection due to difficulty in recognizing the genus. It is known to form part of the normal flora in cattle (D.G. Pitcher, D.H. Lloyd and W.C. Noble, unpublished observations) as well as man (Pitcher and Noble, 1978). It is involved in human foot infection where it causes extensive destruction of the skin of the toeweb by proteolysis and where it results in the cheesy malodour. *Brevibacterium epidermidis* is the species found in man whilst *B. linens* is used in the dairy industry to enhance flavour and odour in cheeses such as Brie and may have originated from cattle skin. Both release the same odorous gas, CH_3SH, as a metabolic endproduct of methionine derived from protein degradation.

Another Gram-positive bacillus which exhibits a rod-to-coccus morphological cycle is *Dermatophilus congolensis*. This is rarely reported as a human pathogen, though occasional infections are reported in persons in contact with animals (Kaminski and Suter, 1976; see also Kaplan (1976) for a review), but has been reported as the cause of pitted keratolysis (Rubel, 1972; Woodgyer *et al.*, 1985) a condition in which erosions develop on the soles of the feet usually associated with excessive sweating. Pitted keratolysis has been described as caused by coryneforms and actinomycetes as well as by *Dermatophilus* but this may merely illustrate the poor state of taxonomy. In animals an entirely different lesion is seen. *D. congolensis* is a well established pathogen of cattle skin and is also found in sheep and goats, more rarely in horses and in many other animal species (see Lloyd and Sellars, 1976). In cattle in the tropics it is a chronic condition which develops from a moist papule to become evident when a thick exudate forms and mats the hair together to give the classic, tufted, paint-brush appearance with a firmly adherent scab. Lesions in sheep are similar. In temperate climates the disease is usually similar though milder. The gross difference between the appearance of the disease in man and animals is almost certainly related to the structure of the hair follicles and perhaps to differences in the secretions which in cattle are of mixed sebaceous and eccrine gland origin but in man of sebaceous origin only. Lloyd and Noble (1982) reported that experimental lesions in hairless mice more nearly resembled those seen in humans that did lesions in haired mice.

In general, coryneform skin diseases in animals have little in common with those in man.

THE STAPHYLOCOCCI

As a result of a more detailed taxonomy, and perhaps because in man and animals staphylococci cause more distinct diseases, much more is known of skin carriage, infection and pathogenicity. Table 2 shows the principal staphylococci recoverable from skin of man and some animals and it is evident that, although there is some species predilection, many staphylococcal species will inhabit the skin of several mammalian hosts. In man the anterior nares form a focus of colonization (Noble *et al.*, 1964) from which dissemination occurs to other body areas, probably via the hands and this is especially a problem where there is a surgical wound or prosthesis (Davies *et al.*, 1989). In animals nasal carriage also occurs but the assessment of infection in the muzzle area in such diverse species as laboratory gerbils (Peckham *et al.*, 1974) or unweaned sheep (Parker *et al.*, 1983) is complicated by the use of the muzzle as an exploratory device.

Table 2 Percentage distribution of staphylococci from skin and nares of man and animals

	Humans	Cattle	Cats	Pigs	Poultry
S. aureus	4.5	–	5	–	–
S. capitis	6	–	1	–	–
S. chromogenes	–	12	–	17	5
S. cohnii	5	6	–	3	5
S. epidermidis	23	29	17	0	2
S. gallinarum	–	0	–	0	11
S. haemolyticus	11	9	3	4	3
S. hominis	30	0	1	0	0
S. hyicus	–	5	1	7	16
S. intermedius	–	–	14	–	–
S. lentus	–	9	–	27	28
S. saprophyticus	7	2	0.5	0	2
S. sciuri	–	3	2	22	9
S. simulans	1.2	7	44	4	3
S. warneri	4	7	2	2	0
S. xylosus	7	10	11	9	11

– = not done (taxonomy not available or coagulase positive not counted).
Based on Kloos *et al.* (1976), Cox *et al.* (1984b), Devriese *et al.* (1985).

In general, the coagulase negative staphylococci do not cause disease in man unless a plastic prosthesis or indwelling catheter has been implanted; the most widely studied current example is peritonitis following exit site infection in continuous ambulatory peritoneal dialysis (CAPD) were *S. epidermis* and to a lesser extent *S. haemolyticus* are implicated (see Spencer, 1988; Dougherty, 1988; for reviews). Skin disease due to the coagulase negative cocci is generally trivial (M. Dahl and W.C. Noble, unpublished; Pospisil *et al.*, 1986). In animals the position may be different, Medleau *et al.* (1986) reported 7% of deep pyodermas in dogs to yield coagulase negative staphylococci, again chiefly *S. epidermis*, and subclinical mastitis in sheep may also be due to coagulase negative staphylococci.

In older literature, *S. aureus* was the only coagulase positive staphylococcus to be recognized and was defined by its ability to coagulate plasma, to produce a heat stable nuclease and to possess protein A. In the last decade however we have come to realise that not only do specific ecovars of *S. aureus* inhabit and infect man, cattle or rabbits but that other distinct species of coagulase positive cocci exist. Table 3 shows that characteristics of the currently accepted species; *S. intermedius* is a well recognized pathogen in dogs (Lloyd and Reyss-Brion, 1984), *S. hyicus* in pigs and other species (Devriese *et al.*, 1985) *S. aureus* var *anaerobius* in sheep (de la Fuente *et al.*, 1985) and *S. delphini* has been reported as a cause of deep furuncle like lesions in dolphins (Varaldo *et al.*, 1988).

In skin infections it is chiefly the coagulase positive species of staphylococci which are involved. In man, *S. aureus* causes two types of infection: one, characterized by the boil or furuncle, is a deep infection probably initiated in a hair follicle, a characteristic shared with many animals (Parker *et al.*, 1983). A battery of enzymes or toxins such as haemolysins, coagulase, leucocidins etc is implicated; surgical wound infection is a similar process. The second type is a more surface phenomenon referred to as impetigo which appears with characteristic honey-coloured stuck-on crusts and in some forms blistering. The latter is known as bullous impetigo and is a mild form of a disease, caused by specific toxins known as epidermolytic toxins, the severe form of which is known as scalded skin syndrome in which the skin peels away in sheets at the stratum granulosum (Melish, 1982). The epidermolytic toxins have a very restricted host and tissue range causing splitting only at the stratum granulosum of the cornified epithelium in man, mouse, hamster and some monkeys (Elias *et al.*, 1976). The rat, rabbit, guinea pig, dog, frog and chicken are known to be unsusceptible to these toxins. It is interesting to note that impetigo in the young dog involves superficial pustules, not involving hair follicles, which rupture and lead to yellow stuck-on crusts and that bullous impetigo in puppies involves sheets of skin which peel away from the bullae (Muller *et al.*, 1989). Love and Davis (1980) described ten greyhounds with a disease which closely resembled staphylococcal scalded skin syndrome. The skin split occurred, as in man, at the stratum granulosum and although staphylococci were recovered from these blisters this may represent secondary contamination. The staphylococci were reported as *S. aureus* but were slide coagulase negative and non-typable using *S. aureus* phages suggesting that they were in fact *S. intermedius*. Since the dog is known to be insusceptible to experimental challenge with *S. aureus* epidermolytic toxin, this suggests that *S. intermedius*, the coagulase positive species found in dogs, may also possess epidermolytic toxins but with a slightly different host range. It is worth noting

Table 3 Some characteristics of coagulase-positive staphylococci

	Coagulase	Clumping factor	Heat stable DNAase	Protein A (bound)	Haemolysin	Enterotoxin	Comments
S. aureus	+	+	+	+	+	+	Man and animals. Widespread; host specific biotypes
S. aureus var *anaerobius*	+	–	+	–	+	–	Sheep
S. intermedius	+	–	+	+	D	+	Dogs, cats
S. hyicus	D	D	+	+	–	–	Pigs, cattle, chickens etc.
S. delphini	+	–	–	ND	+	ND	Dolphins

+ = more than 90% positive; – = less than 10% positive; D: intermediate; ND: not determined.

that the two epidermolytic toxins known to affect man have markedly different structures (Lee *et al.*, 1987) so that other similar proteins may well exist with different host ranges but the same clinical effect. In rabbits exudative lesions resembling impetigo may be caused by *S. aureus* of phage group II (3A/3C/55/71) (Okerman *et al.*, 1984). Group II strains are the most common cause of impetigo in man and also most frequently bear the epidermolytic toxin genes.

A similar disease in some respects, but without direct parallel in humans is the exudative dermatitis of pigs due to *S. hyicus*. This disease also appears to be toxin mediated (Amtsberg, 1979) although presumably different from the epidermolytic toxins described above. Strains of *S. hyicus* known to be virulent for pigs are without epidermolytic activity in mice susceptible to *S. aureus* toxins (W.C. Noble, D.H. Lloyd and R.B. Allaker, unpublished observations, confirming the work of Amtsberg). *Staphylococcus hyicus* is known to produce several proteases (Takeuchi *et al.*, 1987) and also lytic enzymes which destroy other bacteria (Lämmler, 1989) but an epidemolytic toxin has yet to be described. A study of toxic shock toxin or other enterotoxins might be valuable in this disease. It may be relevant to some animal diseases that toxic shock toxin has been reported from coagulase-negative staphylococci, principally *S. epidermidis* (Crass and Bergdoll, 1986) and from *S. hyicus* (Aliu and Bergdoll, 1988) and from a caprine *S. aureus* (Morgan *et al.*, 1986) though *S. aureus* remains the most common source of toxin in strains of human origin. In dogs *S. intermedius* is known to produce enterotoxins, though at a low level and a canine strain of *S. aureus* produced toxic shock toxin (Fukuda *et al.*, 1984; Almazan *et al.*, 1987).

The potential role of staphylococcal protein A in disease seems not to have been explored. In man intradermal injection of small amounts of protein A results in a response very similar to that elicited by an allergen. In normal humans without skin disease there is a weal and flare in 10–15 min disappears at 6 h with a return of the flare at 24 h (White and Noble, 1980, 1985). In patients with atopic dermatitis this response is significantly reduced posing the question: do atopics carry large quantities of *S. aureus* on the skin because of this reduced response or is the response reduced as a result of carriage? The structure of protein A in *S. hyicus* and *S. intermedius* differs from that in *S. aureus* (see Noble, 1990) suggesting a different role but all protein A's examined react with the Fc portion of IgG rather than the Fab fragment.

STREPTOCOCCI

Streptococcal infection of human skin is best classed as a pyoderma, being characterized by a punched out lesion surrounded by erythema. Epidemic streptococcal infection of this type is often superimposed on scabies or on viral infections such as varicella (Svartman *et al.*, 1973). Alternatively a profuse cellulitis is seen as in erysipelas, especially of the face. Erythrogenic toxins are well described (Gerlach *et al.*, 1981). Although principally the Lancefield group A *Streptococcus pyogenes* is involved, groups G and C, both groups including strains usually associated with infection in animals, are prevalent in some localities (Efstratiou, 1989). The most common streptococcal infections in man are those of the throat and differences are evident in the M proteins of throat and skin-infecting strains.

Natural infection in animals does not seem to include skin surface disease. Streptococcal mastitis occurs in sheep and in cattle and is related to colonization of the teat skin (Wilson and Salt, 1978). Streptococcal abscesses occur in pigs affected with swinepox virus (Miller and Olson, 1980) but the histological appearance of these lesions is unlike that in humans. Strangles in horses is caused by *S. equi* and strains known as *S. agalactiae* are the cause of acute or subacute mastitis of cows, both belong to Lancefield group C. In dogs group G is the most common in isolations from the skin, though it is difficult to assess the clinical significance of these isolations (Biberstein *et al.*, 1980). Experimentally however mice and hamsters injected with group A streptococci exhibit pyodermal lesions similar to those seen in man.

EXOTICA

Many bacteria may occasionally cause skin lesions in both man and animals and the list of organisms, especially the anaerobes, is very similar (Meislin *et al.*, 1977; Ghoneim *et al.*, 1981; Berg *et al.*, 1979). Well recognized in humans, and known but less well reported in animals, are the mycobacteria. Apart from *Mycobacterium tuberculosis* and *M. leprae* where skin lesions are usually either secondary to, or the result of, deeper infection, human skin may be infected by *M. marinum*, *M. fortuitum* or *M. chelonei*. *M. marinum*, originally described as a pathogen of fish in the Philadelphia aquarium (Aronson, 1926) is generally associated with water and lesions appear on the elbows and knees in swimmers or on the hands of fish owners or boating enthusiasts (Collins *et al.*, 1985). *Mycobacterium fortuitum* and *M. chelonei* are the taxonomically valid terms which cover a number of organisms often described under other names. In man these are associated with subcutaneous injections, usually of contaminated fluids such as flu vaccine (Grange *et al.*, 1988). A similar picture has been presented in a dog given parvovirus vaccine (Gross and Connelly, 1983).

ANTIBIOTIC THERAPY AND ANTIBIOTIC RESISTANCE

The choice of appropriate antibiotic is a constant preoccupation in human medicine and also among veterinarians. A rational choice for first line therapy before laboratory results are available may be made difficult by a lack of knowledge of the infecting organism and of the local resistance patterns.

Hinton *et al.* (1978) in a study of infection in dogs found that 8% of lesions had a mixed flora of *S. aureus* and β-haemolytic streptococci. The streptococci usually proved to be resistant to antibiotics to which the staphylococci were sensitive. In humans with impetigo the mixed infection rate varies between 6% and 57% with a mean of about 35% (Mobacken *et al.*, 1975).

The proportion of organisms resistant to specific antibiotics varies with species, time and place. Table 4 shows the percentages of staphylococci resistant to a selection of antibiotics. The difficulty of making simple statements on the situation will be appreciated, especially since patterns change over a period of years (Cox *et al.*, 1984a). Most workers agree that the prevalence of antibiotic resistance is a reflection of antibiotic usage. In human microbiology we have been apt to blame the recent high levels of resistance to tetracycline on its extensive use in acne and recent studies on *P. acnes* confirm that the same is true for erythromycin and clindamycin (Eady *et al.*, 1989).

Table 4 Percentage of resistant strains of coagulase-positive staphylococci in dogs and humans

	Dogs				Humans		
	UK	UK	USA	USA	UK	Norway	Japan
Penicillin	69	29	61	83	82	82	29
Tetracycline	30	26	35	53	8	4	24
Erythromycin	7	ND	4	26	2	0	43
Clindamycin	9	6	7	25	0.5	0	ND
Chloramphenicol	0.5	24	2	11	0	1	13

Based on Biberstein *et al.* (1974), Hinton *et al.* (1978), Hassam *et al.* (1978), Dekio *et al.* (1981), Skjervan *et al.* (1982), Medleau *et al.* (1986), deSaxe and Lloyd (1982).

This presumably does not hold true for veterinary medicine where topical agents are less used but equally humans are not given erythromycin or tylosin as a growth promoter. Nevertheless Medleau *et al.* (1986) have shown that dogs previously treated for *S. intermedius* infection more often carried strains resistant to antibiotics that did untreated dogs (Table 5).

Antibiotic resistance may arise in a number of ways. Resistant variants may be selected from microbial populations by small, cumulative changes as a result of chromosomal mutations. Although such variants can be selected in the laboratory they are often less vigorous than naturally occurring variants and the mechanism of resistance may be different (Lacey, 1977). Resistance due to such mechanism is rarely a problem in clinical practice except with fusidic acid and rifampicin (Eng *et al.*, 1985). The most common clinical occurrence is the replacement by, or selection of, a preexisting resistant strain, which originated elsewhere. Genes mediating antibiotic resistance may be chromosomally encoded or, more generally, are borne on plasmids, extrachromosomal DNA which is transferable between microbial species and

Table 5 Effect of previous treatment on antibiotic resistance in *Staphylococcus*

	Percentage of resistant strains in dogs	
	Previously treated	Not previously treated
Penicillin	83	81
Chloramphenicol	15	2
Clindamycin	32	9
Erythromycin	34	9
Tetracycline	56	47

Based on Medleau *et al.* (1986).

sometimes between genera. Chance observation showed that gene transfer may occur on skin surface and this opened up an interesting field of study.

GENE TRANSFER ON THE SKIN

In 1978 we reported studies on two human patients whose underlying skin lesions were infected by *S. aureus* (Naidoo and Noble, 1978), various antibiotics were prescribed over a long period in an attempt to reduce infection and in both patients during the use of topical gentamicin with a minimal inhibitory concentration of over 32 mg/l from an initial value of less than 0.5 mg/l. It was later established that the strains had acquired a plasmid mediating gentamicin resistance (Naidoo and Noble, 1981) and that this plasmid had most probably originated in a strain of coagulase negative staphylococcus (*S. hominis*) which was part of the patients normal flora. Later studies showed that many gentamicin resistant coagulase negative staphylococci were also able to transfer their resistance to coagulase positive and coagulase negative members of the skin human flora (Naidoo and Noble, 1987). The mechanism of transfer is known as 'conjugation' in which the donor and recipient strains must come into stable physical contact. It is assumed that changes in the cell wall occur which are mediated by the plasmid and which enable the plasmid to transfer copies of itself to the recipient cell.

Although most laboratory studies now use filters to bring the organisms into intimate contact, we found that transfer occurred experimentally on human skin and on the skin of hairless mice at the same rates as can be achieved by filters. Experiments using dogs showed that genes would transfer between coagulase negative staphylococci of human origin and *S. aureus* and *S. intermedius* of canine origin (Naidoo and Lloyd, 1984). Plasmids bearing genes for gentamicin, tetracycline, erythromycin or chloramphenicol resistance can also be transferred in this way provided that a conjugative plasmid is present in the donor cell. Recent studies show that other conjugative plasmids, not normally visible in agarose gels, are associated with resistance to mupirocin (Rahman *et al.*, 1989). Equally, although not yet explored *in vivo*, antibiotic resistance may be transferred from *Streptococcus faecalis* to *Staphylococcus aureus* (Schaberg *et al.*, 1982); this route may yield a mechanism by which genes are exchanged between the gut and skin floras. There is then a natural mechanism for gene transfer between members of the skin flora and the potential for transfer of resistance between microorganisms infecting animals and humans, albeit at very low rates, in the absence of antibiotic. Many other virulence factors such as the epidermolytic toxins and enterotoxins are carried on plasmids and therefore also have the potential for transfer between staphylococci and between mammalian hosts.

The skin can be envisaged as a habitat for a variety of organisms which possess antibiotic resistance genes and which form a pool of genes available at least to members of the same genus. The role of antibiotic therapy is to eliminate the sensitive organisms and to select the resistant variants which then proliferate to form the dominant flora. Most of the work on the transfer of genes has been carried out using antibiotic resistance markers since these are relatively easy to manipulate in the laboratory. Modern techniques such as the use of probes should enable us to follow genes which mediate pathogenicity factors and this opens up a new and exciting field of research on the true similarity, or difference, at least in the microbial moiety, between skin diseases of man and animals.

REFERENCES

Aliu, B. and Bergdoll, M.S. (1988). Characterization of staphylococci from patients with toxic shock syndrome. *Journal of Clinical Microbiology* **26**: 2427–2428.

Almazan, J., de la Fuente, R., Gomez-Lucia, E. and Suarez, G. (1987). Enterotoxin production by strains of *Staphylococcus intermedius* isolated from dog infections. *Zentralblatt für Bakteriologie, Mikrobiologie und Hygiene* **A264**: 29–32.

Amtsberg, G. (1979). Demonstration of exfoliation-producing substances in cultures of *Staph. hyicus* of pigs and *Staph. epidermidis* biotype 2 of cattle. *Zentralblatt für Veterinarmedizin* **B26**: 257–272.

Aronson, J.P. (1926). Spontaneous tuberculosis in salt water fish. *Journal of Infectious Diseases* **39**: 315–320.

Ayyagari, A., Agarwal, K.C., Kaur, S., Iyer, R.V. and Kumar, B. (1979). Prevalence of *Corynebacterium diphtheriae* in pyoderma and other skin lesions. *Indian Journal Pathology and Microbiology* **22**: 37–45.

Barton, M.D. and Hughes, K.L. (1980). *Corynebacterium equi*: a review. *Veterinary Bulletin (Weybridge)* **50**: 65–80.

Bedford, C.J. and Young, J.M. (1981). A comparison of comedonal and skin surface lipids from hairless dogs showing clinical signs of acne. *Journal of Investigative Dermatology* **77**: 341–344.

Berg, J.N., Fales, W.H. and Scanlan, C.M. (1979). Occurrence of anaerobic bacteria in diseases of the dog and cat. *American Journal of Veterinary Research* **40**: 876–881.

Biberstein, E.L., Franti, C.E., Jang, S.S. and Ruby, A. (1974). Antimicrobial sensitivity patterns in *Staphylococcus aureus* from animals. *Journal of the American Veterinary Medical Association* **164**: 1183–1186.

Biberstein, E.L., Brown, C. and Smith, T. (1980). Serogroups and biotypes among beta

hemolytic streptococci of canine origin. *Journal of Clinical Microbiology* **11**: 558–561.
Collins, C.H., Grange, J.M., Noble, W.C. andd Yates, M.D. (1985). *Mycobacterium marinum* infections in man. *Journal of Hygiene, Cambridge* **94**: 135–149.
Cox, H.U., Hoskins, J.D., Roy, A.F., Newman, S.S. and Luther, D.G. (1984a). Antimicrobial susceptibility of coagulase-positive staphylococci isolated from Louisiana dogs. *American Journal of Veterinary Research* **45**: 2039–2042.
Cox, H.U., Newman, S.S., Roy, A.F. and Hoskins, J.D. (1984b). Species of *Staphylococcus* isolated from animal infections. *Cornell Veterinarian* **74**: 124–135.
Crass, B.A. and Bergdoll, M.S. (1986). Involvement of coagulase-negative staphylococci in toxic shock syndrome. *Journal of Clinical Microbiology* **23**: 43–45.
Davies, S.J., Ogg, C.S., Cameron, J.S., Poston, S.M. and Noble, W.C. (1989). *Staph. aureus* nasal carriage, exit-site infection and catheter loss in patients treated with continuous ambulatory peritoneal dialysis (CAPD). *Peritoneal Dialysis International* **9**: 61–64.
Dekio, S., Takagaki, K., Yamasaki, R., Hamanaka, K., Ikeda, S. and Onimura, K. (1981). Staphylococci isolated from pyodermas and their sensitivities to antibiotics. *Journal of Dermatology* **8**: 215–221.
Devriese, L.A., Schleifer, K.H. and Adegoke, G.O. (1985). Identification of coagulase-negative staphylococci from farm animals. *Journal of Applied Bacteriology* **58**: 45–55.
Dougherty, S.H. (1988). Pathobiology of infection in prosthetic devices. *Reviews of Infectious Diseases* **10**: 1102–1117.
Eady, E.A., Cove, J.H., Holland, K.T. and Cunliffe, W.J. (1989). Erythromycin resistant propionibacteria in antibiotic treated gene patients associated with therapeutic failure. *British Journal of Dermatology* **121**: 51–57.
Elias, P.M., Fritsch, P. and Mittermayer, H. (1976). Staphylococcal toxic epidermal necrolysis: species and tissue susceptibility and resistance. *Journal of Investigative Dermatology* **66**: 80–89.
Efstratiou, A. (1989). Outbreaks of human infection caused by pyogenic streptococci of Lancefield groups C and G. *Journal of Medical Microbiology* **29**: 207–219.
Ellis-Pegler, R.B., Parr, D.H. and Orchard, V.A. (1983). Recurrent skin infection with Rhodococcus in an immunosuppressed patient. *Journal of Infection* **6**: 39–41.
Eng, R.H.K., Smith, S.M., Tillem, M. and Cherubin, C. (1985). Rifampicin resistance. Development during the therapy of methicillin-resistant *Staphylococcus aureus* infection. *Archives of Internal Medicine* **145**: 146–148.
Freney, J., Brun, Y., Bes, M., Meugnier, H., Grimont, F., Grimont, P.A.D., Nervi, C. and Fleurette, J. (1988). *Staphylococcus lugdunensis* sp. nov. and *Staphylococcus schleiferi* sp. nov., two species from human clinical specimens. *International Journal of Systematic Bacteriology* **38**: 168–172.
Fukuda, S., Tokuno, H., Ogawa, H., Sasaki, M., Kishimoto, T., *et al.* (1984). Enterotoxigenicity of *Staphylococcus intermedius* strains isolated from dogs. *Zentralblatt für Bakteriologie, Mikrobiologie und Hygiene* **A258**: 360–367.
de la Fuente, R., Suarez, G. and Schleifer, K.H. (1985). *Staphylococcus aureus* subsp *anaerobius* subsp. nov.; the causal agent of abscess disease of sheep. *International Journal of Systematic Bacteriology* **35**: 99–102.
Gerlach, D., Knoll, H., Kohlerr, W. and Ozegowski, J.H. (1981). Isolation and characterization of erythrogenic toxins of *Streptococcus pyogenes. Zentralblatt für Bakteriologie, Mikrobiologie und Hygiene* **A250**: 277–286.
Ghoneim, A.T.M., McGoldrick, J., Blick, P.W.H., Flowers, M.W., Marsden, A.K. *et al.* (1981). Aerobic and anaerobic bacteriology of subcutaneous abscesses. *British Journal of Surgery* **68**: 498–500.
Gower, D.B., Nixon, A. and Mallet, A.I. (1988). The significance of odorous steroids

in axillary odour in Perfumery. In: Van Toller, S. and Dodd, G.H., (eds) *The Psychology and Biology of Fragrance* Chapman & Hall, London.

Grange, J.M., Noble, W.C., Yates, M.D. and Collins, C.H. (1988). Inoculation mycobacterioses. *Clinical and Experimental Dermatology* **13**: 211-220.

Gross, T.L. and Connelly, M.R. (1983). Non-tuberculous mycobacterial skin infection in two dogs. *Veterinary Pathology* **20**: 117-119.

Harnish, J.P., Tronca, E., Nolan, C.M., Turck, M. and Holmes, K.K. (1989). Diphtheria among alcoholic urban adults. A decade of experience in Seattle. *Annals of Internal Medicine* **111**: 71-82.

Hassam, Z.A., Shaw, E.J., Shooter, R.A. and Caro, D.B. (1978). Changes in antibiotic sensitivity in strains of *Staphylococcus aureus* 1952-78. *British Medical Journal* **2**: 536-537.

Heffner, K.A., White, S.D., Frevert, C.W. and Jakowski, R. (1988). Corynebacterium folliculitis in the horse. *Journal of American Veterinary Medical Association* **193**: 89-90.

Higgins, R. and Paradis, M. (1980). Abscess caused by *Corynebacterium equi* in a cat. *Canadian Veterinary Journal* **21**: 63-64.

Hinton, M., Marston, M. and Hedges, R. (1978). The antibiotic resistance of pathogenic staphylococci and streptococci isolated from dogs. *Journal of Small Animal Practice* **19**: 229-235.

Kaminski, G.W. and Suter, I.I. (1976). Human infection with *Dermatophilus congolensis. Medical Journal of Australia* **1**: 443-447.

Kaplan, W. (1976). Dermatophilosis in primates. In: Lloyd, D.H. and Sellars, K.C. (eds) *Dermatophilosis in Animals and Man*. Academic Press, London.

Kloos, W.E., Schleifer, K.H. and Noble, W.C. (1976). Estimation of character parameters in coagulase-negative staphylococcus species. In: *Staphylococci and Staphylococcal Diseases. Zentralblatt für Bakteriologie, Parasitenkunde und Infections* krankheiten 1 Abt. (Supopl 5): 25-41.

Krogh, K.V. and Kristensen, S. (1976). A study of skin diseases in dogs and cats. II Microflora of the normal skin of dogs and cats. *Nordisk Veterinaire Medicine* **28**: 459-463.

Lacey, R.W. (1977). Lack of evidence for mutation of erythromycin resistance in clinical strains of *Staphylococcus aureus. Journal of Clinical Pathology* **30**: 602-605.

Lämmler, C. (1989). Characteristic bacteriolytic activities of *Staphylococcus hyicus. Journal of Clinical Microbiology* **27**: 1682-1683.

Lee, C.Y., Schmidt, J.J., Johnson-Winegar, A.D., Spero, L. and Iandolo, J.J. (1987). Sequence determination and comparison of the exfoliative toxin A and toxin B genes from *Staphylococcus aureus. Journal of Bacteriology* **169**: 3904-3909.

Lloyd, D.H. and Noble, W.C. (1982). *Dermatophilus congolensis* as a model pathogen in mice for the investigation of factors influencing skin infection. *British Veterinary Journal* **138**: 51-60.

Lloyd, D.H. and Reyss-Brion, A. (1984). Le peroxyde de benzoyle: efficacite clinique et bacteriologique dans le traitement des pyodermites chronique. *Pratique Medicale et chururgicale de l'animal de compagnie* **19**: 445-449.

Lloyd, D.H. and Sellars, K.C. (1976). *Dermatophilus Infection in Animals and Man*. Academic Press, London.

Love, D.N. and Davis, P.C. (1980). Isolation of *Staphylococcus aureus* from a condition in Greyhounds histologically resembling "staphlyococcal scalded skin syndrome" in man. *Journal of Small Animal Practice* **21**: 351-357.

Medleau, L., Long, P.E., Brown, J. and Miller, N.H. (1986). Frequency and antimicrobial susceptibility of *Staphylococcus* species isolated from canine pyodermas. *American Journal of Veterinary Research* **47**: 229-231.

Meislin, H.W., Lerner, S.A., Graves, M.H., McGhee, M.D., Kocka, F.F.E. *et al.*

(1977). Cutaneous abscesses. Anaerobic and aerobic bacteriology and patient management. *Annals of Internal Medicine* **87**: 145-149.

Melish, M.E. (1982). Staphylococci, streptococci and the skin: Review of impetigo and the staphylococcal scalded skin syndrome. *Seminars in Dermatology* **1**: 101-110.

Miers, K.C. and Ley, W.B. (1980). *Corynebacterium pseudotuberculosis* infection in the horse: Study of 117 clinical cases and consideration of etiopathology. *Journal of the American Veterinary Medical Association* **117**: 250-253.

Miller, R.B. and Olson, L.D. (1980). Experimental induction of cutaneous streptococcal abscesses in swine as a sequela to swinepox. *American Journal of Veterinary Research* **41**: 341-347.

Mobacken, H., Holst, R., Wengstrom, C. and Holm, S.E. (1975). Epidemiological aspects of impetigo contagiosa in western Sweden. *Scandinavian Journal of Infectious Diseases* **7**: 39-44.

Morgan, K.L., Gruffydd-Jones, E., Wieneke, A.A., de Azavedo, J., Carroll, P.J. *et al.* (1986). Staphylococcal toxic shock syndrome. *Veterinary Record* **119**: 559.

Muller, G.H., Kirk, R.W. and Scott, D.W. (1989). *Small Animal Dermatology*. W.B. Saunders Company, Philadelphia.

Naidoo, J. and Lloyd, D.H. (1984). Transmission of genes between staphylococci on skin. In: Woodbine, M. (ed.) *Antimicrobials and Agriculture*, pp. 285-292. Butterworth, London.

Naidoo, J. and Noble, W.C. (1978). Acquisition of antibiotic resistance by *Staphylococcus aureus* in skin patients. *Journal of Clinical Pathology* **31**: 1187-1192.

Naidoo, J. and Noble, W.C. (1981). Transfer of gentamicin resistance between coagulase-negative and coagulase-positive staphylococci on skin. *Journal of Hygiene, Cambridge* **26**: 183-187.

Naidoo, J. and Noble, W.C. (1987). Skin as a source of transferable antibiotic resistance in coagulase-negative staphylococci. *Zentralblatt für Bakteriologie Mikrobiologie und Hygiene* (Suppl) **16**: 225-234.

Nicolaides, N., Fu, H.C. and Rice, G.R. (1968). The skin surface lipids of man compared with those of eighteen species of animals. *Journal of Investigative Dermatology* **51**: 83-89.

Nikkari, T. (1974). Comparative chemistry of sebum. *Journal of Investigative Dermatology* **62**: 257-267.

Noble, W.C. (1981). *Microbiology of Human Skin*. Lloyd Luke, London.

Noble, W.C. (1990). Systematics and the natural history of staphylococci. In: *Staphylococci*. Academic Press, London. (in press).

Noble, W.C., Williams, R.E.O., Jevons, M.P. and Shooter, R.A. (1964). Some aspects of nasal carriage of staphylococci. *Journal of Clinical Pathology* **17**: 79-83.

Nordstrom, K.M. and Noble, W.C. (1985). Application of computer taxonomic techniques to the study of cutaneous propionibacteria and skin-surface lipid. *Archives of Dermatological Research* **278**: 107-113.

Okerman, L., Devriese, L.A., Maertens, L., Okerman, F. and Godard, C. (1984). Cutaneous staphylococcosis in rabbits. *Veterinary Record* **114**: 313-315.

Onon, E.O. (1979). Purification and partial characterization of the exotoxin of *Corynebacterium ovis*. *Biochemical Journal* **117**: 181-186.

Parker, B.N.J., Bonson, M.D. and Carroll, P.J. (1983). Staphylococcal dermatitis in unweaned lambs. *Veterinary Record* **113**: 570-571.

Peckham, J.C., Cole, J.R., Chapman, W.L.Jr, Malone, J.B.Jr, McCall, J.W. and Thompson, P.E. (1974). Staphylococcal dermatitis in mongolian gerbils (*Meriones unguiculatus*). *Laboratory Animal Science* **24**: 43-47.

Pitcher, D.G. and Noble, W.C. (1978). Aerobic diphtheroids of human skin. *In*: Bousfield, I.J. and Callely, A.G. (eds) *Coryneform Bacteria*, pp. 265-287. Academic Press, London.

Pospisil, L., Kabatova, A. and Haklova, A. (1986). Report on isolation of coagulase-negative staphylococci in skin lesion and their special identifications. *Dermatologische Monatsschrift* **172**: 462-467.

Rahman, M., Noble, W.C. and Cookson, B. (1989). Transmissible mupirocin resistance in *Staphylococcus aureus. Epidemiology and Infection* **102**: 261-270.

Richards, M. and Hurse, A. (1985). *Corynebacterium pseudotuberculosis* abscesses in a young butcher. *Australia and New Zealand Medical Journal* **15**: 85-86.

Rubel, L.R. (1972). Pitted keratolysis and *Dermatophilus congolensis. Archives of Dermatology* **105**: 584-586.

deSaxe, M. and Lloyd, D.H. (1982). Antibiotic resistance and other characteristics of *Staphylococcus aureus* isolated from dogs. *Association of Veterinary Clinical Pharmacology and Therapy, Proceedings* **6**: 50-54.

Schaberg, D.R., Clewell, D.B. and Glatzer, L. (1982). Conjugative transfer of R plasmids from *Streptococcus faecalis* to *Staphylococcus aureus. Antimicrobial Agents and Chemotherapy* **22**: 204-207.

Schleifer, K.H., Meyer, S.A. and Rupprecht, M. (1979). Relatedness among coagulase negative staphylococci, deoxyribonucleic acid reassociation and comparative immunological studies. *Archives of Microbiology* **122**: 93-101.

Scott, D.W. and Manning, T.O. (1980). Equine folliculitis and furunculosis. *Equine Practice* **2** (6): 11-32.

Skjerven, O., Melby, K., Dramsdahl, H. and Alvestad, P.M. (1982). Staphylococcal infections among newborn babies in two towns in North Norway. *NIPH Annals* **5**: 51-56.

Somerville-Millar, D.A. and Noble, W.C. (1974). Resident and transient bacteria of the skin. *Journal of Cutaneous Pathology* **1**: 260-264.

Spencer, R.C. (1988). Infection in continuous ambulatory peritoneal dialysis. *Journal of Medical Microbiology* **27**: 1-9.

Svartman, M., Potter, E.V., Poon King, T. and Earle, D.P. (1973). Streptococcal infection of scabietic lesions related to acute glomerulonephritis in Trinidad. *Journal of Laboratory and Clinical Medicine* **81**: 182-193.

Takeuchi, S., Kobayashi, Y. and Morozumi, T. (1987). Proteolytic zymograms of *Staphylococcus hyicus* subsp. *hyicus* isolated from pigs, chickens and cows. *Veterinary Microbiology* **14**: 47-52.

Varaldo, P.E., Kilpper-Balz, R., Biavasco, F., Satta, G. and Schleifer, K.H. (1988). *Staphylococcus delphini* sp. nov., a coagulase positive species isolated from dolphins. *International Journal of Systematic Bacteriology* **38**: 436-439.

White, M.I. and Noble, W.C. (1980). Skin response to Protein A. *Proceedings of the Royal Society of Edinburgh* **79B**: 43-46.

White, M.I. and Noble, W.C. (1985). The cutaneous reaction to staphylococcal Protein A in normal subjects and patients with atopic dermatitis or psoriasis. *British Journal of Dermatology* **113**: 179-183.

Wilson, G.D. and Salt, G.F.H. (1978). Streptococci in animal disease. In: Skinner, F.A. and Quesnel, L.B. (eds) *Streptococci*, pp. 143-156. Academic Press, London.

Woodgyer, A.J., Baxter, M., Rush-Munro, F.M., Brown, J. and Kaplan, W. (1985). Isolation of *Dermatophilus congolensis* from two New Zealand cases of pitted keratolysis. *Australian Journal of Dermatology* **26**: 29-35.

Wong, T.P. and Groman, N. (1984). Production of diphtheria toxin by selected isolates of *Corynebacterium ulcerans* and *Corynebacterium pseudotuberculosis. Infection and Immunity* **43**: 1114-1116.

5.2 Bacterial Interference in the Control of Exudative Epidermitis of Pigs

Robert P. Allaker,[1] David H. Lloyd[2] and Anne I. Lamport

[1]*Research Fellow,* [2]*Senior Lecturer (Dermatology), Dept of Veterinary Medicine & Animal Husbandry, Royal Veterinary College, Hatfield, Herts, UK*

INTRODUCTION

Exudative epidermitis is a sporadic dermatitis of piglets caused by *Staphylococcus hyicus*. The agent commonly resides on the skin (Hooper, 1988) and thus neither infection nor the disease can readily be eradicated. One approach to the control of such infections uses bacterial interference mechanisms involving exposure to inhibitor-producing bacteria or to avirulent strains of the pathogen. In man, for example, the relatively avirulent strain 502A of *Staphylococcus aureus* has been used to protect babies against staphylococcal disease (Aly and Shinefield, 1982).

Gnotobiotic piglets are susceptible to exudative epidermitis after exposure experimentally to *S. hyicus* (Bollwahn *et al.*, 1970). Such susceptibility allowed the development of a model of exudative epidermitis (Lloyd *et al.*, 1990) to study bacterial interactions on the skin and to assess the ability of potential antagonists to prevent disease. It was shown that precolonization with certain inhibitor-producing bacteria can ameliorate the severity of exudative epidermitis (Allaker *et al.*, 1990) and antagonism by an avirulent variant of *S. hyicus* completely inhibited the disease (Allaker *et al.*, 1988). Investigations are now being undertaken to observe the effects of induced colonization by antagonistic bacteria and their ability to inhibit colonization and infection by *S. hyicus* on pigs under farming conditions.

This paper describes a study carried out in three parts:

1. To monitor the acquisition of the normal skin bacterial flora by piglets.

2. To determine the relationship of the skin flora of neonatal piglets to the flora within the birth canal of the sow.
3. To establish a flora to antagonise the colonization of *S. hyicus*.

MATERIALS AND METHODS

Animals

Large White breed gilts and their piglets were used and held in the same farrowing house.

Sampling

Bacterial populations were monitored using swabs (Exogen, Medical Wire Co.) moistened with a buffered Triton X-100 wash fluid (Lloyd, 1984) and rubbed for 15 s over the skin (9 cm^2). The vaginal vestibule was sampled by introducing a moistened swab for 5 s without touching the surrounding skin.

Bacterial counting

Swab tips were cut off and shaken manually in 2 ml of wash fluid for 1 min. Serial dilutions of the resulting suspension were made in diluting fluid (wash fluid diluted 1 in 2 with distilled water). Appropriate dilutions were plated onto agar media and differential colony counts performed after 48 h incubation at 37°c and 24 h at room temperature.

Blood Agar Base (Oxoid, CM 271) with bovine blood (5% v/v) was used for the presumptive differentiation of the staphylococci, micrococci and non-lipophilic coryneforms. A medium incorporating Tween 80 (Devriese, 1977) was also used to allow the differentiation of presumptive *S. hyicus* and the growth of the lipophilic coryneforms.

Bacterial strains and inoculation

A known virulent strain of *S. hyicus* (P411) and a known avirulent strain (SK170) were used. Both strains had been isolated from cases of exudative epidermitis; their virulence had been tested in previous studies in gnotobiotic piglets (Lloyd *et al.*, 1990). The animals were infected approximately 12 h after parturition by rubbing a swab (Exogen, Medical Wire Co.) which had been dipped into an overnight broth culture of the organism, onto 4 cm^2 of skin on both sides of the midline in the sacral region. The skin was sampled and bacteria counted as described previously. Nutrient agar (Oxoid, CM3), incorporating added antibiotic (20 $\mu g/ml$), was used to allow the selective growth of the *S. hyicus* strains. Fusidic acid resistance had been induced in *S. hyicus* strain P411 and rifampicin resistance in SK170.

Sites and times of sampling

Part 1
Three sows were each sampled weekly for 2 weeks before parturition and then, together with three of their piglets (litters 1–3) at 12 h after parturition and at weekly intervals for 5 weeks. In the sows, the skin caudal to the ear, in one axilla, on the udder adjacent to the third and fourth teats from the rear and over the sacrum was sampled. The piglets were sampled in the same way but excluding the udder.

Part 2
The vestibule of five sows was sampled 6 h before parturition and at intervals of 12 h until parturition. Samples were also taken at parturition.

Part 3
Three piglets from each of four litters were sampled at the ear, axilla and sacrum at 12 h after parturition and then inoculated as described previously with antibiotic-resistant *S. hyicus* strains. Two litters (nos. 4 and 5; three piglets per litter) received a virulent strain (P411), while the other litters (nos. 6 and 7; three piglets per litter) received an avirulent strain (SK170). The piglets were then sampled weekly for 3 weeks at the same sites. The sows were also sampled at the same times and at the sites described in Part 1.

RESULTS

Part 1
No significant change in the populations of the coryneforms and micrococci on the sows was observed over the 7-week period (Table 1). However a significant decline ($p < 0.05$) in the number of staphylococci was observed.

Table 1 Mean bacterial populations on the skin of sows, 2 weeks before and 5 weeks after parturition

Week	Populations[a]		
	Coryneforms	Staphylococci	Micrococci
1	6.46 ± 0.26	6.48 ± 0.27	5.68 ± 0.37
7	6.19 ± 0.04	5.41 ± 0.08	4.93 ± 0.11
mean[b]	6.55 ± 0.18	5.92 ± 0.18	5.47 ± 0.21
p[c]	N.S.	<0.05	N.S.

[a] Log colony forming units per swab ± SEM.
[b] Mean of weekly counts (7 weeks).
[c] Regression of weekly counts against time (7 weeks).

The piglets were colonized by a range of bacteria closely similar to that of the sows 12 h after parturition. Although significant short-term fluctuations in populations were then observed, over the 5-week period the populations remained essentially stable (Fig. 1). The micrococci (not shown in Fig. 1) colonized the lower level (mean population: 4.17×10^4) and demonstrated the same weekly trends as the other bacterial groups. Fluctuations in the counts of *S. hyicus* on the piglets and sows tended to follow one another during the study (Fig. 2).

Part 2

Within the vestibule of the five sows sampled *Pasteurella* spp. were the predominant Gram-negative isolates in four of the animals. A coliform

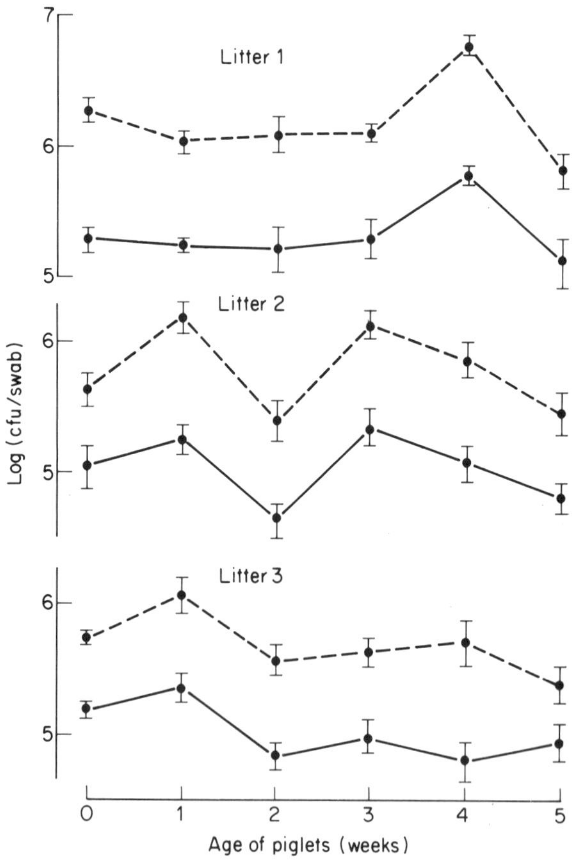

Figure 1 Mean skin populations (± SEM) of staphylococci (•———•) and coryneforms (•— —•) on piglets from three litters (1, 2 and 3) over a 5-week period from parturition.

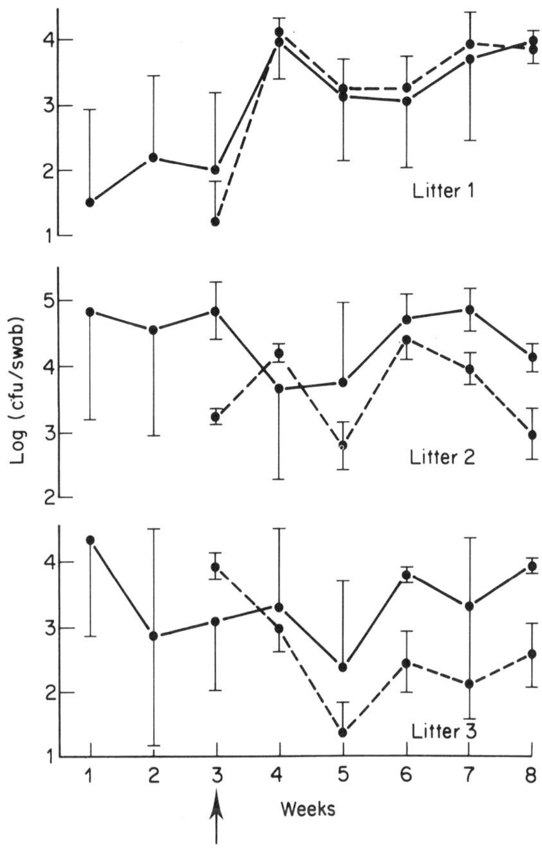

Figure 2 Mean skin populations (± SEM) of *S. hyicus* on sows (•———•) and piglets (•— —•) from three litters (1, 2 and 3) from 2 weeks before parturition (▲) until 5 weeks afterwards.

predominated in the other sow. There was no significant change in the Gram-negative population over the 60-h period before parturition (Fig. 3). Gram-positive bacteria representing those types found on the skin, including *S. hyicus*, were also present. Their populations remained essentially stable until 12 h prior to parturition when there was a dramatic rise in the number of staphylococci ($p < 0.05$) and coryneforms ($p < 0.01$).

Part 3

At 12 h postparturition the populations of staphylococci including endogenous *S. hyicus*, had become established on the skin of the piglets and remained stable thereafter. The mean populations of staphylococci and endogenous *S. hyicus* on the sows and piglets over the 3-week period following parturition are shown in Table 2. However the applied *S. hyicus* strains (P411

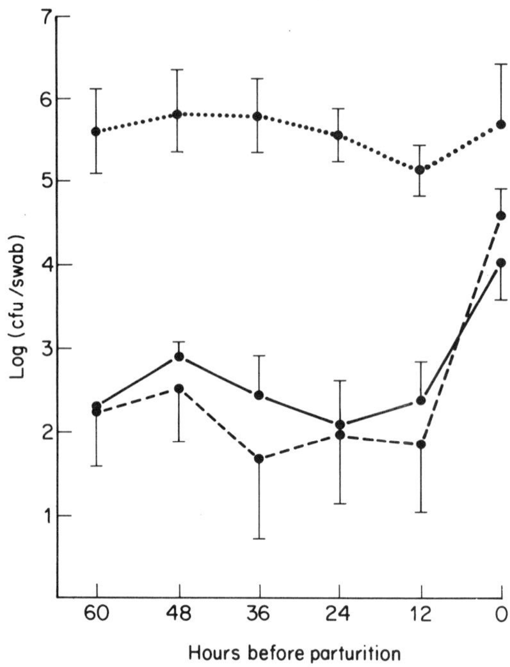

Figure 3 Mean sow vestibular populations (± SEM) of Gram-negative bacteria (•·······•), coryneforms (•— —•) and staphylococci (•———•) in the 60-h period before parturition.

Table 2 Mean populations of staphylococci and endogenous *S. hyicus* on the skin of sows and piglets (0–3 weeks postpartum)

Litters	Animals sampled	Populations[a]	
		Staphylococci	Endogenous *S. hyicus*
4 and 7	Sows	5.68=0.15	3.91=0.49
	Piglets	4.69=0.09	3.27=0.20
6 and 7	Sows	5.62=0.11	3.32=0.42
	Piglets	4.71=0.12	2.14=0.56

[a] Log colony forming units per swab ± SEM.

and SK170) failed to become established and they could only be detected on the piglets at low levels 1 week after inoculation (Table 3). Transfer of the exogenous strains to the sows also occurred. They were detected on the udder at 1 week (SK170) and 2 weeks (P411) following introduction onto the piglets (Table 3).

Table 3 Isolation of exogenous *S. hyicus* strains on the skin of sows and piglets

Litters	Strain inoculated onto piglets	Animals sampled	Isolation of exogenous *S. hyicus*[a] after inoculation		
			Week 1	Week 2	Week 3
4 and 5	P411	Sows	– (1)	+ (1)[b]	–
		Piglets	+ (1)	–	–
6 and 7	SK170	Sows	+ (1)	–	–
		Piglets	+ (3)	–	–

[a] Mean no. of colonies isolated per swab from skin sites sampled on animals; – no colonies isolated; + 1-5 colonies isolated.
[b] ( ) No. of animals colonized.

DISCUSSION

In the field, exudative epidermitis caused by *S. hyicus* infection generally affects piglets up to 5 weeks of age (Jones, 1956). In man, babies are also susceptible to staphylococcal skin disease, caused by *S. aureus*, during the neonatal period. Such infection has been prevented by bacterial interference using an avirulent *S. aureus* strain (Aly and Shinefield, 1982). Our studies using gnotobiotic piglets have shown that it is also possible to prevent exudative epidermiditis using an avirulent *S. hyicus* strain (Allaker *et al.*, 1988).

In man the normal bacterial flora protects against exogenous bacteria; it is often necessary to remove resident *S. aureus* before successful implantation of an avirulent *S. aureus* strain can occur and act as an antagonist (Aly and Shinefield, 1982). The same phenomenon may occur in farm piglets. Our studies have shown that the skin of the piglet is colonized within 12 h of parturition by bacteria, including *S. hyicus*, which represents the spectrum found on the adult. In preliminary studies to determine the pattern of skin colonization from birth it was shown that piglets are born with a flora similar to that found at 12 h after parturition (Allaker and Lloyd, unpublished observations). Gram-negative organisms from the birth canal are also present at birth and are then rapidly lost. Sarkany and Gaylarde (1968) similarly found that the skin of the newborn human baby is not sterile and that it is colonized at the moment of delivery by staphylococci and coryneforms, the two predominant organisms of the skin flora of all ages.

The significant rise in the populations of staphylococci and coryneforms within the vestibule of the sow in the immdediate period before parturition may be associated with nutrient and pH changes. The normal porcine fetus *in utero* is bacteriologically sterile (Tavernor *et al.*, 1971) and since the newborn skin is colonized at birth, it is clear that the flora appears on the skin during transit through the birth canal. Human studies (Sarkany and Gaylarde, 1968) of the flora of the vagina and vulva lend support to this finding since shortly before delivery the vaginal flora consists mainly of staphylococci and there is a predominance of these organisms on the skin of the newborn baby.

If bacterial antagonism of *S. hyicus* infection is to be achieved, the insertion of an antagonistic strain must be induced despite the presence of a normal flora from birth. However, an attempt to introduce exogenous *S. hyicus* strains at 12 h postparturition by contact inoculation was not successful, despite the fact that transfer of the exogenous strains to the sows occurred and they persisted in the environment for at least 2 weeks. Hence other methods to implant an antagonistic strain onto the skin of the pig are required. Modification of the vulval/vaginal flora including the implantation of a potential antagonist may be necessary, to ensure that the piglet skin is colonized by an appropriate flora at the moment of birth.

ACKNOWLEDGEMENTS

This study was supported from a grant from the Wellcome Trust.

REFERENCES

Allaker, R.P., Lloyd, D.H. and Smith, I.M. (1988). Prevention of exudative epidermitis in gnotobiotic piglets by bacterial interference. *Veterinary Record* **123**: 597–598.

Allaker, R.P., Lloyd, D.H., Smith, I.M. and Noble, W.C. (1990). Interaction of *Staphylococcus hyicus* with inhibitor-producing bacteria on the skin of gnotobiotic piglets. *Microbial Ecology in Health and Disease* **3** (accepted for publication).

Aly, R. and Shinefield, H.R. (eds) (1982). *Bacterial Interference.* CRC Press, Florida.

Bollwahn, W., Bähr, K.-H., Hazem, A.S., Amtsberg, G. and Schmidt, U. (1970). Experimentelle Untersuchungen zur Ätiologie des nässenden Ekzems der Schweine. *Deutsche Tierarztliche Wochenschrift* **77**: 601–603.

Devriese, L.A. (1977). Isolation and identification of *Staphylococcus hyicus. American Journal of Veterinary Research* **38**: 787–792.

Hooper, R. (1988). *Staphylococcus hyicus*: studies on its ecology, antigenic structure and haemolysin production. PhD Thesis, University of London.

Jones, L.D. (1956). Exudative epidermitis of pigs. *American Journal of Veterinary Research* **17**: 179–193.

Lloyd, D.H. (1984). Evaluation of a cup-scrub technique for the quantification of the microbial flora on bovine skin. *Journal of Applied Bacteriology* **56**: 103–107.

Lloyd, D.H., Allaker, R.P., Smith, I.M. and Mackie, W.M. (1990). Colonisation of gnotobiotic piglets by *Staphylococcus hyicus* and the development of exudative epidermitis. *Microbial Ecology in Health and Disease* **3** (accepted for publication).

Sarkany, I. and Gaylarde, C.C. (1968). Bacterial colonisation of the skin of the newborn. *Journal of Pathology and Bacteriology* **95**: 115–122.

Tavernor, W.D., Trexler, P.C., Vaughan, L.C., Cox, J.E. and Jones, D.G.C. (1971). The production of gnotobiotic piglets and calves by hysterectomy under general anaesthesia. *Veterinary Record* **88**: 10–14.

5.3 Clinical and Immunological Responses of Dogs with Recurrent Pyoderma to Injections of Staphylococcus Phage Lysate

Douglas J. DeBoer,[1] Kevin T. Schultz,[2] Chester B. Thomas[2] and Karen A. Moriello[1]

[1] *Department of Medical Sciences and* [2] *Department of Pathological Sciences, School of Veterinary Medicine, University of Wisconsin–Madison, USA*

INTRODUCTION

Recurrent superficial pyoderma due to infection with *Staphylococcus intermedius* is a common skin disease of dogs. Though the primary treatment for this disease is antibiotics, other agents such as antibacterial shampoos and immunomodulatory bacterins are frequently used as adjunct treatment. Commercially available bacterin preparations have been recommended for such use for more than 10 years (Scott *et al.*, 1978). These recommendations initially were made based on personal observations and anecdotes, without the benefit of controlled trials. Recently, more controlled studies demonstrating the efficacy of bacterin treatment have been published (Becker *et al.*, 1989; DeBoer *et al.* 1990).

We recently reported results from a double-blind, placebo-controlled trial on the efficacy of a commercial staphylococcal bacterin product (Staphage Lysate [SPL], Delmont Laboratories, Swarthmore, PA USA) as adjunct treatment for idiopathic recurrent superficial pyoderma in dogs. This product, which is made from *Staphylococcus aureus* bacteria, showed significantly greater efficacy in controlling recurrence of disease than did placebo injections (DeBoer *et al.*, 1990); SPL is a product with a variety of demonstrated *in vivo* and *in vitro* immunomodulatory effects. It is unknown which of these effects were responsible for the improvement seen in the patients in this trial.

One possible mechanism of action of SPL is alteration of the amount and/or antigenic specificity of antistaphylococcal IgG in patient sera. The purpose of this study was to characterize the IgG antibody response to staphylococcal antigens in dogs with recurrent pyoderma, and to measure changes in this antibody response with SPL treatment.

MATERIALS AND METHODS

Patients and serum samples

This study utilized canine patients with idiopathic recurrent superficial pyoderma, which were part of an efficacy trial of SPL. The protocol and results of this trial have been described previously (De Boer *et al*, 1990). Briefly, dogs in this trial were treated with oral sodium oxacillin for 6 weeks. Concurrently, dogs received twice-weekly subcutaneous injections of SPL or of a placebo liquid, for 18 weeks. Blood samples were obtained from these patients by jugular venipuncture; samples were taken prior to treatment (pretreatment sample) and at the conclusion of the study (posttreatment sample). The blood was allowed to clot at room temperature, then centrifuged and the serum recovered. Serum samples were stored frozen at −70°C prior to use.

Staphylococcal antigens

SPL antigens were prepared for use in the ELISA and immunoblotting assays by extensive dialysis of SPL against 0.01 M phosphate buffered saline, pH 7.4 (PBS), for 96 h at 4°C. The dialysate was concentrated 100-fold by ultrafiltration on a Spectra/Por Type C cellulose membrane (10 000 molecular weight cut-off, Spectrum Medical Industries, Los Angeles, CA USA), aliquoted, and stored frozen at −70°C. The concentrated solution was thawed and centrifuged at 15 000 × ***g*** for 5 min before use.

Staphylococcus intermedius antigens were prepared from Protein A-free strains of *S. intermedius* isolated from canine skin lesions (a gift from Dr H. Cox, Baton Rouge, LA USA). Bacteria were grown for 24 h in brain-heart infusion broth (Difco, Detroit, MI USA) at 37°C with constant shaking. Cultures were centrifuged to pellet the bacteria. The pelleted bacteria were washed three times with PBS, then resuspended in PBS; 10 ml of the bacterial suspension was mixed with 20 g of sterile glass beads (0.11 mm average diameter), then homogenized in a rotary homogenizer (Model MSK, B. Braun Instruments, Burlingame, CA USA) for 10 min at 4°C. The resulting suspension was centrifuged at 300 × ***g*** for 5 min to pellet debris and glass beads; the supernatant was recovered and centrifuged at 20 000 × ***g*** for 30 min to pellet fine particles. The final supernatant was recovered, sterilized through a 0.2 μm pore size syringe filter, aliquoted, and stored frozen at −70°C until use.

Reference sera

A reference antistaphylococcal antiserum was prepared by hyperimmunization of two normal random-bred laboratory dogs. *S. intermedius* antigens were emulsified 1:1 with incomplete Freund's adjuvant. Each dog was injected with a total of 0.5 cc of the antigen preparation (containing approximately 1.6 mg protein), intradermally in five sites. The immunization was repeated every 2 weeks for a total of six times. One week after the final immunization, the dogs were bled, the serum was recovered and pooled in equal proportions, and stored at −70°C until used. This antiserum was positive on ELISA against *S. intermedius* antigens or SPL antigens at a dilution of 1:4096.

A pooled normal canine reference serum was prepared by bleeding ten normal random-bred laboratory dogs and recovering the serum. Sera were mixed in equal proportions and stored at −70°C until used.

ELISA for antistaphylococcal antibody

The concentrations of IgG antibody against SPL antigens and antibody against *S. intermedius* antigens were measured in the pretreatment and posttreatment serum samples from 19 dogs; 11 of these dogs had received injections of SPL and eight had received injections of placebo.

Antibody concentrations were measured with an ELISA assay and SPL antigens prepared above were diluted 1:1000 in coating buffer (0.1 M Na_2CO_3, pH 9.6) then 100 μl of this solution was transferred to each well of a 96-well microtiter plate (Immulon I, Dynatech, Chantilly, VA USA). Plates were incubated 20 h at 4°C. The wells were then washed six times with washing solution (0.15 M NaCl, 0.05% v/v Tween-20). All serum samples were diluted in serum dilution buffer (SDB [0.15 M NaCl, 0.05 M Tris-HCl, 0.1% v/V Tween 20, 0.1% bovine serum albumin, pH 7.4]). Two-fold serial dilutions of hyperimmune reference serum were prepared, from 1:8 to 1:1024. Pooled normal dog serum and patient samples were diluted 1:64. Duplicate 100 μl portions of sera and buffer blank were transferred to the microplate wells. Plates were incubated at 1 h at room temperature, then washed with washing solution. Rabbit anticanine IgG (peroxidase conjugated; Organon Teknika Cappel, Malvern, PA USA) was diluted 1:400 in SDB and 100 μl was added to each well. After another 1 h incubation at room temperature, the wells were washed six times. 100 μl of freshly prepared substrate solution (0.05 M citrate buffer [pH 4.0], containing 2 M H_2O_2 and 0.2 mM 2,2'-azino-di-(3-ethylbenzthiazoline) sulphuric acid) was next dispensed into each well. Colour development was observed, and after an empirically determined optimal time (approximately 10 min), 50 μl of 0.2 M HF, pH 3.3, was added to each well to stop the reaction. The absorbance of each well was read at 405 nm with a microplate reader (Bio-Tek, Winooski, VT USA), with subtraction of the buffer blank absorbance.

Using absorbance readings from the hyperimmune reference serum dilutions, a standard curve was plotted as ln(absorbance) vs ln(serum dilution). The slope of this curve's linear portion was calculated by linear regression analysis. Antibody concentrations for each of the unknown serum samples was expressed as multiple of normal activity (MONA) using pooled normal canine serum as the normal reference (Tijssen, 1985).

A similar ELISA assay was used to measure the concentration of antibody directed against *S. intermedius* antigens. In this case, microplate wells were initially coated with 100 μl of a solution of *S. intermedius* antigens (10 μg/ml) in coating buffer. Otherwise, the assay was conducted as specified above.

Immunoblotting

To further characterize the antigenic specificities of the antistaphylococcal antibodies formed in patient sera with repeated SPL immunization, protein immunoblotting (Western blot) assays were performed on pre- and posttreatment samples from 15 dogs. Eight of these dogs had received SPL injections, and seven had received placebo injections. Each serum sample was tested individually on a blot of electrophoretically separated SPL antigens.

According to standard techniques SPL antigens were separated by discontinuous vertical slab gel electrophoresis on 14 × 16 cm 10% polyacrylamide-SDS gels under reducing conditions (Laemmli, 1970). Separated proteins were transferred to BA85 nitrocellulose (NC) sheets (Schleicher and Schuell, Keene, NH USA) with a semi-dry electroblotting apparatus (Milliblot SDE, Millipore, Bedford, MA USA) for 55 min at 475 mA constant current. Following transfer, gels were stained with Coomassie blue stain to verify complete transfer of proteins.

The blotted NC sheet was blocked overnight at 4°C with PBS containing 0.1% v/v Tween-20 (PBS-T). The sheet was cut into strips approximately 4 mm wide for further use; NC strips were incubated in a 1:25 dilution of patient serum in PBS-T for 1 h at room temperature with constant rotation. After three 5-min rinses in PBS-T, strips were incubated for 1 h at room temperature in a 1:200 dilution of biotinylated rabbit antidog IgG (Jackson ImmunoResearch, West Grove, PA USA). After three additional 5 min rinses in PBS-T, the strips were incubated for 30 min in preprepared avidin-biotin-peroxidase complex reagent (ABC reagent, Vector Laboratories, Burlingame, CA USA). Following a final three rinses in PBS-T, the strips were developed for 10 min in a substrate solution of 0.06% 4-chloro-1-naphthol with 0.1% H_2O_2 in PBS and dried overnight in a dark room.

The resulting stained strips were scanned with a laser densitometer (Model 2202, Pharmacia LKB Biotechnology, Piscataway, NJ USA). The scan patterns were printed out for reference as well as being stored on magnetic media for further analysis. The area under the curve of each scan tracing was determined by the integration function of the software, and expressed in arbitrary units.

Statistical analysis

Data from the ELISA and immunoblotting assays were analysed with the use of paired or independent *t*-tests, or with linear regression analysis, as appropriate for the comparison being made. All analyses were done using the SYSTAT statistical software package (SYSTAT Inc., Evanston, IL USA).

RESULTS

Antibody against staphylococcal antigens

Preliminary studies showed that the titration curves of the hyperimmune reference serum and patient sera were parallel for both ELISA assays (data not shown). Table 1 and Fig. 1 show the antistaphylococcal IgG antibody concentrations measured in patient sera before and after treatment with SPL or with placebo. Amounts of serum antistaphylococcal IgG present prior to treatment varied widely among individual dogs. There was no significant difference in the concentration of antibody against *S. intermedius* antigens from pretreatment to posttreatment sample, by the paired *t*-test, in either the SPL-treated or placebo-treated group. In contrast, there was a small but significant increase in antibody against SPL antigens in the SPL-treated group, but not in the placebo-treated group ($p < 0.002$).

To test for an association between concentrations of antibody against *S. intermedius* antigens and antibody against SPL antigens, linear regression analysis was used. The measured concentration of antiSPL antibody in each sample was plotted against the concentration of anti-*S. intermedius* antibody in the same sample (Fig. 2). Regression analysis showed a significant association between these two antibody measurements ($p < 0.001$). The coefficient of determination (R^2) was 0.41, indicating that 41% of the

Table 1 Mean antistaphylococcal antibody in patient sera prior to and after treatment with 18 weeks of injections of either SPL or placebo

		Antibody measured (as MONA)	
Antibody against	Treatment group	Pretreatment	Posttreatment
S. intermedius antigens	Placebo	2.00 ± 2.39	1.89 ± 2.35
	SPL	1.27 ± 1.16	1.53 ± 1.40
SPL antigens	Placebo	0.87 ± 1.15	0.57 ± 0.41
	SPL	0.57 ± 0.34	0.89 ± 0.54*

Data are expressed as mean ± SD
*$p = 0.017$

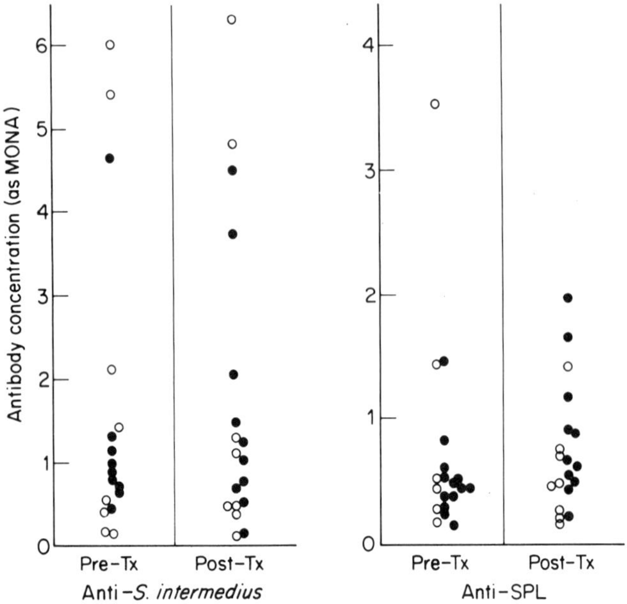

Figure 1 Antistaphylococcal antibody in individual dog sera, before and after treatment with injections of SPL or placebo.

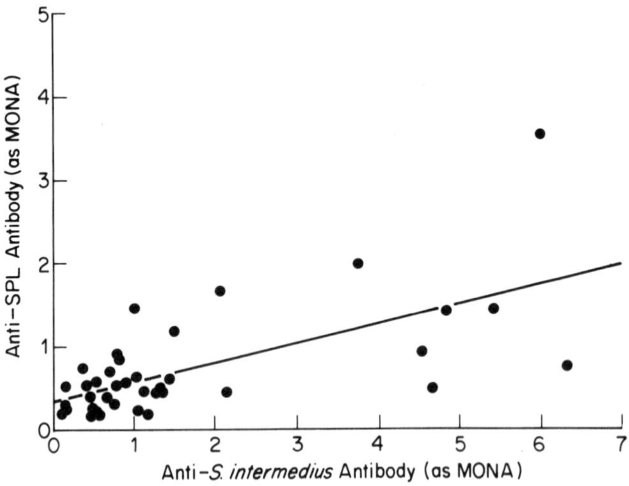

Figure 2 Correlation between concentrations of anti-SPL antibody and anti-*S. intermedius* antibody in individual serum samples. Regression analysis showed a significant association between the two parameters ($p < 0.001$, $R^2 = 0.41$).

variation in the anti-SPL antibody concentration could be attributed to variation in anti-*S. intermedius* antibody concentration. An additional point of interest on this graph was the presence of several serum samples with very high concentrations of anti-*S. intermedius* antibody, but low concentrations of anti-SPL antibody (data points in the lower right-hand region of the graph in Fig. 2).

Immunoblotting studies

Empirical inspection of the densitometer scan tracings indicated that the antibody peaks could be divided roughly into four molecular weight ranges (Fig. 3). These ranges were named Range 1, 2, 3, and 4, and corresponded to

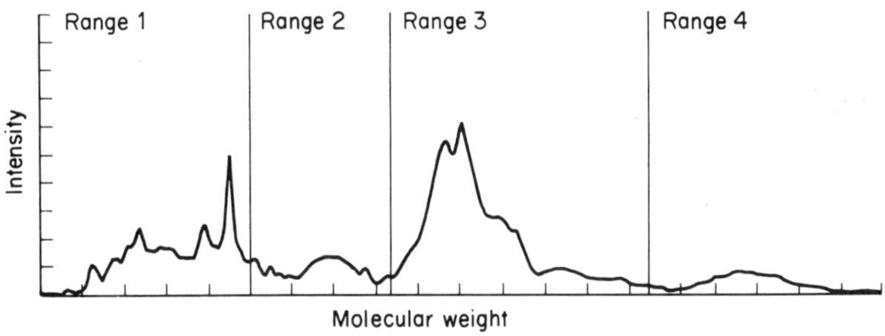

Figure 3 Typical densitometer scan tracing from an immunoblotting assay. Note that the peaks tend to occur in four major molecular weight ranges (Ranges 1–4).

molecular weight of greater than 100 000 daltons (Range 1), 60 000–100 000 daltons (Range 2), 40 000–60 000 daltons (Range 3), and less than 40 000 daltons (Range 4). Moreover, there appeared to be differences in the scan tracings between pretreatment and posttreatment samples within Range 1 and Range 2. An example of these observed differences is shown in Fig. 4.

To test for significant differences in the scan patterns, the portion of the integrated area under the scan tracing curve corresponding to each molecular weight range was calculated and expressed both in arbitrary units and as a percentage of the total area under the curve. These values were grouped according to treatment (SPL vs placebo) and time (pretreatment vs posttreatment) and mean values were calculated (Table 2). Differences between pretreatment and posttreatment samples were analysed with the paired *t*-test. In the group of dogs that received placebo injections, there were no significant differences between the pretreatment and posttreatment samples by this criterion. In the SPL-treated dogs, there was a significant increase in the area under the densitometer tracing in Range 1 and Range 2 only. In Range 2, both the absolute area and percentage of total area were significantly higher

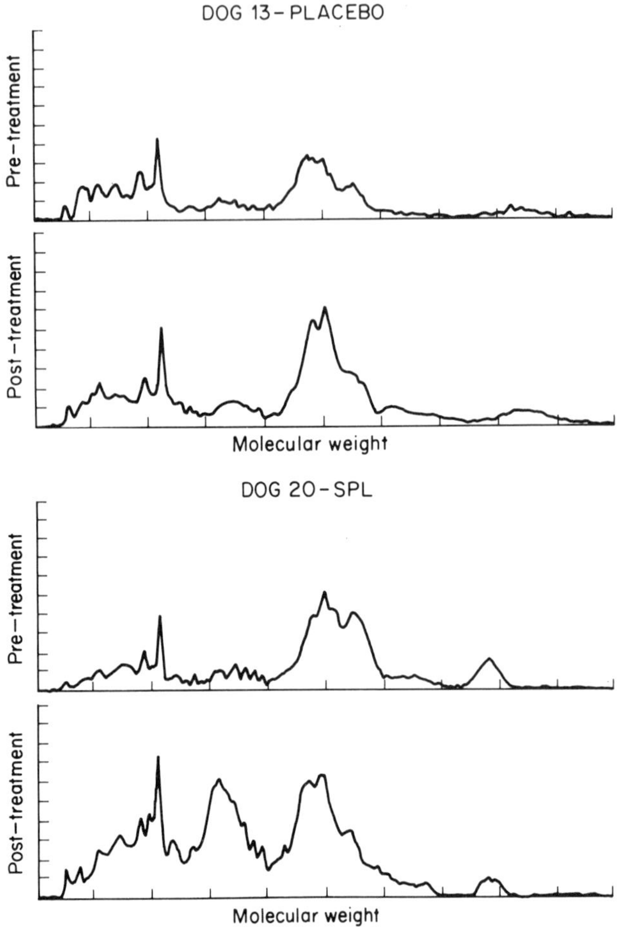

Figure 4 Typical pre- and posttreatment densitometer scan tracings from a dog treated with placebo injections (above) and from a dog treated with SPL injections (below). Note that the tracings from the placebo-treated dog change little before and after treatment; those from the SPL-treated dog appear to have higher peaks in the Range 1 and Range 2 regions.

in the posttreatment sample. Range 1 showed a significant increase in the absolute area only.

The same data set was analysed by dividing the data into placebo and treatment groups, and by dividing into groups based on good or poor response to treatment as originally defined in the clinical trial. When comparing the SPL-treated group as a whole to the placebo-treated group as a whole in the independent *t*-test, Table 2 shows that there was a significant difference in the total area under the curve (all ranges taken together), as well as in Range 2, for

Table 2 Mean integrated areas under densitometer scan tracing of immunoblots. The tracings were divided into four ranges based on molecular weight (see Fig. 3)

Treatment	Sample	Mean area under curve (in arbitrary units and % of total area)				
		Range 1	Range 2	Range 3	Range 4	All ranges
SPL	Pretreatment	12 236 (17.0%)	7 225 (10.1%)	37 981 (51.0%)	18 470 (21.9%)	75 914
(n = 8)	Posttreatment	18 495* (20.6%)	15 693** **** (17.9%)*	40 549 (43.0%)	18 070 (18.5%)	92 809***
Placebo	Pretreatment	12 697 (23.7%)	6 820 (11.2%)	33 800 (51.7%)	10 601 (13.4%)	63 920
(n = 7)	Posttreatment	16 251 (25.3%)	7 262 (10.8%)	33 117 (50.8%)	9 428 (13.1%)	66 059

* Significant difference vs pretreatment sample ($p < 0.02$) with paired t-test.
** Significant difference vs pretreatment sample ($p < 0.01$) with paired t-test.
*** Significant difference vs placebo group ($p < 0.05$) with independent t-test.
**** Significant difference vs placebo group ($p < 0.02$) with independent t-test.

the posttreatment samples. Pretreatment samples did not differ significantly between these groups, nor did posttreatment samples in other ranges. When the data was divided into groups based on treatment response (11 responders, four non-responders), significant differences in the densitometer tracings could not be demonstrated between these groups, either in the total area or in individual ranges (data not shown).

DISCUSSION

The bacterin product, SPL, is prepared by lysis from whole *Staphylococcus aureus* bacteria by polyvalent bacteriophage. As obtained from the manufacturer, it contains antigenic components of *S. aureus*, virulent bacteriophage, and medium components. It was originally recommended for use in human *S. aureus* infections (Salmon and Symonds, 1963), atopic eczema (Epinette, 1988), and hidradenitis suppurativa (Kress, 1981). SPL has several demonstrable immunomodulatory effects *in vivo* and *in vitro*. It can affect both the humoral and cellular aspects of the immune system, and its effects include both antigen-specific and non-specific phenomena. Its efficacy in a given disease has not been definitively attributed to a specific action or actions. Canine pyoderma is caused by *S. intermedius*, not *S. aureus*. Though there is likely some antigenic cross-reactivity between these two bacterial species, an *S. aureus*-based bacterin may not be ideal for treating an *S. intermedius* infection in dogs.

It has been reported that SPL augments the antibody response to specific antigen in mice (i.e. increase antigen-specific IgG) in an adjuvant-like action, as well as to non-specifically increase serum IgG (Esber *et al.*, 1985). It was therefore possible that the beneficial actions of SPL in canine pyoderma are partly a result of stimulation of the IgG antibody response against staphylococcal antigens. Our results show that repeated injection of dogs with SPL did not cause significant increases in the serum concentrations of IgG antibody directed against *S. intermedius* antigens. Treatment with SPL did result in significant increases in anti-SPL IgG from pretreatment to posttreatment sample; placebo treatment did not yield similar increases. Differences in IgG concentration, though significant, were small. An increase in anti-SPL IgG is not surprising; with repeated injections of any foreign protein substance into an immunocompetent animal, some increase in antibody against that substance would be expected. Our data suggest that, in the case of canine pyoderma, the mechanism of action of SPL is not simply augmentation of the antibody response to produce much higher titers of antistaphylococcal IgG.

The amounts of antistaphylococcal antibody present in pretreatment sera of all dogs in this study were quite variable (Fig. 1), ranging from less than one MONA to greater than six. This corresponds to a difference of more than five two-fold dilutions in the titer of the sera from weakest to strongest. Halliwell

(1987) also reported wide variation in antistaphylococcal IgG among dogs with recurrent pyoderma, and was unable to relate this variation to disease severity or clinical status of the dog. Our results are in agreement with these observations, and provide additional evidence that serum antistaphylococcal IgG concentrations are unrelated to disease state or resistance to recurrent infection.

We did find a significant association between concentrations of serum IgG antibody against SPL antigens and antibody against *S. intermedius* antigens. Antigenic cross-reactivity between other staphylococcal species, such as between *S. aureus* and *S. epidermidis*, is well documented (Espersen *et al.*, 1981). It is reasonable to presume that there is also antigenic cross-reactivity between *S. intermedius* and *S. aureus*, which would explain this result. However, several serum samples contained very little anti-SPL antibody, yet high amounts of antibody directed against *S. intermedius* antigens. This indicates the presence of antigenic differences between SPL and our *S. intermedius* antigen preparation. These differences may be inherent in the bacteria themselves, or may be related to the method of antigen preparation. If there are marked antigenic differences between *S. intermedius* and SPL, a bacterin containing the complete spectrum of *S. intermedius* antigens could be more desirable as a treatment for canine pyoderma.

Results from the immunoblotting studies showed that the increase in anti-SPL IgG in posttreatment samples was largely due to increases in IgG specific for antigens in the molecular weight range from 60 000 daltons to greater than 100 000 (Ranges 1 and 2). This finding is interesting, as the majority of the components of SPL have been reported to be less than 50 000 daltons in molecular weight by gel filtration analysis (Miyakoshi *et al.*, 1981). Our data would suggest that the majority of the antigenic activity in SPL is concentrated in a relatively small portion of its components. The many components of SPL have not been well characterized biochemically nor immunologically, though Miyakoshi *et al.* (1981) reported that the molecular weight of the mitogenic fraction is approximately 25 000 daltons.

When this immunoblotting data was grouped based solely on patient response to treatment (good response vs poor response—regardless of whether the treatment was SPL or placebo), there were no significant differences found in the densitometer tracings between the two groups. It therefore appeared that a good clinical response (i.e. lessening of recurrence of the pyoderma) was not correlated with development of increased amounts of IgG specific for SPL antigens. However, our poorly responding group was small (n = 4), and it is possible that evaluation of larger numbers of sera would yield significant differences.

We conclude that treatment of dogs with recurrent staphylococcal pyoderma with injections of SPL bacterin does not result in dramatic increases in total serum antistaphylococcal IgG. Small but significant increases in IgG specific for SPL antigens does occur with SPL treatment, and these IgG antibodies are primarily directed against SPL antigens above 60 000 daltons in mol. wt. We were unable to show that these increases in IgG concentration correlate with response to SPL treatment. Similar studies might be undertaken to characterize the antistaphylococcal IgE response in dogs with recurrent pyoderma treated with SPL, and to further define antigenic differences between *S. intermedius* and SPL.

ACKNOWLEDGEMENTS

This study was supported by grants from the American College of Dermatology/Combe, Inc. fund and the American Veterinary Medical Association Foundation. The authors thank Michael Ortengren for technical assistance.

REFERENCES

Becker, A.M., Janik, T.A., Smith, E.K., Sousa, C.A. and Peters, B.A. (1989). *Propionibacterium acnes* immunotherapy in chronic recurrent canine pyoderma. An adjunct to antibiotic therapy. *Journal of Veterinary Internal Medicine* **3**: 26–30.

DeBoer, D.J., Moriello, K.A., Thomas, C.B. and Schultz, K.T. (1990). Evaluation of a commercial staphylococcal bacterin for management of idiopathic recurrent pyoderma in dogs. *American Journal of Veterinary Research* **51**: 636–639.

Epinette, W.W. (1988). Treatment of atopic eczema with staphylococcal toxoid. *Journal of the Americal Medical Association* **259**: 2759–2760.

Esber, H.J., Ganfield, D. and Rosenkrantz, H. (1985). Staphage Lysate: an immunomodulator of the primary immune response in mice. *Immunopharmacology* **10**: 77–82.

Espersen, F., Hertz, J.B. and Hoiby, N. (1981). Cross-reactions between *Staphylococcus epidermidis* and 23 other bacterial species. *Acta Pathologica et Microbiologica Scandinavia Section B*, **89**: 253–260.

Halliwell, R.E.W. (1987). Levels of IgE and IgG antibody to staphylococcal antigens in normal dogs and in dogs with recurrent pyoderma. *Abstracts of the American Academy of Veterinary Dermatology/American College of Veterinary Dermatology Annual Meeting, Phoenix, 1987.*

Kress, D.W. (1981). A preliminary report on the use of Staphage Lysate for treatment of hidradenitis suppurativa. *Annals of Plastic Surgery* **6**: 393–395.

Laemmli, U.K. (1970). Cleavage of structural proteins during the assembly of the head of bacteriophage T4. *Nature* **227**: 608–685.

Miyakoshi, H., Aoki, T. and Mizukoshi, M. (1981). Mitogenic substances in Staphage Lysate. *Biomedical Research* **2**: 629–638.

Salmon, G.G. Jr and Symonds, M. (1963). Staphage Lysate therapy for chronic staphylococcal infections. *Journal of the Medical Society of New Jersey* **60**: 188–193.

Scott, D.W., MacDonald, J.M. and Schultz, R.D. (1978). Staphylococcal hypersensitivity in the dog. *Journal of the American Animal Hospital Association* **14**: 777–779.

Tijssen, P. (1985). *Practice and Theory of Enzyme Immunoassays*, pp. 403–406. Elsevier, Amsterdam.

5.4 The Bacteriology and Pathogenesis of Fleece Rot and Associated Myiasis; Control of these Diseases with *Pseudomonas aeruginosa* Vaccines

D.H. Burrell

CSIRO Division of Animal Health, McMaster Laboratory, New South Wales, Australia

INTRODUCTION

Flystrike currently may cost the Australian wool industry up to $\$200 \times 10^6$ annually. In the case of myiasis of the body of sheep, the prophylactic use of insecticides is the common common method for control. However, the development of resistance to insecticides has occurred and there is environmental concern about their use. An understanding of the pathogenesis of flystrike may indicate alternative methods for control.

There are essentially three schools of thought expressed in the literature as to the common mechanism for pathogenesis of body strike. Two of these purport that fleece rot is the common predisposing condition for body strike but differ in their view of the importance of bacteria in development of fleece rot (either a causal or merely a secondary role). The third school of thought purports that flystrike can occur irrespective of any predisposing condition provided there is sufficient moisture for survival of fly larvae. The authors representing these views are given in Table 1.

The role of fleece rot in predisposition to body strike has already been substantiated by extensive field observation (although not reported in detail) by Belschner (1937) and Seddon (1937) and more recently by Murray (1980), Murray and Ninnes (1980) and Murray and Wilkinson (1980) by questionnaire survey of wool growers. Sandeman *et al.* (1987) base their conclusion that

Table 1

Role of fleece rot in body strike	Role of bacteria in fleece rot	Proponent authors
Predisposition	causal	Belschner (1937) Seddon (1937) (Mackeras 1936)
Predisposition	secondary (odour, colour)	Hayman (1953) Nay and Watts (1977) Merritt and Watts (1978a,b)
Not mandatory	not relevant	Sandeman *et al.* (1987) (Mackerras 1936)

fleece rot is not mandatory for development of body strike on laboratory experimental application of fly larvae on a small number of sheep.

The proponents for a causal role by bacteria (Belschner, 1937; Seddon, 1937) based their conclusions on knowledge of the multiplication of bacteria (including *P. aeruginosa*) on the wet skin of sheep during the development of fleece rot. They assumed that a bacterial dermatitis was involved but did not report any experiments concerning active production of dermatitis in sheep with any species of bacteria isolated from fleece rot lesions.

The proponents for bacteria having only a secondary role (by way of producing colouration of the fleece or odour for attraction of the blowfly) assumed that the fleece rot lesion develops primarily as a result of the action of water on the skin. Examination for an active role by bacteria in production of the lesion was neglected. The studies of Hayman (1953), Nay and Watts (1977) and Merritt and Watts (1978a,b) culminated in the hypothesis that serious exudation preceded bacterial growth.

Mackerras (1936) has been included in Table 1 under two categories because, not only had he accepted the extensive evidence for predisposition to body strike by fleece rot, but also had shown that by artificial wetting and exposure to flies in the insectory or by placing eggs or first stage larvae on wet skin, flystrike could occur in the absence of fleece rot. He held a conservative view of the role of bacteria since an essential relationship between bacterial activity in the fleece and flystrike had not been proved to exist, nor had any evidence been obtained that particular species of bacteria were causal.

This paper summarizes progress in recent studies of the pathogenesis of fleece rot and associated flystrike. These have involved a bacteriological survey of fleece rot and flystrike lesions, characterization of organisms for virulence factors which may cause dermatitis, their use in experimental production of dermatitis and examination of the effect of vaccination (in particular with *P. aeruginosa*) on the development of fleece rot and associated body strike.

MATERIALS AND METHODS

Bacteriological survey

Bacteriological examination of fleece rot and flystrike lesions has continued from 1979 to the present. Collection of material has been accompanied by clinical examination of the lesions in order to record the extent of exudation, colouration and stage of development of the lesion. A substantial part of the survey has involved the periodic inspection of tagged sheep during the course of development of fleece rot in order to determine the relationship between fleece rot and body strike. Material from more than 1000 cases of stained wool, fleece rot wool, fleece rot lesions which had been flystruck and 59 unaffected fleece rot samples were collected from 18 different properties in New South Wales. Methods included direct swabs of affected areas when sufficiently moist or placement of clipped fleece samples in sterile swab tubes. In the latter case a suspension of bacteria was obtained by the addition of 1 ml of sterile distilled water to each tube followed by vigorous agitation with the swab stick. Skin washings were also obtained by repeatedly flushing the skin with 1 ml of distilled water from a sterile pasteur pipette within a 4 cm length of 5 mm internal diameter sterile rubber tubing.

The scheme generated for bacteriological examination of fleece rot and flystrike lesions was based essentially on the methods of Cowan (1974) and consisted of obtaining separate colonies then pure cultures of the bacteria by conventional and selective media, Gram stain and morphological examination, followed by the use of standard identification tests which were greatly facilitated by the use of API Systems (Carter Wallace Australia Pty Ltd, French's Forest, New South Wales).

Since certain species of bacteria appeared in fleece rot lesions only after flystrike had occurred, the bacteria shed by adult *L. cuprina* and larvae were examined. Wild, trapped flies and artificially reared flies (Ciba Geigy Australia Ltd), and larvae from either lesions or artificial sources were placed in petri dishes on conventional and selective media. Bacteria growing on the media were identified using the scheme described above.

Characterization of fleece rot bacteria

Isolates of *P. aeruginosa* from sheep were characterized in terms of biochemical reactions, serological typing, the production of the enzymes exotoxin A, protease, keratinase, elastase, phospholipase, lipase and deoxyribonuclease, pigment production, colony morphology and production of antibacterial substances.

In addition to the methods previously described (Burrell and MacDiarmid, 1983), isolates were screened by the technique of Elek (1948) for production of exotoxin A using sheep and rabbit antisera raised against purified toxin kindly supplied by Dr Olgerts Pavlovskis. Phospholipase C was assayed by the method of Berka *et al.* (1981) using *p*-nitrophenylphosphorylchloline. Methods for assay of alkaline phosphatase, hyaluronidase and chondroitin sulphatase have been described previously (MacDiarmid and Burrell, 1986). The antibacterial effects of *P. aeruginosa* were studied by observation and adjacent cultures of other bacteria on solid medium and the effect of addition of *P. aeruginosa* supernatant fluids to broth cultures of other fleece bacteria.

Several commonly recurring Gram-negative fleece rot bacteria were also characterized for comparison with *P. aeruginosa* isolates as potential causal organisms. These included *Pseudomonas maltophilia* (MacDiarmid and Burrell, 1986), *P. putida*, *P. stutzeri*, *P. fluorescens*, *P. cepacia*, *P. oryzihabitans*, *P. diminuta*, *Moraxella urethralis*, *Alcaligenes faecalis* and *Flavobacterium* sp. (API 20NE profile 0410004). Of the Gram-positive bacteria, *Bacillus* spp., *Staphylococcus* spp., *Micrococcus* spp. and *Corynebacterium* spp. have also been the subject of a preliminary examination for potential virulence factors.

Experimental production of dermatitis

The method for attempted experimental production of dermatitis with various fleece rot bacteria was that described previously for *P. aeruginosa* (Burrell *et al.*, 1982). In addition to *P. maltophilia*, P. stutzeri and *P. putida*, enzyme deficient biotypes of *P. aeruginosa* were also examined. The methods used for histological examination of vertical sections of skin affected by experimental and natural dermatitis have been previously described (Burrell *et al.*, 1982).

The effect of vaccination with *P. aeruginosa*

Immunization of sheep against experimental dermatitis and natural fleece rot and associated body strike has been previously described (Burrell, 1985). In a large-scale field trial of a prototype commercial vaccine (Biotechnology Australia Pty Ltd), 2548 sheep located in three different areas of New South Wales were exposed to natural fleece rot and flystrike for approximately 5 months from December 1983 to April 1984. The vaccine was prepared from *P. aeruginosa* strain 88 (Difco serotype 6) of the McMaster collection. Half of the total number of sheep were vaccinated. The development of fleece rot and flystrike was recorded during regular inspections and bacteriological examination of lesions was carried out.

RESULTS

General clinical examination of fleece rot and flystrike

Fleece rot presented clinically as an exudative dermatitis on the body of sheep which develops following wetting of the fleece by rain. Practically all cases of body strike developed in preexistent fleece rot lesions during the exudative phase. Conditions of the fleece such as mere colouration, non-palpable bands of discoloured material washed from the skin and fleece ('water stain'), and old bands of exudate which had grown outwards with the fleece did not predispose to flystrike. Exudation was almost always associated with colouration (green, yellow-brown or red-brown) or discolouration (dirty yellow-brown) of the fleece at skin level or extending the full length of the staple. In some cases there was a clean break in the wool fibres within the band of exudate.

Flystrike almost always commenced with one female *L. cuprina* laying one mass of eggs on the outer staple or near the base. Multiple masses of eggs were never observed at the initiation of strikes. In many cases of fleece rot examined daily for flystrike, flystrike arose without any eggs being previously observed, so few were the numbers of eggs required to initiate flystrike. It appeared that if a few first, then second stage larvae were able to further cause irritation of the skin (observed as a small patch of inflamed and weeping skin) for a few hours, or even survive in the fleece for a few hours, then the site suddenly became more attractive for further egg laying by other *L. cuprina*. Only after this stage were numerous and large egg masses found on the fleece. Once strikes had become established, the surrouding fleece always developed a damp and khaki coloured appearance. Second- and third-stage larvae were found in large numbers in pockets of the exudate-matted fleece as well as feeding directly on the flystrike wound.

Strike wounds tended to follow tracks of exudate down the sides of the neck, shoulder and flank. Some sheep which had developed strikes and had evaded regular, but not close, inspections by the farmers, died between weekly close inspections. Severely struck sheep, if treated, still lost condition and often suffered a complete break in the wool evident within a month of the strike occurring.

Histology

Vertical sections of skin from cases of colouration without exudation differed little from sections of normal skin. There was sometimes thickening of the cornified layer of the epidermis and the living keratinocyte layer. In sections from cases of active exudation, varying degrees of dermatitis ranging from mild to ulcerative dermatitis were observed. At later stages presumably coincident with the drying of skin and fleece after cessation of rain, areas of epidermis affected by dermatitis had formed a slough leaving small scabs made up of parakeratotic mounds and scales, and masses of polymorphonuclear cellular materials. Such scabs were also observed macroscopically.

In areas of maggot infestation the picture was that of an open wound, the areas being denuded of epidermis. Extensive polymorphonuclear cell infiltration of the dermis and necrosis of cells near the exposed surface of the dermis were observed.

Bacteriological examination of fleece rot and associated flystrike

The bacteriological composition of samples was variable between sites on the one sheep, between different sheep on the one property, between sheep from different properties, between different years on the one property, before and after flystrike, and after different management procedures such as jetting were carried out. A total of 32 Gram-negative species of bacteria were isolated from cases of normal fleece, fleece rot lesions and lesions of flystrike. The genera *Pseudomonas*, *Alcaligenes*, *Acinetobacter*, *Moraxella*, *Flavobacterium*, *Pasteurella*, *Agrobacter*, *Enterobacter*, *Providencia*, *Proteus* and *Citrobacter* were all represented. Of an additional 114 isolates of non-fermentative Gram-negative bacteria, 26 were also classified within these genera by the API Profile Recognition Program (computer search). Profiles of unidentified isolates are recorded for future corroboration. Of the 32 Gram-negative species, each was represented by several different biotypes occurring either on the same property or on different properties.

A total of 22 different Gram-positive bacteria were isolated from the fleece and skin and consisted of up to ten different species of *Staphylococcus* (the species *cohnii* and *xylosis* were recognized), two different species of *Micrococcus*, at least six different biotypes or species of *Corynebacterium* and four *Bacillus* species.

Following flystrike of fleece rot lesions, a consistent change in the bacterial population took place. *Proteus mirabilis* was always recovered from fresh flystrike lesions but rarely prior to flystrike. *Providencia stuartii* and *Providencia rettgeri* were also frequently recovered from flystrike while *Alcaligenes faecalis*, although most commonly recovered from flystrike lesions, was occasionally recovered from fleeces not flystruck.

Flies and larvae of *L. cuprina* were confirmed as a source of these species when the latter were isolated from wild and artificially reared flies. The transition from fly to egg, first, second and third stage larvae, pupa and fly was completed within the petri dish upon a lawn of mixed bacterial culture which had originated from the fly. A *Bacillus* sp. and a *Microccus* sp. were also isolated from the fly.

The data obtained for frequency of isolation of the various bacterial species from fleece rot lesions and sequential changes in the populations of bacteria during development of fleece rot is complex in that within a particular flock of sheep, the outcome was highly depdendent upon the virulence of the indigenous biotypes of *P. aeruginosa* (see below under Characterization. Multiplication of both Gram-positive and Gram-negative bacteria followed wetting of the fleece. In early stages of wetting, *Bacillus cereus* was frequently prominent but within 48–72 h had generally disappeared. Continued multiplication of *Staphylococcus* spp. and *Micrococcus* spp. occurred in the absence of *P. aeruginosa*. *Corynebacterium* spp. appeared unaffected by *P. aeruginosa* and usually were the most numerous species. Depending on the predominance of particular species, horse blood agar plates sewn from fleece rot lesion material could be classified into six different categories on gross appearance:

1. Plates sewn from coloured fleece rot were usually predominant in *P. aeruginosa* colonies, darkly coloured and produced the perfume-like odour characteristic of *P. aeruginosa*. In cases of yellow fleece rot the numbers of colonies of *P. aeruginosa* were relatively fewer.
2. Plates obviously bearing *B. cereus* (characteristically grey-green dull, rapidly spreading colonies extending for up to 1 cm from the edge of heavily sewn material and streaks).
3. Plates with a preponderance of darkly coloured colonies but *P. aeruginosa* and *B. cereus* not evident. The appearance of these plates was due to the large numbers of *P. maltophilia* commonly isolated from cases of yellow fleece rot.
4. Plates with *Pseudomonas stutzeri* or crinkly CDC group VE colony types predominant. The white or cream colour of culture was also due to the prevalence of *Staphylococcus*, *Micrococcus* and *Corynebacterium* spp.
5. Plates with mostly white or cream coloured culture were predominantly *Staphylococcus*, *Micrococcus* and *Corynebacterium* spp. with smaller numbers of crinkly pseudomonads or CDC types. Very few of the darkly coloured pseudomonads such as *P. maltophilia* were present although other non-coloured species such as *Pseudomonas diminuta* could be present in large numbers.
6. Plates with mostly pink colonies of *Moraxella urethalis*. Generally observed only after flystrike, a seventh category consisted of plates containing any of the above species but completely overgrown by swarming culture of *P. mirabilis*. In general, the occurrence of all Gram-positive genera other than *Bacillus* was consistent throughout the six fleece rot categories listed above whereas the populations of the Gram-negative bacteria were variable and formed the basis of the categorization.

Of the above categories, only 1 and 2 were associated with predisposition to flystrike, that is, fleece rot lesions predominant in either *P. aeruginosa* or *P. maltophilia*. These organisms were associated with relatively severe degrees of exudation.

Characterization of fleece rot bacteria

Ovine isolates of *P. aeruginosa* were capable of rapid growth on minimal nutrient media and produced the enzymes exotoxin A, proteases (three including elastase), phospholipase, lipase and DNAse, and the pigment pyocyanin, with some variation in quantities according to different biotypes. Evidence for production of antibacterial substances was obtained for most isolates when supernatants were used in combination with culture of other species (Table 2). The isolates of *P. aeruginosa* shown in Table 2 originated from different flocks of sheep. Coloured fleece rot was prominent in the flock where isolate 106 was indigenous whereas yellow fleece rot was prominent in the flock where isolate 117 was indigenous. On solid media, the only species conspicuously affected by adjacent growth of most isolates of *P. aeruginosa* was *B. cereus*.

Table 2 *In vitro* growth inhibitory effect of *Pseudomonas aeruginosa* in organisms isolated from field fleece rot lesions

P. aeruginosa isolate %	*P. malto-philia* %	*P. putida* %	*P. stutzeri* %	*Alcaligenes* faecalis %	*P. fluorescens* %
106	100[a]	59	59	66	86
117	12	31	31	33	71
38	75	71	33	29	71
39	50	0	0	0	29

[a] Percentage reduction in opacity (as measured by Wellcome opacity tubes) compared to control cultures.

Of the other Gram-negative species examined, only *P. maltophilia* exhibited a similar enzyme profile (excluding exotoxin A). No evidence for the production of antibacterial substances by this organism was obtained. It required more complex media for growth than *P. aeruginosa* and culture for 72 h was necessary in order to achieve a culture mass equivalent to 24 h growth of *P. aeruginosa*. A *Flavobacterium* sp. was the only other Gram-negative species found to be elastolytic.

Gram-positive organisms such as *B. cereus* and *Staphylococcus* spp. produced proteases and phospholipases; *S. cohnii*, the *Micrococcus* spp. and two *Corynebacterium* spp. were particularly productive of lipases. All of the *Corynebacterium* spp. produced phospholipases.

Experimental production of dermatitis

A subacute dermatitis featuring parakeratosis and formation of micro-abscesses could be produced with ovine isolates of *P. aeruginosa* but not with biotypes deficient in the enzymes protease, elastase and DNAse. These biotypes were capable of producing phospholipase and exotoxin A.

Of the other Gram-negative species so far examined, namely *P. maltophilia*, *P. putida* and *P. stutzeri*, only *P. maltophilia* was capable of producing dermatitis. The use of such other pseudomonads in experimental infection was occasionally complicated by the adventitious appearance of *P. aeruginosa* at experimental infection sites.

The effect of vaccination with *P. aeruginosa*

The results of a field trial using a monovalent vaccine are summarized in Fig. 1. Significant levels of protection ($p < 0.05$) against flystrike of the body of

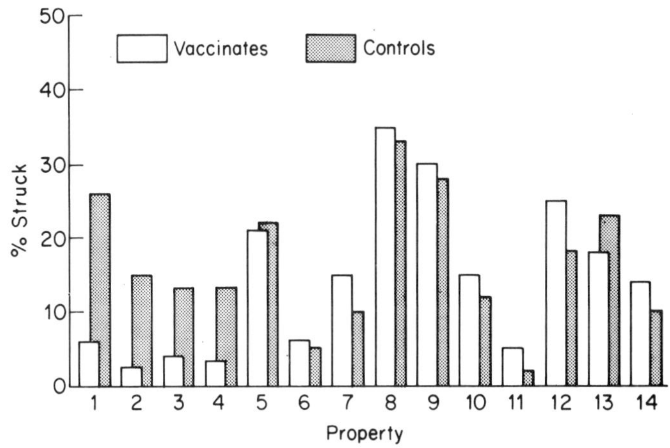

Figure 1 Field trial of *P. aeruginosa* vaccine against natural body strike.

sheep were obtained where the homologous serotype of *P. aeruginosa* was indigenous (properties 1–4) while no protection was evident where heterologous challenge occurred (properties 5–14). The sheep on property 11 were accidentally jetted with Vetrazin® (Ciba Geigy Pty Ltd) before fly activity had commenced. The prevalence of body strike in this flock was comparable to that in vaccinated sheep under homologous challenge.

Three vaccinates and three control sheep from flock 13 were challenged by experimental induction of dermatitis. There was no evidence for protection against challenge with the homologous strain 88 in the vaccinated sheep.

DISCUSSION

The diseases fleece rot and associated myiasis on the body of sheep represent a remarkable complex of interactions between bacteria, between bacteria and the sheep, and between the bacteria/sheep complex and a potentially lethal ectoparasite *Lucilia cuprina*. It would appear that a particular dermatitic bacterial species must first achieve a pathogenic biomass in competition with many other bacterial species before producing an exudative dermatitis and simultaneously liberating odours preferentially attractive to *L. cuprina*, the primary sheep blowfly in Australia.

Pseudomonas aeruginosa possesses characteristics which would permit such a causal role. The ability to grow rapidly under conditions of minimal nutrition, to produce factors inhibitory for the growth of other species of bacteria, to produce a variety of toxins or enzymes with known dermal-necrotizing activity and to produce odours attractive to *L. cuprina* (the latter demonstrated by Merritt and Watts (1978a) and Emmens and Murray (1982,

1983) all support the potential for a causal role by *P. aeruginosa* over and above other bacterial species present. A consideration of the action of *P. aeruginosa* exoproducts in relation to the structure of sheep skin as described by Lloyd *et al.* (1979) has been presented elsewhere (Burrell, 1988). *Pseudomonas maltophilia* possessed an enzyme profile similar to that of *P. aeruginosa* but exhibited slower growth and an apparent lack of any comparable bacterial inhibitor. Any ability to produce comparably attractive odours awaits examination. The Gram-positive organisms isolated from fleece rot which were capable of producing lipases and phospholipases may contribute to pathogenesis and deserve further study.

Previous production of experimental dermatitis with *P. aeruginosa* (Burrell *et al.*, 1982) and presently with *P. maltophilia* and the association of these species with exudative dermatitis occurring in fleece rot provides further incrimination of these organisms. The failure of protease deficient biotypes of *P. aeruginosa* to produce experimental subacute dermatitis suggests that these enzymes may be of particular importance in pathogenesis. The failure of wetting alone, in the presence of a bacteriostatic compound, to induce a comparable dermatitis (Burrell *et al.*, 1982) also suggests that activity by bacteria may be required for development of an exudative dermatitis.

That fleece rot and myiasis on the body of sheep are indeed associated (Seddon, 1931; Seddon, 1937; Belschner, 1937) was confirmed in the present field survey. Fleece rot was clearly the major predisposing factor for body strike under natural conditions. While artificial strikes can be produced readily in the absence of fleece rot (Mackerras, 1936; Sandeman *et al.*, 1987), the extrapolation that preexistent fleece rot is not mandatory for natural flystrike on the body of sheep by Sandeman *et al.* (1987) is supported neither by the early surveys of Seddon (1931, 1937) nor the present study.

A role for fly-borne bacteria in the pathogenesis of flystrike of the body of sheep has not previously been described. Following oviposition in the fleece rot lesion, the newly hatched larvae appeared to have been sustained by the preexistent exudate until development to the second and third stages which have abrasive mouthparts. Coincident with the development of the larvae, several bacterial species were apparently contributed to the lesion by the larvae or the fly itself. The most prominent of these were *Proteus mirabilis*, *Providencia* spp. and *Alcaligenes faecalis*. *P. mirabilis* in particular overgrew the original bacterial population and this appeared to have dramatically potentiated the odour attraction of other *L. cuprina* thus resulting in a rapid increase in the number of larvae in the strike wound. A synergistic attraction *in vitro*, for oviposition by *L. cuprina*, between *P. aeruginosa* and *P. mirabilis* has been observed previously by Emmens and Murray (1983). According to Erdmann (1987) *P. mirabilis* is an endosymbiont of screwworms and several blowfly species. *P. mirabilis* may inhibit potential larval pathogens and serve as a food for the larvae.

Protection obtained against *P. aeruginosa* experimental dermatitis, natural fleece rot dermatitis and associated flystrike of the body by immunization with

P. aeruginosa provides confirmation of the causal role suggested for this organism in fleece rot; also that bacteria (in particular *P. aeruginosa*) are an essential component in the development of exudative dermatitis that constitutes fleece rot; also that fleece rot is a major predisposing factor to body strike. According to these results, fleece rot could be considered essentially as a bacterial dermatitis such as proposed originally by Seddon (1931) and Belschner (1937).

The close dependence of myiasis of the body of sheep upon preexistent fleece rot means that the two dermatoses can be controlled by the one vaccine, namely a bacterial vaccine based on the causal organisms of fleece rot. So far it appears that *P. aeruginosa* is the most important causal organism of fleece rot with regard to predisposition to flystrike of the body of sheep.

An outstanding feature of the field vaccine trial results was that protection was achieved in every flock where the resident serotype of *P. aeruginosa* was homologous with the vaccine strain.

Pseudomonas maltophilia was often recovered from fleece rot lesions in company with *P. aeruginosa* in these flocks. Since the *P. aeruginosa* vaccine was effective it may be concluded that *P. maltophilia* was not an essential component in the development of fleece rot and predisposition to flystrike. Whether other organisms may cause milder types of fleece rot which are not predisposing to flystrike is the subject of continuing field studies.

The prototype commercial vaccine used in the field trial failed to protect sheep against experimental dermatitis and has been shown (results in preparation) to have lacked the antigens responsible for such protection previously obtained against homologous and heterologus experimental and field challenge (Burrell, 1985). Whereas the latter vaccines afforded heterologous protection by antibody-mediated neutralization of dermal necrotoxins (results in preparation), the protection dependent on homology of serotype exhibited in the present trial suggests that only bacteriostatic or bactericidal mechanisms of protection were in operation.

ACKNOWLEDGEMENTS

Gratitude is expressed to the Australian Wool Corporation for continuing support of these studies.

REFERENCES

Belschner, H.G. (1937). In Studies of the sheep blowfly problem. II. Observations on fleece rot and body strike in sheep, particularly in regard to their incidence, type of sheep susceptible and economic importance. *Scientific Bulletin of the Department of Agriculture, New South Wales* **54**: 61-87.

Berka, R.M., Gray, G.L. and Vasil, M.L. (1981). Studies of phospholipase C (heat-labile haemolysin) in *Pseudomonas aeruginosa. Infect. Immun.*, **34**: 1071-1074.

Burrell, D.H. (1979). *Annual Report* - McMaster Laboratory, Division of Animal Health, CSIRO. pp. 29-30.
Burrell, D.H. (1988). *Bacteriology and pathogenesis of fleecerot and flystrike. Sheep health and production.* The T.G. Hungerford Refresher Course for veterinarians. 110th proceedings. University of Sydney. pp. 231-246.
Burrell, D.H. and McDiarmid, J.A. (1983). The role of *Pseudomonas aeruginosa* in pathogenesis of fleece-rot and indirect control of body strike by immunisation. Sheep blowfly and flystrike in sheep. Proc. 2nd Nat. Symp., University of New South Wales, Australia. pp. 283-291.
Burrell, D.H., Merritt, G.C., Watts, J.E. and Walker, K.H. (1982). Experimental production of dermatitis in sheep with *Pseudomonas aeruginosa. Australian Veterinary Journal* **59**: 140-144.
Cowan, S.T. (1974). *Cowan and Steel's Manual for the Identification of Medical Bacteria.* 2nd ed. Cambridge University Press, Cambridge.
Elek, S.D. (1948). The recognition of toxigenic bacterial strains *in vitro. British Medical Journal* **1**: 493.
Emmens, R.L. and Murray, M.D. (1982). The role of bacterial odours in oviposition by *Lucilia cuprina* (Wiedemann) (Diptera: Calliphoridae), the Australian sheep blowfly. *Bulletin of Entomological Research* **72**: 367-375.
Emmens, R.L. and Murray, M.D. (1983). Bacterial odours as oviposition stimulants for *Lucilia cuprina* (Wiedemann) (Diptera: Calliphoridae), the Australian sheep blowfly. *Bulletin of Entomological Research* **73**: 411-415.
Haymann, R.H. (1953). Studies of fleece-rot of sheep. *Australian Agricultural Research* **4**: 430-468.
Lloyd, D.H., Amakiri, S.F. and McEwan Jenkinson, D. (1979). Structure of the sheep epidermis. *Res. Vet. Science.* **26**: 180-182.
MacDiarmid, J.A. and Burrell, D.H. (1986). Characterisation of *Pseudomonas maltophilia* isolates from fleece rot. *Appl. Environ. Microbiol.* **51**: 346-348.
Mackerras, I.M. (1936). In *The Sheep Blowfly Problem in Australia. Pamp. Counc. Scient. Ind. Res. Aust.* No. 66, pp. 1-39.
Merritt, G.C. and Watts, J.E. (1978a). An *in vitro* technique for studying fleece-rot and fly strike in sheep. *Australian Veterinary Journal* **54**: 513-516.
Merritt, G.C. and Watts, J.E. (1978b). Changes in protein concentration and bacteria of fleece and skin during the development of fleece-rot and body strike in sheep. *Australian Veterinary Journal* **54**: 517-520.
Murray, M.D. (1980). Blowfly Strike of sheep in southern Australia. 3. Victoria. *Agricultural Record* **7**: 54-58.
Murray, M.D. and Ninnes, B.A. (1980). Blowfly strike of sheep in southern Australia. 1. Kangaroo Island, South Australia. *Agricultural Record* **7**: 44-49.
Murray, M.D. and Wilkinson, F.C. (1980). Blowfly strike of sheep in southern Australia. 2. Western Australia. *Agricultural Record* **7**: 50-53.
Nay, T. and Watts, J.E. (1977). Observations on the wool follicle abnormalities in Merino Sheep exposed to prolonged wetting conducive to the development of fleece-rot. *Australian Journal of Agricultural Research* **28**: 1095-1105.
Sandeman, R.M., Collins, B.J. and Carnegie, P.R. (1987). A scanning electron microscope study of *L. cuprina* larvae and the development of blowfly strike in sheep. *International Journal of Parasitology* **17**: 759-765.
Seddon, H.R. (1931). Conditions which predispose sheep to blowfly attack. *Agricultural Gazette, New South Wales* **42**: 581-594.
Seddon, H.R. (1937). In studies on the sheep blowfly problem. III. Bacterial colouration of wool. *Scientific Bulletin of the Department of Agriculture, New South Wales* **54**: 96-110.

5.5 New Approaches to Footrot Vaccination and Diagnosis Utilizing the Proteases of *Bacteroides nodosus*

D.J. Stewart,[1] A.A. Kortt[2] and G.G. Lilley[2]

[1]*CSIRO Divisions of Animal Health and* [2]*Biotechnology, Parkville, Victoria 3, Australia*

INTRODUCTION

Ovine footrot is a contagious, chronic, bacterial infection causing inflammation of the epidermal tissues of the hoof which is characterized by separation of the horn of the hoof progressing from an initial interdigital dermatitis. The essential causative agent of ovine footrot infection is the anaerobic Gram-negative bacterium *Bacteroides nodosus* (Beveridge, 1941). The disease is of considerable economic significance throughout the temperature areas of the world where sheep are raised. In Australia alone the estimated losses due to footrot amount to millions of dollars annually in terms of decreased productivity and labour intensive treatment.

Classification of strains of *B. nodosus* into serogroups and subgroups (Claxton *et al.*, 1983) is based on pili or fimbriae which induce a high level of protection in vaccinated sheep against homologous serogroups of *B. nodosus* (Stewart 1978; Every and Skerman, 1982; Stewart *et al.*, 1982b, 1983a,c, 1986a). The current commercial vaccines contain killed whole cells of 8–10 well piliated strains representative of all the known serogroups (Claxton *et al.*, 1983). These vaccines are more expensive than other vaccines used in sheep due to the need for the incorporation of a multiple number of strains in the vaccine, the fastidious growth requirements and relatively sparse growth of *B. nodosus* in liquid media. Pilus expression tends to be variable in *B. nodosus* and, especially with some strains, the irreversible loss of pili from cells following subculture in liquid medium is a major problem to manufacturers. A collaborative research program at CSIRO (Divisions of Animal Health and Biotechnology) and the University of Sydney in conjunction with Arthur

Webster Pty Ltd and Biotechnology Australia Pty Ltd has been undertaken to develop a genetically engineered *B. nodosus* pili vaccine. This followed expression in *Pseudomonas aeruginosa* of pili from a prototype strain of *B. nodosus* (Elleman *et al.*, 1986; Mattick *et al.*, 1987) and successful vaccination experiments with a monovalent recombinant pili vaccine (Egerton *et al.*, 1987; Stewart and Elleman, 1987). However, a commercial recombinant DNA produced pili vaccine still needs to be multivalent since pili induce only serogroup specific immunity.

Although homologous protection is superior to that obtained against heterologous strains, nevertheless some cross-protection against heterologous serogroups has been obtained with whole cell vaccines (Thorley and Egerton, 1981; Stewart *et al.*, 1983a, 1985, 1986a,b). The identification of the nature and location of the cross-protective antigens shared by strains from different serogroups may facilitate the rational selection of a reduced number of vaccine serotypes based on the presence of serogroup-specific pilus antigens and cross-protective non-pilus antigens. Alternatively vaccination of sheep with cross-protective antigens may enable a high level of protection to be induced against a wide range of serogroups.

Bacteroides nodosus elaborates extracellular proteases which are used in diagnostic tests to differentiate virulent and benign strains of the organism. Polyacrylamide gel electrophoresis (PAGE) of *B. nodosus* culture supernatants has shown the presence of a mixture of protease isoenzymes which can be separated into four to five unique bands (Every, 1982; Kortt *et al.*, 1982) on the basis of differences in ionic charges present, on 5–7% polyacrylamide gels using the non-dissociating buffer system of Davis (1964). The proteases are detected by their activity using the zymogram technique (Every, 1982; Kortt *et al.*, 1983).

The protease isoenzyme patterns can be differentiated from those produced by benign strains (Every, 1982; Stewart *et al.*, 1982a, 1983b, 1986c; Kortt *et al.*, 1983; Stewart 1983; Gordon *et al.*, 1985). The disadvantage of this test is that it does not discriminate between virulent strains and strains of intermediate virulence (Stewart *et al.*, 1986c). The elastase test (Stewart, 1979) is a reasonably reliable method for differentiating the more virulent strains from benign and can differentiate at least some strains of intermediate virulence. However, this test is slow, requiring a minimum of 28 days to obtain a result.

The purification and properties of the extracellular protease isoenzymes have been described previously (Kortt *et al.*, 1982, 1986). These serine protease isoenzymes of *B. nodosus* are promising candidates as cross-protective antigens since they have been shown to provide protection against a number of different heterologous strains (Stewart *et al.*, 1986b). The results indicate that the development of a vaccine for ovine footrot based on the extracellular proteases of *B. nodosus* as the sole protective antigen or in combination with selected pili antigens may overcome some of the difficulties associated with the production of multivalent pili vaccines.

Recently a new protease, which had not been previously recognized in the cultures of *B. nodosus*, was isolated and purified to homogeneity.

The similarities and differences for the novel protease and the protease isoenzymes are shown in Table 1. The novel protease and the protease isoenzymes do not show any preference for cleavage at specific amino acid residues and may, therefore, be described as non-specific proteases.

Table 1 Properties of *B. nodosus* extracellular proteases

Novel protease		Protease isoenzymes
Apparent M_r	37 000	40 000–42 000
Serine protease	+	+
pI	≈ 9.0	4.9–6.0
Calcium for stability	+	+
Specificity	Non-specific	Non-specific
Virulent strains	+	+
Benign strains	+	+

The proteases are completely inhibited by phenylmethylsulphonyl fluoride (PMSF) and they are also inhibited by the metal ion chelator EDTA indicating that they are serine proteases which also require a divalent ion such as calcium for activity. The novel protease has been isolated from *B. nodosus* cultures of virulent strains 198 (serogroup A), 234 (B), 265 (H) and intermediate strain 332 (I); however, this novel protease was not found in *B. nodosus* cultures of benign strain 305 (C). Furthermore, ELISA and agar gel immunodiffusion demonstrated that the novel protease of *B. nodosus* is serologically distinct from the protease isoenzymes and like the latter possesses common antigenic determinants shared by strains from the different serogroups.

This paper describes the results obtained with this novel protease as a vaccine for inducing both protection and cure in sheep against footrot and as a diagnostic test for discriminating virulent from benign footrot.

MATERIALS AND METHODS

Vaccine efficacy experiment

Vaccine groups

1. Strain 183 (serogroup B2) recombinant pili
2. Strain 198 (serogroup A1) native novel protease
3. Strain 198 (serogroup A1) broth grown recombinant novel protease
4. Strain 198 (serogroup A1) agar grown recombinant novel protease
5. Strain 198 (serogroup A1) modified native novel protease
6. Unvaccinated controls

Experimental design and assessment of lesions

The experiment was conducted on irrigated pasture at the CSIRO Werribee Field Station utilizing flood irrigation to provide sufficient moisture for pasture growth and continuous transmission of footrot. Merino sheep were ranked on body weight and randomly distributed to groups of 12. Four donors infected with pure cultures of *B. nodosus* strain 334 (serogroup B2) by the method of Egerton and Roberts (1971) were introduced into the experimental flock at the time of the first vaccination. The feet of all sheep were inspected at 0, 33 and 53 days after the first vaccination and the lesions were evaluated by the scoring system of Stewart *et al.* (1983c),

Vaccine preparation

The native novel protease was purified from *B. nodosus* strain 198 (serogroup A1) grown in trypticase-arginine-serine (TAS) broth and was heterologous to the challenge strain (334, B2).

Strain 183 recombinant pili, prepared from *P. aeruginosa* harbouring a plasmid containing the pilin gene of *B. nodosus* strain 183 and controlled by a strong prokaryotic promoter, was provided by Dr T.C. Elleman.

For the broth grown recombinant novel protease one litre of Luria Bertani (LB) broth plus ampicillin innoculated with *Escherichia coli* containing the plasmid pPR322 with a cloned gene insert, was grown for about 20 h at which time the culture supernatant contained proteolytic activity. The *E. coli* cells were removed by centrifugation at 10 000 × ***g*** for 60 min and the supernatant concentrated on an ultrafiltration cell (Amicon). The concentrated supernatant was frozen and following thawing was clarified by a further centrifugation.

For the agar grown recombinant novel protease 100 LB agar plates containing 100 μg/ml ampicillin and 10% skim milk powder were innoculated to give confluent growth using *E. coli* containing pBR322 with the cloned insert. The plates were harvested after 24 h at 37°C when clearing of the skim milk by protease was complete. The protease was extracted from the agar by high speed centrifugation at 23 000 × ***g*** for 60 min and clarified by additional centrifugation. The supernatant was then concentrated on an ultrafiltration cell. The concentrated supernatant was frozen and following thawing clarified by a further centrifugation.

The protein content of the recombinant pili was estimated by SDS-PAGE. Amount of novel protease in the respective vaccines was estimated by a sandwich ELISA (Fahey *et al.*, 1983). Purified strain 198 novel protease was used as a standard. The amount of protein in the native novel protease vaccines was also estimated by absorbance at 280 nm. The aqueous phase of the vaccines mixed with an equal volume of Alhydrogel and tween 80 (1% of final vaccine volume) was emulsified with incomplete Freund's adjuvant (Difco) in the ratio 1:2.

Vaccination

The sheep received two doses of 2 ml subcutaneously on opposite sides of the neck. The second dose of vaccine was administered to the appropriate group 33 days after the first.

Serology

Sheep were bled at the first and second vaccination and 20 days after the second (53 days after the first). An ELISA (Fahey *et al.*, 1983; Emery *et al.*, 1984) and a microtitre plate agglutination test were used to assess antinovel protease and pilus agglutinating antibody titres respectively.

Diagnosis

Detection of novel protease antigen

A sandwich ELISA (Fahey *et al.*, 1983) incorporating a monoclonal antibody was used to detect novel protease in either *B. nodosus* broth cultures or in swabs containing exudate from footrot lesions. The swabs were taken on two separate occasions (34 and 42 days) in a pen experiment from *B. nodosus* lesions in groups of sheep which had been challenged separately with different isolates of *B. nodosus* representative of virulent, intermediate and benign strains. The amount of mouse Ig binding to the novel protease was then detected using horse radish peroxidase conjugated sheep antimouse Ig antiserum and the addition of substrate (5-aminosalicylic acid/H_2O_2). After incubation for 1-2 h the optical density of each well was read on an ELISA autoreader spectrophotometer at a wavelength of 450 nm.

Detection of antinovel protease antibody

An ELISA (Fahey *et al.* 1983; Emery *et al.*, 1984) was used to determine the serum antinovel protease responses in unvaccinated sheep infected with virulent, intermediate and benign strains of *B. nodosus*.

RESULTS

Vaccination experiment

Vaccine efficacy

When inspected 53 days after initiation of natural challenge and vaccination the native and recombinant novel protease vaccines induced substantial heterologous protection against all categories of footrot lesions and this was most marked against lesions of severe footrot (Fig. 1). Of the novel protease vaccines the modified native protease vaccine induced the highest level of protection which was comparable to that induced by the homologous recombinant pili vaccine.

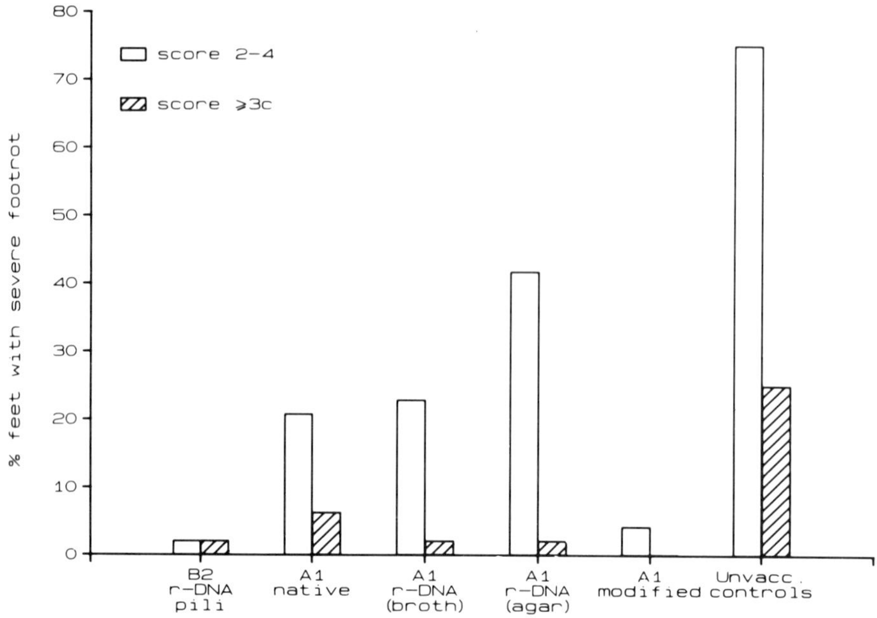

Figure 1 Percentage of feet affected with all categories of footrot (lesion score ≥ 2) or severe footrot (scores ≥ 3c) in groups of sheep immunized with either homologous pili or various heterologous novel protease vaccines and challenged from the time of the first vaccination.

Serology

Pilus agglutinating antibody titres

The mean titres of the groups of sheep vaccinated with the native and recombinant novel protease vaccines after the second dose (≤48) were similar to the unvaccinated controls (≤85). By comparison the mean titres of the group immunized with the recombinant pili vaccine after the first and second doses were 5702 and 28 735 respectively.

Mean ELISA antibody titres

After the first and second doses the mean titres of the group vaccinated with modified native novel protease were substantially higher than those vaccinated with unmodified native or recombinant novel protease vaccines (Fig. 2). As expected there was no antiprotease response following vaccination with recombinant pili.

For the agar grown recombinant novel protease vaccine after the first dose there was a smaller antibody response in comparison to the broth grown recombinant and unmodified native protease vaccines. After the second dose this difference was no longer evident.

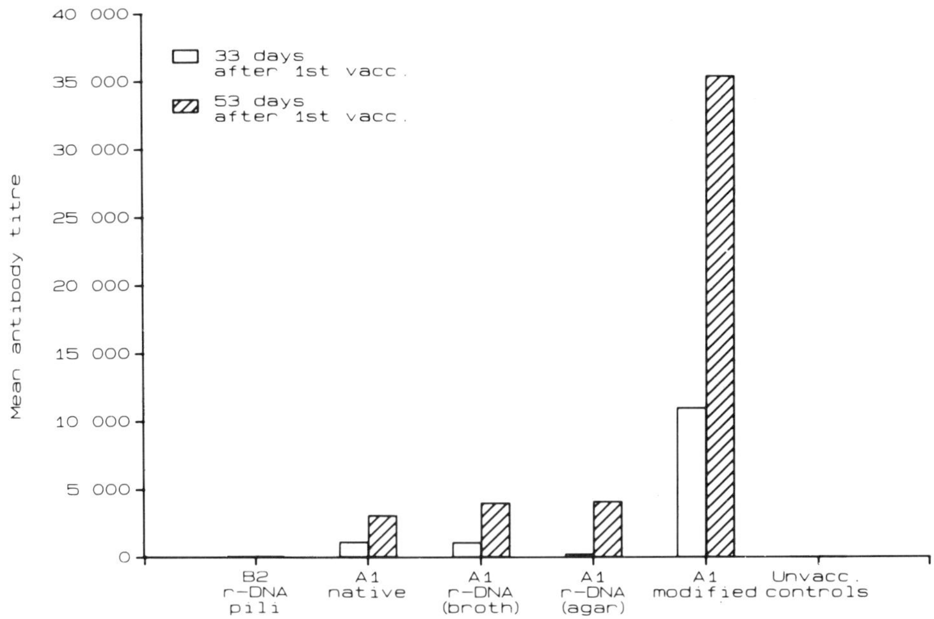

Figure 2 Mean ELISA antibody titres to the *B. nodosus* novel protease in groups of vaccinated sheep.

Diagnosis

Detection of novel protease antigen

Broth cultures of virulent and intermediate strains contained much more novel protease as detected by ELISA than benign strains (Table 2). In all, 23 of the 24 swabs of exudate from lesions of virulent and intermediate footrot contained substantial amounts of novel protease in contrast to the negligible quantity in the swabs from the benign footrot lesion.

Table 2 An ELISA for detecting the novel protease in *B. nodosus* broth cultures

Strain	Serogroup	Virulence	ELISA titre	ELISA titre per 10^8 cells
1	G1	Virulent	100	125
2	A1	Benign	6	5
3	A1	Virulent	260	217
4	B1	Benign	5	6
5	B1	Benign	<5	<5
6	G1	Virulent	100	100
7	C2	Benign	8	10

Detection of antinovel protease serum antibody

The two most virulent strains induced a substantially greater antibody response than any of the other strains and this was evident 39–42 days after challenge. Seven out of eight sheep (titre range 65–650) and eight out of eight sheep (titre range 78–1650) in each of the groups challenged with the two virulent strains developed a marked increase in antibody titre after challenge when compared to preinfection antibody levels.

By contrast, only two sheep in each group of eight challenged with the three intermediate strains developed antibody titres greater than 50 (titres 83 and 93, 50 and 475, 104 and 275 respectively). None of the sheep challenged with the benign strain developed titres above 40 with six out of eight sheep having titres <25. Thus the ELISA serum antibody test using the novel protease of *B. nodosus* may be useful for screening flocks for the presence of virulent footrot.

DISCUSSION

In two previous field experiments the novel protease vaccine induced marked curative and protective effects against natural challenge with heterologous serogroups of *B. nodosus* (unpublished). Furthermore protection and cure were similar in groups vaccinated with either homologous or heterologous novel protease indicating the presence of a common protective epitope. These experiments also demonstrated that monovalent pili vaccines performed better than protease vaccines when the challenge is homologous. By comparison, a heterologous pili vaccine was ineffective in marked contrast to the results obtained with a heterologous novel protease vaccine.

The results of the most recent vaccination trial with the novel protease of *B. nodosus* have been most encouraging in that they establish, for the first time, that a heterologous modified native novel protease vaccine can be as effective as an homologous monovalent pili vaccine. Furthermore the mean antiprotease antibody titre of the group of sheep vaccinated with the former was 10-fold higher than that induced by the unmodified native novel protease vaccine. This level of protection and antibody response demonstrates the feasibility of developing a single antigen, cross-protective vaccine for ovine footrot. Protection and ELISA antibody titres induced by recombinant DNA produced novel protease in *E. coli* were comparable to unmodified native protease. Because of the relatively low yield of *B. nodosus* proteases obtained conventionally and to enable development of a commercial vaccine it is proposed to achieve high level expression of the gene for novel protease in a suitable alternative host. The recombinant product will then require modification prior to testing for vaccine efficacy in comparison with *B. nodosus* modified native novel protease.

Our research has also demonstrated the great value of monoclonal antibodies for a rapid diagnostic test for footrot. Conventional diagnostic tests require the culture of *B. nodosus* which can take several weeks before a result can be obtained. Using lesion material from footrot and a monoclonal antibody to the novel protease, virulent and intermediate strains can be discriminated from benign strains, without resorting to culture, within a few hours of obtaining the sample from the field. The novel protease has also been found to be useful in an immunoassay for detecting antibodies in sheep serum resulting from infection of sheeps' feet with virulent *B. nodosus*. Thus the novel protease has considerable potential not only as a vaccine against ovine footrot but also as the basis of a rapid diagnostic test since it is produced by virulent and intermediate but not benign strains. The availability of rapid and definitive tests for differentiating virulent, intermediate and benign strains of *B. nodosus* will greatly assist eradication of footrot, particularly in areas of Australia where regional strategic control programmes have been introduced.

REFERENCES

Beveridge, W.I.B. (1941). Foot-rot in sheep: a transmissible disease due to infection with *Fusiformis nodosus* (n.sp.). *Bulletin No. 140* Council for Scientific and Industrial Research (Australia).

Claxton, P.D., Ribeiro, L.A. and Egerton, J.R. (1983). Classification of *Bacteroides nodosus* by agglutination tests. *Australian Veterinary Journal* **60**: 331-334.

Davis, B.J. (1964). Disc electrophoresis-II. Method and application to human serum proteins. *Annals of the New York Academy of Sciences* **121** (Art.2): 404-427.

Egerton, J.R. and Roberts, D.S. (1971). Vaccination against ovine foot-rot. *Journal of Comparative Pathology* **81**: 179-185.

Egerton, J.R., Cox, P.T., Anderson, B.J. *et al.* (1987). Protection of sheep against foot-rot with a recombinant DNA-based fimbrial vaccine. *Veterinary Microbiology* **14**: 393-409.

Elleman, T.C., Hoyne, P.A., Stewart, D.J., McKern, N.M. and Peterson, J.E. (1986). Expression of pili from *Bacteroides nodosus* in *Pseudomonas aeruginosa. Journal of Bacteriology* **168**: 574-580.

Emery, D.L., Clark, B.L., Stewart, D.J., O'Donnell, I.J. and Hewish, D.R. (1984). Analysis of the outer membrane proteins of *Bacteroides nodosus*, the causal organism of ovine footrot. *Veterinary Microbiology* **9**: 155-168.

Every, D. (1982). Proteinase isoenzyme patterns of *Bacteroides nodosus*: distinction between ovine virulent isolates, ovine benign isolates and bovine isolates. *Journal of General Microbiology* **128**: 809-812.

Every, D. and Skerman, T.M. (1982). Protection of sheep against experimental footrot by vaccination with pili purified from *Bacteroides nodosus. New Zealand Veterinary Journal* **30**: 156-158.

Fahey, K.J., McWaters, P.G., Stewart, D.J., Peterson, J.E. and Clark, B.L. (1983). Quantitation by ELISA of pili and sheep antibodies to the pili of *Bacteroides nodosus. Australian Veterinary Journal* **60**: 111-116.

Gordon, L.M., Yong, W.K. and Woodward, C.A.M. (1985). Temporal relationships and characterisation of extracellular proteases from benign and virulent strains of *Bacteroides nodosus* as detected in zymogram gels. *Research in Veterinary Science* **39**: 165-172.

Kortt, A.A., O'Donnell, I.J., Stewart, D.J. and Clark, B.L. (1982). Activities and partial purification of extracellular proteases of *Bacteroides nodosus* from virulent and benign footrot. *Journal of Biological Sciences* **35**: 481-489.

Kortt, A.A., Burns, J.E. and Stewart, D.J. (1983). Detection of the extracellular proteases of *Bacteroides nodosus* in polyacrylamide gels: a rapid method of distinguishing virulent and benign ovine isolates. *Research in Veterinary Science* **35**: 171–174.

Kortt, A.A., Caldwell, J.B., Burns, J.E., Guthrie, R.E. and Stewart, D.J. (1986). Characterisation and substrate specificity of the extracellular proteases of *Bacteroides nodosus* from virulent and benign ovine isolates. In: Stewart, D.J., Peterson, J.E., McKern, N.M. and Emery, D.L. (eds) *Footrot in Ruminants: Proceedings of a Workshop, Melbourne 1985*, pp. 237–243. CSIRO Division of Animal Health and Australian Wool Corporation, Glebe, NSW.

Mattick, J.S., Bills, M.M., Anderson, B.J. *et al.* (1987). Morphogenetic expression of *Bacteroides nodosus* fimbriae in *Pseudomonas aeruginosa. Journal of Bacteriology* **169**: 33–41.

Stewart, D.J. (1978). The role of various antigenic fractions of *Bacteroides nodosus* in eliciting protection against foot-rot in vaccinated sheep. *Research in Veterinary Science* **24**: 14–19.

Stewart, D.J. (1979). The role of elastase in the differentiation of *Bacteroides nodosus* infections in sheep and cattle. *Research in Veterinary Science* **27**: 99–105.

Stewart, D.J. (1983). Review of footrot-diagnosis and the role of vaccination. In: *Refresher course for veterinarians, Proceedings No. 67: Sheep Protection and Preventive Medicine*, pp. 487–491. University of Sydney, Post Graduate Committee in Veterinary Science, Sydney.

Stewart, D.J. and Elleman, T.C. (1987). A *Bacteroides nodosus* pili vaccine produced by recombinant DNA for the prevention and treatment of foot-rot in sheep. *Australian Veterinary Journal* **64**: 79–81.

Stewart, D.J., Clark, B.L. and Jarrett, R.G. (1982a). Observations on strains of *Bacteroides nodosus* of intermediate virulence to sheep. *Australian Advances in Veterinary Science*, pp. 219–222. Australian Veterinary Association.

Stewart, D.J., Clark, B.L., Peterson, J.E., Griffiths, D.A. and Smith, E.F. (1982b). Importance of pilus-associated antigen in *Bacteroides nodosus* vaccines. *Research in Veterinary Science* **32**: 140–147.

Stewart, D.J., Clark, B.L., Emery, D.L., Peterson, J.E. and Fahey, K.J. (1983a). A *Bacteroides nodosus* immunogen, distinct from the pilus, which induces cross-protective immunity in sheep vaccinated against footrot. *Australian Veterinary Journal* **60**: 83–85.

Stewart, D.J., Clark, B.L. and Kortt, A.A. (1983b). Differentiation of *Bacteroides nodosus* infections in sheep and cattle. *XXII World Veterinary Congress, Perth, WA, 1983*. Summaries, p. 145.

Stewart, D.J., Clark, B.L., Peterson, J.E. *et al.* (1983c). Effect of pilus dose and type of Freund's adjuvant on the antibody and protective responses of vaccinated sheep to *Bacteroides nodosus. Research in Veterinary Science* **35**: 130–137.

Stewart, D.J., Clark, B.L., Peterson, J.E. *et al.* (1985). The protection given by pilus and whole cell vaccines of *Bacteroides nodosus* strain 198 against ovine foot-rot induced by strains of different serogroups. *Australian Veterinary Journal* **62**: 153–159.

Stewart, D.J., Clark, B.L., Emery, D.L. *et al.* (1986a). Cross-protection from *Bacteroides nodosus* vaccines and the interaction of pili and adjuvants. *Australian Veterinary Journal* **63**: 101–106.

Stewart, D.J., Clark, B.L., Emery, D.L., Peterson, J.E. and Kortt, A.A. (1986b). The phenomenon of cross protection against footrot induced by vaccination of sheep with *Bacteroides nodosus* vaccines. In: Stewart, D.J., Peterson, J.E., McKern, N.M. and Emery D.L. (eds) *Footrot in Ruminants: Proceedings of a Workshop, Melbourne, 1985*, pp. 185–192. CSIRO Division of Animal Health and Australian Wool Corporation, Glebe, NSW.

Stewart, D.J., Peterson, J.E., Vaughan, J.A. *et al.* (1986c). The pathogenicity and cultural characteristics of virulent, intermediate and benign strains of *Bacteroides nodosus* causing ovine foot-rot. *Australian Veterinary Journal* **63**: 317–326.

Thorley, C.M. and Egerton, J.R. (1981). Comparison of alum-absorbed or non-alum-absorbed oil emulsion vaccines containing either pilate or non-pilate *Bacteroides nodosus* cells in inducing and maintaining resistance of sheep to experimental foot rot. *Research in Veterinary Science* **30**: 32–37.

5.6 Factors Influencing the Penetration of Bacterial Antigens through Canine Skin

Ian S. Mason[1] and David H. Lloyd[2]

[1]*Leverhulme Resident in Veterinary Dermatology; and* [2]*Senior Lecturer in Veterinary Dermatology, Department of Veterinary Medicine & Animal Husbandry, Royal Veterinary College, Hatfield, Herts., UK*

INTRODUCTION

It is generally accepted that canine pyoderma occurs as a sequel to some other underlying disease such as hypersensitivity (Ihrke, 1987). In dogs there is a high incidence of pyoderma in atopic individuals (Scott, 1981; Willemse, 1984) and similar observations have been made in man (Dahl, 1983). Although the mechanisms linking hypersensitivity with pyoderma have not been fully elucidated, it has been suggested that local cutaneous hypersensitivity reactions may promote the penetration of bacterial antigens from the stratum corneum into the dermis so leading to cutaneous damage (Blaylock, 1976; Parish *et al.*, 1976; Welbourn *et al.*, 1976; Gabrielsen and Brantzaeg, 1985; Hauser *et al.*, 1985; Mason and Lloyd, 1986, 1989). Such penetration is limited in normal individuals by physical and immunological defence mechanisms and bacterial skin disease occurs if these mechanisms are compromised (Noble, 1975; Jenkinson, 1980).

The epidermis is a major barrier preventing penetration of microorganisms and their metabolites from the skin surface (Lai a Fat and Van Furth, 1974). However, studies of the histology and ultrastructure of the mammalian epidermis have revealed morphological differences between the dog and other mammals. The stratum corneum is thinner and more compact than that of other species and may contain less intercellular material (Lloyd and Garthwaite, 1982; Mason and Lloyd, in prep.). Furthermore, there is no obvious lipid seal at the hair follicle infundibula as is present in ruminants (Mason and Lloyd, in prep.). It has been proposed that the intercellular material of the mammalian stratum corneum is an emulsion of immunologically active proteins with sebaceous lipid and may have an important role in cutaneous defence (Lloyd *et al.*, 1979; Lloyd and Garthwaite, 1982). Hence, it is possible that cutaneous defences may be less well developed in dogs than in other species so that canine skin is inherently more permeable to bacterial antigens and therefore more susceptible to bacterial skin disease. These observations may explain the high incidence of pyoderma in dogs.

In man, studies of percutaneous absorption of one important bacterial product, staphylococcal protein A, have indicated that the intact stratum corneum is an important barrier preventing the penetration of this substance (White and Noble, 1985). In dogs, investigations involving autoradiography have shown that radiolabelled polyvalent staphylococcal antigens and protein A can penetrate normal skin following intradermal injection of the mast cell degranulating agent compound 48/80 (Mason and Lloyd, 1989) but this has not been studied quantitatively.

In this study penetration of radiolabelled protein A through canine skin is evaluated quantitatively under conditions of experimentally induced inflammation.

MATERIALS AND METHODS

The ventral abdomens of three beagle bitches were clipped (No. 40 blade, Oster) and six treatment sites marked with a waterproof pen. Injections of 5 μg histamine (0.01% w/v, Hal), 5 μg compound 48/80 (0.01 w/v, Sigma) and 50 μl PBS (0.01 M PO_4, 0.15 M Cl, pH 7.2) were made intradermally using 0.4 mm by 12 mm (25 gauge by 5/8 inch) needles and 1 ml syringes. Each solution was injected at two sites within each dog. Fifteen minutes after injection 10 μl (15.9 KBq) of tritiated protein A (Amersham) or 10 μl unlabelled protein A (100 mg/ml; Pharmacia) was applied to the sites. The distribution of treatment sites was randomized within each dog (Fig. 1): 17 mm Finn chambers (Epitest)

Inject PBS Apply Protein A	Inject PBS Apply Tritiated Protein A
Inject Compound 48/80 Apply Protein A	Inject Compound 48/80 Apply Tritiated Protein A
Inject Histamine Apply Protein A	Inject Histamine Apply Tritiated Protein A

Figure 1 Summary of treatments used in the study. Each rectangle represents a treatment site on the canine ventral abdomen.

were placed over each treatment site and held in place with a pad of cotton wool, conforming bandage and adhesive surgical tape. Euthanasia was performed 5 h later and skin samples were collected with 6 mm circular biopsy punches. Specimens were placed in aluminium foil containers with fresh egg albumin and frozen using liquid nitrogen. They were held at $-20°C$ before being cut in a cryostat at 10 μm. Frozen sections were mounted onto glass slides, then dipped in molten Ilford K2 autoradiographic emulsion in a darkroom. They were allowed to gel on a cold tray for 3 h, packed in light-proof boxes and incubated at 4°C for 60–90 days (Fukuyama, 1985) before being developed in Kodak D19 developer and fixed in Amfix (May and Baker). Haematoxylin and eosin (HE) or celestine blue were used as counterstains. Specimens were coded and examined blind. In each specimen the numbers of exposed silver granules in the emulsion in 20 random circular microscope fields (0.02 mm in diameter) immediately below the dermal–epidermal junction were counted. Student's unpaired *t*-test was used to compare differences in results between each treatment.

RESULTS

No evidence of erythema or oedema was present at any of the injection sites 5 h after topical application of protein A.

Highly significant differences ($p < 0.001$) were present between the numbers of silver granules in specimens from sites to which tritiated protein A had been applied ('labelled' sites) compared with sites to which unlabelled protein A had been applied ('unlabelled' sites). Counts from 'labelled' sites previously injected with compound 48/80 and PBS were not significantly different, but counts from 'labelled' sites previously injected with histamine were significantly greater ($p < 0.001$) than those from 'labelled' compound 48/80 and PBS treated sites (Fig. 2).

DISCUSSION

These results indicate that radiolabelled staphylococcal protein A can be detected within the superficial dermis of normal dog skin 5 h after topical application. Absorption of protein A was enhanced by prior injection of histamine intradermally supporting the hypothesis that release of inflammatory mediators from mast cells during hypersensitivity reactions may facilitate percutaneous absorption of staphylococcal products leading to the development of pyoderma. However, injection of compound 48/80 did not promote penetration of protein A, suggesting that it may form a less useful model of cutaneous hypersensitivity in dogs than previous studies have indicated (Mason and Lloyd, 1986, 1989). It is possible that the response of

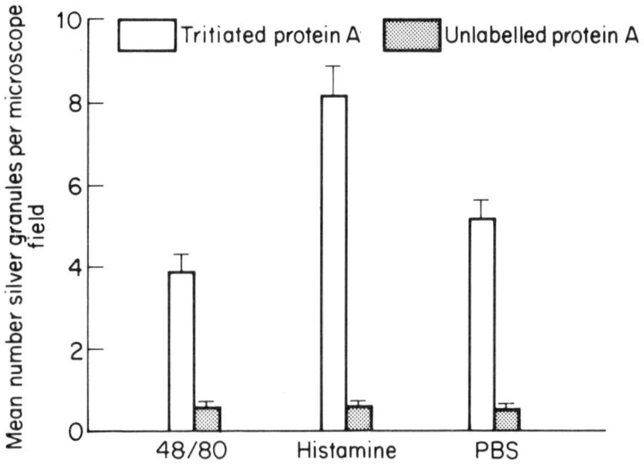

Figure 2 Histogram of results obtained in the study. Mean number of exposed silver granules counted in random microscope fields is plotted for each treatment.

individual dogs to intradermal injection of compound 48/80 varies or that canine mast cells are less sensitive to the effects of this substance than that of other species. Hence, a higher dose may have facilitated greater absorption of protein A from the skin surface.

The mechanisms by which hypersensitivity can lead to altered epidermal barrier function are unknown. Within the lesions of hypersensitivity changes in blood flow, blood vessel permeability and rate of sweat production occur which may have an effect on local cutaneous permeability. Moreover, such changes may affect the cutaneous microenvironment (temperature, humidity and nutrient availability) and promote a shift in the skin flora in favour of coagulase-positive staphylococci so increasing the concentration gradient of staphylococcal metabolites across the epidermis so promoting absorption. Cutaneous hypersensitivity is characterized by pruritus and resultant self trauma may lead to epidermal damage and enhanced penetration of such metabolites.

Mast cell degranulation and the release of inflammatory mediators is only one aspect of hypersensitivity. In human atopic dermatitis the stratum corneum of affected individuals is thinner and contains fewer cell layers and less lipid than that of normal people (White *et al.*, 1987). Although no similar studies have been performed in dogs, it is possible that similar structural abnormalities to those reported in human atopics may be present in canine atopy.

REFERENCES

Blaylock, W.K. (1976). Atopic dermatitis: Diagnosis and pathobiology. *Journal of Allergy and Clinical Immunology* **57**: 62–79.

Dahl, M.V. (1983). *Staphylococcus aureus* and atopic dermatitis. *Archives of Dermatology* **119**: 840–846.
Fukuyama, K. (1985). Autoradiography. In: Skerrow, D. and Skerrow, C.J. (eds) *Methods in Skin Research*, pp. 71–89. John Wiley, Chichester.
Gabrielson, T.O. and Brantzaeg, P. (1985). Enzyme-linked immunosorbent assay (ELISA) for isotype-specific quantitation of antibodies to *Staphylococcus aureus* in patients with atopic dermatitis. *Acta Dermato-venereologica (Stockholm)* (Suppl) **114**: 61–66.
Hauser, C., Wuethrich, B., Matter, L., Wilhelm, J.A. and Schopfer, K. (1985). The immune response to *S. aureus* in atopic dermatitis. *Acta Dermato-venereologica (Stockholm)* (Suppl) **114**: 112–118.
Ihrke, P.J. (1987). Overview of bacterial skin disease in the dog. *British Veterinary Journal* **143**: 112–118.
Jenkinson, D.M. (1980). Topography, climate and chemical nature of the mammalian skin surface. *Proceedings of the Royal Society of Edinburgh* **79B**: 3–22.
Lai a Fat, R.F. and Van Furth, R. (1974). The role of the skin & adjacent mucous membranes in host defense. *Journal of Cutaneous Pathology* **1**: 61–70.
Lloyd, D.H. and Garthwaite, G. (1982). Epidermal structure and surface topography of canine skin. *Research of Veterinary Science* **33**: 99–104.
Lloyd, D.H., Dick, W.D.B. and Jenkinson, D.M. (1979). Structure of the epidermis in Ayrshire bullocks. *Research in Veterinary Science* **26**: 172–179.
Mason, I.S. and Lloyd, D.H. (1986). The influence of allergic factors on the penetration of staphylococcal antigens through skin. *Tijdschrift voor Diergeneeskunde* **111** (Suppl)1: 14S.
Mason, I.S. and Lloyd, D.H. (1989). The role of allergy in the development of canine pyoderma. *Journal of Small Animal Practice* **30**: 216–218.
Noble, W.C. (1975). Skin as a microhabitat. *Postgraduate Medical Journal* **51**: 151–155.
Parish, W.E., Welbourn, E. and Champion, R.H. (1976). Hypersensitivity to bacteria in eczema. IV. Cytotoxic effect of antibacterial antibody on skin cells acquiring bacterial antigens. *British Journal of Dermatology* **95**: 493–506.
Scott, D.W. (1981). Observations on canine atopy. *Journal of the American Animal Hospital Association* **17**: 91–100.
Welbourn, E., Champion, R.H. and Parish, W.E. (1976). Hypersensitivity to bacteria in eczema. I. Bacterial culture, skin tests and immunofluorescent detection of immunoglobulins and bacterial antigens. *British Journal of Dermatology* **94**: 619–632.
White, M.I. and Noble, W.C. (1980). Skin response to Protein A. *Proceedings of the Royal Society of Edinburgh* **79B**: 43–46.
White, M.I. and Noble, W.C. (1985). The cutaneous reaction to staphylococcal protein A in normal subjects and patients with atopic dermatitis or psoriasis. *British Journal of Dermatology* **113**: 179–183.
White, M.I., Jenkinson, D.M. and Lloyd, D.H. (1987). The effect of washing on the thickness of the stratum corneum in normal and atopic individuals. *British Journal of Dermatology* **116**: 525–530.
Willemse, A. (1984). Investigations on canine atopic dermatitis PhD thesis, University of Utrecht.

5.7 Controlled Trial of Ethyl Lactate and Benzoyl Peroxide Shampoos in the Management of Canine Surface Pyoderma and Superficial Pyoderma

F. Ascher,[1] L. Maynard,[2] J. Laurent[3] and B. Goubet[4]

[1]Doctor in Veterinary Medicine, and Clinical Research Manager; [2]Doctor in Veterinary Medicine, VIRBAC Laboratories, Carros, France; [3]Doctor in Veterinary Medicine, Saint-Avold, France; [4]Doctor in Veterinary Medicine, Chateau Renard, France

INTRODUCTION

A 10% alcoholic solution of ethyl lactate was first used by Swanbeck (1972) in the treatment of acne in man and his results were confirmed by Gloor (1977) and Grosshans *et al.* (1978). The mode of action of ethyl lactate was described by Prottey *et al.* (1984). Once ethyl lactate has penetrated the hair follicles and sebaceous glands, it is hydrolysed locally into lactic acid and ethanol. The free lactic acid lowers the cutaneous pH. This inhibits bacterial lipases, thereby exerting a bacteriostatic or bactericidal activity. Ethanol renders fats soluble and lowers sebaceous secretions.

Because of its properties, ethyl lactate, or etilac, was assessed for veterinary use for the treatment of pyodermas. In order to avoid interference from antibiotics which would be required for the treatment of deep pyoderma, the trial was limited to the treatment of canine surface and superficial pyodermas.

MATERIAL AND METHODS

Products

Etiderm® is a shampoo containing 10% etilac. Its activity was compared to that of another shampoo containing 2.5% benzoyl peroxide. The antiseptic properties of benzoyl peroxide have already been described (Ihrke, 1983; Lloyd and Reyss-Brion, 1984) and the clinical efficacy demonstrated.

The shampoos were applied on wet hair and massaged to produce a lather. Etiderm was left on the hair for 10 min before being washed off. Once the first application of the benzoyl peroxide shampoo had been rinsed off, a second application of the same shampoo was left on the hair for 10 min before being carefully washed off. Each shampoo was applied three times a week, for 4 weeks.

Test animals and treatment regimens

Forty-six dogs of random breeds and ages were selected; 33 were treated with etilac, and 13 with benzoyl peroxide. The animals were suffering from either a surface or a superficial pyoderma, defined as follows:

Surface pyoderma

This involves bacteria localized in crusts, on the skin surface or within the stratum corneum (fold pyodermas or intertrigo, pyotraumatic dermatitis or hot spot).

Superficial pyoderma

This involves bacteria within the epidermis but below the stratum corneum or within the hair follicles (impetigo, papulopustular pyoderma (PPP) or non-specific superficial pyoderma (NSP)).

Assessment of the therapeutic response

The animals were examined three times at 14-day intervals, with the final examination on day 28 occurring 48 h after the last shampoo.

At each presentation, all animals were subjected to a full clinical examination. Bacteriological cultures were taken from involved areas at day 0 and day 28 after clipping the hair. Bacterial species present were identified and the density was assessed semi-quantitatively.

RESULTS AND DISCUSSION

Clinical results

Interpretation of data

A grade (G) was assigned to each clinical sign according to its degree of severity, before treatment, during the first visit (Day 0), and after the treatment (Day 28). In order to take into account the relative importance of the 11 clinical signs considered, a coefficient (C) was assigned to each of them. The severity at Day 0 and at Day 28 are represented by a value corresponding to the sum of the grades (G × C) specifically assigned to each clinical sign. The efficacy rate of the treatment was calculated as follows:

$$\frac{\text{Grade at Day 0} - \text{Grade at Day 28}}{\text{Grade at Day 0}} \times 100$$

80–100% excellent
60–80% good
40–60% fair
0–40% poor to null

Results

There were 40 interpretable clinical results, 30 from the etilac group and 10 from the benzoyl peroxide group. The six non-interpretable cases included four dogs who did not complete the trial and two who received additional treatment.

Etilac had an 'excellent and good' efficacy rate of 90%, whereas benzoyl peroxide had an 'excellent and good' rate of 70% (Table 1). This difference was not statistically significant ($\chi^2 = 1.046$).

Table 1 Clinical results (only interpretable cases)

	Etilac						Benzoyl peroxide					
	Results						Results					
Pyodermas	G		F		Total		G		F		Total	
	Nb	(%)	Nb	(%)	Nb	(%)	Nb	(%)	Nb	(%)	Nb	(%)
Surface												
intertrigo	4	(100)	–	–	4	(100)	1	(50)	1	(50)	2	(100)
hot spot	2	(67)	1	(33)	3	(100)	1	(100)	–	–	1	(100)
Total	6	(86)	1	(14)	7	(100)	2	(67)	1	(33)	3	(100)
Superficial												
impetigo	4	(80)	1	(20)	5	100)	–	–	–	–	–	–
PPP	5	(83)	1	(17)	6	(100)	–	–	–	–	–	–
NSP	12	(100)	–	–	12	(100)	5	(72)	2	(28)	7	(100)
Total	21	(91)	2	(9)	23	(100)	5	(72)	2	(28)	7	(100)
OVERALL TOTAL	27	(90)	3	(10)	30	(100)	7	(70)	3	(30)	10	(100)

G: excellent + good (60–100% decrease of the clinical signs on Day 28).
F: fair + poor + null (0–60% decrease of the clinical signs on Day 28).
(%) percentage relative to the total number of cases considered within the same category and treated with the same product (horizontal reading).

Bacteriological results

Bacterial agents isolated at Day 0

Bacteriological studies were undertaken on Day 0 of 34 samples taken from active lesions. A total of 60 bacteria were isolated representing 1.8 per culture taken (Table 2). The pathogenic coagulase positive staphylococci (C + staph) are predominant and represent 43% of the isolates. The techniques employed did not permit distinction between the coagulase positive *S. aureus* and *S. intermedius*. The *Bacillus* species was the next most frequent (18%), followed by *S. epidermidis*, a coagulase negative staphylococcus (12%). *S. epidermidis*, streptococci, *Acinetobacter* and *Micrococcus* are all considered as part of the natural cutaneous flora in dogs. *Pseudomonas*, *Proteus*, *Enterobacter*, *Klebsiella*, *Aeromonas* and *Citrobacter* are all considered as pathogenic when found on skin and represented 23% of the isolates. Furthermore, C + staph are found in association with other bacterial species in 59% of the samples. However, the association of more than two isolates was not often encountered (9% of the samples). In 45% of the samples where multiple bacterial species were identified within the same sample, the C + staph isolates was found in association with *Bacillus*.

Table 2 Distribution of the bacterial agents identified on Day 0 (all samples)

Bacterial agents identified on Day 0	Etilac	Benzoyl peroxide	Total Nb	(%)[a]
Pathogenic				
Coagulase + staph.	15	11	26	(43)
Enterobacter	3	1	4	(7)
Proteus	2	1	3	(5)
Citrobacter	2	1	3	(5)
Pseudomonas	1	1	2	(3)
Aeromonas	1	–	1	(2)
Klebsiella	1	–	1	(2)
Non-pathogenic				
Bacillus	6	5	11	(18)
S. epidermidis	5	2	7	(12)
Group D strep.	1	–	1	(2)
Acinetobacter	1	–	1	(2)
OVERALL TOTAL	38	22	60	(100)

[a] (%) percentage relative to the total number of isolated germs (60).

Clinical evolution and infection

When considering the clinical evolution of the pyoderma with regard to the bacterial agents identified on Day 0 (disregarding both their pathogenic or saprophytic character and disappearance or persistence at the end of the treatment) it is possible to reach conclusions as to the products' efficacy when used to treat an infected skin (Table 3).

Table 3 Clinical evolution with regards to bacteria on Day 0 (interpretable cases only)

	Etilac				Benzoyl peroxide			
Bacterial agents identified on Day 0	Clinical results G		F	Total	Clinical results G		F	Total
Pathogenic								
Coagulase + staph	11	(85)	2	13	5	(62.5)	3	8
Entercbacter	2		1	3	0		–	–
Proteus	2		1	2	–		–	–
Citrobacter	2		0	2	–		1	1
Pseudomonas	1		0	1	0		1	1
Aeromonas	–		–	–	–		–	–
Klebsiella	1		0	1	–		–	–
Non-pathogenic								
Bacillus	5	(83)	1	6	4	(80)	1	5
S. epidermidis	3		0	3	1		0	1
Group D strep.	1		0	1	–		–	–
Acinetobacter	–		–	–	–		–	–
TOTAL	28	(87.5)	4	32	10	(62.5)	6	16

G: excellent + good.
F: fair + poor + null.
( ) percentage relative to the total number of cases within the same category and treated with the same product (horizontal reading).

When all bacteria are considered, etilac has a favourable clinical evolution of 87.5%, compared with the 62.5% recorded with benzoyl peroxide. However, this difference is not statistically significant ($\chi^2 = 1.92$). Etilac has an efficiency rate of 85% on skin infected with C + staph.

Antibacterial efficacy

Interpretation of the data. The antibacterial efficacy can be guaged by the reduction in number of pathogenic bacteria that were isolated on Day 0. The saprophytes were disregarded in the evaluation of the results. A difference was made between the C + staph and the other pathogenic bacteria as the healthy skin of a dog often harbours the former whereas the latter are absent from normal skins. C + staph can be held responsible for the infection only when a great number of them is found in lesions.

Therefore, the efficacy of the product was measured according to whether or not there was a decrease in the colony density of C + staph. Bacteriological results were considered poor when the density of the colonies did not decrease.

With regard to other pathogens (*Pseudomonas*, *Proteus*, *Klebsiella*, *Enterobacter* and *Citrobacter*), the products were considered efficaceous when the bacteria were no longer recoverable after treatment.
Results. Posttreatment cultures were taken on Day 28 in 21 cases. Thirty-two pathogens were isolated, representing a mean value of 1.5 isolates per sample (Table 4).

Table 4 Comparison of the antibacterial efficacy of etilac and benzoyl peroxide

	Etilac				Benzoyl peroxide			
Pathogenic agents isolated on Day 0	Bacteriological results G	(%)	P	Total	Bacteriological results G	(%)	P	Total
Coagulase + staph.	11	(85)	2	13	6	(75)	2	8
Enterobacter	1		2	13	-		-	-
Proteus	2	(100)	0	2	-		-	-
Citrobacter	12	(100)	0	2	1		0	1
Pseudomonas	0		1	1	0		1	1
Klebsiella	1		0	1	-		-	-
OVERALL TOTAL	17	(77)	5	22	7	(70)	3	10

G: good.
P: poor.
(%) percentage calculated according to the category and product considered (horizontal reading).

Etilac. On Day 28 *Proteus*, *Klebsiella* and *Citrobacter* were not isolated and the efficacy rate was 85% on C + staph. Clinically, we observed the same efficacy rate and we can therefore conclude that there is a good correlation between the clinical response and the antibacterial activity. When considering all the pathogens involved, etilac has an antibacterial efficacy rate of 77%.
Benzoyl peroxide. The efficacy rate was 75% on C + staph and 70% when all pathogens are considered. It must be noted that the presence of *Pseudomonas* persisted in the samples (one case in each group). However, the clinical result obtained with the use of etilac was excellent, whereas it was poor in this instance with benzoyl peroxide.

Etilac seems to be a more potent product than benzoyl peroxide, namely when infections involve C + staph. However, the difference is not statistically significant.

Cosmetic value of the products

The veterinarians noted that the skin and coat, as well as the odour of the animal, were improved (Table 5). In 74% of the cases in which Etiderm was used, the response was good or excellent. Benzoyl peroxide, on the other hand, only had a 50% rate of success.

Table 5 Cosmetic virtues of the products (improvement of skin and coat aspect)

Etilac			Benzoyl peroxide		
Cosmetic results			Cosmetic results		
G	F	Total	G	F	Total
All pyodermas considered					
23 (74)	8	31	5 (50)	5	10

G: excellent and good.
F: fair and poor.
( ) percentage referring to each product.

CONCLUSION

When treating surface or superficial pyoderma, ideally the drug should be applied topically, rather than orally or parenterally. Topical formulations such as ointments or creams are of little practical value in dogs and cats, and shampoos seem more appropriate. Shampoos facilitate the removal of the debris, crusts and scale, and thus enable better access of the antibacterial agent. The coat's appearance and the odour resulting from an infected skin are very important to the owner of the animal. When the treatment is effective and also improves the outward appearance of the animal, this will encourage the owner to pursue the treatment until the animal has recovered.

Clinical trials have revealed the potential of a new shampoo for treating surface and superficial pyoderma. With its use the infection is reduced and locally accumulated fatty acids are eliminated. These characteristics have been demonstrated namely on infections arising from C + staph.

The formulation of the shampoo also contributes to the treatment, as it restores the coat's natural beauty.

REFERENCES

Amine-Khodja, C.A., Pellerin, J.L., Chantal, J. and Milon, A. (1983). La flore microbienne des pyodermites et des otites suppurées du chien. *Revue de Médecine Vétérinaire* **134** (5): 307–312.

Gloor, M. (1977). Uber die Reduktion der freien Fettsäuren in den Hautoberfläche-Lipiden als Kriterium für die therapeutische Wirksamkeit antimikrobieller Aknetherapeutika. *Arzneim-Forsch/Drug. Res.* **27** (11): 2179–2181.

Grosshans, E., Fourtanier, A. and Guibaud, B. (1978). Evaluation clinique d'un traitement local de l'acné juvénile par le lactate d'éthyle. *Ann. Dermatol. Venereol.* **105**: 833–838.

Ihrke, P.J.B. (1983). The management of canine pyodermas. In: *Current Veterinary Therapy* Vol. VIII, pp. 505–517. W.B. Saunders Company, Philadelphia.

Lloyd, D.H. and Reyss-Brion, A. (1984). Le péroxyde de benzoyle: efficacité clinique

et bactériologique dans le traitement des pyodermites chroniques. *Pratique Médicale et Chirurgicale de l'Animal de Compagnie* **19** (4): 445–449.
Prottey, C., George, D., Leech, R.W. *et al.* (1984). The mode of action of ethyl lactate as a treatment for acne. *British Journal of Dermatology* **110**: 475–485.
Swanbeck, G. (1972). A new principle for the treatment of acne. *Acta Dermatovener* **52**: 406–410.

PART 6

WORKSHOP REPORTS

Workshop Report 1

Avian Dermatology

M. Muller and J.E. Cooper

Institut für Tierpathologie, Universitaet Bern, Bern, Switzerland; and The Royal College of Surgeons of England, London, UK

Max Muller *Bern, Switzerland* emphasized that in all species the integument is very important. The feather has a particularly complex and fascinating structure, showing variety in shape, construction and function. It is divided into a compact part, the flag, a downy part and a quill.

Before investigating feather disorders and avian dermatology one has to be able to tell what is normal and what is pathological. The crowned crane (*Balearica pavonia*) for example, has special feathers on its head: these are quite normal but might be thought to be pathological.

Feathers show great variety of colours. The physical principal is the reflection and absorption of light of specific wavelengths.

A transverse section through a ramus shows that it consists of melanin, keratin and gas. Melanin is arranged in five different ways: small filaments, large filaments, gas-filled tubes, compact sheets and segmented, gas-filled, sheets. There are 19 different types of arrangement in birds. The more regular the layers of melanin are, the more shiny is the feather.

One must not forget the special down plumage of nestlings. This is important in avian paediatrics and in diagnostic work. Sometimes a decision has to be made as to whether feathers are normal or their appearance is indicative of juvenile French moult disease.

Alopecia is a common problem in parrots. A bald head is a characteristic sign of social aggressive interaction, usually because of insufficient space in the cage. Generally the rest of the body is not affected.

Feather-chewing may be a consequence of pruritus with various aetiologies including viral infection, mycosis and parasitism. Feather-chewing in individual parrots is often a sociopsychological problem in which case the feathers on the head are untouched.

A contact dermatitis in the axilla may be secondary or, as in eczema syndrome of budgerigars (*Melopsittacus* spp.) and lovebirds (*Agapornis* spp.) (see later), a primary disease.

Abnormal moulting in more or less naked cockatoos is well recognized and known as psittacine beak and feather disease (PBFD) (see later).

Feather cysts are an example of a genetic feather disorder. In juvenile canaries (*Serinus canaria*) and budgerigars many feathers are affected, whereas *Hypopteronosis cystica* in adult parrots usually involves only one follicle. Automutilation and/or secondary bacterial infection may occur.

Insofar as viral infections are concerned cutaneous avian pox is particularly prevalent. In Europe it is a frequent problem in canaries.

Marek's disease is a Herpes virus-induced disease of the feather follicular epidermis. There is a nodular enlargement of feather follicles, often with ulceration. Numerous cells in the outer layers of the feather follicle epidermis contain nuclei with amorphous amphophilic inclusion bodies. Perifollicular aggregation of lymphoid cells is prominent. Sometimes the nodules are confluent. Differential diagnoses in galliform birds include mycoplasmosis and avian tuberculosis. In the latter there may not be any granulomas: however, a massive accumulation of macrophages is usually a feature. Whether or not there is necrosis depends on the severity of the lesion. In HE-stained material avian macrophages are faintly basophilic and in ZN-stained sections acid-fast organisms are visible.

Examples of feather abnormalities were then given, illustrated with slides. The following is a summary.

A feather-chewing *Eclectus* parrot (*Eclectus roratus*): careful examination of feathers reveals signs of automutilation.

Clubbed down feathers, a disorder of moulting in a budgerigar: individual feathers on the head are affected. The colour is white. A sample shows the feather resting in the keratin sheath and haemorrhage in the quill.

Histological sections of candidiasis show hyphae between the quill and sheath. Massive hyperkeratosis is pathognomonic.

The most common parasitic disease affecting the skin of budgerigars is *Cnemidocoptes* mite infestation. The typical lesion is a hyperplasia of the cere, eyelid and legs. There is only mild inflammation. If a scraping is taken the mites can be seen.

Mites of feathers are not so conspicuous. There is a brownish patchy discolouration of the rami. But they may cause pruritus and automutilation.

Subcutaneous oedema may be a sign of anasarca. However, if localized on the wings or the abdomen, it is often an indication of *Trombicula* infestation. White nodules under the skin in the area of joints are strongly suggestive of articular gout.

Neoplasms are often seen in budgerigars (see later). A less common lesion was observed on the tarsus of a passerine: the swelling was well localized, firm, elevated and brown in colour. The cyst-like proliferation of the stratum spinosum and the massive hyperkeratosis led to a diagnosis of acanthoma.

M. Muller concluded by reminding his audience that changes in the skin and feathers may assist in general diagnosis. For example, dirty feathers around the cloaca are a sign of diarrhoea, around the beak indicative of vomiting.

J.E. Cooper *London, UK* discussed the laboratory investigation of feathers. He stressed that diseases of the skin of birds, including feathers, could be classified on the basis of their aetiology (e.g. infectious or non-infectious), the structure affected (beak, feet, claws etc.) or specific syndromes (e.g. French Moult, Feather Cysts, Psittacine Beak and Feather Disease).

The taking of material for laboratory investigation could be divided into a) sampling, b) transportation, and c) processing. At each stage problems could arise and complicate the investigation. A systematic approach was therefore required and the use of standard protocols was advisable. Examination of feathers and other material should first be with the naked eye, followed by use of a hand lens and, where appropriate, light microscopy and transmission and scanning electron microscopy (SWM). Microbiological culture and other techniques could be performed as necessary.

Scanning electron microscopy was proving very useful in the study of feather abnormalities, the investigation of the lines of weakness commonly called fault bars or fret marks and in the differential diagnosis of conditions causing damage to barbs and barbules. Transmission electron microscopy (TEM), on the other hand, was a valuable tool in the detection of virus particles and, in conjunction with histopathology, the investigation and diagnosis of pathological changes in the feather follicle.

Ulrich Rytz *Bern, Switzerland* then discussed tumours. He pointed out that the typical clinical features of a skin tumour are a white or yellowish mass, that can be localized or invasive, flat or raised, soft or firm.

Illustrated examples followed, starting with a soft mass on the sternum of a budgerigar. The cytological diagnosis of this tumour was a lipoma. Macroscopical differential diagnosis of such a tumour would include a xanthoma (see later).

Histopathological examination of a mixed lipoxanthoma revealed adipose tissue, a granuloma with many vacuolated macrophages, multinucleated giant cells and typical cholesterol clefts. Xanthomatosis is not a true neoplasm but a tumour-like lesion which presents as diffuse thickening of the skin.

A raised nodular mass on the skull of a lovebird proved histopathologically to be diffuse lymphoid tissue. Lymphoid leukosis, cutaneous or visceral, may appear anywhere in birds. A white firm mass on the wing with a central cavity of necrosis may be a fibroma or a fibrosarcoma.

Ulcerative dermatitis is not infrequently seen under the wings, the axilla or the neck of budgerigars and lovebirds. Automutilation often aggravates the lesion and severe blood loss is possible.

A condition called eczema syndrome occurs in budgerigars and lovebirds. A histopathological section shows loss of the epidermis in the centre of the lesion, hyperkeratotic thickening of the epidermis on the edge and a necrotic dermatitis. Bacterial or mycotic infection is likely to be secondary rather than primary. Stress factors probably play a major role in this condition, but Dr Muller has seen several cases with similar clinical signs that proved to be squamous cell carcinomas. In these, the characteristic features are irregular islets of keratinizing epidermal cells with keratin pearls, frequent intercellular bridges and mitoses.

In budgerigars neoplastic involvement of the gonads and the kidney may be reflected as a colour change in the cere due to hormonal changes. The cere is generally blue in male budgerigars. A male individual with a brown, hyperkeratotic cere may have a neoplasia of the testes.

Nadia Zangger *Bern, Switzerland* discussed psittacine beak and feather disease syndrome (PBFD), a well known disease complex in parrots.

The beak lesions in PBFD are characterized by progressive elongation, breakage and weakening. The quantity, as well as the quality, of the feathers is reduced. Contour feathers may be replaced by down feathers. Characteristic features of feather disorders are a retained feather sheath, circumferential constriction and small clubbed feathers. Macrophages laden with multiple basophilic inclusions in the cytoplasm are pathognomonic for PBFD.

Haemorrhage in feathers may be a consequence of necrosis of the epidermis and pulp. Examination of cases with the electron microscope has revealed crystalline hexagonal particles with a diameter of 17–22 nm which are typical of a parvovirus-like particle.

French moult disease (FMD) is also called Budgerigar fledgling disease. Loss of contour feathers in the wings and tail of subadult and adult birds is the characteristic feature. In juvenile budgerigars Dr Zangger has found a new feature of FMD: all growing feathers of the body have a retained sheath (Plate 26). As in PBFD the feather quantity and quality are reduced. One may see feathers clubbed to different degrees. There is haemorrhage in the pulp. Necrosis of follicle epidermis, intracellular eosinophilic inclusion bodies in ballooning cells and haemorrhage in the pulp are typical histological features. Dr Zangger and her colleagues have never seen inclusions in macrophages as in PBFD.

The aetiology of FMP is a polyoma virus, measuring 40–45 nm. The virus particles are disseminated or partly arranged in a crystalline array in the nucleus of the cell.

An endemic papillomatosis affected different species of waterfowl in the zoological garden of Basle. The lesions were located on the side of the feet, especially at the articulations. The surface was often ulcerated. There was close resemblance to bumblefoot (Plate 27). In longitudinal sections massive fibrosis and extensive hyperkeratosis were the main feature. Intranuclear basophile inclusions were seen in the inner layers.

Using electron microscopy hexagonal virus particles, 50–55 nm in diameter, could be demonstrated in the nucleus.

Pox infection has been reported in nearly 70 species of birds, but appears never to have been described in storks. In 1988, an endemic cutaneous avian pox affected young white storks (*Ciconia ciconia*) and black storks (*Ciconia niqra*) in a restocking station in Switzerland. The typical verrucous efflorescences were located on legs, feet, upper back and eyelids. Histological sections revealed a papilliform proliferation of the epidermis with necrosis of the surface. The cells of the stratum germinativum were ballooned and contained eosinophilic lipophilic intracytoplasmic inclusions. Ultrastructural examination revealed filaments and inclusions (400–1600 nm) in the cytoplasm. Mature viruses measuring 340 of 150 nm were located on the periphery of the inclusion.

M. Muller, the Chairman, *Bern, Switzerland* finally covered moulting problems. One condition, called 'stuck in the moult', is a feather disorder with worldwide distribution characterized by an interrupted moult and feather replacement cycle. In the literature this is described as a miscellaneous disorder, the aetiology being as yet unknown.

In the zoological garden, Basle, three hermit ibises (*Geronticus eremita*) showed ulceration on the back and widespread alopecia resulting from automutilation: the speaker interpreted this as a sign of pruritus. The feathers had a clubbed down appearance, and the keratin sheath was elongated and thickened.

Histological features were hyperkeratosis of the sheath, a lymphocytic inflammatory reaction, and intracytoplasmic and intranuclear basophilic inclusions of different sizes in the follicular epidermis.

Similar lesions, but more acute, were seen in a sunbittern (*Eurypyga* sp.) in Walsrode, Germany. A haemorrhagic quill was a feature. The syndrome has also been reported in other species—for example, sparrows (*Passer* spp.).

Two questions arise over this condition: 1) If it is worldwide, is it an infectious disease? 2) Are sparrows the reservoir of the infectious agent? Dr Muller suggested that this might be a paramyxovirus-like infection (Plate 25).

In April 1989 the *National Geographic Magazine* carried an article entitled 'Loon Cries for Help'. This described loons (divers—Gaviidae) in Canada which showed signs of abnormal moult. Water pollution (intoxication) was suspected. Is it possible that this was a form of French moult? Could it have been a paramyxovirus infection or was it really intoxication and water pollution?

A lively discussion period ensued, with questions or comments from **Drs D. Deboer**, **R. Aronson**, **J.D. Conroy**, **C. Alderman**, **J. Bainbridge**, **J.E. Cooper** and **F. Laval**. Topics covered included sources of information on avian dermatology, the possible value of *Hibiscus* leaves in the treatment of self-mutilating parrots, the diagnosis of feather disorders, the possibility that hypersensitivity might play a part in avian skin diseases, the role of local anaesthesia in the taking of skin biopsies and the best diagnostic approach to the feather-picking bird.

The session provided an excellent opportunity for those with an interest in birds to meet and exchange views. There have been many exciting advances recently in our understanding of avian diseases and dermatological aspects have not been neglected: the field is ripe for further research.

REFERENCES

Cooper, J.E., Gschmeissner, S. and Ion, F. (1989). The laboratory investigation of feathers. *Proceedings of 2nd European Symposium on Avian Medicine and Surgery, Utrecht, 1989.*
Hillyer, E.V., Quesenbery, K.E. and Baer, K. (1989). Basic avian dermatology. *Proceedings of the Association of Avian Veterinarians. Seattle, Washington, September 1989.*
Pass, D.A. (1989). The pathology of the avian integument: a review. *Avian Pathology* **18**: 1–72.

Workshop Report 2

Equine Insect Hypersensitivity

Valerie A. Fadok and Carol S. Foil

National Jewish Center for Immunology and Respiratory Medicine, Denver, Colorado, USA; and School of Veterinary Medicine, Louisiana State University, Louisiana, USA

Valerie A. Fadok *Denver, Colorado, USA* Insect hypersensitivity is a common cause of pruritic dermatitis in horses throughout the world. Allergy to *Culicoides* species is the best documented equine insect hypersensitivity; the role of other insects, including black flies, and stable flies, remains to be determined. The purpose of this workshop was to discuss the *Culicoides* species involved in causing disease, the clinical syndromes associated with this disease, the benefit of intradermal skin testing, and potential therapy with hyposensitization. Additionally, seasonal dermatoses other than those known to be associated with *Culicoides* hypersensitivity were discussed in an attempt to determine whether insect hypersensitivity was a probable cause. The immunologic and inflammatory pathogenic mechanisms of insect hypersensitivity in the horse are largely unknown; however, the potential role of platelet activating factor as an inflammatory mediator in equine insect hypersensitivity was addressed.

Culicoides hypersensitivity (CHS) has been described classically as a pruritic dermatosis affecting primarily the dorsal midline. With my colleague, Dr Ellis Greiner, I evaluated 101 seasonally pruritic Florida horses. Three clinical syndromes were seen: dorsal midline dermatitis, in approximately 20% of the horses, ventral midline dermatitis, in approximately 30% of the horses, and dermatitis affecting both the dorsal and ventral midline, in 50% of the horses. These horses were skin tested with commercially available insect, pollen, and mold extracts; additionally, an extract not commercially available was prepared from a colony of *C. variipennis*. Reactions were read at 30 min, 6 h, and 24 h. Reactions to pollens and molds occurred in a few horses; however, no trends were seen that enabled the correlation of these reactions with the seasonality of disease or location on the body. Several horses, however, reacted to multiple insect extracts. When compared by their ability to respond to a particular concentration (PNU/ml) of antigen, more affected horses reacted to *Culicoides* extract than to black fly, horse fly, or mosquito extracts. Regardless of which clinical syndrome they manifested, 80% of horses in each group showed significant positive reactions at 30 min to *Culicoides* extract; 50% of all horses reacted to *Culicoides* at 6 h and 20% reacted at 24 h.

Of the 59 horses biopsied, 85% had eosinophilic and mononuclear superficial and deep perivascular dermatitis, supportive of a diagnosis of insect hypersensitivity. The biopsy results, in conjunction with the skin testing data, suggested that Florida horses were allergic to *Culicoides*, and that CHS could be associated with significant ventral midline dermatitis. Trapping of insects off the horses and in their environment confirmed this hypothesis, and implicated *C. insignis* and *C. stellifer* as the primary causes of insect hypersensitivity in Florida horses.

In conclusion, skin testing horses with commercially available insect extracts seemed of questionable value, particularly in determining to what insect the horse was actually allergic. Because the horses reacted to *C. variipennis*, a species not commonly found in Florida, we believe that the majority of horses were reacting to a major antigen found in all *Culicoides* species. Additionally, there may be a generic or cross reacting insect antigen, which would explain the positive reactions seen to black fly extract, an insect also relatively uncommon in Florida.

Carol S. Foil *Baton Rouge, Louisiana, USA* presented skin testing data obtained from horses seen in Louisiana, in which *Culicoides* hypersensitivity presented primarily as a dorsally distributed disease. Two horses with CHS were donated to the university because of unmanageable and unsightly dermatitis. These animals were skin tested with extracts derived from multiple species of *Culicoides*, at dilutions ranging from 1:20 to 1:6400; control groups consisted of horses not affected with skin disease, and specific pathogen free ponies raised in an environment free of endo- and ectoparasites. The species from which extracts were prepared included laboratory-raised and wild-caught *C. varriipennis*, male *C. variipennis*, *C. biguttatus*, *C. obsoletus* complex, *C. stellifer*, *C. venustus*, and four species of *Culicoides* from Israel, including one species not known to feed on mammals.

Skin test results were read at 30 min, 4-6 h, 24 h, and 48 h. In general, the horses affected with insect hypersensitivity showed more responsiveness, particularly at the lower dilutions of the extracts, than the normal horses. It was noted, however, that two of the ponies never exposed to insects reacted to *Culicoides* extracts at 1:400 dilution, suggesting an irritant or cross-reacting factor present in the extract. Reactions at 48 h seemed to show the most sensitivity and specificity, as they separated the normal horses from the affected horses, at dilutions greater than or equal to 1:800. All the control horses reacted to some extracts, often at very low concentrations, at the 30 min and 4-6 h readings. The most important finding was that skin testing was unable to predict to which insects the animals were allergic, as the affected horses reacted to extracts from *Culicoides* not found in Louisiana.

Lane Foil *Baton Rouge, Louisiana, USA* presented data from insect trapping done in the environment and off the horses affected with CHS in Louisiana. One horse afflicted with a dorsally distributed pruritic dermatitis was seen to improve significantly when moved to a different farm in the same vicinity. Light traps were set in the locale in which the horse was affected, and in the locale in which he was not affected. No one species was absent from the farm where the horse remained symptom free. On both farms *C. obsoletus* and *C. biguttatus* could be trapped off the horse on some occasions. Probably the most important factor in limiting this animal's disease was that the second farm was better drained and had a more windy exposure, allowing the horse to find protection from fly attack. Confirmation of *C. obsoletus* and *C. biguttatus* as the cause of *Culicoides* hypersensitivity in Louisiana horses was obtained by trapping flies directly off of affected horses from other farms in the same parish. Further confirmation came when two affected horses from other parts of the state were taken at sunset to a locale where *C. biguttatus*, a diurnal feeder, was known to be present in high numbers: one animal began to scratch immediately, whereas the other horse began to scratch at 3 to 4 h after exposure. These results suggested that the immunopathogenesis for each horse differed. The first horse showed signs compatible with an immediate IgE mediated hypersensitivity reaction; the second horse showed signs compatible with a late phase IgE response, or possibly the cutaneous basophil hypersensitivity reaction, as seen in dogs with flea allergy dermatitis.

Marianne Sloet *Utrecht, Holland* discussed equine insect hypersensitivity seen in Holland. This disease was diagnosed primarily in Icelandic ponies, and to a lesser extent, in Shetland and Welsh ponies. It was rarely seen in warm blooded breeds or in stabled ponies or horses. The affected horses were known to come from those geographic areas in which standing water is available for the life cycle of the insects. Ponies were often treated with long acting injectable corticosteroids, which induced laminitis in some patients. Effective treatment of CHS in Holland has consisted of the use of insecticides and repellents, particularly cattle ear tags attached to the halter or braided into the mane and tail. The major problems associated with this disease in Holland were in the area of client education: should affected animals be eliminated from the breeding program, and if so, how could they be reliably identified?

Discussion at this point centered around the issue of treatment, particularly stabling at night. It was noted that in many parts of the world, animals had no access to stables, or had access to an open building consisting of a roof only. The general consensus was that a solid barn with four walls provided the physical barrier required to keep *Culicoides* out, as they were easily trapped from the open barns described above. Dr Foil and Dr Fadok suggested that control in open barns could be accomplished with the use of fans, which provided a breeze significant enough to inhibit the flight of *Culicoides*.

Anthony Stannard *Davis, California, USA* presented examples of seasonal pruritic dermatoses seen in California, that did not conform to the insect hypersensitivities described in the literature. Many of these diseases had eosinophils in the biopsy, suggesting that they might be associated with an ectoparasite. The first syndrome was pruritic intermandibular dermatitis, seen alone as an individual entity, or as part of a more generalized pruritic dermatitis. This disease has been attributed to black fly allergy, although this has never been confirmed. Comments from the audience suggested that this disease was seen in other parts of the USA, in association with *Culicoides* hypersensitivity lesions, but not as a single entity. No one from Europe or Australia had seen it. This area on the horse was aspirated for *Culicoides* in the Florida study; only one insect was ever trapped. This could have been due to the technical difficulties associated with trapping from an area interfered with by a standard halter. Additional comments from the audience suggested that the lesions in the intermandibular area did not look clinically like those associated with classical black fly dermatitis.

The second syndrome was an intensely pruritic papular dermatitis seen only on the masseter areas of the face. The only geographic areas in which this disease has been seen, according to the participants, was California and Australia. It was suggested that perhaps this lesion *might* be associated with lice; cattle are known to have lice restricted to the head, and it has been observed by Dr Lane Foil that biting lice on horses have spread from mane to the face at night. This does not account completely, however, for the restriction of the lesions to the masseter area, as there is no equine louse that is restricted to the head. Perhaps food allergy might be worth pursuing in these horses.

The third syndrome was the extremely well delineated circular area on the chest characterized by alopecia and crusting, colloquially called 'hole in the chest'. Dr Stannard observed that this lesion has disappeared since ivermectin came into common use, suggesting onchocerciasis as the probable cause. The participants who had seen this disease concurred. *Culoicoides* hypersensitivity that occurs on the chest is never so clearly delineated.

Discussion at this point centred on the role of insects such as black flies and stable flies in causing equine skin disease. All the participants agreed that aural plaques, attributed in the past to black fly bites, were unlikely to be a manifestation of insect hypersensitivity, as the histopathology of these lesions is more compatible with a virus-induced disease. Dr Lane Foil reported that he has observed blackflies feeding inside the forelegs and in the ears of horses, causing lesions. *Stomoxys* as a cause of ventral midline dermatitis was discussed. These insects feed primarily on the legs; most participants noted foot stamping as a clinical sign. Dr Lane Foil suggested that these insects will feed on the neck and shoulders when population numbers are high. Their true role in the aetiology of equine insect hypersensitivity remains to be determined.

Most of the information available on *Culicoides* hypersensitivity concerns the entomology and clinical signs. The pathogenesis, from an immunologic and inflammatory point of view, has only been examined tentatively in the past; however, this is beginning to change.

Adrian Foster *Hatfield, Herts, UK* presented some preliminary data on the potential role of platelet activating factor (PAF) in the pathogenesis of *Culicoides* hypersensitivity. This lipid mediator has been shown to be involved in the pathogenesis of several human inflammatory dermatoses. Mr Foster had injected PAF intradermally into the skin of normal and affected horses, and found that this lipid mediator could induce wheal formation in both groups that peaked at 30 min, and that wheal formation increased with increasing concentrations of PAF. These data suggest that PAF can induce vascular permeability in the skin of the horse, and, therefore, that it is worth investigating as a putative mediator in the pathogenesis of insect hypersensitivity. Future areas of work could include the effect of PAF antagonists on the ability to induce skin test reactions in allergic horses to *Colicoides* extracts, further analysis of PAF injected sites by histopathology and determination of the ability of equine neutrophils, eosinophils, and other inflammatory cells to produce and/or respond to PAF.

Kenneth Baker *Dublin, Ireland* concluded the meeting with a discussion of the potential role for hyposensitization in the treatment of CHS. Because much information has been gathered already on the entomology, clinical signs, and skin test reactivity of affected horses, he suggested that research efforts in the area of CHS now should be directed toward the development of a viable antigen for treatment, as owners frequently had trouble complying with stabling regimens or frequent insecticide applications. Also, the potential hazards of glucocorticoid therapy are well known. Other non-steroidal antiinflammatory agents, such as evening primrose oil (EPO) have been tried; however, the minimal effective dose for the horse of 5 g is prohibitively expensive. The ideal antigen for hyposensitization would consist of salivary extracts; whole body extracts have not been successful in the treatment of venomous insect hypersensitivities in man, or flea allergy in dogs and cats. Dr Baker has been able to generate a flea extract with increased salivary components by placing the fleas in a glass tube and rolling them to induce salivation. It would be worthwhile to see if such a procedure would be effective for *Culicoides* flies, also. If a viable treatment extract can be obtained, horses ideally would be given immunotherapy prior to the onset of the insect season.

WORKSHOP CONCLUSIONS

1. *Culicoides* hypersensitivity in horses is seen throughout the world primarily as a dorsally distributed pruritic dermatitis. It can, however, be the cause of significant ventral midline dermatitis also. Development of ventral midline dermatitis may relate, in part, to the feeding behaviour of *Culicoides* species in the particular geographic area. There may be other host factors, including behavioural factors or mast cell reactivity or distribution, that influence disease distribution as well.
2. Intradermal skin testing, while suggesting reactivity to *Culicoides*, does not enable the determination of which species is actually causing the allergy. Commercially available whole body insect extracts, such as those of black fly, horse fly, or mosquito, may contain irritants or a generic insect antigen that cross-reacts with antigens found in

Culicoides; their use in intradermal skin testing is of questionable value at this time. The ideal skin testing antigen for insects would be a salivary extract. Some researchers have suggested that the 48-h reaction is more specific for *Culicoides* hypersensitivity than the 30-min reaction.

3. The role of black flies and stable flies in the induction of equine insect hypersensitivity remains unclear; entomologic studies, such as those performed for *Culicoides*, must be done. Drs Carol and Lane Foil have tested horses with stable fly, tabanid, and mosquito extracts, and have seen no significant reactions; other workers have reported skin test reactivity to these extracts. This issue needs to be resolved.

4. Platelet activating factor has been shown to induce vascular permeability in the skin of normal and allergic horses. This mediator, as well as others, should be examined further, so that a clearer picture of the immunologic and inflammatory mechanisms associated with equine insect hypersensitivity will emerge.

5. In spite of the poor response of flea allergic dogs and cats to flea antigen hyposensitization, this type of therapy for insect hypersensitivity in horses should be pursued. Venomous insect hypersensitivity in man has been treated successfully with hyposensitization using salivary extracts. If an extract enriched for salivary antigens could be made from *Culicoides*, hyposensitization would provide specific therapy for a disease frustrating to owner and veterinarian alike. If a major protein allergen could be identified, current recombinant DNA technology could allow for the cloning and expression of the gene in large quantities. The major issue at this point is financial: who will pay for the development of such a vaccine?

Workshop Report 3

Pigmentary Disturbances

E. Guaguere and Z. Alhaidari

Clinique Vétérinaire Saint Bernard, Lomme, France; and Clinique Vétérinaire, Roquefort Les Pins, France

E. Guaguere *Lomme, France* Disorders of melanin pigmentation are very common in many canine and feline dermatoses. Their aetiologic diagnosis often requires a very methodical clinicopathologic approach. A careful history and physical examination will permit the clinician to establish an inclusive differential diagnosis, which will determine the laboratory tests used. The topics of this workship will cover some new aspects of these disorders.

LENTIGO IN DOGS AND CATS

D.W. Scott *Ithaca, New York, USA* Lentigines are common lesions in dogs and are seen mostly in orange cats (Plate 28). Lentigo means lentil shaped spot. In man, there are three types of lentigo—lentigo simplex (a common form, and the only one recognized in animals), solar lentigo (lentigo senilis) (arises in sun-exposed skin), and lentigo maligna.

Lentigosis is a marker for genetic abnormalities such as: Leopard syndrome associated with abnormalities of heart, lungs and gastrointestinal tract and transmitted as an autosomal dominant trait; Lamb syndrome associated with multiple lentigines with visceral abnormalities; Peutz-Jeghers syndrome associated with multiple lentigines with multiple polyps of the gastrointestinal tract. These syndromes may exist in animals, but have not been recognized.

In veterinary medicine, lentigines have been described on dogs' teats, in a litter of pugs on the ventrum and extremities and on the lips, nose, and eyelids of orange cats.

Lentigo lesions are well demarcated melanocytic macules (1–10 mm diameter), not variable with the sun exposure.

In orange cats, lentigines are seen on the nose, lips and eyelids. The lesions gradually enlarge, and increase in number with time. There is no transition to melanoma. Diagnosis is based on history (young adult onset); physical examination (symmetrical, multiple lesions, melanotic macules); histology (sudden transition to heavily melanized epidermis and increased number of melanocytes with increased overload in epidermal cells). There is no therapy.

HISTOPATHOLOGICAL AND ULTRASTRUCTURAL STUDY ON THE BLUE DOBERMAN SYNDROME

E. Guaguere and A. Janin *Lille, France* The purpose of this study is to characterize the histological and ultrastructural features of pigmentary disturbances associated with the blue doberman syndrome (Plate 29).

The histopathological features reveal:

A superficial and follicular hyperkeratosis, with follicular cysts. Hair follicles are small and inactive (telogen).

A homogenous distribution of melanocytes with a melanosomic overload.

The presence of large aggregates of melanin within the hair cortex and medulla.

Melanin-laden cells in the base of the external root sheath and hair bulb.

Dermal macrophages (melanophages), sometimes surounding the base of the follicle.

A pigmentary incontinence (Plate 30).

Examination of affected hair reveals numerous large melanin aggregates, association with deformation and fracture of the hair cortex. These abnormalities seem to contribute to hair loss.

The ultrastructural study shows:

A normal number of melanocytes with a moderate activity. Their melanocytic dendrits are infrequent. The melanosomic overload of the melanocytes is very important.

A normal maturation of melanosomes. Melanosomes of stages 1, 2, 3, 4 can be observed, but there is an accumulation of the melanosomes at stage 4.

A variable size of the melanosomes. Small and large melanosomes (macromelanosomes) can be observed. The aspect of some macromelanosomes suggest a fusion of melanosomes.

The presence of vacuoles in the melanocytes, which shows an alteration of the cellular activity.

A defect in transfer of the melanosomes to the keratinocytes.

The presence of melanophagic cells and a pigmentary incontinence with macromelanosomes which proceeds from the death of the melanocytes.

The excessive melanin overload with mature melanosomes of variable size in the melanocytes and the small concentration of melanosomes in the keratinocytes suggests a defect in transfer of the melanosomes to the keratinocytes. It is difficult to know if the abnormalities of the melanosomes (macromelanosomes) are the cause or the consequence of the transfer defect.

ULTRASTRUCTURAL STUDY OF THE HUMAN AND CANINE ACANTHOSIS NIGRICANS

Z. Alhaidari *Roquefort les Pins, France*; **J.P. Ortonne** *Nice, France* In human acanthosis nigricans, the most obvious feature is the presence of large vacuoles inside the keratinocytes. It is associated with other degenerative changes characterized by a fragmentation of the keratin filaments which are packed and marginated. The melanocytes appear hyperactive and contain a large number of melanosomes at every step of maturation. The frequent presence of these melanosomes in the stratum corneum suggest a defect in their process of degradation.

In canine acanthosis nigricans, we also find signs of diskeratinization with fragmentation and margination of the tonofilaments but no vacuolization. The melanocytes are active and contain numerous mature melanosomes, which are found at all the levels of the epidermis. There is no present explanation for the presence in the basal layers of dendritic cells, with sometimes a very well developed endoplasmic reticulum, and no specific organelles.

The conclusions are:

Acanthosis nigricans is associated with an epidermal hypermelanosis related to a hyperstimulation of melanocytes.

The number of melanocytes is not increased.
A slight pigmentary incontinence is also present probably as a consequence of the overproduction of melanin.
Acanthosis nigricans is associated in both species with severe signs of dyskeratinization.
In man, the tritiated thymidine labelling index of epidermal keratinocytes is increased in acanthosis nigricans involved skin.
The hyperstimulation of melanocytes probably represents a secondary event due to a disruption of the homeostasis in the epidermal unit.

PATHOGENIC HYPOTHESIS OF PRIMARY ACANTHOSIS NIGRICANS

B. Hubert *Beziers, France* Two elements could be implicated in the pathogenesis of acanthosis nigricans: the propiocortine, a melanin precursor and the APUD system.

Propiocortine is a precursor of various hormones and neurotransmitters (ACTH, lipotrophic hormone, and MSH, endorphine). It is secreted by the hypothalamic and pituitary neurons in physiological conditions, and by the APUD cell system in pathological conditions as a consequence of the loss of the regulatory mechanism, which normally inhibits the production of propiocortine in these cells.

This regulation is under genetic and cellular control, loss of genetic control could be an explanation for primary acanthosis nigricans in the daschhund.

Clinical cases have often shown the link between acanthosis nigricans and tumours. So investigations have to be done and plans for future are to measure the level of propiocortin metabolites in cancerous animals, and to discover if the tumoural tissue is secreting such metabolites by itself or if it activates the APUD system.

GENETIC HYPOMELANOSIS AND AMELANOSIS

Albinism

E. Guaguere Albinism is an autosomal recessive disorder, described in several dog breeds. The pathogenic mechanism is a defect in the melanization of the melanosomes. In humans, recessive oculocutaneous albinism is divided into tyrosinase negative albinism and tyrosinase positive albinism. Albino dogs have a normal number of melanocytes, but they lack tyrosinase to produce melanin. Clinically, it is expressed by a generalized amelanosis of the skin, hair, and mucous membranes. Ocular manifestations are milder in dogs than in humans: blue eyes (rarely pink) and slightly modified visual acuity.

Ophthalmoscopic examination reveals a normal yellow tapetal fundus, but no pigment in the nontapetal fundus. The choroidal vessels are prominent against the white scleral background. Other patients may have no colour in the tapetum and bright orange colour of the fundus. Albino animals should not be used for breeding.

Chediak–Higashi syndrome

This disorder is an autosomal recessive, reported in humans and blue-smoke Persian cats. This hereditary abnormality is characterized by a generalized hypomelanosis (pigmentary dilution) and visual disorders such as photophobia and hypochromia of the irides. Increased susceptibility to infection is secondary to decreased chemotactic and bacteriocidal properties of leucocytes and is responsible for early death. Leucocytes, melanocytes, and many other cell types (kidney, liver) contain enlarged lysosomal granules. Gigantic melanosome complexes are also present in the phagosomes in melanocytes and keratinocytes. It is not clearly established if the complexes are synthesized as such, or result from the abnormal combination of melanosomes. Ultrastructural aspects suggest that hypomelanosis is secondary to an accelerated degradation of the melanosomes. There is no effective treatment, and affected cats should not be used for breeding.

Waardenburg-Klein syndrome

This syndrome is characterized by a hypomelanosis or amelanosis, a blue homochromia or heterochromia of the irides, and deafness. This association of genetically determined hearing loss and hypomelanosis or amelanosis had been described in humans, cats and several genotypes of mice. Hereditary deafness and pigmentation abnormalities, such as white spotting or the merling trait, are also found in many breeds of dogs: bull terrier, Sealyham terrier, collie and Dalmatian. Abnormalities of the inner ear responsible for the deafness are as follows: reduction in the number of cochlear coils, reduction of the saccular lumen, and retraction of the tectorial membrane (cats). The pathogenic mechanism is dual: a defect in the migration of the melanoblasts or their inability to survive in the skin and a defect in the differentiation of melanoblasts into melanocytes. In cats, this syndrome is transmitted as an autosomal dominant trait with incomplete penetrance. Affected animals should not be used for breeding.

Vitiligo

Vitiligo is an autosomal dominant hypomelanosis in humans, with a variable expressivity. In humans, three pathogeneses are commonly proposed: autoimmune, neurogenic, or hereditary. Vitiligo has been described in Belgian shepherds, German shepherds, collies (Plate 31) and a Siamese cat. In the USA, canine vitiligo is most commonly observed in rottweilers and doberman pinschers. The gradual depigmentation is more or less symmetric and appears generally before the age of 3 years and in various sites (nose, lips, oral mucosa and eyelids) (Plate 32). Poliosis (leukotrichia), focal or widespread, can be seen. The evolution is very unpredictable. Leukoderma, leucotrichia, or both, are often permanent. In some cases repigmentation is possible. Histologically, the condition is characterized by an absence of melanocytes and the absence of inflammation or other dermatohistopathological abnormalities.

Workshop Report 4

Nutrition and Skin Disease

Peter J. Ihrke and Candace A. Sousa

School of Veterinary Medicine, University of California, Davis, California, USA and Elvas Avenue Animal Hospital, Sacremento, California, USA

The broad topic of nutrition and skin disease can encompass nutritional skin diseases *per se* and the use of nutritional supplementation for the treatment of skin diseases. Controversy exists in both of these fields of study. Nutritional skin diseases may be caused by a dietary deficiency, dietary excess, or nutrient imbalance leading to differential absorption or metabolic utilization. Nutritional supplements may be used to correct a deficiency or for a pharmacologic effect. Supraphysiologic doses of dietary supplements such as fatty acids have been used recently in human and veterinary medicine as drugs to modulate the inflammatory response.

The frequency of occurrence of nutritional skin disease is controversial. In parts of the world where animals are fed either good quality food developed and manufactured for a specific species of animal or food prepared for human consumption, nutritional skin diseases are uncommon. In other circumstances, nutritional skin diseases may be a more common occurrence. Fat deficient rations, especially those packaged as dry dog foods, are possible because fat is the most expensive ingredient used in the manufacture of these diets. With storage they are subject to rancidity and leakage into the packaging material which may further reduce their content in the diet.

Previously published clinical reports of nutritional skin diseases should be critically scrutinized. Much of the work done in this area may be open to question. Specific nutrient deficiencies are difficult to prove biochemically. Clinical and histologic corroborating evidence also is difficult to obtain since the skin has only a limited number of potential reaction patterns.

Most reports of nutritional skin diseases may be categorized as fatty acid deficiencies, protein deficiency, vitamin deficiencies, mineral imbalances, or combined deficiencies. At Cornell Univeristy, vitamin E deficient diets have been shown to have an effect on the immune system. Animals followed for 2 years were found to have defects in their T-lymphocytes. Dogs that were fed vitamin E deficient diets for 4–6 weeks developed a light, non-adherent scaliness on the face and pinnae that overlay erythema and inflammation. After 6 months, the dogs became greasy and developed alopecia, especially over the face, pinnae and extremities. Histopathology showed a mononuclear, lymphocytic, perivascular dermatitis with mild epidermal hyperplasia and mild focal parakeratosis. When the dogs were again fed a diet containing vitamin E, there was a rapid regression of the lesions. Within 8 weeks, they were returned to immunologic normality. (This study has been previously reported in the *Journal of Companion Animal Practice* in 1987.)

In Sweden, many cases were noted several years ago of a dermatosis in large-breed puppies fed a soy-based dry dog food at the time of weaning. The animals developed thick crusting periorally, periocularly, over the elbows, hocks, abdomen, and between the pads on the ventral paws. When treated with zinc sulphate at 1–2 mg/kg daily without a diet change, all skin lesions resolved within 1 week. It is speculated that the high soy content of the diet impaired zinc absorption. Since then, the soy content of these diets has been lowered from 13.5% to almost zero, another vegetable source has been used, the meat content has been increased from 11 to 15% and the zinc content has been increased from 40 to 70 mg/kg.

In Siberian huskies, a similar clinical syndrome is seen that will occasionally respond to zinc therapy. There is strong evidence for a genetic predisposition. During lactation, but not gestation, the clinical signs worsen. It is not known conclusively if this is due to a primary alimentary problem.

In California several years ago, a series of 13 dogs with a mean age of 1 year also developed a similar clinical pattern after being fed a poor quality, corn-based generic dog food. The dogs were depressed, had a low-grade fever and enlarged peripheral lymph nodes. Histopathology of the lesions showed both surface and follicular parakeratosis, mild dyskeratosis and a diffuse mixed cellular superficial dermal infiltrate. The diet contained 55 mg/kg of zinc but its bioavailability could not be assayed. There was a rapid clinical improvement once the dogs were fed a diet that met NRC requirements and was complete and balanced.

Foods such as soy and corn, which are high in phytates, can bind zinc and impair its absorption. Zinc also interacts with calcium and copper.

The term nutrient-responsive dermatosis has become popular as a descriptive disease label and has been used to encompass syndromes characterized by nutrient deficiency, nutrient imbalances or the genetic inability of an animal to absorb or metabolize a nutrient. Vitamin A has been used to treat seborrhoeic disorders but its close relationship to synthetic retinoids may be the reason for its effectiveness.

It has been observed clinically that animals treated with the addition of fats to their diets seem to get better. Recent work has shown that supplying these animals with N6 fatty acids (gamma linolenic acid, linoleic acid) improves their coats. Fish oil has also been shown to participate in the arachidonic acid cascade to inhibit the production of the two series prostaglandins, thromboxanes and leukotrienes. Future treatment of atopy in the dog and other imflammatory skin disease may involve the use of more fatty acid supplementation.

Workshop Report 5

Ticks: Immunity to Ticks and Tick-borne Diseases

J.P. Opdebeeck and S. Merchant

Department of Parasitology, University of Queensland, St Lucia, Brisbane, Australia; and School of Veterinary Medicine, Louisiana State University, Louisiana, USA

Ticks attach mechanically to their host by inserting their mouthparts to variable depths in the skin; some ticks also secrete a cement-like substance in the shape of a cone, to strengthen their attachment. A cavity forms in the vicinity of the mouthparts and this fills with tissue fluids, leucocytes and whole blood. The dominant cell types in the infiltrate are neutrophilic leucocytes and monocytes in naive hosts (Tatchell and Moorhouse, 1968). Numerous basophilic leucocytes are found in the feeding lesion in hosts previously exposed to ticks and appearance of these cells coincides with development of antigen specific responses by lymphocytes (Wikel *et al.*, 1978) and resistance. Treatment of the host with antisera against basophilic leucocytes causes a decrease in resistance whereas antisera against eosinophilic leucocytes does not depress immunity significantly (Brown *et al.*, 1982).

Saliva injected in by feeding ticks contains substances which are active in the host. The saliva of *Ixodes dammini*, a tick which transmits Lyme disease in the USA, has antihaemostatic, antiinflammatory, and immunosuppressive activity in its host (Ribeiro *et al.*, 1985). Immunosuppression of the host by feeding ticks has mainly been assayed by the responses of lymphocytes to mitogens. Cells collected from guinea pigs infested with *Dermacentor andersoni* had depressed responses to T-lymphocyte mitogens but not to B-lymphocyte mitogens (Wikel, 1982). However, we found no effect on the response of bovine lymphocytes to Concanavalin A in lymphocyte blastogenesis assay following infestation with up to 160 000 *Boophilus microplus* (Opdebeeck and Daly, submitted). *Amblyomma variegatum* appears to have more effective life-cycle on goats after they have been infested 11 times, implying immunosuppression of the host may be occurring (Barré, reported in this workshop). It has also been suggested that *Babesia bovis*, a piroplasm that causes disease in cattle, suppresses its host against *B. microplus*, its tick vector (Callow and Stewart, 1978); the advantages of suppression for both parasites are obvious.

Acquired immunity, resulting from repeated infestation with ticks, has been described in several experimental model systems and also in natural host-parasite systems e.g. cattle with *B. microplus*, and African ticks; the acquisition of resistance by cattle with *Bos indicus* genes is more rapid and effective than by those with *Bos taurus* genes (Rechav, 1987). Because of the development of an acquired immunity, much effort has been directed towards the development of vaccines against ticks using antigens extracted from salivary glands. The protection provided by these vaccines has, however, been disappointingly low (e.g. 24% greater rejection of ticks from vaccinated animals compared to control animals) (Brown, 1986).

The focus of work in tick vaccination has shifted, therefore, towards attempts to generate protective immune responses against so-called concealed antigens (see review by Willadsen and Kemp, 1988). These concealed antigens are believed to be unavailable to drive the immune system of the host during a natural infestation; however immunization with these concealed antigens generates immune responses which may subsequently be delivered to an appropriate site in the tick via the blood meal and there cause damage to the tick (Plate 33). This principle was exploited when crude extracts of guts from haematophagous ectoparasites were used to provide significant protection against ticks, mosquitoes, and stable flies. Subsequently, we showed that Hereford cattle, immunized with membrane extracts purified from the midgut of *B. microplus*, were protected (>90% decrease in tick egg production) against challenge with 60 000 larval ticks (Opdebeeck *et al.*, 1988a). The protection was clearly associated with the membrane fraction of the gut and this has been confirmed in more recent work. Immune responses to a vaccine prepared from synganglia (nervous tissue) alone did not damage feeding ticks (Opdebeeck *et al.*, 1988b) despite the fact that host immunoglobulins pass intact across the gut of ticks (Ackerman *et al.*, 1981) and may bind specifically to internal organs.

The levels of antibodies induced by vaccination with gut membrane (GM) are significantly correlated to protection (Wong and Opdebeeck, 1989) and are higher than the levels induced by repeated infestation. Antibodies in the sera of vaccinated and infested cattle recognized extracts of salivary gland, gut and larvae, implying that GM is not a concealed group of antigens, although its protective component(s) may well be concealed (Opdebeeck and Daly, submitted).

Recently, extracts from larval ticks, purified by immunoaffinity chromatography, using as ligands immunoglobulins from an immune steer vaccinated with tick midgut antigens, provided significant protection (>80%) against challenge with ticks (Opdebeeck *et al.*, 1989). Contrary to previous popular opinion, protective gut antigens are not unique to the developing midgut of rapidly engorging ticks, but are also common to the unfed larval tick.

Protective antigens are being purified from whole adult tick extracts (Willadsen *et al.*, 1988) and from tick gut (Wong and Opdebeeck, 1989). However, great individual variation in protective responses has been shown to be associated with crude and partly purified vaccines. This variation is at least partly related to genetic variation in cattle and the role of the major histocompatibility complex (MHC) in regulating immune responses is well known. The presence of three MHC antigens (MB5, MB14, MB20) had significant effects on the immunity induced by GM vaccines in 43 cattle (Wong and Opdebeeck, 1989) and an effective tick vaccine will likely be multicomponent in order to stimulate immunity in those cattle which may otherwise develop a poor response to a single component. Multicomponent vaccines would also decrease the likelihood of resistance developing in ticks.

Tick vaccines are unlikely to be made of native antigen, mainly because availability of antigen is limited, despite the efficiency of low levels of antigen in stimulating effective immune responses (Jackson and Opdebeeck, 1990). Possibilities for scaling up production of antigens for practical use include recombinant DNA technology, surrrogate antigens, tissue culture of cells, chemical synthesis and the use of vector viruses. The first three methods are currently being investigated to produce protective tick antigens. Surrogate antigens can be made by using protective antibodies to form antiidiotypic antibodies which mirror the image of the inducing antigen and these antiidiotypic antibodies can therefore be used as antigen in the host. This form of antigen production is particularly useful where it is desirable to generate an immune response against a carbohydrate epitope.

The effect of tick vaccines on the transmission of tick-borne diseases, e.g. arboviruses, is currently being studied. Interference with feeding of ticks which cause tick paralysis may affect the disease because the severity of the paralysis is proportional to the time the tick feeds. Decreasing the population of ticks where the tick acts as a vector of a disease e.g. babesiosis would likely decrease the prevalence of the disease. Nonetheless, it is most probable that tick-borne diseases will have to be controlled by either a specific pathogen vaccine or by its combination with tick vaccines rather than by a tick vaccine alone.

Some cross-reactive/common antigens between tick species have been reported but the possibility of cross protection between economically important species such as *B. microplus* and African ticks has yet to be addressed.

REFERENCES

Ackerman, S., Clare, F.B. and McGill, T.W. (1981). Passage of host serum components, including antibody, across the digestive tract of *Dermacentor variabilis* (Say). *Journal of Parasitology* **67**: 737–740.

Brown, S.J. (1986). *Amblyomma americanum*: Physiochemical isolation of a protein derived from the tick salivary gland that is capable of inducing immune resistance in guinea pigs. *Experimental Parasitology* **62**: 40–50.

Brown, S.J., Galli, S.J., Gleich, G.J. (1982). Ablation of immunity to *Amblyomma americanum* by anti-basophil serum: Cooperation between basophils and eosinophils in expression of immunity to ectoparasites (ticks) in guinea pigs. *Journal of Immunology* **129**: 790–795.

Callow, L.L. and Stewart, N.P. (1978). Immunosuppression by *Babesia bovis* against its tick vector, *Boophilus microplus. Nature* **272**: 818–819.

Jackson, L.A. and Opdebeeck, J.P. (1990). The effect of antigen concentration and vaccine regimen on the immunity induced by membrane antigens from the midgut of *Boophilus microplus. Immunology* (in press).

Opdebeeck, J.P. and Daly, K.E. Immune responses of infested and vaccinated Hereford cattle to antigens of the cattle tick, *Boophilus microplus.* (Submitted)

Opdebeeck, J.P., Wong, J.Y.M., Jackson, L.A. (1988a). Hereford cattle immunized and protected against *Boophilus microplus* with soluble and membrane-associated antigens from the midgut of ticks. *Parasite Immunology* **10**: 405–410.

Opdebeeck, J.P., Wong, J.Y.M., Jackson, L.A. (1988b). Vaccines to protect Hereford cattle against the cattle tick, *Boophilus microplus. Immunology* **63**: 363–367.

Opdebeeck, J.P., Wong, J.Y.M. and Dobson, C. (1989). Hereford cattle protected against *Boophilus microplus* with antigens purified by immunoaffinity chromatography from larval and adult ticks. *Immunology* **67**: 388–393.

Rechav, Y. (1987). Resistance of Brahman and Hereford cattle to African ticks with reference to serum Gamma globulin levels and blood composition. *Experimental & Applied Acarology* **3**: 219–232.

Ribeiro, J.M.C., Makoul, G.T., Levine, J. (1985). Antihemostatic, anti-inflammatory and immunosuppressive properties of the saliva of a tick, *Ixodes dammini. Journal of Experimental Medicine* **161**: 332–344.

Tatchell, R.J. and Moorhouse, D.E. (1968). The feeding processes of the cattle tick *Boophilus microplus* (Canestrini). Part II. The sequence of host-tissue changes. *Parasitology* **58**: 441–459.

Wikel, S.K. (1982). Influence of *Dermacentor andersoni* infestation on lymphocyte responsiveness to mitogens. *Annals of Tropical Medicine and Parasitology* **76**: 627–632.

Wickel, S.K., Graham, J.E. and Allen, J.R. (1978). Acquired resistance to ticks. IV. Skin reactivity and *in vitro* lymphocyte responsiveness to salivary gland antigen. *Immunology* **32**: 257–263.

Willadsen, P. and Kemp, D.H. (1988). Vaccination with 'concealed' antigens for tick control. *Parasitology Today* **4**: 196–198.

Willadsen, P., McKenna, R.V. and Riding, G.A. (1988). Isolation from the cattle tick, *Boophilus microplus*, of antigenic material capable of eliciting a protective immunological response in the bovine host. *International Journal for Parasitology* **18**: 183–189.

Wong, J.Y.M. and Opdebeeck, J.P. (1989). Protective efficacy of antigens solubilized from gut membranes of the cattle tick, *Boophilus microplus. Immunology* **66**: 149–155.

Workshop Report 6

Dietary Allergy

Stephen D. White and Ian S. Mason

Veterinary Teaching Hospital, Colorado State University, Fort Collins, Colorado, USA; and Albert Animal Hospital, Springwood, Queensland, Australia

Stephen D. White *Fort Collins, Colorado, USA* Dietary allergy or hypersensitivity in dogs and cats has no age, sex or breed predilection. A recent change of diet is unusual; most affected animals have been fed the offending diet for 2 years or more. In dogs, the clinical signs commonly include pruritus, erythema and a papular eruption although epidermal collarette formation, seborrhoea, otitis externa and pododermatitis are occasionally seen. In cats, pruritus, alopecia, papular eruptions and eosinophilic plaques may be present and in around 45% of cases papular and crusting lesions will be localized to the head (Plates 34, 35 and 36).

Restriction diets should be tailored to the individual and should contain, if possible, sources of food which are novel to the animal. The diet should be fed *exclusively* for at least 3 weeks and no chewy toys, snacks or palatable medications given during this period. Cats should be kept indoors during the dietary trial.

Due to the problems associated with the use of elimination diets in the diagnosis of food allergy (prolonged duration [> 3 weeks], compliance problems, expense) an *in vitro* test has been sought. A radioallergosorbent test (RAST) has been developed in the USA to detect IgE against dietary allergens but a number of problems have been recorded.

IgE to food allergens has been detected in clinically normal dogs.
Only IgE to allergens containing amino acids can be assayed.
The accuracy of the test varies between antigens.
Antigens are poorly characterized.
Results vary with seasonal and other factors.

RAST was performed on blood samples from dogs with food allergy, healthy dogs and dogs with skin disease unrelated to diet. All of the healthy dogs and 75% of the dogs with other skin diseases had antibody to dietary allergens. The dogs with confirmed dietary allergy also had IgE towards food allergens but in most instances the substances implicated by the test were not the ones which initiated the disease. Hence, there is a poor correlation between RAST results and clinical response in dogs and at present no substitute for the use of elimination diets and provocative exposure in the diagnosis of food hypersensitivity.

Lowell Ackerman *Toronto, Canada* The terminology pertaining to adverse reactions to foods is confusing. Hypersensitivity implies that an immune-mediated (Type I, II or IV) reaction has occurred which is unrelated to any physiological effect of the food. Dietary ingredients inducing such reactions include: beef, pork, chicken, milk, whey, eggs and fish. The antigenic constituents of these foods are poorly characterized glycoproteins (molecular weight 18–36 kDaltons). Cooking and processing may alter the antigenic make-up of a diet.

In man, reactions to food are often not immune-mediated, such dietary intolerances may result from idiosyncratic reactions, toxicological and pharmacological effects and metabolic defects.

Idiosyncratic reactions: can be initiated potentially by any product in a sensitive individual.

Toxic effects: e.g. botulism, shellfish poisoning and additives (tartrazine, sulphites).

Pharmacological effects: some foods contain vasoactive amines (e.g. tyramine in some cheeses or histamine in scromboid fish), lectins, mast-cell degranulating agents, etc. may induce a 'mock' allergic reaction.

Metabolic defects: individuals may have enzyme deficiencies (e.g. lactase deficiency leading to milk intolerance) or gastrointestinal problems such as ulceration which leads to intolerance of certain foods.

Clinical signs of food intolerance vary and can mimic many other diseases.

In order to diagnose dietary hypersensitivity or intolerance a hypoallergenic diet should be administered for at least 4 weeks. If clinical improvement occurs then provocative challenge with the original diet should be undertaken to eliminate the possibility of spontaneous recovery. Following diagnosis, 80% of dogs can be maintained on commercially prepared 'hypoallergenic' diets.

Ewan Ferguson *London, UK* In cases of suspected food hypersensitivity the animal's original diet should be carefully examined to facilitate avoidance of possible offending allergens when formulating an elimination diet. Such diets should be based on a single novel protein source and, in dogs, a single novel carbohydrate source. More than 70% of 84 dogs seen as dermatology referrals were fed canned diets with mixer (kibble) biscuits. In the UK such diets may contain beef, chicken, lamb, flours, vegetable oils, binders, supplements and occasionally horse meat and cereals. Mixer biscuits may contain chicken, beef, wheat, sunflower oil and glucose. Furthermore, many dogs receive home cooked meats, complete diets, vegetables, table-scraps and nutritional/vitamin supplements. From these observations it is recommended that in most instances elimination diets may be based on pork, rabbit and fish in dogs and on pork and rabbit in cats. Compliance problems arise as owners feel that such dietary restriction implies a 'rejection' of their pet and a denial of its status within a household.

In the UK canned commercial 'hypoallergenic' diets contain rice, vegetable oils and binding agents with either chicken or lamb. Many pets receive such products in their normal ration and so canned diets cannot be used for diagnosis but should be evaluated for use in maintenance.

Ulla Petersson *Sparsor, Sweden* Following the diagnosis and successful stabilization of dogs with food allergy, relapses may occur. In some instances another disorder may have developed such as ectoparasitism, pyoderma or atopic dermatitis. It is not inconceivable that dogs with an immunological defect towards one source of allergens (the gastrointestinal tract) may become sensitized to allergens from other sources such as the respiratory tract. Of 72 dogs with confirmed atopic dermatitis, 7% had concomitant dietary hypersensitivity and required both elimination diets and hyposensitization.

Isabelle Remy *Belgium* Dietary hypersensitivity was diagnosed in 43 dogs and 10 cats. No breed or age predisposition was observed. The age range of onset of signs was 4 months to 5 years (mean: 2.4 years) in dogs and 6 months to 10.5 years (mean: 4 years) in cats. Female animals accounted for 60% of the feline cases and 39% of the canine cases. In 23 dogs, beef was the food responsible for the condition. Pruritus was the major clinical feature in both species. In dogs folliculitis, seborrhoea, lichenification, hyperpigmentation, pyotraumatic dermatitis and otitis externa were also recorded. In two dogs chronic enteritis was present. Intradermal skin tests were performed in 42 of the dogs. In six dogs a positive response was observed suggesting that concomitant atopic dermatitis may be a feature of this disease. In cats miliary dermatitis, psychogenic alopecia, crusting of head and neck, eosinophilic plaques and linear granuloma were observed. In both species glucocorticoids were less effective than anticipated in controlling pruritus.

Candace Sousa *Sacramento, California, USA* A food eruption affecting three dalmatians was reported. It was characterized by facial and groin pruritus with no primary lesion and responded to elimination diets.

Philippe Denerolle *Le Seyne-Sur-Mer, France* Two cases of feline dietary hypersensitivity were reported. The diagnosis was said to be difficult to achieve as cats may show reluctance to eat elimination diets due to low palatability. Both cases appeared to be poorly responsive to glucocorticoids.

Workshop Report 7

Dermatophilosis

N. Barré and S. Woodman

Institut d'Elevage et de Médecine des Pays Tropicaux, Guadeloupe, French West Indies; and Station de Pathol.-Immunol., Centre INRA de Tours-Nouzilly, Monnaie, France

N. Barré *Guadeloupe, France* Dermatophilosis is a widespread disease occurring in regions of permanent or seasonal high humidity and is particularly common in West Africa and the Caribbean. The disease, which is caused by the filamentous bacterium *Dermatophilus congolensis*, can be described as a chronic exudative dermatitis and is characterized by often spectacular clinical lesions composed of thick scabs. Dermatophilosis, although found in many species, primarily affects herbivores particularly cattle. It seems that natural selection has occurred since African Zebu in endemic areas are much more resistant than imported Brahman-type Asian Zebu. Losses through dermatophilosis vary but, in exotic breeds, morbidity of 100% is not rare and mortality is often around 60% (Plates 37–40).

One of the more curious aspects of the disease is the impossibility of reproducing severe, generalized dermatophilosis by experimental application of *D. congolensis*, although lesions are easily induced they are always mild and heal rapidly. In contrast, natural transmission can induce a variety of forms including a subclinical carrier state which can be detected by serological or bacteriological methods. At the other end of the disease spectrum animals are affected by chronic and widespread lesions. These generalized cases arise following development of primary persistant lesions which usually commence at sites of skin damage.

The first question I would like to introduce is that of the mode of transmission. We do not know if the only source of infection is the scabs of affected animals or whether the skin or fleece of subclinical carriers can act as the source. Also, perhaps biting arthropods can retain *D. congolensis* for a long time and the bacterium may be able to survive long periods in the soil. The actual mode of transmission is also unclear; it may occur via direct contact, biting arthropods, thorn scratches, soil etc. In Guadeloupe we suspect the role of biting insects such as *Culicoides*. In contrast, it seems unlikely that *Amblyomma variegatum* is involved in direct transmission since we have not found *D. congolensis* present in the next life-cycle of the tick following feeding on infected animals. We have noted primary lesions on animals in Guadeloupe at various sites of skin damage. These include tick attachment sites and the preferential biting sites of *Stomoxys*, mosquitos and *Culicoides*. Lesions can also often be seen spreading from scratches caused by thorns and, in breeds with areas of white skin, sun burn irritation can favour the spread of *D. congolensis*.

Probably the least understood aspect of the pathogenesis of the disease is how it becomes generalized to affect the whole of the body thus inducing loss of condition and even mortality. We know that this generalization does not occur following experimental infection even when factors considered to be involved in the aetiology of the disease, such as rain or tick infestation, are reproduced. Furthermore, generalization does not occur in certain breeds although we do not know if this resistance is a result of a better immune response, either local or general, to infection or of the physical characteristics of the skin such as the thickness of the *Stratum corneum* and the sebaceous film or the presence of a competitive microflora.

On susceptible animals, generalization to the severe form of the disease occurs during humid periods and nearly always on grazing animals; those kept indoors are usually not seriously affected. The lesions tend to spread preferentially over certain anatomical sites such as the back, sides and sacrum of cattle; one must remember that these are not the preferential tick attachment sites. The progression of the disease to a generalized state is probably due to a host imbalance which favours the growth of the pathogen. We can hypothesize that the imbalance is induced by factors affecting local skin resistance such as water, immunological inhibitors found in tick saliva and/or factors affecting the general immune response. Thus, for example, *D. congolensis* could itself be immunosuppressive or tick saliva may have immunosuppressive properties. Alternatively, certain viruses may be inoculated into the animals along with the tick saliva. Finally, a disturbance in the regulation of the immune responses may bring about a tolerant state, dominance of T-suppressor cells, the occurrence of blocking antibodies or an autoimmune disorder all or which may favour progression of the disease.

In conclusion, I would like to highlight three linked areas which are poorly understood and are much in need of further investigation. These are the role of arthropods in the transmission of *D. congolensis*, the immune response in experimental dermatophilosis and in particular the cellular and humoral mechanisms which are involved in rapid healing and, finally, the reasons for the failure of the immune response in natural cases leading to generalization of infection.

D. Jenkinson *Edinburgh, UK* How frequently do you see parapox and pox infections in association with dermatophilosis in the tropics?

N. Barré They are present in some cases.

D. Jenkinson So it is possible that a regular association exists?

N. Barré Yes.

O.O. Oduye *Ibadan, Nigeria* The occurrence of pox virions in *D. congolensis* lesions has already been noted by Isitor and there is no doubt that there is an association but we do not know if such observations would be repeated in every case.

D. Jenkinson Orf virus is very often present in dermatophilosis cases in Scotland but this fact is often missed since the virus has latent periods when you would not be able to find it even if you were looking for it.

V.A. Fadok *Denver, Col., USA* We have observed that horses and cattle in Florida which are heavily parasitized by gastrointestinal worms seem to develop the most severe cases of generalized dermatophilosis. Have others made this observation and is there data to support the hypothesis that gastrointestinal parasites are immunosuppressive? We have also noted that dermatophilosis is often associated with lymphosarcoma in horses.

O.O. Oduye *Dermatophilus congolensis* on its own causes no problems; generalized infections are invariably associated with predisposing factors such as orf or pox infections, trypanosomiasis, babesiosis or anaplasmosis. In fact 50–70% of cattle in Nigeria are infected with trypanosomes.

D.H. Lloyd *London, UK* We looked at theileriosis in St Kitts and Nevis and found no correlation between *Theileria* and dermatophilosis.

O.O. Oduye Which *Theileria*, *annulata* or *parva*?

D.H. Lloyd *Theileria mutans*.

O.O. Oduye But *mutans*, although widespread, is supposed to be a non-pathogen.

Chermette *Masons-Alfort, France* What about the survival of *D. congolensis* in pastures? We found infected animals surrounded by apparently healthy ones in adjacent fields so where did the infection come from?

D. Martinez *Guadeloupe, France* The resistance of *D. congolensis* depends on the soil type and the water content; it can survive at least two months in the clay soils we have in Guadeloupe.

C.B. Hart *London, UK* Were you looking at filament or zoospore survival? The filaments are killed easily whereas the zoospores are much more resistant.

D. Martinez We did not differentiate between the two.

O.O. Oduye The cocci are protected as long as they remain in filaments in the scab; in fact, isolates made by Stableforth in 1938 and kept in the scab were still viable in 1970.

D. Martinez Yes, but the scabs must be kept dry.

S. How *London, UK* *D. congolensis* is certainly viable after 10 years if kept dry.

D.H. Lloyd There is also the complicating factor of subclinical infection to consider. One of the biggest surveys, which was carried out on sheep by Hart, found extensive occurrence of *D. congolensis* but this was subclinical. This fact is also brought out by the frequent observations made by tanners of hide damage whereas infections were never noticed whilst the animals were still alive. It is also worth pointing out that small mammals can carry *D. congolensis*.

M. Sloet *Utrecht, Holland* Cases of dermatophilosis in horses are often referred to us at Utrecht University. These animals present with characteristic, painful lesions usually on the dorsal surface and sacrum. The cases are most frequently seen in the spring and autumn which are the wettest seasons and occur in horses which have been kept outside. We diagnose dermatophilosis on the basis of clinical symptoms, on cultures of smears made from scab material and on Gram stains. Our treatment consists of keeping the animals in a clean, dry stable and clipping the affected areas which are then washed every other day with Povidone iodine (Betadine®) shampoo. The shampoo is left on the skin for 15–30 min and then the scab pulled off. We find this treatment very successful and hardly ever have to use antibiotics. For animals with particularly deep lesions we also apply pure Betadine after the shampooing but we never use the Betadine scrub because this has an alcohol base which can cause allergic reactions in some horses.

We find it very interesting that cross-infection never occurs between the affected animals and other horses even though they are kept in close contact. Another point is that we have not noticed an association between dermatophilosis and parasite infections.

N. Barré Have you tried corticosteroid treatment?

M. Sloet No but all our cases are referred to us and have often been treated, unsuccessfully, beforehand with corticosteroids or even antimycotics.

D.H. Lloyd Are the limbs usually affected?

M. Sloet No, sometimes the infection does spread to the legs but we have never seen it solely in this region.

D. Martinez In the Caribbean we have observed a geographical correlation between the occurrence of *Amblyomma variegatum* ticks and that of severe dermatophilosis. This association has also been noted in Africa. We tested the hypothesis that *A. variegatum* may be a vector for dermatophilosis by allowing the ticks to feed on infected animals and then examining them for the presence of *D. congolensis*. We were unable to isolate the bacterium from either engrossed larvae or from nymphs or, indeed, from the male ticks which emerged from the nymphs. In contrast, we did isolate *D. congolensis* from the male ticks which had directly fed on the animals. However, since the males die after feeding they can hardly act as vectors for the disease.

In another experiment we kept 20 goats, imported from a tick-free and dermatophilosis-free island, in a tick-free environment and found that after 3 weeks 20% were seropositive for *D. congolensis* and after 8 weeks 70% were seropositive. Furthermore, again using previously unexposed goats, we allowed 12 *A. variegatum* females to attach to the animals and found that all the goats soon showed high antibody titres to *D. congolensis*. Eventually, all the animals died of dermatophilosis. In contrast, those goats which were kept free of ticks did not develop lesions although they did have high *D. congolensis* antibody titres. So, it is obvious that a close association exists between *A. variegatum* ticks and the occurrence of severe dermatophilosis. However, the relationship is not a simple one since *D. congolensis* lesions are most commonly found on the upper part of the body whereas the ticks preferentially attach to the lower parts.

S. How We have been working on the possibility of protecting against dermatophilosis by vaccination. We compared three different types of vaccine: 1) a 1:1 mixture of killed, whole *D. congolensis* cells and incomplete adjuvant 2) live *D. congolensis* and 3) an immunostimulatory complex (ISCOMS) vaccine. ISCOMS are 20 nm particles made of antigen and Quill A® adjuvant and theoretically give a prolonged stimulation to the immune system. For each type of vaccine, six female New Zealand White rabbits were given two doses separated by 4 weeks. The animals were then challenged with between 10^2 and 10^8 *D. congolensis* zoospores and the resulting lesions scored by the same observer. We noted a clear, dose-dependent response to infection. On control animals the lesions had resolved by Day 28 with the peak of infection occuring around Day 8.

For rabbits which had been vaccinated with whole killed cells in incomplete Freunds adjuvant we observed a reduction in the severity of the lesions and an increase in the dose required to produce noticeable lesions as compared with controls. We also found that the infection resolved more quickly than those of controls with the peak occurring on Day 2.

In contrast, there was no marked difference in the infective dose required for rabbits vaccinated with live *D. congolensis* than for controls. However, a reduction in the severity of lesions did occur and these also resolved more quickly with the peak of infection occurring between Days 2 and 4.

Rabbits vaccinated with ISCOMS also required the same infective dose as controls. However, the lesions did resolve more quickly and there was some reduction in severity but this was not as marked as for the other types of vaccine.

Thus, we can produce a degree of protection by vaccination but the immunity is not complete. However, we were giving extremely high challenge doses e.g. 10^8 zoospores over a 2 cm^2 area, which would presumably not be encountered in the field, so I do think that this is a promising avenue of research.

C.B. Hart I would like briefly to describe a treatment which I found to be successful some years ago. Having heard that *D. congolensis* zoospores lose their flagellae after treatment with trivalent metals, we tried dipping naturally infected sheep, just once, in potassium aluminium sulphate solution. We found that the lesions disappeared whereas they persisted on the sheep which we had not dipped.

O.O. Oduye It is most important to stress that *D. congolensis* is an opportunist. As Dominique Martinez has just shown us, animals exposed only to *D. congolensis* do not develop generalized lesions whereas this does occur if ticks are present. It is certainly essential that the skin is damaged for an infection to occur and progress. Dermatophilosis is a major problem in developing countries; for example, an entire stock of 500 Fresians was wiped out in Nigeria a few years ago. In fact, there are no exotic breeds surviving in Nigeria and our own breeds are poor milk producers. What intrigues me most is that *D. congolensis* infections only seem to become fatal if the animal's legs are affected.

N. Barré In Guadeloupe the local Zebu breed, which was imported from Africa about 200 years ago along with the tick, is completely resistant to dermatophilosis whereas imported breeds are susceptible. Also, *Amblyomma* only reached Martinque recently and the Creole Zebu breed there is just as susceptible as the European breeds.

D. Jenkinson If it is a question of whether *D. congolensis* is transmitted by *Amblyomma* or *Culicoides* this could be easily determined by looking for the presence of the organism on the arthropods using anti-*D. congolensis* mononclonal antibodies.

O.O. Oduye Oppong has already found evidence of *D. congolensis* in ticks but this does necessarily mean that enough is present for an infective dose and after a tick has fed it falls off the animal and does not get the chance to feed again.

D.H. Lloyd Similar work was done by Richard who showed that *Musca* and *Stomoxys* flies can transmit *D. congolensis*. On another subject, I would like to ask who prefers topical and who prefers systemic treatment?

V.A. Fadok We use both for the treatment of cattle and this is very successful even when there is lower limb involvement.

At this point the workshop ran out of time and was concluded by Dr Lloyd's comment that the dermatophilosis conference held in Nigeria several years ago had also had to stop before the discussion had finished and that was after several days rather than just one hour.

REFERENCES

Isitor, G.N., Kazeem, H.N., Njoku, C.O., Adegboye, D.S. and Dellmann, H.D. (1988). Frequency of involvement of pox virions in lesions of bovine dermatophilosis. *Tropical Animal Health and Production* **20**: 2–10.

Richard, J.L. and Pier, A.C. (1966). Transmission of *Dermatophilus congolensis* by *Stomoxys calcitrans* and *Musca domestica. American Journal of Veterinary Research* **27**: 419–423.

Workshop Report 8

Otitis Externa

Beat Bigler and Sandra R. Merchant

Kleintierpraxis Laupeneck, Bern, Switzerland; and School of Veterinary Medicine, Louisiana State University, Lousiana, USA

Beat Bigler *Berne, Switzerland* A recommended source of reference on ear diseases is *The Veterinary Clinics of North America, Small Animal Practice* July 1988; **18**: 4, Diseases of the Ear Canal.

It is critical to remember that the term 'otitis externa' means inflammation of the external auditory canal, without implying any underlying cause; therefore patients treated symptomatically, with no attempt to address the causative factor(s), are likely to have a relapse or recurrences of the problem.

Causative factors of otitis externa include:

Primary factors: parasites, foreign bodies, hypersensitivity diseases, disorders of keratinization and autoimmune diseases.

Predisposing factors: conformation, ear canal maceration, climatic variation, treatment errors, obstructive ear disease, anal sac disease, pyrexia and systemic disease.

Perpetuating factors: bacteria, yeast, otitis media and progressive pathologic changes.

Of the hypersensitivity diseases causing otitis externa, 50% of the atopic dogs and 50% of the dogs suffering from food allergic dermatitis will have evidence of otitis externa. A few of these dogs will have otitis externa as the only evidence of their allergic disease. Less often flea bite allergy will have concomitant otitis externa. Contact allergy and drug eruptions are also hypersensitivity diseases that can cause otitis externa.

Otitis externa will be seen in more than 90% of the cases of seborrhoea caused by a disorder in keratinization. Auto-immune disease can affect primarily the pinna with extension down the ear canal. These include systemic lupus erthematosus, pemphigus vulgaris and pemphigus foliaceus.

Bacteria found in otitis externa ears include *Staphylococcus*, *Pseudomonas*, *β-Streptococcus*, *Proteus*, *Enterococcus*, *E. coli* etc.. The role of *Malassezia canis* = *Pityrosporum pachydermatis* in otitis externa has been controversial. It can be found in 20–50% of the ears of normal dogs and 25% of the ears of normal cats. It is found in 50–75% of the dogs with otitis externa often in conjunction with *Staphylococcus intermedius*.

In diagnosing otitis externa, a history is very important to include exposure to other dogs and cats, metabolic or endocrine problems, familial (breed) problems, pruritus, previous treatment of otitis externa, recurrent infections, and seansonal versus non-seasonal occurrence. Cytologic evaluation of the otic exudate may be helpful in defining appropriate treatment for the otitis externa.

If an underlying cause of the otitis externa can be elucidated then appropriate treatment for the underlying disease can be instituted. Any secondary or perpetuating factors must also be treated. Questions to be answered in the therapy of otitis externa are many including: are antibiotics needed, what cleaning solutions are best to use, what are the drugs of choice and which ones are to be avoided in certain situations?

Appropriate therapy includes topical medication for yeast, bacteria, parasites, and associated inflammation. Systemic medication may be warranted in cases of otitis media or when the animal is systemically ill.

Sandra R. Merchant *Baton Rouge, USA* This portion of the workshop will be to report on the results of a study funded by Solvay Veterinary Incorporated on the quantitative and qualitative comparison of bacteria and yeast from normal canine ears versus ears with otitis externa, with evaulation of various treatment regimens.

The purpose of the first part of the study was to quantitate and qualitate the microflora from normal canine ears including serial recovery for validation and to classify the otic microflora present as resident versus transient based on numbers recovered per cm^2 surface area.

Conclusions from the study are as follows: dependent ears have a larger number of microflora; only 4% of the microflora isolated were considered resident flora (greater than $1000/cm^2$ surface area); percent incidence is as previously reported with *Bacillus*, *Staphylococcus intermedius*, non *Staphylococcus intermedius* staphylococci and *Corynebacterium* being isolated most often and, when isolated, these bacteria composed between 35 and 80% of the microflora of the individual ear.

The purpose of the second part of the study was to quantitate and qualitate the microflora from canine otitis externa ears and evaluate various topical treatment regimes. Included in the study were 87 ears (47 dogs) with non-parasitic otitis externa. These samples were obtained at weekly intervals to characterize the microflora responsible for the otitis.

The dogs were randomly placed in one of five treatment groups: (1) Panalog®, Squibb (neomycin, thiostrepton, triamcinolone acetonide and nystatin in a polyethylene and mineral oil base); (2) neomycin and thiostrepton; (3) triamcinolone acetonide; (4) neomycin, thiostrepton and triamcinolone acetonide and (5) Panalog® vehicle. Treatment was initiated with 0.5 ml twice daily of the assigned medication; An otic examination was performed initially and once weekly and a subjective grading system, including owner's observation, was employed to note a change in the clinical disease. This was a double-blind study.

Conclusions from the second part of the study are as follows: the percent incidence and composition of microflora agreed with previous studies; significantly greater numbers of *Malassezia canis* were found in normal ears as compared to ears with otitis externa; clinical improvement of otitis externa was found to be equal for the following treatment groups: the antibiotic steroid combination, the antibiotic combination and the Panalog® solution; the subjective scoring of an ear's response to medication did not always correlate with posttreatment bacterial counts; Kirby-Bauer disc sensitivities showed that the greatest number of bacteria isolated from cases of canine otitis externa were sensitive to tobramycin; and of the currently available antibiotics in otic preparations, neomycin showed the greatest bactericidal activity.

The discussion of this paper gave the additional information that a few dogs had a pure yeast otitis externa.

In many instances cytology will be helpful when a culture can be misleading e.g. with a pathogen found in smaller numbers overgrowing a pathogen that is the major problem in the ears. In this study cytology was not performed but quantitative analysis was performed.

Kathleen Vlaminck *Beerse, Belgium* Predominant microbial ear flora in healthy ears includes staphylococci, micrococci, *Malassezia canis*. Predominant microbial ear flora in otitis includes staphylococci, streptococci, *Malassezia canis*, *Pseudomonas* spp., *E. coli*.

Surolan® contains: miconazole: antifungal, antiyeast (*P. pachydermatis*), antibacterial (Gram-positive); polymyxin B: antibacterial (Gram-negative): prednisolone: antiflammatory. Therefore Surolan® combines a broad antimicrobial spectrum with antiinflammatory properties.

The fungicidal effect of miconazole, nystatin and thiabendazole against *Malassezia canis* has been compared *in vitro*. Miconazole was the most potent of the three (0, 01–01 μg/ml). Nystatin was fungicidal at 1–10 μg/ml and thiabendazole at 100 μg/ml.

The discussion of this paper gave the additional information that in the cases the author investigated and in which *Proteus* was one of the isolates, there was a good response to Surolan® treatment.

Bruce Hornstein *Baltimore, USA* Ivermectin (1% bovine preparation) was given to felines over 6 months of age for ear mite infestation (*Otodectes cynotis*). Felines over 10 lb in weight were given 0.15 ml^2 - those under 10 lb, 0.10 ml^2. Retreatment was repeated 3 weeks later, if needed.

There were no reactions, except for animals accidentally given intradermal injection. These showed ulcerations at the point of injection.

Success in house cats, not exposed to other animals was over 90% after one treatment. Felines permitted to roam outdoors or exposed to other animals had frequent reinfections. I have only treated cats over 6 months old with invermectin but it was reported at the workshop that other practitioners had treated cats as young as 4 months. Animals less than that age are reported to be prone to convulsions. It is also recommended that all cats in a household be treated to prevent reinfection.

Animals treated with invermectin should also receive appropriate treatment for ensuing otitis externa.

Edmund J. Rosser *East Lansing, USA* A 4-year-old, castrated, male, West Highland white terrier was presented to the hospital for pruritus of the ears and excess paw licking that first developed at 1 year of age (a non-seasonal pruritus of 3 years duration). The dietary history indicated that the dog was fed primarily Purina Dog Chow in various forms and flavours since puppyhood, with occasional table scraps. Upon physical examination there was erythema of both pinnae with some mild proliferative changes of the external ear canal, interdigital erythema and salivary staining of the hairs over all four feet. Previous treatment included the intermittent use of either Panalog® or Gentocin® otic topically into the external ear canals. Initial screening tests included; skin scrapings, cytology of otic exudate and intradermal skin testing to airborne allergens. The skin scrapings and intradermal skin tests were negative. Cytology of the otic exudate revealed numerous yeast organisms with occasional cocci.

Highest on the differential diagnosis was a food allergy and the owners were instructed to feed the dog an elimination diet of home cooked lamb and rice for up to 60 days. To symptomatically relieve the pruritus and to reduce the proliferative changes in the external ear canal, the dog was placed on prednisolone at a dosage of 0.5 mg/kg twice daily, for 7 days, the 0.5 mg/kg six times daily for 7 days, the 0.5 mg/kg every 48 h for 1 week given orally. Both ear canals were first cleaned with Clearx® ear cleansing solution (dioctyl sodium sulphosuccinate, ureaperoxide and lidocaine hydrochloride). Topical treatment of the external ear canals included the instillation of four drops of Tresaderm® (each cc contains 40 mg thiabendazole, 1 mg dexamethasone, and 3.2 mg neomycin) followed by four drops of Otic Domboro® solution (2% acetic acid in aluminum acetate) twice daily for 21 days.

Initial response to symptomatic treatment was very good, but $4\frac{1}{4}$ weeks into the diet trial (or $1\frac{1}{4}$ weeks after stopping the symtomatic treatment) there was a return of erythema and pruritus to both pinnae and a return of the paw licking. The dog was placed in an Elizabethan collar and socks were put on all four feet and changed daily. After 7 weeks of feeding the elimination diet, there was a spontaneous resolution of clinical signs. The dog was then re-fed the previous diet of Purina Dog Chow and the clinical signs of head shaking, ear scratching and paw licking returned within 48 h. The dog was then put back on home cooked lamb and rice and there was clinical improvement in 10 days. The dog was then fed Hill's D/D canned dog food diet and pruritus returned once again within 48 h. The dog was then put back on home cooked lamb and rice and there was a clinical improvement in 10 days. The dog was then fed Wysong's Anergen kibbled lamb diet and has been free of pruritus and ear disease for the past 2 years.

This case demonstrates a primary diagnosis of food allergy that was referred primarily because of a chronic otitis externa of 3 years duration. Further history taking and physical exam also indicated the concurrent presence of excess licking of all four feet.

The discussion of this paper gave the additional information that the current recommended duration of elimination diet testing in both dogs and cats is up to 60 days; otitis externa as the sole or predominant chief complaint in a patient with a food allergy is a common finding; and it currently is Ed Rosser's impression that otitis externa as the sole manifestation of an allergic state is more common in patients with food allergy than it is in patients with atopy.

Craig E. Griffin *San Diego, USA* Soft rubber feeding tubes are valuable aids for flushing external ear canals and the middle ear. A variety of sizes are kept in a cold sterilizer. They have been cut to several different lengths and can help flushing ears. The bulb syringe technique of infusion and aspiration of water with the syringe and feeding tube is often effective in removing more debris. This technique is especially helpful in cleaning the middle ear. Since the flushing and tube placement is completed under visualization through a surgical otoscopic head, this technique is helpful in assessing the integrity of the tympanic membrance.

Malassezia canis though controversial as a pathologic agent is felt to be a secondary pathogen in some cases. The diagnosis is usually limited to those cases when smears show numerous yeast with minimal numbers of bacteria present and WBCs are present. In mixed infections the yeast appear to be less important. When the tympanic membrane is ruptured and yeast are numerous within the middle ear the systemic ketoconazole (10–15 mg/kg) once daily is especially effective in eliminating the secondary yeast infection.

The discussion of this paper gave the additional information that for ear cytology the rapid modified Wrights stain is preferred (Diff Quik® by Herle Co.). Normally the middle ear needs flushing at least 3 times a day. Also, in cases where the client is willing and the pet will allow the clients will be taught to use a bulb syringe. A variety of products are recommended for ceruminous cases where the client can do a good job. Clearx cleanser (DVM), a combination of dioctyl sodium sulphosuccinate (DSS) and carbamide peroxide is very effective. In some cases 6.5% carbamide peroxide without DSS is used. Usually rinsing with white vinegar and water mixed equally works quite well.

REFERENCES

Ascher, F. *et al.* (1988). A new formulation for the treatment of external otitis in dogs and cats. 1. Epidemiological and aetiological survey. 2. Therapeutic results. *Practique Medicale & Chirurgicale de l'Animal de Compagnie* **23**: 267–272; 278–279.

August, J. (1988). Otitis externa: a disease of multifactorial etiology. *The Veterinary Clinics of North America* **18**: 731–742.

Hajsig, M. *et al.* (1985). Malassezia pachydermatis in dogs: significance of its location. *Veterinarsky Arhiv* **55**: 259–266.

Lorenzini, A. *et al.* (1984). Further studies on the activity of antifungal agents on *Malassezia* spp. *Atti della Societa italiana delle Scienze Veterinarie* **39**: 379–391

Stellmacher, W. *et al.* (1986). Results of microbiological studies of ear swabs from dogs. *Monatshefte für Veterinärmdedizin* **41**: 416–417.

Wooley, R.E. *et al.* (1988). Treating canine otitis externa with EDTA-TRIS-SDS combination. *Veterinary Medicine* **10**: 1088–1091.

Workshop Report 9

Parasiticidal Agents

J.M. MacDonald and G.A. Kunkle

Small Animal Surgery and Medicine, Auburn University, Auburn, Alabama, USA; and College of Veterinary Medicine, University of Florida, Gainesville, Florida, USA

DEMODICOSIS

Neil McEwan *Glasgow, Scotland* Dr McEwan discussed 19 cases of adult onset canine demodicosis observed at the University of Glasgow. All cases were referred over a 5-year period. Cases were classified as adult onset if the dogs were at least 3 years of age before demodicosis or any other skin disease was noted. The Yorkshire terriers, West Highland white terriers, and shihtzus were represented more than other breeds when compared to juvenile onset dogs and the general hospital population. Pododermatitis was the most common presenting complaint. More than 50% had pyoderma. Association of underlying disease(s) revealed the following: three dogs had low thyroid tests which may have represented sick euthyroid, two dogs had diabetes mellitus, one had lymphoma and one had atopy. Twelve dogs had no identifiable underlying problem. Eleven of the 19 cases had history of glucocorticoid therapy.

Dr McEwan reported that a good prognosis may be given for adult onset demodicosis. Ten of the nineteen cases had a permanent cure (negative scrapings and clear of symptoms for 1 year). Five had a partial cure, two were euthanatized (one lymphoma and one poor response), one died suddenly before therapy and one was lost to follow-up. Most were treated with rotenone and alcohol dips. Three were treated with weekly amitraz. The average therapy was 4 months.

In a discussion regarding hormone therapy, it was felt that oestradiol would not be helpful in the treatment of demodicosis (although this is a treatment utilized in some areas) since relapse or disease intensification is often associated with natural oestrus. Comparably, glucocorticoid therapy should be avoided. It was stated that glucocorticoid therapy is a main contributing factor to the occurrence of adult onset demodicosis in the southeastern USA. Amitraz was used as a demodicide by all participants of the workshop. Organophosphates such as Ronnel® or trichlorfon were not conventionally used by attendees. The attributes of antibiotic therapy were discussed when treating the demodicosis case with coexistent pyoderma.

A discussion ensued concerning the occurrence, diagnosis and treatment response of the shar pei breed. Approximately one-third of the attendees observe shar peis with demodicosis. A case report was presented by Dr Ashley Wilson (UK) of a 10-month-old shar pei with generalized demodicosis revealing numerous adult mites following rotenone therapy and six weekly amitraz dips. Chronic demodicosis had been observed by other attendees affecting the shar pei breed. A discussion of difficulties in acquiring positive scrapings from shar peis with demodicosis resulted in the observation that demodex mites may not be obtained from skin scrapings in some cases therefore requiring more radical diagnostic pursuit such as a skin biopsy. A statement of difficulty in attaining positive scrapings in this breed may be a result of the increased mucin in the skin. Monitoring the therapy of demodicosis cases was discussed with specific reference to the association of dead/live mite counts with effective therapy. Many veterinary dermatologists monitor patients by this technique. A statement was made concerning the importance of waiting appropriate intervals (4–6 weeks) to assess mite counts while continuing therapy. Performing scrapings to determine mite counts was advised to be done at similar times after dips. An attendee stated that his routine course of treatment included continuation until all lesions cleared and then restarted only when new lesions develop.

FLEAS

Roy Aronson *South Africa* Dr Aronson reported that Cape Town, South Africa has the most optimum breeding and growth conditions for *Ctenocephalides felis*. In 5 years of practice they have had to change therapeutic remedies eight or nine times. They use dips, sprays, systemics, Tiguvon®, Supona® and Grenade®. Even the topical application of cattle dip has become ineffective. Steroid therapy is the only treatment that gives the flea-allergic pet relief. A question of insecticide preferences indicated the majority used organophosphates with only six attendees routinely using pyrethrin-containing products.

The use of systemics was discussed with data presented by Dr MacDonald (USA) showing the effect of fenthion (10 mg/kg) on flea control on dogs in a natural flea infested environment. Twelve dogs were used in the study (8 = treated; four = untreated controls). All treated dogs had a flea infestation at each collection time which minimizes the effectiveness of this product in controlling flea allergy dermatitis. In a study of 16 dogs with pyrethrin or phosmet treatment, there was an effective control of fleas for approximately 3 days.

A discussion of environmental treatment included the use of insect growth regulators such as benzyl phenyl ureas (demilin) and fenoxycarb in inhibiting earlier stages of the life-cycle than the adult. A statement was made of research currently being conducted in California, USA, in the development of a flea vaccine. Comments concerning the association of flea induced dermatitis referenced Dr Richard Halliwell indicating the necessity of a flea hypersensitivity to elicit the development of an inflammatory cutaneous reaction. Insecticide studies performed in the southeastern USA were also referenced where individual non-flea allergic dogs harbouring as many as 1500 fleas showed minimal pruritus and no dermatitis. A consensus felt that predilection for flea allergy seems to occur and is most common in atopic dogs. German shepherds were mentioned by several attendees as chronic flea allergy dermatitis cases.

SCABIES (SARCOPTIC MANGE)

Canine scabies was discussed with consideration of the difficulties in diagnostic confirmation by skin scraping. Dr MacDonald reported that in a study of 134 dogs with scabies in which a maximum of 25 skin scrapings were performed per dog, positive scrapes were observed in only 50%. Ivermectin therapy (200–300 μg/kg) given twice at 2-week intervals was stated as a common therapy. In some areas of USA, amitraz is not effective as a scabicide. The safety of ivermectin was discussed. One attendee reported a case of ataxia in a cat treated with ivermectin and another reported a guinea pig death after three treatments. It was stated that ivermectin is widely used in the treatment of exotic animals with minimal side-effects observed.

MISCELLANEOUS PARASITES

A question was asked if anyone had experience with the use of Pro-Spot® (fenthion) or Tiguvon® to prevent reinfestation of chiggers. No comments were made.

Workshop Report 10

Dermatoses of Claws, Nails and Hoof

Carol S. Foil and James Conroy

School of Veterinary Medicine, Louisiana State University, Louisiana, USA; and Mississippi State University College of Veterinary Medicine, Mississippi, USA

Diseases of the nail, claw and hoof have to some extent been neglected by veterinary dermatologists except as an element of more widespread skin disease. Particularly, diseases of the hooves of large animals have been left to our colleagues who deal with lameness in these species, while veterinary dermatology has concerned itself more with afflictions of the coronary band in hoofed animals.

As the germinative epithelium and its specialized keratinized products—the claw and hoof—and the supportive connective tissues are a part of the integumentary system, it is logical that diseases affecting these structures are classified in the way that other cutaneous diseases have been classified. A brief overview of the various categories of diseases of claws and hooves was given with examples of several, e.g. *Developmental*—epidermolysis bullosa; *Traumatic*—the most common cause of claw/hoof loss; *Infectious*—many examples, best studied category (dermatophytosis of claws is a rare disease in dogs and cats); *Valscular disease*—laminitis, DIC, cold agglutinin disease. (This category may be important in many 'idiopathic' small animal cases.)

Another classification of claw and hoof disease is the distinction between those that are associated with more widespread dematopathies and those that involve only the claws or hooves. The latter category has been particularly difficult to deal with on an aetiological basis and many such cases remain idiopathic. This is partly due to the difficulty in making histopathologic specimens from affected tissue (see below). Many dermatologists have theorized that there exists, especially in dogs and horses, claw or coronary band 'dystrophy/dysplasia' which accounts for some of the idiopathic cases. Further study of these cases is certainly warranted.

James Conroy *Mississippi, USA* The tissue in question involves haired skin, dense collagen, fat, bone and hard keratin. This makes for difficulty in processing as each tissue type is normally handled by a specific process, and the variation in density leads to knife-induced artifacts. Clinicians who are investigating diseases of the claws often submit either an amputated digit or the claw itself. The hard keratin is the most difficult to process.

There are some techniques which are helpful in the analysis of hard keratin. The claws can be thinly shaved in cross-section using a scalpel blade. This will allow visualization of pathogens and cellular infiltrates, but of course does not allow examination of intact corium and other supportive structures. Alternatively, the claw can be soaked overnight in plain or soapy water or can be processed in depilatory solutions. Then the softened keratin can be sectioned. This also damages the associated soft tissue structures. One other technique available to some laboratories involves plastic embedding with glycol methacrylate which gives a substrate for the microtome which is as hard as the keratin itself.

Other participants suggested that once a section of hoof horn or claw is embedded in a block, the block face can be soaked in fabric softener or wool softening agent which will allow subsequent sectioning.

AUTOIMMUNE SKIN DISEASES

Peter Ihrke *Davis, USA* It is rare to identify an autoimmune disease which affects the claw alone, although many claw 'dystrophies' are referred as potential autoimmune diseases. The important diseases which involve the feet are *systemic lupus erythematosus*, *pemphigus vulgaris*, and *pemphigus foliaceus*. The lesions are dermoepidermal which includes the corium and hard nail junction of the claw.

In *pemphigus vulgaris*, pad ulcerations and ulcerations of the ungual fold are common. *Pemphigus foliaceous* is the most common autoimmune skin disease of the foot. It can be strictly localized to the digits. In 10 years, at the University of California, Davis, there have been six cases restricted to the feet. Vasculitis can also affect the claws, but is most often identified by looking at other affected tissues. The audience was asked if they had identified cold agglutinin disease affecting the nails. Dr Thierry Olivry from France had seen one case.

Some breeds of dogs (e.g. Siberian huskies) seem prone to claw problems. This may represent a breed-associated nail dystrophy or dysplasia. Dr Olsen from Sweden cited evidence that some may represent a biotin deficiency. Dr Ihrke cited a colleague who has successfully treated nail 'dystrophy' with gelatin supplementation.

DISEASES OF THE EQUINE CORONARY BAND

Tony Stannard *Davis, USA* Horses not infrequently present with coronitis and no other signs of skin disease. Typically, the lesions are flaking and crusted and do not become exudative. A characteristic observation is the winging out or lifting up of the hair of the coronary band. The frog is often affected. Chronic coronary band disease leads to hoof wall defects.

Unfortunately, biopsy of the coronary band may cause a hoof wall defect, so the clinician is forced to sample the heel bulb. A superficial shave biopsy just to the depth of the dermis may be obtained from this site without adverse consequences. After studying several similar cases, no agent or aetiology has been found; this may represent a coronary band dysplasia/dystrophy.

Pemphigus foliaceous in the horse may affect just the coronary band as well as the ergot and chestnut. A shave biopsy of the heel is also used for diagnosis in these cases.

Another disease is termed 'hepatocutaneous syndrome'. There is erosive, ulcerative and exudative coronitis which becomes necrotizing and may lead to sloughing of the hoof wall. It is associated with liver pathology.

NEOPLASMS OF THE CLAWS

Emily Walder *Los Angeles, USA* Epithelial neoplasms include inverted squamous papillomas, subungual keratoacanthomas, squamous cell carcinomas and eccrine carcinomas. All present similarly with swollen painful toes with radiographic evidence of bone lysis.

Subungual keratoacanthomas are complex lesions. Bone lysis is caused by pressure. In squamous cell carcinoma of the dog, amputation should be curative; the bad reputation of this tumour is undeserved. In the cat, however, this is a very aggressive malignancy. Eccrine carcinomas are aggressively malignant neoplasms seen in cats.

Other neoplasms of the subungual tissues include malignant melanomas of dogs, which are very malignant, and osteosarcomas in both dogs and cats.

Dr Walder had some comments on the preparation for histopathologic analysis of amputated digits. The ideal is a midsagittal plane of an entire digit. First, parasagittal sections are cut as close to phalangeal bones as possible on either side. These are used for soft tissue sections. Then, the claw and the footpad are removed and the phalangeal tissue is decalcified for midsagittal sectioning.

QUANTITATIVE ANALYSIS OF CLAWS AND HOOVES

Christopher Chesney *Exeter, UK* Clinicians and academicians need to study claw and hoof problems more quantitatively. We need to record parameters such as elasticity, stiffness, harness (scratchability, compressibility, extensibility), and permeability. Only then will we be able to understand such 'syndromes' as dystrophy/dysplasia, biotin deficiency, etc. In therapeutics, there is much room for quantification and analysis of similar factors as well.

PEMPHIGUS-LIKE DRUG ERUPTION IN A CAT

Neil Smart *Hythe Southampton, UK* The case was a DSH cat which presented 2 days after an application of an ear drop (dichlorophen, propylene glycol, terpanil). The cat had crusting of the pinna, nose and chin. There was a caseous paronychia of two digits without lameness. Workup revealed no mites nor fungi. A biopsy demonstrated urticaria-like changes. Direct immunofluorescence was negative. Ear drops were withheld and corticosteroids and antibiotics were given. By Day 5, there was complete resolution of the ungual disease. The hair of the pinnae regrew within 2 months. It was later determined that the cat had a probable exposure to dichlorophen (for tapeworms).

Workshop Report 11

Skin Diseases of Laboratory Animals

John E. Harkness and Julie A. Yager

College of Veterinary Medicine, Mississippi State University, Mississippi, USA; and Department of Pathology, Ontario Veterinary College, University of Guelph, Guelph, Ontario, Canada

DEMODEX IN HAMSTERS

Demodex mites probably accompanied hamsters from the wild into domestication. *Demodex aurati* is found more often than *D. criceti* and in larger numbers on male hamsters. *Demodex aurati* is a long, slender (183–192 mm × 21 × 23 mm) and, like *D. folliculorum*, is a follicular mite. *Demodex criceti* is smaller and rounded (87–103 mm × 32–32 mm) and lives in epidermal folds or pits down to the *stratum germinativum*. Mouth parts of all stages are directed toward the dermis. *Demodex aurati* resides in the pilosebaceous system at or above the sebaceous canal opening. Immature forms may penetrate follicular epithelium.

Transmission is by direct contact, and factors predisposing to infection are stress, age, debilitation, intercurrent infection, hyperadrenocorticism, sex, and long-term carcinogen exposure.

Diagnosis involves plucking hair for adult *D. aurati*. Dorsal skin from adult male hamsters should be digested in 10% KOH and filtered on 80 mesh brass wire.

Demodex spp. in hamsters rarely causes tissue pigmentation or tissue reaction. Follicles may be filled with debris and mites and have small inflammatory foci.

Prevention is to minimize stress, provide good sanitation, and remove infected animals.

Three to six topical treatments with amitraz 14 days apart will eliminate mites. The dog product is diluted 5×.

REFERENCES

Nutting, W.B. (1961). *Demodex aurati* sp. nov. and *D. criceti*: ectoparasites of the golden hamster. *Parasitology* **51**: 515–522.

Nutting, W.B. and Ranch, H. (1963). Distribution of *Demodex aurati* in the host (*Mesocricetus auratus*) skin complex. *Journal of Parasitology* **49**: 323–329.

Owen, D. and Young, C. (1973). The occurrence of *Demodex aurati* and *Demodex criceti* in the Syrian hamster in the United Kingdom. *Veterinary Record* **92**: 282–284.

ULCERATIVE DERMATITIS IN RATS

Staphylococcus aureus of lytic groups I and III of several phage types are involved; *S. aureus* is a common inhabitant of the rat oropharynx and intestinal tract, is present in or on many colony rats, and is spread by contact. Human carriers of involved phage types may occur. An allergic reaction to some antigen or irritation accompanying sialodacryoadenitis may provide the pruritic stimulus that leads to self-traumatization. Moist skin lesions, crusty and without hair from a few mm to 3 cm diameter are found on the shoulders and side of neck. Ulcers occur within the first week of scratching, and lesions may last several months. Scab formation indicates healing. Epidermal ulceration, necrolysis, purulent reaction, and chronic and acute inflammation characterize the lesion. Acanthosis and hyperkeratosis occur.

Trimming toenails promotes healing in 2-5 weeks. Transmission of various *S. aureus* phage types between species is possible.

REFERENCES

Ash, G.W. (1971). An epidemic of chronic skin ulceration in rats. *Laboratory Animals* **5**: 115-122.

Fox, J.G., Niemi, S.M., Murphy, J.C. and Quimby, F.W. (1977). Ulcerative dermatitis in the rat. *Laboratory Animal Science* **27**: 671-678.

Wagner, J.E., Owens, D.R., LaRegina, M.C. and Vogler, G.A. (1977). Self trauma and *Staphylococcus aureus* in ulcerative dermatitis in rats. *Journal of the American Veterinary Medical Association* **171**: 839-841.

TRIXACARUS CAVIAE IN GUINEA PIGS

Trixacarus caviae is burrowing/non-burrowing; the female has a dorsal anus unlike the terminal anus in *Sarcoptes. Trixacarus* has pointed, dorsal scales, and is smaller than *Sarcoptes* (females 200 μ vs 400 μ).

Deep skin scrapings with warmed 10% KOH digestion are the methods of diagnosis. Transmission is by direct contact with infected animals or contaminated cage or bedding. There are no breed, sex, and probably age predispositions. Predisposing factors include infected cagemates, environmental stressors, and perhaps dietary deficiencies (e.g., ascorbic acid). Scratching is obvious and intense 11-15 days postexposure.

Gross signs (Plate 41) begin on areas of contact: face, ears, outside legs, and back as flaking skin and extend over back, neck, and entire animal, except lower legs may be spared. Lesions are denuded, red, thickened, wrinkled with grey crusts, which may be greasy or dry. Hair is matted to crust. The condition is highly pruritic. Hyperesthesia results from handling: spasms, seizures, running in circles, and banging into objects.

Histologic signs include acanthosis, hyperkeratosis, with mites embedded in epidermal folds, hair follicles and in caverns attached to follicles, and in tunnels in hyperkeratotic tissue. Mites do not penetrate the stratum granulosum.

Treatment includes ivermectin 200-400 μg/kg; lime-sulphur dip once a week; lindane dip 0.07%-1% three weekly baths; or trichlorphon 0.15% washing over 15 days.

Shampooing of guinea pig before treatment may be advised. Recovery occurs over 3-4 weeks.

REFERENCES

Beresford-Jones, W.P., Fain, A. and Thoday, K.L. (1976). Further observations relating to *Trixacarus caviae* in guinea-pigs. *Acta Zoologica et Pathologica Antverpiensia* **64**: 33-36.

Dorrestein, G.M. and Van Bronswijk, J.E.M.H. (1979). *Trixacarus caviae* as a cause of mange in guinea-pigs and papular urticaria in man. *Veterinary Parasitology* **5**: 389-398.

Fain, A., Howell, G.J.R. and Hyatt, K.H. (1972). A new sarcoptid mite producing mange in albino guinea-pigs. *Acta Zoologica et Pathologica Antverpiensia* **56**: 73-82.

Kummel, B.A., Estes, S.A. and Arlian, L.G. (1980). *Trixacarus caviae* infestation of guinea pigs. *Journal of American Veterinary Medical Association* **177**: 903-908.
McDonald, S.E. and Lavoipierre, M.J. (1980). *Trixacarus caviae* infestation in two guinea pigs. *Laboratory Animal Science* **30**: 67-70.
Zajac, A., Williams, J.F. and Williams, C.S.F. (1980). Mange caused by *Trixacarus caviae* in guinea pigs. *Journal American Veterinary Medical Association* **177**: 900-903.
Zenoble, R.D. and Greve, J.H. (1980). Sarcoptid mite infestation in a colony of guinea pigs. *Journal of American Veterinary Medical Association* **177**: 898-900.

NASAL DERMATITIS IN GERBILS

The condition, also called 'sore nose' or 'bald nose', occurs in postpubertal gerbils at reported incidences from 5-18.1%. Higher incidences exist in caged groups. The skin lesion results from irritation by the porphyrins in tears followed by self-traumatization (scratching or rubbing) and, in some cases, bacterial (*Staphylococcus* spp.) infection (Plate 42). The animal scratches with the front legs. The porphyrin (or lacrimal) deposits derive from failure to groom away or hypersecretion of the Harderian gland sections. Blocking grooming increases porphyrin deposits but reduces self-traumatization. Stress may cause Harderian hypersecretion. The condition does seem to be contagious, to some extent. *Staphylococcus aureus*, *epidermidis*, and *saprophytus* have been recovered from the lesions. Transmission is by direct contact. First lesion appearance is of crusty red scabs and alopecia ventral to external nares (end of a lacrimal drainage path). The lesion spreads laterally and dorsally and may extend to forepaws (grooming) and periorbital areas. Lesions are usually dry, but they may progress to a moist, ulcerative dermatitis. Up to 80% of affected animals may recover without treatment over a several-week period. Epidermal changes include acanthosis, mild hyperkeratosis, and diffuse inflammatory cell infiltration. Adenomatous hyperplasia of Harderian glands has been reported. Attempted treatments using antibiotics are usually not curative, but oral chloramphenicol or tetracycline may help. Provision of a sand bath allows removing of prophyrin from hair, and increasing environmental temperature may stimulate grooming. Harderian gland removal leads to remission of signs and hair regrowth within a few weeks. Characteristic signs and fluorescense of protoporphyrins under long wave ultraviolet light confirm diagnosis. Culture will indicate degree of secondary infection.

REFERENCES

Bresnahan, J.F., Smith, G.D., Lentsch, R.H., Barnes, W.G. and Wagner, J.E. (1983). Nasal dermatitis in the Mongolian gerbil. *Laboratory Animal Science* **33**: 258-263.
Farrar, P.L., Opsomer, M.H., Kocen, J.A. and Wagner, J.E. (1988). Experimental nasal dermatitis in the Mongolian gerbil: Effect of bilateral Harderian gland adrenectomy on development of facial lesions. *Laboratory Animal Science* **38**: 72-76.
Peckham, J.D. and Cole, J.R. (1974). Staphylococcal dermatitis in Mongolian gerbils (*Meriones unguiculatus*). *Laboratory Animal Science* **24**: 43-44.
Thiessen, D.D. and Pendergrass, M. (1982). Harderian gland involvement in facial lesions in the Mongolian gerbil. *Journal of American Veterinary Medical Association* **181**: 1375-1377.

Workshop Report 12

Cutaneous Drug Eruptions

Kenneth Y. Mason and Edmund J. Rosser

Albert Animal Hospital, Springwood, Queensland, Australia; and College of Veterinary Medicine, University of Michigan, East Lansing, Michigan, USA

Kenneth Y. Mason *Springwood, Australia* The criteria for making a diagnosis of a drug eruption are (1) a history of exposure to the drug, (2) a physical examination demonstrating clinical signs consistent with a drug eruption, (3) biopsy with histopathological features of a drug eruption, (4) withdrawal of the drug inducing resolution of the dermatitis, (5) a negative challenge with other concurrently in use drugs and the appropriate ruling out of other causes. The value and need to challenge with the suspected drug must be weighed against the risk of potential for worsening of clinical signs even the potential for a lethal outcome. The situation of life being dependent on the suspected drug and there being no other available drug would warrant special consideration. However, some types of eruptions have a low risk of lethal sequence if challenged with the offending drug. These considerations will be canvassed further here.

Urticaria and angioedema are possibly the most common types of reaction encountered. Vaccines, levamisole, antibiotics and barbiturates are, in my practice, the most common causes. The histopathology features dermal oedema with lymphocytes and eosinophils as the inflammatory cell type seen. The pathophysiology usually involves a Type 1 hypersensitivity reaction. However, we reported one case due to a barbiturate, in which no previous exposure to that drug was known. This caused us to speculate that the drug induced an anaphylactoid reaction by either alternate complement pathway activation or by a direct action on basophils and/or mast cells causing degranulation. The dog in question had systemic signs of shock as well as cutaneous oedema.

Exfoliative dermatitis also called erythroderma and exfoliative erythroderma is also associated with drug eruptions as well as many other causes. I present a case here that was induced by lincomycin but have seen similar cases associated with levamisole. The main clinical feature is an intensive erythroderma, best appreciated by looking at non-haired skin especially the inside of ears. Painful skin and systemic signs may be features also. Other allergies for example atopy, food allergy, as well as superficial pyoderma and mycosis fungoides may present similarly.

Fixed drug eruptions are one of the more interesting and rarer of the types of drug eruptions. I reported two cases caused by the heartworm prophylactic drug diethylcarbamazine citrate (DEC) in which the feature was ulceration of a well demarcated area on the scrotum (Plate 43). On withdrawal of the drug the area became hyperpigmented and healed. Challenge with DEC caused vesiculation then ulceration of the exact same area of scrotal skin. That is the feature of fixed drug eruptions: only a fixed piece of skin is sensitized. In general, fixed drug eruptions are not dangerous to challenge, however, in the human literature there is a variant called bullous fixed drug eruption in which the histology has a toxic epidermal necrolysis-like feature.

In the area of drug eruptions the French have performed some very daring experiments to answer some important fundamental questions. There is a report of a series of human cases of erythema multiforme (EM) fixed eruption and toxic epidermal necrolysis (TEN) being challenged up to 2 years later with the suspect drug. Interestingly not all individuals were still sensitive. Regarding the histology of fixed drug eruption, it is essentially very similar to EM with the possible feature of a deeper dermal inflammation. Necrotic keratinocytes, vesiculation, dermoepidermal disruption by inflammatory cells and satellitosis are features shared with EM.

Erythema multiforme as the name implies has a variable clinical manifestation. It can be macular, papular, urticarial, vesicular and bullous. Illustrated (Plate 44) is a macular case caused by levamisole, and another case featuring depigmentation and erythema of the nose and lips, and a bullous type seen here on the ventral abdomen. Levamisole and potentiated sulphonamides are among the more common causative drugs. The histology of EM like the fixed type is necrotic keratinocytes with attached lymphocytes like an octopus, the so-called satellitosis. Necrotic keratinocytes are a dermatopathological clue to look for a drug cause. There is also a vacuolar alteration of basal cells and a lichenoid infiltrate which contains neutrophils and lymphohistiocytes.

Tony Stannard *Davis, USA* What about those eosinophils in that section?

Ken Mason I see a few eosinophils in EM, however, I have not been willing to comment. I think that eosinophils can, like they do in humans, indicate a drug reaction. The couple of EMs I have shown here are what I would classify as EM minor. The animals are bright and happy apart from the dermatitis. However, some more severe ulcerative cases, especially when involving mucocutaneous junctions and more obvious systemic illness I would classify as EM major. Danny Scott and I agree that affected animals are often bright and happy despite the extensive mucocutaneous ulceration.

The histology of EM major has interesting features. There is a spectrum of individual keratinocyte necrosis through to coalescing keratinocyte necrosis with a lymphocytic intraepidermal infiltrate resulting in intraepidermal cleft formation. There can also be extensive, almost full thickness necrosis. Is this EM or TEN? Some pathologists would tend to call this TEN because as you follow it further the epidermis becomes pink and lifts off the dermis. In my opinion, provided you can find individual cell necrosis and some healthy epidermis and inflammation of the dermis it should be called EM major.

Tony Stannard Is TEN by definition cell rich or cell poor?

Ken Mason That is difficult. I say it is cell poor and it is full thickness necrosis. It is confusing because in the cases we were discussing with cell rich and extensive epidermal necrosis but the basal cell layer is often intact are often reported as TEN.

Tony Stannard Do you think that it is critically important that we all agree, if you have individual cell necrosis coalescing before you get the majority of, if not all, the epidermis in a necrotic state? As a pathologist it seems to me there are those that are cell rich and then there is a necrotizing process of the epidermis and follicular wall, and those that are cell poor even acellular with necrosis until it ulcerates. I believe a cell-rich necrotizing process cannot be TEN.

Valerie Fadok *Denver, USA* I think that is a really important point to make from a pathogenesis point of view, because if you are going to involve the immune system as a cause you really should have T-cells in the area and it is hard to conceive of TEN as a cell poor process being an immunological reaction in a total absence of inflammatory cells. It would be hard to believe that cytokines could selectively kill off the epidermal cells and not damage the surrounding dermis. I imagine it is possible and certainly there is data to suggest that lymphokines have different effects on different cell types. I would think if TEN is an immunological disease you should have T-cells in the area.

Ken Mason Returning to EM, I have done immunofluorscence on a number of cases with Michael Day. We did not find dramatic or consistent immunoglobulin deposits. However, pressing forward let us now look at some cases of TEN. I will show slides of TEN due to penicillin (case of Richard Halliwell or one of his residents), levamisole and adriamycin—note the ease with which the epidermis lifts off (Plate 45). The histopathology features, as has already been discussed, full thickness epidermal necrosis and no dermal or epidermal inflammatory infiltrate i.e. cell poor epidermal necrosis. I have seen some dermal thrombosis. The immunofluorescence of these cases shows a dramatic deposit of immunoglobulin around the basal keratinocytes. A feature also noted in the human literature.

Valerie Fadok The presence of immunoglobulin in the tissue could be a normal phenomenon and not the cause.

Ken Mason Yes that is the question. However, remember dogs with TEN do not live very long. Death often occurs within 2 days. The problem is as Tony Stannard has alluded, what the criteria is to differentiate EM from TEN, because to look into the literature when immunological studies have been performed reveals that there is confusion as to which case is EM and which is TEN making it difficult to make sense of these studies. I go through and readjust the diagnosis according to my criteria, so all the cases of TEN associated with graft vs host I will call EM major associated with G vs H. Tony Stannard will discuss this because he has some special insight into this area.

Now pressing on to drug-induced subepidermal bullous eruption. I have seen a case associated with triamcinolone injection. There were distinct bullae in the mouth as shown, the ears and axilla as well as foot pad ulceration. The histology was identical to bullous pemphigoid. This section could be labelled bullous pemphigoid.

Edmund J. Rosser *East Lansing, USA* Have you special-stained these to show that the basement membrane is on the bottom of these splits when you say it is BP-like?

Ken Mason Yes. A PAS stain revealed that there was vacuolar alteration only affecting the basement membrane and that the cleft formed within it or between the basal keratinocytes and the basement membrane. No acantholysis is seen. Rare necrotic basal cells were observed.

Tony Stannard The point you just made is absolutely critical to this discussion. For years many dermatopathologists have taken cases with splits affecting the subepidermal basal layer or region especially if it has oral cavity lesions and mucocutaneous junctions and have lumped them together as bullous pemphigoid.

Ken Mason Some are easy and some are difficult to treat.

Tony Stannard Yes, two groups of bullous pemphigoid: those that are easy to treat—which I think is prima facie evidence that they are drug eruptions—and then the difficult ones. We should go back and regard some pemphigoids with the deep suspicion that we have, in fact, been talking about drug eruptions.

Ken Mason I agree. Look at the immunofluorescence on this dog with subepidermal bullous eruption, basement membrane deposits of immunoglobulins are very dramatic and clear.

Peter Ihrke *Davis, USA* May I muddy the water with an additional differential of basement membrane splitting. We have seen one sheltie at Davis with dermoepidermal splitting and follicular atrophy very similar to canine dermatomyositis but without EMG changes. We think that there may be an adult onset dermatomyositis-like disease.

Ken Mason Drugs may also induce a pemphigus foliaceous (PF)-like eruption. I present two cases here: one I have published involves a cat on ampicillin and there is an identical case in the *Journal of Small Animal Practice* caused by cimetidine. The clinical signs are subcorneal pustules on an erythematous base (Plate 46). The histopathology is similar to PF with subcorneal splitting, neutrophils and acanthocytes. It may involve the hair follicle. Immunofluorscence as demonstrated in this slide is similar with intraepithelial deposits of immunoglobulin. Both cases in the literature also describe a vasculitis which is different from typical autoimmune PF. This PF-like drug eruption is well recorded in the human literature most often associated with penicillamine. The human literature reports PF as well as pemphigus vulgaris-like eruption with the penicillamine reaction. So in human dermatology there are two groups of pemphigus—those that are drug induced and those that are autoimmune.

Peter Ihrke Are these animals sore? Humans often complain of pain in association with drug eruption.

Tony Stannard What are we talking about? Are we talking about drug-induced disease that is sore? Do pemphigus foliaceous go sore? Do pemphigus vulgaris? Or are we talking about drug-induced pemphigus foliaceous or pemphigus vulgaris? From a pathologists point of view if the histogenesis looks identical we are probably talking about a very similar, if not the same, disease. Although the vasculitis might be different, the prognosis I think we would agree, is vastly different in drug-induced cases. Perhaps this is a fine point.

Ken Mason Oh no it is not a fine point. What is autoimmune? Is it when we do not know the cause? In these cases of drug-induced pemphigus we know the cause.

Valerie Fadok If the drug fixed itself to the outer membrane of keratinocytes it might be difficult to tell the difference between the two. Now that in human medicine they are characterizing proteins against which antisera will react it might be possible to tell the difference.

Ken Mason As I understand it, some penicillamine-induced pemphigus do not resolve immediately the drug is withdrawn. The disease lasts for long periods like the autoimmune disease. They believe that penicillamine induces pemphigus foliaceus. Do these drugs expose some sequestered antigen that then induces the autoantibody production along the line of the work discussed earlier?

Tony Standard You know that there is literature on drug-induced lupus erythematosus.

Ken Mason Returning to the immunofluorescence of this cat with ampicillin-induced pemphigus foliaceus, there are immunoglobulin deposits in the spaces between keratinocytes.

Ed Rosser Where is the basement membrane and are there desposits there?

Ken Mason Your comment is relevant; there are interkeratinocyte deposits but also what appears to be a basement area deposit. I have not yet sorted that question out with Michael Day who does my immunofluorescence.

Just before I conclude I would like to show cases in which the skin was not directly involved. There is a case of a dog with a potentiated sulphonamide-induced thrombocytopenia and subsequent cutaneous haemorrhage; also a dog dying from disseminated intravascular coagulation (DIC) secondary to repeated blood transfusions and demonstrating the haemorrhage in the gums signifying the presence of coagulopathy.

Tony Stannard I have been asked to present a graft vs host in the dog. It has similarities with cell-rich erythema multiforme which many people have remarked upon when looking at the pathogenesis of both. I have been fortunate to see a case of graft vs host in a beagle undergoing bone marrow transplantation. The striking feature, clincially, is generalized multifocal alopecia. There is some scaling and crusting. The clinical differential diagnosis might be dermatophytosis, demodicosis or a low grade pyoderma. Histologically in the beagle graft vs host disease is a follicular disease. You will notice some epidermal hyperplasia and hyperkeratosis but the striking feature is in the areas of alopecia in which virtually every follicle is in telogen or undergoing some type of degenerative process. The other feature is a rather noticeable semi-lichenoid infiltrate particularly hugging the follicular wall and the base of the hair follicle. The pattern observed was reminiscent of alopecia areata. Necrotic keratinocytes are present in the follicular wall and some have a small nucleus hugging dead cells. This lymphocyte attached to and killing the keratinocyte is a feature called satellitosis but is not universally demonstrated on all necrotic keratinocytes. In contrast, these changes are more evident in the epidermis than the follicular wall in EM.

Ken Mason I have seen a case of a drug eruption due to levamisole which I classified as an EM which clinically presented as generalized alopecia and primarily showed a follicular disrupting process like the one you described here for graft vs host.

Tony Stannard The question that I would ask Valerie Fadok is to comment on the alopecia areata-like cell-rich lymphocyte reaction around the hair follicle bulb.

Valerie Fadok Immunologically, you can make a beautiful case for cytoxic T-cells killing off individual keratinoctyes. You do not necessarily have to see lymphocytes attached to keratinocytes. *In vitro*, cytotoxic T-cells will only need transient contact, and pull away having activated the target cells' own death programme. In the case of alopecia areata, I think there must be some abnormal follicular antigen or a cross-reaction with some other antigen to which the immune system is sensitized.

Peter Ihrke We saw a case that really makes sense, in accordance with Valerie Fadok's comments. We saw an alopecia areata-like case in a dog where only one hair colour was affected and not the other hair colours. It was symmetrical on the face of a doberman-like dog with a brown face and black body.

Valerie Fadok I would like to discuss why some animals might have drug reactions, and others might not, to the same drug? An area that is very exciting in immunology now is that some researchers are identifying what they call super antigens. These super antigens, for example, staphylococcal exotoxins, stimulate a reaction only in certain individuals who have the correct gene in their genetic pool. These individuals, regardless of their MHC association, form a certain kind of T-cell receptor that the toxin can activate. Are drugs doing the same?

Ewan Ferguson *London, UK* Is there any link between the persistent autoimmune reactions thought to be induced in man by penicillamine and HLA groups—HLAB27?

Ken Mason In the human literature there are papers indicating some individuals or families have a genetic predisposition to getting TEN and EM, in particular to some individual drugs for example sulphonamides. I am not aware of the association you propose, there is a dermatologic clinics on the subject.

Gail Kunkle *Gainesville, USA* In looking back through my records of drug eruptions at Florida I was amazed to find that schnauzers were overrepresented in our series. The drugs causing these reactions included potentiated sulphonamide and gold salts.

Dominique Heripret *Paris, France* I wish to present you with a few cases of EM and TEN seen in our practice in Paris. The first was a 4-year-old German shepherd presenting with ulceration of the facial skin and mucocutaneous junction. The patient was systemically ill. The skin lesions resolved on withdrawing tetracyclines but the dog died of lung problems. The histology was of epidermal necrosis of the cell rich variety and our final diagnosis was drug-induced EM major. We have seen TEN in a cat, extensive investigation of infective agents were negative and we concluded it was from griseofulvin. The skin lifted off the entire body, the ears were crusted. There was positive immunofluorescence on skin samples. We diagnosed EM in a 4-year-old male dachshund that was treated with two different antibiotics. Thus it was difficult to identify the causative agent; we suspect erythromycin. The animal also had bullous lesions and pancytopenia and thrombocytopenia. We classified it as EM major. We have seen two cases of TEN in cats treated with ampicillin.

Ken Mason I would like to introduce Julie Yager from Ontaria, Canada who will show us another way in which medications can cause cutaneous reactions.

Julie Yager *Guelph, Canada* I would like to present a cutaneous reaction to the administration of killed (not modified live) rabies vaccine in poodles. The most common presentation is a single focal alopecic hyperpigmented patch over the caudal lateral thigh, the site of administration of the vaccine. We suspect patients had received the vaccine subcutaneously, rather than intramuscularly. The time elapsed from the date of vaccination to the development of the cutaneous reaction was variable from 3 to 6 months. This reaction has now also been observed in other breeds including Lhasa apsos, bichon frise, shihtzus and Bedlington terriers. The histopathological changes included lymphocytic panniculitis, oedema within the dermis that often stained positive for the presence of mucin, the so-called faded follicles appeared in a highly characteristic atrophic stage (not a normal telogen), the epidermis may show hydropic interface lesions. There was an increased density of connective tissue collagen around hair follicles, atrophy of sebaceous glands, a vasculitis of both small arterioles and venules indicated by necrosis of mural cells and occasional intramural mononuclear cells. Occasionally there was a florid lymphocytic panniculitis that resembled lupus profundus in man. The rabies antigen can be demonstrated by fluorescent antibody technique in vessel walls and hair follicles.

Tony Stannard I have noticed a similar looking lesion clinically and histologically, in dogs given depo-type injections i.e. methylprednisolone acetate. The follicular changes are very similar and very frequently there is a granulomatous panniculitis possibly due to the vehicle. This would be a differential diagnosis both clinically and histologically.

Ken Mason I recognize the same reaction in silkie terriers, Yorkshire terriers and poodles. In what breeds do you see this reaction?

Peter Ihrke Poodles and little fuzzy terriers. The other clinical point is there is no hyperpigmentation in the depo drug reaction which is different to the vaccine type. The breeds, for example the poodle are the same, why?

Julie Yager I think the pathogenesis of what we are describing is probably a very low-grade vasculopathy and a resulting anoxic lesion.

Peter Ihrke I have two cases to present that have a bearing on the previous discussion. One is a dog with a drug reaction to tribrissen that looks both clinically and histologically identical to *pemphigus foliaceous*. The first was a dachshund that was clinically and histologically compatible with *pemphigus foliaceous* in every way yet the animal responded to withdrawal of a trimpethoprim–sulphonamide combination. I do not believe that there was any way besides withdrawal of the drug that we could have determined that this was different from the usual *pemphigus foliaceous*. The second case, a German shorthair pointer was presented with erythematous and urticarial looking lesions with extreme cutaneous tenderness or pain. In man this type of cutaneous pain is associated with drug eruptions and viral infections. This 13-year-old German shorthair pointer was on procainamide plus other cardiac medications. The symptoms settled in 4 days and by 2 weeks was normal upon withdrawing the procainamide. Histologically there were features of *pemphigus foliaceous*, but the acanthocytes were not as rounded as we would like to see for true *pemphigus foliaceous*. Other sections showed a more prominent epidermal spongiotic pustule without much evidence of cleavage. We did not identify single cell neurosis.

Pascal Prelaud *Paris, France* I would like to repeat what I said in the general session on the value of the *in vitro* basophil degranulation test for allergy in dogs; this might also be useful to detect drug allergy. It is used for this in human medicine.

Roy Aronson *Brighton, UK* On numerous occasions I have been presented with a cat that has a large focal area of alopecia and pruritus at the back of its neck. These lesions really take a long time to heal and are a source of frustration to both owner and practitioner. One common factor is that the lesion seemed to arise shortly after the cat had been seen by a vet and had been injected with penicillin. It was proposed that the drug had been injected intradermally and had caused its problem in this fashion. I must say that I find it hard to accept so many intradermal injections by so many competent practitioners.

We took biopsies from a few of these lesions over a number of cases and the diagnosis returned by the histopathologist was one of necrotic vasculitis probably of allergic origin. From this we concluded that the problem arose probably as a straightforward penicillin sensitivity and that penicillin sensitivities were a lot more common than is generally thought. The most interesting examples we have seen of this type of suspected allergy have been: 1) Loss of all front claws from both feet of a cat. They became necrotic and just fell off. Once again, histopath was done on selected pieces and the diagnosis of necrotic vasculitis of allergic origin was returned. 2) Another cat presented with necrotic spots in its ears which eventually progressed to being holes through its ear pinna. Both pinnae were affected and the holes were through the entire pinna. In all cases the lesions seemed to be bilateral and symmetrical. I feel that penicillin sensitivities based on these and other colleagues' observations of a similar nature are a lot more common than we give credit for and I would like to know if anyone has had similar experiences.

Tony Stannard You have hit on a frustrating problem we have observed over many years. Often referred to as suckers disease, it being postulated that the mother cat or some other cat sucked the area. What explanation do you have for the fact that only one injection of penicillin or at times no history of prior exposure to drugs can be elicited on history?

Roy Aronson On investigation in South Africa we found that some vaccines are preserved with penicillin.

Kenneth Mason: Summary
There was a universal consensus that drug eruptions are pleomorphic by nature and should be considered as a differential diagnosis for any unusual clinical syndrome as well as those known to be drug associated. The forms that drug eruption take and which were mentioned in this workshop were (1) urticaria angioedema and anaphylaxis (2) exfoliative dermatitis and erythroderma (3) fixed drug eruption (4) erythema multiforme (5) toxic epidermal necrolysis (6) pemphigus foliaceus, vulgaris and bullous pemphigoid or any autoimmune disease (7) vasculitis and mention was made of secondary skin involvement in more systemic drug-induced illnesses like disseminated intravascular coagulation and thrombocytopenia. Not discussed because of time constraints but also recognized were lupus-like drug eruption and the sulphadiazine eruption in dobermans where joint, eye, kidney, haematological, as well as a poorly defined skin rash occurs.

The histological features of drug eruption can also be pleomorphic. However, findings of individual cell necrosis of keratinocytes should invoke a search for a drug cause as well as any histopathological features of classical autoimmune disease. One histopathology controversy for which there was world wide consensus in those participating at this workshop was the separation of cell-rich epidermal necrosis with a good prognosis on early drug withdrawal from cell-poor epidermal necrosis with serious systemic signs often leading to death. The former was universally labelled erythema multiforme major by participants and the latter toxic epidermal necrolysis. The similarity between graft vs host disease and erythema multiforme was considered striking enough for both to be considered of a similar immunological process. Toxic epidermal necrolysis was concluded to be unlike graft vs host disease but the pathophysiological cause remains a mystery.

Workshop Report 13

Shampoos and other Topical Therapy

Candace A. Sousa and Kenneth W. Kwochka

Elvas Avenue Animal Hospital, Sacramento, California, USA; and The Ohio State University Veterinary Hospital, Columbus, Ohio, USA

Candace A. Sousa *Sacramento, USA* opened the workshop with an overview of topical therapy in veterinary dermatology. Topical medicaments may be used as sole treatment of some disorders such as ectoparasitism, as adjuncts to systemic therapy in dermatoses such as dermatophytosis, and as strictly symptomatic therapy in some idiopathic conditions such as canine seborrhoea. Topical therapeutics are chosen based on type of lesion, vehicle, and active ingredients. Commonly used vehicles include shampoos (medicated and non-medicated), rinses (antiseborrhoeic, antiparasitic, antifungal), ointments, creams, gels, sprays, powders, soaks, and wet dressings. Active ingredients include steroids, antibiotics, antiseborrhoeics, antimycotics, antiparasitics, and combinations. Percutaneous penetration characteristics are important and are affected by particle size, particle coefficient, partition coefficient, drug solubility in the vehicle, and viscosity. Dr Sousa indicated that most topical agents are chosen by trial and error and clinical impressions. She, along with all participants in the workshop, very strongly stressed the need for more basic research and better controlled clinical studies on topical therapeutics.

Christopher Chesney *Broadclyst, UK* presented an overview of the microclimate of the skin and changes in this 'microworld' with various dermatoses and topical therapeutics. Deep in the hair coat near the skin surface the temperature is high at 37°C, but in the sun this temperature rises even further to 43°C. The pH of the skin surface in the dorsal lumbosacral area of 40 kennel dogs was found to range from 6.0 to 10.0. The skin surface appears to be a very moist area with ambient relative humidity affected by many factors including rain, sun, wind, saliva, glandular secretions, and accumulated foreign material.

Amy Trettien *Nutley, USA* discussed the importance of developing safer topical glucocorticoid preparations and the results of a study on a steroid-containing shampoo. Topical steroids are generally considered safer alternatives to systemic glucocorticoids and are indicated when a patient has a health problem which precludes systemic steroids, when the steroid will need to be used for long periods of time, and in an animal which has endogenous Cushings disease. However, even topical steroids (cutaneous, ophthalmic, otic) may have side-effects including suppression of the hypothalamic-pituitary-adrenal axis. A shampoo containing 0.1% fluocinolone acetonide was evaluated for safety. Seven dogs were bathed for 15 min for 5 consecutive days in the shampoo and three control dogs were bathed in the vehicle. All dogs were evaluated pre- and posttreatment with CBCs, serum biochemical profiles, baseline cortisols, and ACTH stimulation tests. No differences were noted between the two populations. In a preliminary clinical trial on dogs with generalized pruritic and inflammatory dermatoses, 75% of dogs showed beneficial response. This shampoo is not commercially available at this time.

Zeineb Alhaidari *Roquefort Les Pins, France* discussed the clinical use of antibacterial shampoos. These shampoos offer the first line of treatment in pyoderma and contain various active ingredients including quaternary ammonium compounds, chlorhexidine, phenols, salicylates and carbanilides, alcohols, aldehydes, oxidizing agents, acids, heavy metals, and dyes. The three most useful clinical formulations include chlorhexidine, benzoyl peroxide, and povidone iodine. Chlorhexidine is bactericidal with a Gram-positive and negative spectrum and is fungistatic. It is not sporicidal or virucidal, stable, nor very effective against mycobacteria. It is non-irritating, rarely sensitizing, and is available in emollient vehicles. Benzoyl peroxide has a similar spectrum of activity to chlorhexidine but is also keratolytic, degreasing, follicular flushing, and antipruritic. It is stable but may be irritating and potentially sensitizing. For this reason formulations over 5% should not be used in dogs or cats. Povidone iodine is bactericidal with a Gram-positive and negative spectrum and efficacy against mycobacteria. It is also sporicidal, fungicidal, and virucidal. It is stable but organic products will reduce activity. Povidone iodine may be irritating and should be avoided in cats and on the scrotum and in the external ear of dogs.

Kenneth W. Kwochka *Columbus, USA* presented the results of a study comparing prophylactic efficacy of four antibacterial shampoos against *Staphylococcus intermedius* in the dog. Ten beagles were used and a laboratory controlled quantitative technique was employed. The antibacterial agents in the shampoos were 3.0% benzoyl peroxide, 0.5% chlorhexidine acetate, 1.0% available iodine as a polyalkyleneglycol-iodine complex, and a combination of 0.5% triclosan, 2.0% sulphur, and 2.0% salicylic acid. All four shampoos demonstrated significant prophylactic activity against *S. intermedius* over 5 h. Also, the antibacterial agents are listed above in decreasing order of efficacy.

Manfred Kietzmann *Hannover, West Germany* stressed the need for basic research on pharmacokinetics of topical therapeutics. He indicated that compounds such as tar, sulphur, and benzoyl peroxide are active and that their pharmacokinetics must be evaluated in different species and different body regions. Such factors as number and frequency of baths may be important for metabolism. Benzoyl peroxide is metabolized in the epidermis and may be concentrated in the canine epidermis.

Claudia von Tscharner *Bern, Switzerland* reported on the use of topical tretinoin for aural plaques in horses. She identified two clinical forms including seborrhoeic-type lesions and depigmented hyperkeratotic plaques. Histologically there is a lack of a granular layer in the epidermis and many mitotic figures in the basal cell layer. Topical 0.05% tretinoin applied to the pinnae resulted in complete clearing of the condition in two horses. Four months after discontinuation of therapy lesions returned but again responded when treatment was resumed. No side-effects have been noted.

Stephen White *Fort Collins, USA* gave an overview on the clinical use of topical steroids. Some common applications include control of pruritus associated with allergies in local sparsely haired areas, focal nasal or facial lesions such as those associated with pemphigus or lupus, and focal idiopathic conditions such as nasal pyoderma and sterile cutaneous granulomas. Dr White stressed that the pathogenesis of nasal pyoderma is controversial and that antibiotics should be tried before topical or systemic controls. Problems with topical steroids include client compliance (too frequent application and too messy) and patient compliance (irritability and ingestion). Side-effects may include iatrogenic hyperadrenocorticism, dermatophytosis, demodicosis, pyoderma, epidermal atrophy, and allergic reactions, usually to something in the base. Before topical steroids are used for any condition, scrapings should be performed, fungal cultures should be taken, and other infections should be eliminated from consideration.

Workshop Report 14

Skin Diseases of Zoo and Wild Animals

J.E. Cooper and M. Muller

The Royal College of Surgeons of England, London, UK; and Institut für Tierpathologie, Universitaet Bern, Bern, Switzerland

INVESTIGATION OF SKIN DISEASES IN ZOO AND WILD ANIMALS

J.E. Cooper *London, UK* Information on skin diseases in zoo and wild animals is scattered in the literature in the form of papers and chapters. Because of the lack of a textbook on dermatology of exotic animals, this workshop was a chance to provide a summary of the subject.

No research is possible without an understanding of comparative pathology. We have to remember the great number of species of animals. Warm-blooded animals consist only of mammals and birds; reptiles, amphibians and fish are ectothermic; 97% of all species are invertebrates. Often the most difficult problem in this chapter of dermatology is how to catch the wild exotic animal and to carry out examination on the lesion.

The reaction of the cutis of exotic mammals is often comparable to that of domestic animals. In birds most lesions are manifested in damage to the plumage. Reptiles are characterized by the presence of scales, in some species in the form of ossified plates, coupled with shedding of skin (ecdysis). As a consequence, a number of skin diseases in reptiles are unknown in other species. The epidermis of amphibians has only a few layers and the skin is often thin. Large number of mucous glands are a characteristic. Before metamorphosis, the integument of the immature amphibian bears some resemblance to the fish skin. The origin of the scales in fish is the mesoderm.

Little is known about dermatology of invertebrates. Insects are important in research and are bred in laboratories. Skin diseases of such species are not uncommon but few people (and virtually no veterinarians) take a specific interest in this subject.

DERMATOLOGY OF AMPHIBIANS

D.L. Williams *Newmarket, UK* An understanding of amphibian dermal pathology can only be achieved when the anatomy and physiology of the amphibian integument have been studied and related to disease processes in the integument and their effect on the entire organism. No one was more aware of the importance of the link between structure, function and pathology in lower vertebrates than Edward Elkan, one of the pioneers of reptile and amphibian pathology.

The skin of amphibians varies between genera but in general the epidermal layer is between two and twelve cells thick with large number of mucous and poison glands. Neuromasts and chromatophores are often present, as are tactile papillae in some areas. The amphibian integument is important in gaseous exchange. Maintenance of the water content of the skin is facilitated by the mucopolysaccharide ground substance found in the dermis of many amphibians. The skin of the immature tadpole stage resembles the fish skin in a number of respects and similar factors can be involved in disease. The amphibian skin is protected by the mucous layer and the antibacterial glands.

The inflammatory response in the skin is an eosinophilic and heterophilic cell infiltrate followed by a lymphocytic response and ultimate granuloma production or fibrosis. The response is temperature-dependent and in hibernating animals infection is more likely. The most important bacterial skin disease of amphibians is 'red leg'. The aetiological agent is *Aeromonas hydrophila*, a classic opportunist pathogen, infecting stressed animals. Aggressive necrotic lesions on the whole body and claw loss are typical findings. Primary chronic cutaneous mycobacteriosis is common in debilitated amphibians but dissemination is rare. Nests of foamy macrophages with intracellular acid-fast organisms can be seen in granulomatous tubercle formation. These become surrounded by a histiocytic zone, within which numerous heterophils migrate. 'Molchpest' of newts is characterized by hyperaemia and inflammation of the skin with dermal abscesses and ventral abdominal oedema, incomplete skin shedding and systemic debilitation. Often fungal infection supervenes.

Of the fungal dermatoses the most important is chromomycosis (family Dermatiaceae). Transmission of the organisms is presumed to be through small skin lesions. Ulceration, vesicles or hard tumour-like nodules are typical findings. Death occurs as a result of systemic spread of fungul granulomas (Plate 48). The disease is a zoonosis and thus handlers of sick animals should take precautions. *Saprolegnia*, a common fungal organism in fish, can cause deep dermal ulceration in amphibia kept in highly contaminated environments.

A number of protozoa cause lesions in skin but diagnosis must take into account that large numbers of purely commensal organisms can be found in scrapings. The dinoflagellate *Oodinium* has been regularly reported in fish, axolotls and tadpoles. Clinically a grey film covers the animal. An important sporozoan parasite is *Dermocystidium*. Of the ciliates, *Trichodina*, a common parasite of the fish integument, is found on axolotls and tadpoles.

Larvae (metacercariae) of certain trematodes occur as pigmented cysts, generally around the neuromasts. Microfilariae cause ischaemic necrosis of areas of integument. Leeches are common ectoparasites of free-living amphibians. In some tree frogs, larval mite infestation is not uncommon.

Very little is known about nutritional influences on the amphibian integument. Environmental factors such as humidity, temperature and pH are very important. Neoplasia is not commonly reported. Squamous cell carcinomas, adenomas of skin glands, fibromas, papillomas, chondromas and melanoma are described. The skin of amphibians has been a neglected area in comparative dermatology. It has intrinsic interest as a model of dermal reactions to external insults and of the development of the lower vertebrate inflammatory response.

THE SKIN OF REPTILES IN HEALTH AND DISEASE

J.E. Cooper; M.P.C. Lawton *London, UK* The Class Reptilia is primarily divided in snakes, lizards and chelonians (turtles, terrapins and tortoises). Each group shows specific structure in the skin. Temperature is very important in ectothermic animals.

The most common aetiology of skin lesions in reptiles is the 'maladaptation syndrome'. Skin responses are temperature related: they consist of cellular infiltration, degeneration and proliferation.

The most common bacterial infection is the well-circumscribed abscess. 'Scale-rot' (necrotic dermatitis) is often seen in snakes. Fungi are important aetiological agents in superficial and deep dermatitis (Plate 47).

In captivity, burning of the skin may be a result of a suboptimum environment. *Pseudomonas* and *Aeromonas* spp. may gain access. Often fibrosis leads to difficulty in skin-shedding (dysecdysis). Viral papillomatosis has been reported in green lizards (*Lactera viridis*). Other neoplasms seen include fibrosarcomas and basal cell carcinomas.

The shedding of the skin is very important and its frequency and quality have to be taken into account in veterinary dermatology. Dysecdysis is common, but the factors responsible are not yet all known.

CONCLUDING SUMMARY

The guiding principle in dermatological work in zoo and wild animals must be to conserve tissue samples and to ensure that data are collated and published.

The audience at this workshop emphatically endorsed the proposal that dermatology of zoo and wild animals should have a permanent place in the programmes of the ESVD.

REFERENCES

Collins, B. (1987). Dermatologic disorders of common small non-domestic animals. In: Nesbitt, G.H. (ed.) *Dermatology*. Livingstone, New York.

Cooper, J.E. and Hutchinson, M.F. (eds) (1985). *Manual of Exotic Pets*. British Small Animal Veterinary Association, Cheltenham, UK.

Gabrisch, K. and Zwart, P. (eds) (1987). *Krankheiten der Wildtiere*. Schlütersche, Hannover.

Jenkinson, D.M. and Roberts, R.J. (eds) (1980). Surface Eco-systems and the Interactions within them which overcome Skin Defence. *Proceedings of the Royal Society of Edinburgh*, 79B.

Workshop Report 15

Pathogenesis and Histopathology of Newly Recognized Dermatoses

Emily Walder and Luis Ferrer

Los Angeles, California, USA; and Facultad de Veterinaria, Universidad Autonoma, Barcelona, Spain

Emily Walder *Los Angeles, USA* Veterinary dermatopathology is a very young discipline which is still in a phase of rapid expansion. Just in the last 2 years we have recognized or increased our understanding of numerous clinical entities. In the neoplastic disease category: we have confirmed the high incidence and generally benign behaviour of canine cutaneous plasma cell tumours; we have learned that the syndrome of multiple cutaneous haemangiosarcomas in white thin-skinned dogs is yet another manifestation of chronic solar damage; we have begun to recognize epitheliotropic cutaneous T-cell lymphomas in cats and horses. In the category of inflammatory diseases: Lyme's disease, a tick-borne zoonosis, has been recognized to produce skin lesions in addition to systemic manifestations in dogs; we are still trying to elucidate the subcategories and aetiologies of the granulomatous dermatitides, especially sebaceous adenitis. In the disorders of hair growth: the keratin defect associated with colour mutant alopecia has recently been recognized; the various endocrine alopecias appear to have histologic clues which allow them to be diagnosed with greater specificity by biopsy; a form of mechanical alopecia similar to traction alopecia has recently been recognized in dogs; we are discovering subtle congenital follicular dysplasias in more breeds of dogs. In the metabolic disease category: a new mutant, the flaky skin mouse, has been proposed as a model for human psoriasis; we have recognized a clear association between liver disease and highly specific cutaneous lesions identical to necrolytic migratory erythema in man. Additional discoveries include a newly recognized variant of mechanobullous disease in dogs and the pathogenetic mechanism for linear granuloma in cats.

CUTANEOUS LESIONS OF BORRELIOSIS (LYME'S DISEASE)

Claudia von Tscharner *Bern, Switzerland* This disease was first described in Lyme, Connecticut in 1975, and since then numerous cases have been reported in humans and dogs in many countries. The main clinical signs in dogs are skin lesions and lameness. A 9-year-old male golden retriever was presented with an area of acute moist dermatitis on the face which did not respond to antibiotics and corticosteroids. Biopsy revealed nodular-to-diffuse lymphoplasmacytic dermatitis with some pyogranulomas in the deep dermis. Antibody titres against *B. burgdorferi* was 1:160. The lesion responded completely to tetracyclines. I have also observed a second histologic pattern, resembling acral lick dermatitis, in occasional cases of canine borreliosis.

SEBACEOUS ADENITIS IN A DOG

Marjana Savic *Guelph, Canada* A 7-year-old neutered male dog presented with non-pruritic, patchy alopecia on the forehead and digits. Biopsy showed perifollicular granulomas at the level of sebaceous glands and complete absence of sebaceous glands. Macrophages in the granulomas contained PAS-positive material. Possible pathogeneses for idiopathic granulomatous sebaceous adenitis include autoimmune disease, altered lipid metabolism or genetic disease (the disease is most prevalent in poodles and akitas). Treatments which have had reported success are corticosteroids, isotretinoic acid, and antiseborrhoeic shampoos.

SUPERFICIAL NECROLYTIC DERMATITIS

This disease, which shares signs with necrolytic migratory erythema of human beings, has been described recently in the dog under several different names, including hepatocutaneous syndrome and diabetic dermatopathy. The main clinical signs in the series of cases we have investigated are erythema and ulceration of the lips and vulva and erythema and crusting of the ears and footpads. Exudative lesions appear on the ventral abdomen in long-standing cases. All affected animals had severely elevated hepatic enzymes; occasional cases had non-ketoacidotic diabetes mellitus, and some had hyperglucagonaemia. The main histologic lesions are epidermal hyperplasia with parakeratosis and crusting and a zone of reticular degeneration in the upper third of the epidermis. Secondary superficial pyoderma, dermatophytosis and *Malassezia* infection can occur. Liver biopsies showed severe fatty vacuolation of hepatocytes with lobular collapse but no true cirrhosis. The aetiopathogenesis of both the skin and liver lesions remains obscure, but amino acid metabolism may play a role. Hyperglucagonaemia promotes inappropriate gluconeogenesis in the liver, resulting in intense amino acid consumption; this is one possible pathway for decreased amino acid activity availability to the skin.

EPIDERMOLYSIS BULLOSA DYSTROPHICA IN BEAUCERONS

Hans Koch *Birkenfeld, FRG*; **Emily Walder** *Los Angeles, USA* Similar lesions were observed in multiple pups in three litters of Bergers de Beauce (Beaucerons), one in Germany, one in Brussels and one in France. Affected animals had areas of alopecia, erosion and crusting around mucocutaneous junctions and pressure points. Defects in tooth enamel, sloughing of nails, retarded growth and abnormal stance were also noted. Biopses revealed occasional foci of dermoepidermal cleft formation with a suggestion of basal cell vacuolation. Extensive ulceration, suppuration and dermal scarring were also present. Clinical and histological findings were felt to be remarkably similar to EBD in man. EBD is a severe hereditary mechanobullous disease in which bullae form as a result of abnormal dermal anchoring fibrils and possibly elevated collagenase levels. Electron microscopy would be helpful in confirming the diagnosis.

TRACTION ALOPECIA IN THE CANINE

Craig Griffin, Wayne Rosenkrantz *Garden Grove, USA*; **Emily Walder** *Los Angeles, USA* Four dogs of varying ages and breeds presented with discrete foci of non-inflammatory alopecia on the top of the head or on the pinnae. All dogs had had rubber bands or barrettes repeatedly placed at these sites by groomers. Histologic changes included follicular atrophy, hyperkeratosis, trichomalacia, drop-out of folliculosebaceous units, dermal fibrosis and minimal inflammation. Follow-up of three out of four cases revealed permanent alopecia. This is different from traction alopecia in man, which is almost always temporary. Possible mechanisms for permanent alopecia in these dogs include: differences in dermal vasculature, allowing more severe ischaemic compromise of the follicles; more prolonged and repeated tension on hair in the same site; removal of rubber bands during repeated grooming may add a component of traumatic hair removal, as is observed in trichomalacia.

CUTANEOUS T-CELL LYMPHOMA IN A HORSE

James Conroy *Starkville, USA* A 10-year-old male quarterhorse presented with a chronic dermatosis characterized by numerous, macular-to-nodular, coalescing, alopecic lesions. Biopsy revealed diffuse infiltration of the epidermis, moderate infiltration of follicular epithelium and mild infiltration of the dermis by large lymphoid cells. Pautrier's microabscesses were not observed. Immunocytochemical studies were negative for immunoglobulins, and electron microscopy confirmed convoluted nuclei in the neoplastic lymphocytes. Necropsy examination revealed neoplastic lymphocytes in lungs, lymph nodes and bone marrow. The final diagnosis was epitheliotropic T-cell lymphoma with features of Sezary's syndrome. The early cutaneous lesions were also consistent with the Worringer-Kolopp variant of mycosis fungoides, in which neoplastic lymphyocytes are confined to epidermis and adnexal epithelium and are not found in the dermis.

APPENDIX

ABSTRACTS OF POSTERS AND FREE COMMUNICATIONS

Abstracts of Free Communications

ADENOCARCINOMAS DERIVED FROM SPECIALIZED CUTANEOUS DIVERTICULA (ANAL SAC) IN DOGS ASSOCIATED WITH PERSISTENT HYPERCALCAEMIA: CLINICAL, PATHOLOGICAL, ULTRASTRUCTURAL, IMMUNOHISTOCHEMICAL STUDIES

T.J. Rosol, J.I. Merryman, S.L. Martin[1] and C.C. Capen *Departments of Veterinary Pathobiology and Clinical Sciences[1] Ohio State University, Colombus, Ohio, USA*

Humoral hypercalcaemia of malignancy (HHM) was investigated in aged predominantly female dogs with a naturaly occurring adenocarcinoma derived from apocrine glands of the anal sac (CA) and persistently elevated blood calcium (15.7 $\pm$ 0.56 mg/dl). The hypercalcaemia and hypophosphataemia returned to normal following surgical excision of the tumour. All tumours had acinar and solid areas with histologic features of malignancy, and over 90% metastisized to regional lymph nodes. Bone mestastases were present only rarely. Plasma immunoreactive parathyroid hormone (iPTH) in dogs with CA were not significantly different from normocalcaemic tumour controls and clinically normal dogs.

A transplantable tumour line (CAC-8) has been developed in nude mice that presently is in the 25th passage. Tumour-bearing mice developed persistent hypercalcaemia and hypophosphataemia, elevated serum 1,25 dihydroxyvitamin D levels, increased urinary excretion of cyclic AMP, hydroxyproline and calcium, and had histomorphometric evidence of increased bone resorption and formation. Immunoreactive C-terminal PTH levels were decreased ($p < 0.01$) in nude mice with mild (11.3 mg/dl) and marked (15.7 mg/dl) hypercalcaemia compared to control nude mice (8.6 mg/dl). Hypercalcaemic nude mice with transplanted CAC-8 fed a low calcium ($p < 0.01$%) diet had a significant reduction ($p < 0.05$) in serum calcium (14.0 $\pm$ 0.9 mg/dl on day 0 and 12.5 mg/dl on day 14); however, serum calcium was not returned to the normal range (8.5 $\pm$ 0.4 mg/dl).

Tumours grown subcutaneously in nude mice were stained immunohistochemically for human PTH-related protein (PTHrP) (1–34) using rabbit polyclonal antiserum to PTHrP at dilutions of 1:10 and 1:20. Four of 10 tumours had areas of positive staining for PTHrP that varied in intensity. Tumours from normocalcaemic dogs were consistently negative (10 of 10 dogs) for PTHrP. Normal apocrine glands of the anal sac were negative but the adjacent skin was positive for PTHrP.

CAC-8 tumour extract stimulated *in vitro* bone resorption in mouse calvaria and adenylate cyclase in osteoblast (UMR-106, ROS 17/2.8) and renal (OK) cell lines that was inhibited by the PTH receptor antagonist [^{8,18}Nle, ^{34}Tyr] bPTH (3–34) amide. This suggests that bone resorption induced by the tumour is due, at least partially, to factors which bind to the PTH receptor. The cancer cells also produce transforming growth factor (TGF) α and β, which can be separated from the PTH-like activity by sequential cation exchange and reverse phase HPLC. Northern blot analysis of mRNA from CAC-8 demonstrated multiple mRNA transcripts for PTH-related protein of similar size as those from human tumours. This unique animal model of HHM will be useful in clarifying the interrelationship of PTHrP, TGF alpha, and TGF beta in the complete expression of cancer-associated hypercalcaemia in human and animal patients.

RE-ESTABLISHMENT OF HAIR GROWTH, SKIN PLIABILITY AND APPARENT RESISTANCE TO BACTERIAL INFECTION AFTER DOSING FISH OIL IN A DOG WITH SEBACEOUS ADENITIS

Claire Marshall and June Williams *Department of CAM & S, Medical University of Southern Africa, South Africa*

Sebaceous adenitis is a primary inflammatory disorder of sebaceous glands in dogs characterized by a dull, dry, brittle hair coat which epilates easily. Generalized scaling and hyperpigmentation occur with or without pruritus. The disease is progressive and symmetrical and may involve the entire body. Recurrent secondary bacterial infection is common. The cause of the disease is unknown.

This report describes sebaceous adenitis in a 4-year-old mixed breed male dog which presented with progressive, symmetrical, non-pruritic alopecia, hyperpigmentation and scaling. Initially being limited to the trunk and legs, it progressed to complete loss of the pelage. On presentation the skin was greasy and odorous and secondary staphylococcal infection was present.

Following successful treatment of this infection the odour disappeared and the skin became extremely dry. Histopathology revealed a granulomatous inflammatory infiltration into, and destruction of, the sebaceous glands. Electron microscopy, tissue cultures, direct immunoflorescence, serum chemistries, hormone assays and haemograms were performed. The dog was treated with high empirical dosages of purified fish oil. After 1 month, hair growth had occured over the dorsum and was commencing elsewhere. The skin was soft and pliable with a few localized areas of scaling. Secondary bacterial infection had not recurred despite a lack of antibiotic prophylaxis. Skin biopsy showed a complete absence of sebaceous glands and inflammatory cells.

Sebaceous gland secretions constitute 90% of the surface lipid film, the remainder being formed from contents of epidermal cells and the apocrine glands. Although regeneration of sebaceous glands after destruction cannot occur, it seems that nutritional supplementation with fish oil somehow ameliorates the lipid deficiency.

CLINICAL AND HISTOPATHOLOGICAL CHANGES AS SEEN IN SIBERIAN HUSKY FOLLICULAR DYPLASIA

Klaas Post, Mary A. Digneau, Edward G. Clark *Department of Veterinary Internal Medicine (Post) and Department of Veterinary Pathology (Dignean, Clark) Western College of Veterinary Medicine, University of Saskatchewan, Canada*

We previously reported hair follicle dysplasia in a Siberian husky dog. Subsequently, we examined skin sections from four Siberian huskies, two English springer spaniels and one Rottweiler with similar clinical signs, and compared the histologic skin changes. The dogs when examined were young adults and included 6 males and 1 female. The clinical presentation was failure to completely shed the puppy coat, breakage and loss of guard hairs and reddish discolouration of the remaining coat. This presentation suggests an endocrinopathy and histologic features of orthokeratotic and follicular keratosis, accompanied by epidermal and adnexal atrophy seem to be shared. Distinctive features are primary and secondary follicle asynchrony, with primary follicles seemingly arrested in catagen, normally a transient phase. These follicles, referred to as 'flame follicles' are characterized by elongated spikes of tricholemmal keratin projecting outward in an exaggerated sun-burst arrangement, accompanied by a thickened and convoluted glassy membrane. This feature is shared with adult onset growth hormone responsive dermatotis, though involvement of both primary and secondary follicles results in total body alopecia.

The pathogenesis remains unclear, though hormonal imbalance is suggested by sex ratio of affected dogs. A heritable predisposition has been proposed.

THE EFFICACY OF ETRETINATE (TEGISON®) IN THE TREATMENT OF KERATINIZATION DISORDERS IN DOGS

Helen T. Power *Veterinary Medical Teaching Hospital, University of California, Davis, California, USA*

The synthetic retinoid drugs, isotretinoin (Accutane®) and etretinate (Tegison®) are both vitamin A analogues, but have marked differences in efficacy in different diseases. We have completed a 4-month open clinical trial evaluating etretinate (Tegison®) therapy in dogs with primary keratinization disorders. We are also utilizing etretinate treatment in a group of dogs with solar induced dermatitis with preneoplastic or early squamous cell carcinoma lesions.

For the study evaluating etretinate therapy for primary keratinization disorders, 25 dogs (cocker spaniels, West Highland white terriers, basset hounds) were selected based on history, physical examination and histopathologic findings. The dogs were evaluated monthly for response to etretinate therapy and for side-effects. Evaluation included physical examination, owner conference and clinical pathological testing (complete blood count, serum chemistry profiles, triglycerides, urinalysis). Skin biopsy specimens and photographs were obtained pretrial and on trial days 60 and 120.

Etretinate therapy was beneficial for cocker spaniels. Specific changes noted were: a softening and thinning of affected skin; decrease to disappearance of keratin deposits and seborrhoeic plaques; decrease in odour and pruritus. In the West Highland white terrier and the basset hound similar changes were seen, but not of adequate magnitude to consider etretinate an appropriate therapy for these breeds.

Five dogs with solar induced dermatitis were treated with etretinate. They were evaluated and monitored as the group with primary keratinization disorders. These dogs had a marked decrease in erythema and induration of affected skin. One dog developed additional squamous cell carcinoma lesions in the first 3 months of therapy. Another dog continued to develop furunculosis, responsive to antibiotic therapy, while receiving etretinate therapy.

Side-effects have been seen in some dogs and include reluctance to chew hard food or chewies (three dogs); transient period of increased pruritus (four dogs); generalized joint stiffness (two dogs); vomiting and conjunctivitis (one dog); eosinophilic histiocytic furunculosis (one dog). These effects have all been tolerated. Although the relationship between the etretinate and the eosinophilic histiocytic furunculosis is not clear, the drug was discontinued in this dog. Laboratory data: No significant changes have been noted.

In conclusion, it appears that etretinate may be an effective therapy for the keratinization disorder of the cocker spaniel and in the management of solar induced dermatitis. Subsequent clinical studies utilizing double-blind crossover techniques are needed to confirm these initial findings. Minimal effective dose, duration of therapy, and potential long-term side-effects need to be determined.

MICROSCOPY OF COLOUR MUTANT ALOPECIA

Michel M. Brignac, Carol S. Foil, Fahri A. Kareem Al-Bagdadi and John Kreeger
Louisiana State University, Baton Rouge, Louisiana, USA

Alopecia associated with diluted coat colour was observed in dogs with bi- and tri-colour dilute and white coats. The purpose of this study was to characterize the histologic features of colour mutant alopecia in dilute and white dogs.

Surgical biopsies and hair samples were collected from clinically abnormal diluted coat colour areas and from normal-appearing white coat colour areas. Biopsy specimens were fixed in neutral-buffered 10% formalin, processed routinely, embedded in paraffin, sectioned at 4μm, and stained with haematoxylin and eosin. Hair samples mounted in potassium hydroxide (KOH) and in mineral oil were examined at 0, 12 and 24 hours. Scanning electron microscopy (SEM) was performed on skin biopsies and hair samples.

All dogs had similar lesions. Biopsies from both dilute coloured areas and white areas revealed superficial and follicular hyperkeratosis, follicular dilation, follicular cysts, and normal to decreased size and number of sebaceous glands. Additional changes in dilute coloured areas were the presence of large aggregates of melanin within the hair cortex and medulla melanin-laden cells in the base of the external root sheath and hair bulb, dermal melanophages surrounding the base of the follicle, large clumps of free melanin pigment in addition to the broken hair shafts and keratin within dilated and cystic follicles, and variable degrees of follicular atrophy. Direct examination of mineral oil-and KOH-mounted dilute coloured hair samples revealed numerous melanin aggregates associated with deformation and fracture of the hair cortex. Entire hair shafts were often devoid of cuticle. Hair shaft abnormalities were observed in both dilute and white hairs using SEM.

Colour mutant alopecia may affect dogs with bi- and tri-coloured dilute and white coats. Fragility and breakage of hair shafts at the site of large melanin aggregates in the hair cortex appear to contribute to hair loss in colour mutant alopecia. The presence of superficial and follicular hyperkeratosis and follicular dilation in both dilute coloured and white haired areas may reflect a generalized defect of epithelialization that is most completely manifested in regions with pigmented hair. Alternatively, a multifactorial epithelial maturation defect may be responsible for expression of colour mutant alopecia. It is interesting to note that the gene responsible for the colour mutant or Maltese dilution does not appear to be associated with cutaneous pathology in mice and domestic cats.

CUTAENOUS LASER DOPPLER VELOCIMETRY IN NINE MAMMALIAN SPECIES

T.O. Manning, N.A. Monteiro-Riviere, D.G. Bristol and J.E. Riviere *Cutaneous Pharmacology and Toxicology Center, College of Veterinary Medicine, North Carolina State University, Raleigh, North Carolina, USA*

Laser doppler velocimetry (LDV) is a non-invasive method for assessing blood flow (F), volume (V), and velocity (VL) in the skin. It has been used to assess the vascular response to acute physiologic and pharmacologic stimuli. The objective of this study is to establish baseline values in nine species and five anatomical sites for (F), (V) and (VL). The following species were used: mouse, rat, rabbit, cat, dog, monkey, pig, cow and horse (n = 6/group). Anatomical sites consisted of the skin above the buttocks, ear, shoulder joint, thoracolumbar, and abdominal areas. Significant differences in (F), (V) and (VL) were noted between species and sites within species. The abdomen had the highest relative blood flow across all species except the monkey. Although the values obtained with LDV are proportional to the physiological parameters, they do not represent absolute values. Changes in these parameters may affect percutaneous penetration/systemic absorption of topically applied drug, and the outcome of wound healing studies. This data provides a foundation for future comparative studies where different species and/or body sites are used.

GENETIC ASPECTS OF GERMAN SHEPHERD DOG PYODERMA

M. A. Wisselink *Department of Clinical Sciences, University of Utrecht, The Netherlands*

German shepherd dog pyoderma (GSP) has been defined as a chronic skin disorder of middle-aged German shepherd dogs, that is characterized by multiple deep-seated skin lesions with a typical morphology and distribution. So far the pathogenesis of GSD is not clear. However, since the disease is restricted to pure-bred or cross-bred German Shepherd dogs, genetic transmission of causative or predisposing factors has to be considered. To study this hypothesis the pedigrees of 42 German shepherd dogs with GSP were analysed. Parents, littermates and offspring of the affected dogs were traced and the owners were questioned on characteristic skin lesions. Suggestive evidence was found for an autosomal recessive trait. Breeders are advised to exclude affected animals and their relatives from further breeding.

SELECTION OF TREATMENTS OF BACTERIAL AND MYCOTIC OTITIS EXTERNA IN DOGS AND CATS IN THE CLINIC

Luc Desplenter and Robert Marsboom *Janssen Research Foundation, Beerse, Belgium*

Various bacterial and fungal pathogens are responsible for clinical otitis externa: Gram-positive bacteria (*Staphylococcus* spp. and *Streptococcus* spp.), Gram-negative bacteria (*Pseudomonas* spp. and Coliforms) and yeasts (*Pityrosporum* spp.). A single pathogen is identified in 26.1%, whereas two or more pathogens are involved in 73.9% of the clinical cases, mostly complicated by a muco-purulent inflammatory reaction and pruritus.

Surolan® (Janssen Pharmaceutica) is a combination product for topical application, containing:

Miconazole-nitrate 23 mg/ml: a synthetic imidazole derivative with antifungal activity against dermatophytes and yeasts, and an activity against Gram-positive bacteria.

Polymyxin-B 5000 U/ml: a broad-spectrum polypeptide antibiotic with bacterial activity against Gram-negative bacilli.

Prednisolone 5 mg/ml: A 1-glycosteroid with antiphylogistic activity.

The key compound is miconazole. Its biochemical mode of action and the induced morphological changes are demonstrated. Yeasts and dermatophytes are completely inhibited *in vitro* at concentrations of 0.1–10 μg/ml. Miconazole is cidal for *Pityrosporum pachydermatis* (*P. canis*) at 0.01–0.1 μg × ml, which is at least 100 times more potent than nystatin. In contrast to nystatin, spontaneous resistance induction is not reported. The antibacterial MIC-values for both *Streptococcus* and *Staphylococcus* spp. are below 6 μg/ml.

The *in vitro* antibacterial effect of Polymyxin-B is obtained at MIC of 1–5 μg/ml. The combination of miconazole and Polymyxin-B demonstrates a slight synergistic effect. The presence of prednisolone offers an immediate antiphlogistic effect and relief of symptoms and discomfort.

As none of the active ingredients is absorbed, systemic effects are absent and a maximal local effect is maintained. In view of the activity of miconazole against dermatophytes, it is also indicated for localized dermatophytic skin lesions, which are often complicated by secondary bacterial infections. As such, the combination of an antimycotic, a Gram-positive and Gram-negative antibacterial and an antiphlogistic treatment is a useful therapeutic for the practitioner.

TREATMENT OF ANAEROBIC INFECTIONS WITH CLAVULANATE POTENTIATED AMOXYCILLIN AND METRONIDAZOLE

R.J. Bywater and M. Bartlett *Beecham Pharmaceutical Research Division, Surrey, UK*

The activities *in vitro* of potentiated amoxycillin and metronidazole were assessed against a series of obligate anaerobes ($n = 231$) isolated from bacterial diseases in dogs and cats. Of the strains examined, *Bacteroide* spp. represented 59% of all the bacteria involved. β-lactamase production was found in 30% of all anaerobic organisms but in the case of *Bacteroides fragilis* the proportion producing β-lactamase was 91%. Amoxycillin and metronidazole were active *in vitro* against most of the anaerobes isolated. For *Bacteroides fragilis* ($n = 70$) the MIC90 was 1.0 μg/ml for both antibiotics. However, against *Bacteroides melangenicus* ($n = 67$) the MIC90 for clavulanate-potentiated amoxycillin was 1.0 μg/ml, while that for metronidazole was 8.0 μg/ml.

A clinical study was carried out in cases of gingivitis and anal sacculitis in dogs and cats, where alternate cases were treated with either clavulanate potentiated amoxycillin or with metronidazole. Of 130 cases treated, the overall cure rate was 83% and there were no statistically verifiable differences between the results for the two treatments.

It was concluded that clavulanate-potentiated amoxycillin and metronidazole were both effective treatments for anaerobic infections whether judged by *in vitro* or *in vivo* criteria.

THE USE OF CLOFAZIMINE IN THE TREATMENT OF THREE CASES OF FELINE LEPROSY

A.C. Mundell *Veterinary Medical Teaching Hospital, University of California, Davis, California, USA*

The purpose of this clinical trial was to determine the safety and efficacy of a medical therapy for non-surgical cases of feline leprosy.

Three domestic short-haired cats were evaluated at the University of California Veterinary Medical Teaching Hospital. The cats had a history of having had multiple dermal and subcutaneous nodules ineffectually treated with a variety of medical and surgical therapies. On physical examination, nodules varied from truncal to truncal-extremity to lip-perioral. The nodules were non-ulcerated and dermal and subcutaneous in orientation. Laboratory evaluations (CBC, serum profile, urinalysis, FeLV, FIV) were normal or negative except for a slight elevation of alanine aminotransferase (ALT) in one cat. Surgical biopsies were submitted for cytology, histology, culture, and laboratory animal inoculation (one cat only). Feline leprosy was diagnosed based on the history, physical examination, cytology, histology, and culture results.

Clofazimine, a drug used in the treatment of human leprosy, was administered to one cat at an oral dose of 8 mg/kg once daily for 6 weeks and then twice weekly for an additional 6 weeks. Clofazimine was administered to 2 cats at an oral dose of 2–3 mg/kg once daily for 5 and 8 months. The drug was continued for 6–12 weeks after the palpable disappearance of lesions. Routine laboratory test values (CBC, serum profile, urinalysis) were periodically monitored. The laboratory tests were normal except for a transient eosinophilia and a sharply elevated ALT at the end of therapy in the cat receiving the 8 mg/kg dose. One cat receiving the 2–3 mg/kg dose briefly developed a slight elevation in ALT when the owner overdosed the medication (approximately 10 mg/kg orally daily for 7 days). The laboratory tests were normal at the end of therapy in the cats receiving the 2–3 mg/kg dose and within 1 month following the discontinuance of therapy in the cat receiving the 8 mg/kg dose. The cats remain free of lesions 3, 6 and 12 months following the cessation of therapy.

RESULTS OF TREATMENT OF ATYPICAL MYCOBACTERIOSIS

K.V. Mason[1] **and G.T. Wilkinson**[2] [1]*Albert Animal Hospital, Springwood;* [2]*University of Queensland and Zeta Blacklock, State Health Laboratory, Brisbane, Australia*

Lesions from 14 cats with cutaneous mycobacterium infections were cultured. Five were found to have *Mycobacterium smegmatis*, seven *M. fortuitum* and two *M. chelonae*. The *in vitro* susceptibilities of the organisms were found to correlate sufficiently well with the organism isolated to make the antibiotic resistance and susceptibility pattern a reliable and simple means of organism definition.

Characteristically *M. smegmatis* is an antibiotic-sensitive organism, while *M. fortuitum* is in general resistant to most antibiotics but sensitive to amikacin and fluroquinolones, whereas *M. chelonae* apart from being sensitive to amikacin, is resistant to most common antibiotics including the new fluroquinolones. Treatment consisting of chemotherapy, based on *in vitro* sensitivity and surgical debulking was proposed to the owners of the affected cats. The five cats from which *M. smegmatis* was isolated, four with *M. fortuitum* and one with *M. chelonae* were included in the treatment trial. The remaining cats were either euthanazed (three), given no treatment or lost to follow-up (one).

Treatment of *M. smegmatis* infections with 10–12 weeks of tetracycline (one) or doxacycline (four) resulted in marked reduction in lesion size and closing over of discharging sinuses. For 3 days prior to the day of debulking and for 3 days after, gentamycin replaced the tetracycline or doxacycline, after which time the original antibiotic was recommenced. Of the five cases treated, three were successfully cured (follow-up period 4, 3, 6 years), one died before recovering from surgery and one owner removed the cat from the trial before completion of treatment. On the basis of the *in vitro* sensitivity, cats with *M. fortuitum* were treated with doxacycline (preferred) (two), ciprofloxacin and enrofloxacin separately (one) or trimethoprim-sulphadimidine mixture (one). Treatment periods and surgery were similar to that for *M. smegmatis*. However, the original oral antibiotic was given with the gentamycin in three cases and in one case gentamycin only was administered during surgical debulking. Three cats with *M. fortuitum* infections were cured—two of which were treated with doxacycline according to antibiotic sensitivity and one with trimethoprim–sulphadimidine. A fourth cat, currently being treated with enrofloxacin still has an open granulating wound about 4 × 3 cm in the inguinal region which does not conern its owners. There are no other signs of the original infection. The one cat with *M. chelonae* had less extensive lesions and was successfully treated with wide marginal surgical excision. In general, we feel that prolonged inappropriate treatment with ineffective antibiotics (i.e. ampicillin) and/or megestrol acetate and/or corticosteroids contributed to a poorer prognosis because delay in effective chemotherapy and the use of these immunosuppressive drugs allowed the infection to spread beyond that which surgery could effectively help.

If atypical mycobacteria are demonstrated to be susceptible to doxacycline by *in vitro* tests, then prolonged courses (4–5 months) of this antibiotic at 5 mg/kg twice per day may prove useful.

REFERENCES

Wallace, R.J., Nash, O.R., Tsukamura, N., Blackfoot, Z. and Silcox, V.A. (1988). A human disease due to *Mycobacterium smegmatis*. *Journal of Infectious Diseases* **158**: 52–59.

Swenson, J.M., Wallace, R.J., Silcox, V.A. and Thornsberry, C. (1985). Antimicrobial susceptibility of five subgroups of *Mycobacterium fortuitum* and *Mycobacterium chelonae*. *Antimicrob. Agents Chemother.* **28**: 806–811.

VARIATION AMONG MERINO SHEEP IN RESPONSE TO EXPERIMENTAL FOOTROT AND SUBSEQUENT VACCINATION WITH *Bacteroides nodosus*

H. W. Radsma, J. R. Egerton, P. Outteridge, S. C. Brown and F. W. Nicholas
Department of Animal Health, The University of Sydney, Australia

We have observed variation in natural resistance of Merino sheep to a contagious, bacterial dermatitis, footrot, under field conditions and following experimental infection. Exploitation of naturally occurring variation in both prevalence and severity of infection may be a suitable long-term option for reducing the impact of this important disease. An experiment was designed to test the hypothesis that there is a genetic basis for this resistance and that it is specifically linked with Class T genes of the ovine major histocompatibility complex (MHC).

Matings were established involving 16 sires from two bloodlines of Merino sheep which were mated in single sire mating groups to approximately 21 ewes/sire.

Both sires and dams were allocated on the basis of their ovine lymphocyte antigen (OLA) type to increase the frequency of six OLA antigens (SY1b, 2, 5, 6 and 9) which were believed to be associated with resistant or susceptibility to infection with footrot.

Eighty-four male progeny from these matings were challenged with a virulent isolate of serogroup B1 *B. nodosus*. Clinical signs of infection were recorded at 9 and 12 weeks after infection with a homologous, recombinant DNA vaccine preparation from the same serogroup used in the challenge.

The prevalence of footrot was 80%, 82% and 81% at 3, 6 and 9 weeks after infection. At 3, 6 and 15 weeks following initial vaccination (12, 15 and 24 weeks after infection) the prevalence of infection was 70%, 35% and 5% respectively. Prior, to vaccination, the sheep expressing the SY1b antigen had less footrot than those in which the SY1b antigen was absent. Further differences between bloodline of Merino and sireline of the progeny were evident and form the basis of a more comprehensive study to evaluate the genetic basis of resistance to footrot in Merino sheep.

DERMATOPHYTOSIS IN ANIMALS: TOPICAL TREATMENT AND ENVIRONMENTAL CONTROL WITH ENILCONAZOLE

Luc Desplenter *Veterinary Clinical Research, Janssen Research Foundation, Beerse, Belgium*

Dermal fungal infections, caused by *Microsporum* spp. or *Trichophyton* spp. can mostly be treated successfully in the individual farm or pet animal by means of a topical or systemic antifungal agent. The final cure rate of this conventional treatment is however rather limited in a heavily contaminated environment or in animal populations which are continuously exposed to reinfections. An optimal result can only be obtained by a simultaneous treatment of the individual animal and of the contaminated environment.

Enilconazole, a β-substituted imidazole, has been developed as a topical and environmental fungicidal product, both by its direct effect and by its vapour phase activity. The topical formulation (Imaverol) is applied as a 0.2% spray or solution directly to the dermatophytic lesions of horses, cattle and dogs. The risk of reinfections from the environment is reduced by the application of enilconazole as a spray formulation (Clinafarm Spray) or as a smoke generator (Clinafarm Smoke). For the prevention of dermatophytosis, the environment as a source of (re)infection and as a target for treatment, is defined in its broader sense:

Farm animals: stable walls and floor, bedding, equipment, belts and saddles, toiletting equipment.

Pet animals: kennels, catteries, nesting material, toiletting equipment.

Rabbits: stable walls and floor, battery cages.

Especially in stress-susceptible animals such as cats and rabbits, the unwanted side-effects of a topical treatment for dermatophytosis control can be avoided. The treatment of the environment reduces the contamination pressure by the fungicidal effect of enilconazole on the fungal spores and the different vegetative stages. This is clearly demonstrated by the morphological changes at the fungal cell membrane level and by the reduction of the fungal spore count and the incidence of clinical lesions. The possible applications of enilconazole as a spray or vaporization or as a smoke formulation in the prevention of dermatophytosis in the various animal species are discussed.

It is clear that this specific antifungal disinfection creates new possibilities for the prevention and/or treatment of dermatophytosis in animals.

BACTERIAL ADHERENCE TO CANINE CORNEOCYTES

Neil A. McEwan *Department of Veterinary Medicine, University of Glasgow, Glasgow, UK*

The ability of bacteria to adhere to epithelial surfaces has been recognized as an important factor in both the colonization process and the pathogenicity of various bacteria. In man it has been shown that pathogenic staphylococci readily colonize the skin of patients suffering from atopic dermatitis. It has also been demonstrated that pathogenic staphylococci adhere more avidly to skin cells (corneocytes) from atopic humans than to corneocytes from normal individuals.

An adherence assay has been developed to examine the ability of *Staphylococcus intermedius* to adhere to canine corneocytes. Using this assay the adherence by pathogenic staphylococci has been compared in normal individuals, dogs suffering from atopic dermatitis, idiopathic seborrhoeic dermatitis and pyoderma.

Corneocytes were incubated with a pathogenic staphylococcus then, using light microscopy, 100 corneocytes counted and the numbers of adherent cocci noted. The adherence index (AI) is defined as the percent of corneocytes with 20 or more adherent cocci. The mean AI for atopic dogs was 36.6 ± 15.7& (n = 15), pyoderma 34.0 ± 8.8% (n = 5), seborrhoea 18.3 ± 12.0% (n = 8) and normal dogs 19.0 ± 15.0% (n = 13). No significant difference was determined between normal dogs and seborrhoeic dogs. Significant difference ($p < 0.005$) did exist between normal dogs and atopic dogs.

This increased adherence may explain why, as in man, the skin of the atopic dog is heavily colonized by pathogenic staphylococci.

THE MICROFLORA OF NORMAL PIG SKIN

V.K. Sieber, S.W. Ketteridge,[1] A.B. Spicer,[2] M.R. Rhymes[2] and S.G. Mann[2] *CRC Normal Tissue Radiobiology Research Group, The Research Institute, Churchill Hospital, Oxford; [1]School of Biological Sciences, Queen Mary and Westfield College, London; [2]Department of Biological and Molecular Sciences, Oxford Polytechnic, Oxford, UK*

The normal microflora of the skin surface of healthy pigs, maintained under standard animal house conditions, was examined over a period of 2 years. Bacterial species were isolated prior to surface disinfection and from the bulbs of plucked hairs following surface disinfection of the skin.

Three techniques for sampling the skin microflora were used; wiping with a sterile alginate swab, adhesion onto contact plates (containing Columbia Blood Agar) and the cub-scrub method. Bacterial isolates were cultured on Columbia Blood Agar (CBA) or on Brain Heart Infusion Agar containing 0.5% Tween 80 (BHIA). Incubation was at 37°C either in air or anaerobically in jars gassed with hydrogen containing ± 10% CO_2.

The bacteria isolated from the skin surface of pigs were mostly *Staphylococcus* spp. with relatively few species of *Streptococcus*. Aerobic spore formers (*Bacillus* spp.) were isolated occasionally, whilst bacteria generally regarded as indicators of faecal pollution (*Enterococcus* spp.) were isolated at low frequencies. Coryneform bacteria were also isolated infrequently. No *Propionibacterium* spp. were isolated from pig skin although they were isolated from human skin with the procedures used in this study.

The skin surface was disinfected using each of four commonly used agents and the numbers of microorganisms recovered following each treatment were compared. No appreciable numbers of bacteria were recovered following treatment with chlorhexidine gluconate in either alcohol or water. The surface microflora was reduced but not eliminated by Betadine®, an iodinate surgical scrub, whilst there was no marked reduction in the number of bacteria recovered following treatment with hydrogen peroxide (1%w/v).

Following skin surface sterilization, bacteria were recovered from deep within the follicle by incubating plucked hairs on CBA or BHIA. Bacterial colonies grew from the hair bulb from 5–15% of the plucked hairs. The range of species isolated from the base of plucked hairs was comparable to those recovered from the skin surface. However, micrococci and coryneforms were apparently isolated more frequently from hair bulbs than from the skin surface.

Although no significant numbers of bacteria were recovered from the skin surface following surface disinfection, bacteria could still be recovered from the bases of plucked hairs. The follicle is considered to be a specialized habitat; it is, however, difficult to understand how bacteria might colonize the hair bulb. One possibility is that bacteria are able to pass between the follicle and the hair during those phases of the hair growth cycle during which the hair is loosely attached within the follicle. Residual bacteria within the follicle may represent a possible source of infection. Isolation of bacteria from plucked hairs is a simple and non-invasive method for sampling the microflora at depth in skin.

CHANGES IN THE HOOF HORN OF PIGS WITH LAMINITIS: A SCANNING AND TRANSMISSION ELECTRON MICROSCOPIC STUDY

Susan A. Kempson[1] and A. M. Johnston[2] *[1]Royal (Dick) School of Veterinary Studies, Edinburgh, UK; [2]Royal Veterinary College, North Mymms, Hatfield, Herts, UK*

The hoof horn from a group of pigs with a high incidence of lameness was compared to a similar group with no foot problems. Two vertical cuts 1 cm apart were made in the medial digit of one front foot, from the hairy skin proximal to the coronary band to the palmar surface. Two equidistant horizontal cuts were then made, providing three blocks of tissue incorporating the full length of the wall. The blocks were carefully removed from the digit leaving as much of the underlying soft tissues as possible attached to the horn. The specimens were then prepared for scanning and transmission electron microscopy.

The observations reported were made on the middle block which incorporated the sensitive laminae. In the scanning electron microscope the sensitive laminae of the lame pigs were elongated and showed a loss of organized structure. In one specimen disruption of the laminae was more acute, with separation of the epidermis from the underlying connective tissue of the corium. The other conspicuous feature of the affected feet was the presence of small, round tubules in the normally non-tubular band of horn adjacent to the sensitive laminae.

Transmission electron microscopy revealed different degrees of disruption of the laminae epidermis in the lame pigs. Enlarged intercellular spaces, containing dense granular material were common. The intercellular material was also present in the differentiated horn, pushing adjacent cell membranes apart. Structures resembling red blood cells were present in the intercellular spaces. The horn of the stratum medium of the lame pigs was of poor quality with gaps and irregularities. Many of the changes in the structure of the hoof horn in the affected pigs were the same as those seen in horses and dairy cattle with chronic laminitis.

ANGORA RABBIT MYXOMATOSIS

J. P. Ganiere, J. M. Gourreau, J. Chantal, D. Montabord and M. Rive *Ministere de l'Agriculture et de La Foret, Centre National d'Etudes Vétérinaire et Alimentaires, Laboratoire Central de Recherches Vétérinaires, Maisons-Alforts, France*

A special form of myxomatosis called "maladie des boutons rouges" is described in Angora rabbits. The disease occurs 8–10 days after the depilation and myxomas are limited to the depilated skin area (cephalic and genital localizations are observed only in 25% of the cases). These myxomas are flat, with coin aspect, first reddish then necrotic and reach a size which varied from some mm to 2 or 3 cm. The disease does not occur during the cold season. Only some rabbits are affected (incidence below 20%) and occasionally fibroma virus vaccinated animals.

The aetiology is confirmed by several investigations: microscopical structure of lesions; viral particles visualization *in situ* by electron microscopy; experimental transmission to Angora and New Zealand rabbits by using a needle previously pricked in a myxoma; viral isolation in cell culture (RL cells).

These observations raise two questions:

Does the depilation play a major role in disease emergence?

What is the viral strain? Classical or specific Angora rabbit adapted strain?

ID inoculation 1000 D150 of an Angora rabbit isolated strain was performed in Angora and New Zealand rabbits. Primary myxoma (flat myxoxma) becomes visible at 6 or 7 days postinoculation and is followed by classical generalization in cephalic and genital areas among all inoculated rabbits. It is a Type III myxomatosis. Most Angora rabbits, but few New Zealand rabbits exhibit flat and necrotic myxomas on the scrotum. Frequent rhinitis occurs 10–20 days postinoculation; mortality caused by pasteurellosis or staphylococcus complications is observed 1–2 months postinoculation in some rabbits.

Depilation, if practiced before secondary myxomas development, produces natural disease feature, with similar lesions in depilated areas. In the natural disease, vector insect bites are probably enhanced by bare skin and the trauma of depilation induces local development of secondary myxomas in these skin areas.

Similar pattern with classical strain of myxomatosis virus and comparative analysis of restriction profiles of Angora strain DNA are now presented to complete these first studies.

AZATHIOPRINE TOXICITY IN THE DOMESTIC CAT

Karin M. Beale *College of Veterinary Medicine, University of Florida, Gainesville, Florida, USA*

Cytototoxic drugs are often used in combination with glucocorticoids in the treatment of immune-mediated diseases in domestic animals. Antimetabolites such as azathioprine have become popular immunosuppressive drugs because of their low overall toxicity. In dogs, dosages of 2.2 mg/kg daily or every other day are generally regarded as safe. The principal toxicoses are haematologic and gastrointestinal. The cat however appears to be more readily susceptible to haematologic toxicity. In one study, four of eight cats given 1.1 mg/kg azathioprine in combination with prednisone for the treatment of pemphigus foliaceous developed leukopenia after a mean of 8.25 doses (Caciolo *et al.*, 1984).

In this study, the toxic effects of azathioprine were evaluated in the domestic cat. Seven cats were included in the study. Azathioprine was administered to cats 1–5 (2.2 mg/kg/every other day) in a suspension of water, cologel and syrup; cats 6 and 7 served as controls and were administered the suspension without the azathioprine every other day. Complete blood counts, serum alkaline phosphatase, ALT, AST and bilirubin were monitored weekly. Bone marrow aspirates were performed and evaluated every 3 weeks. The cats were maintained for 9 weeks on medication after an initial acclimatization period of 10 days.

The granulocytes appeared to be most affected by the drug. All of the treated cats became neutropenic ($< 500/\mu l$) after 20 doses (mean 15.4 doses). Four of the five treated cats became leukopenic (WBC $< 3000/\mu l$) after a mean of 21 doses. Two treated cats developed upper respiratory infections, and one of them eventually developed pneumonia and was euthanized. There were no significant changes in the serum chemistries in the treated vs control cats. The bone marrow aspirates revealed granulocytic hypoplasia, which was not observed in the control cats. Both groups of cats had evidence of bone marrow fibrosis at the end of the study. In summary, azathioprine at 2.2 mg/kg every other day is myelotoxic in cats and should not be recommended for use.

REFERENCE

Caciolo, P.L., Nesbitt, G.H. and Hurvitz, A.I. (1984). Pemphigus foliaceus in eight cats and results of induction therapy using azathioprine. *Journal of the American Animal Hospital Association* **20**: 571-577.

EFFECTS AND METABOLISM OF BENZOYL PEROXIDE IN MURINE EPIDERMIS

M. Kietzmann,[1] D. Lubach[2] and J. Henkemeyer[1] *Institute für Pharmakologie, Toxikologie und Pharmazie, Tierärztliche Hochschule, [1]Hautklinik Linden Medizinische Hochschule, [2]Hannover, FRG*

Benzoyl peroxide is a keratolytic, antibacterial, degreasing and antipruritic agent. Because of these qualities, it is used to treat canine seborrhoea. Benzoyl peroxide containing formulations are gels or shampoos. In mice, a study was performed to demonstrate epidermal effects of benzoyl peroxide. The incorporation of thymidine triphosphate into DNA and of leucine and histidine into protein was measured using ^{3}H-labelled thymidine triphosphate and ^{3}H-labelled amino acids. Histometric data completed this study. Also the ability of epidermal cells to metabolize benzoyl peroxide was assessed.

It was found that benzoyl peroxide induces the development of a retention acanthosis. The thymidine triphosphate incorporation rate was diminished. This is consistent with the results, which show a decreased mitotic activity in benzoyl peroxide treated epidermis. While the histidine incorporation remained nearly unchanged (demonstrating a lacking influence in the keratinocyte differentiation), the leucine incorporation, localised in basal proliferating epidermal layers, was decreased. The effects were more prominent in the ear than in tail epidermis, which normally shows, different from other body regions, orthokeratotic and parakeratotic areas.

Using thin layer chromatography, it could be shown that benzoyl peroxide, while penetrating epidermal layers, is nearly completely metabolized to benzoic acid. This is in agreement with results from *in vitro* studies in human and canine skin.

ORTHOKERATOSIS—AN UNEXPLAINED EPIDERMAL RESPONSE TO RESIDENT ARTHROPOD ECTOPARASITES

A.N. Sinclair *Seaforth, New South Wales, Australia*

Epidermal stratum corneum is formed by an inner dense stratum compactum and an outer loose stratum disjunctum. The former is easily seen in paraffin-embedded vertical skin sections but the stratum disjunctum is better seen in vertical frozen sections of skin biopsies cryofixed in liquid nitrogen.

Hyperkeratotic stratum corneum may be orthokeratotic, with morphologically normal unnucleated cells, or parakeratotic, with cells containing pyknotic nuclei. These are considered to be a new level of homeostasis in the chronically stimulated epidermis. That situation exists in infestations by resident arthropod ectoparasites which complete their life-cycle on the same host, typically lice and mites. When fixed *in-situ* by liquid nitrogen some species have been shown to feed superficially without piercing the epidermis.

A model of epidermis from uninfested European sheep shows mean dimensions as: outer lipid layer -9 μm; stratum disjunctum -16 μm; stratum compactum -16 μm. Uninfested Australian merino sheep show mean dimensions as: combined lipid layer and stratum disjunctum -14 μm; stratum compactum -2 μm. By contrast, merino sheep infested by the chewing louse *Damalinia ovis* show mean dimensions as: combined lipid and stratum disjunctum -24 μm; stratum compactum -7 μm. The general appearance, either in paraffin sections (mostly compactum) or in frozen sections, is one of a reasonably consistent thick orthokeratosis. *Damalinia ovis* feeds superficially on loose scurf and the stratum disjunctum.

Sheep infested by the mite *Psorergates ovis* show orthokeratosis of reasonably consistent thickness in the compactum, but the disjunctum, seen in frozen sections is very irregular with heaped masses of orthokeratotic material. The thickness of compactum varies with the season of the year, probably reflecting seasonal fluctuations in mite populations. *Psorergates ovis* penetrates to the inner surface of the stratum compactum and is thought to feed there as well as at the follicle mouth.

Paraffin sections of pups infested by *Sarcoptes scabei* show a slightly orthokeratotic compactum.

Literature on human scabies, particularly the Norwegian form, shows that the mite burrows as deeply as the basal layer of the epidermis. Also, when mites were in uncornified epidermis the response was parakeratotic, whereas, when mites were in stratum corneum the response was orthokeratotic. The evidence from ectoparasite feeding levels suggests that orthokeratosis is a response to damage of the stratum corneum. Possible mechanisms of its formation are increased proliferation, increased squame retention, or both acting together. There are no obvious indications of major increases of cell divisions in the epidermis of sheep infested by lice or mites. It is thought that increased retention of squames may be the main mechanism of orthokeratosis formation. It is speculated that the increased retention could arise if intercellular binding compounds in stratum compactum remain unaltered, either due to abnormal structure not being degraded by normal enzymes, or that there are enzymic deficiencies. The stimuli could be chronic irritation by ectoparasite feeding activities. Alternatively the orthokeratotic response could be part of an immune reaction to antigenic stimuli from ectoparasites, possibly in saliva.

FURTHER INVESTIGATIONS ON THE USE OF NON-STEROIDAL AND STEROIDAL ANTIINFLAMMATORY AGENTS IN THE MANAGEMENT OF CANINE PRURITIS

Manon Paradis and Danny W. Scott *University of Montreal, Faculty of Veterinary Medicine, Quebec, Canada*

Although glucocorticoids are highly effective in managing pruritus due to many hypersensitivity disorders, the serious side-effects stimulate constant investigations for alternative drugs or methods that will allow the avoidance of, or a reduction in, glucocorticoid administration. The purpose of this presentation is to report the results of a trial conducted at the small animal hospital of the Faculté de Médecine Vétérinaire of the University of Montreal.

Thirty dogs with pruritus due to atopy, flea-bite hypersensitivity and idiopathy were treated, in a double-blind, placebo-controlled trial, with a series of six drugs with potential antipruritic action: astemizole, clemastine, doxepin, trimeprazine, trimeprazine plus prednisone, and prednisone.

As expected, glucocorticoid-containing products were the most effective in controlling pruritus. The trimeprazine-prednisone combination product controlled pruritus in 76.7% of the dogs, while prednisone alone was satisfactory in 56.7%. Trimeprazine, in spite of a very low success rate of 3.3% when used alone, decreased the glucocorticoid requirement by an average of 30% in nine of 12 dogs (75%). Clemastine was, by far, the most effective antihistamine, controlling pruritus in 30% of the dogs. Astemizole, like trimeprazine was effective in only 3.3% of the dogs. Doxepin and the placebo were ineffective in all 30 dogs.

The results of this study confirm that antihistamines alone can be effective in the management of canine pruritus, and that antihistamines can significantly reduce necessary glucocorticoid doses in many dogs.

EFFECTS OF SULPHUR AND COAL TAR IN EPIDERMAL METABOLISM

M. Kietzmann,[1] D. Lubach[2] and J. Henkemeyer[1] *Institute für Pharmakologie Toxikologie und Pharmazie, Tierärztliche Hochschule, [1]Hautklinik Linden Medizinische Hochschule, [2]Hannover, FRG*

Because of their keratoplastic and keratolytic as well as their sebosuppressive effects, sulphur and coal tar are widely used in topical formulations for treatment of different canine skin disorders. Antibacterial, antifungal and antiparasitic effects are described also. The substances are used, mostly as shampoos, in concentrations of 1–10%. The study, described here, demonstrates effects of sulphur and coal tar in epidermal metabolism and histology. Twice daily the tail skin of laboratory animals (NMRI-mice) was treated topically with 10% sulphur or coal tar containing oily formulations. Using ^{3}H-labelled precursors, the incorporation rate of thymidine triphosphate into DNA and of leucine and histidine into protein was measured at the end of the treatment period.

Simultaneously, the epidermal thickness and cell count were measured.

After 8 days of sulphur treatment an increased epidermal thickness and cell count was found. The incorporation of thymidine triphosphate into DNA and of leucine and histidine into protein decreased. Because of these changes the development of a retention acanthosis is concluded.

After treatment with coal tar for 14 days there was a slight increase in tail skin epidermal thickness, while the cell count was unchanged. The thymidine triphosphate remained unchanged, while the leucin incorporation rate decreased. Since leucin is incorporated into the proliferating basal cell layer, it can be concluded that coal tar influences the keratinocyte proliferation. Because of the unchanged histidine incorporation rate into the upper epidermal layers, an effect of coal tar on differentiation is unlikely.

CULTURE AND CHARACTERIZATION OF PORCINE KERATINOCYTES

K. Hancock, H. A. Navsaria, M. E. J. Hackett and I. M. Leigh *Regional Burns Unit St Andres Hospital, Billericay, Essex and Department of Experimental Dermatology, The London Hospital, Whitechapel, London, UK*

Attempts have been made to grow human skin for over 20 years. In 1975 Rheinwald and Green described a culture system using a single cell suspension of epidermal keratinocytes which permitted the serial generation of keratinocytes through multiple passages. Pig skin has long been considered the best animal model for the study of human skin and culture of porcine keratinocytes has been described using different methods. Once it was possible to grow keratinocytes in substantial amounts it then became possible to study the factors controlling growth and differentiation of the keratinocyte alone or in combination. Keratinocyte culture systems were initially developed to study keratinocyte biology but clinical applications were soon recognized.

This study describes our own method of culture using a modified Rheinwald and Green technique. The keratinocytes grown in this way have been used for wound healing and skin grafting projects in the pig. Characterization of the cultured porcine keratinocytes has been studied using immunocytochemical techniques with a battery of monoclonal antibodies known to be reactive against human keratins.

The study presents our culture methodology and the characterization results for porcine keratinocytes.

THE BIOLOGY OF *Ctenocephalides canis* IN IRELAND: ITS SUSCEPTIBILITY TO MARKET INSECTICIDES

K. P. Baker and S. El Harram *Faculty of Veterinary Medicine, University College, Ballsbridge, Dublin, Ireland*

There have been few studies of the biology of fleas on dogs, yet flea hypersensitivity is the commonest cause for consultation in this faculty.

Ctenocephalides canis is easily the most common flea found in dogs in Ireland; a colony has now been established in this faculty. The domestic cat is an unsuitable host. Breeding adults are maintained on dogs and the ideal temperature and relative humidity for breeding is 22°C and 75% relative humidity, when the life cycle is completed in 25 days.

Contrary to several reports in the literature, adult fleas remain on dogs; significantly greater numbers are found on the dorsal mid-line.

When the intradermal reaction to whole flea extract and rolled flea extracts was studied, the latter gave greater reactions.

There are no significant regional differences in reactions to flea extracts in hypersensitive dogs.

The mortality of adult fleas was compared on normal dogs when washed with a placebo, one containing pymethrin and a second containing phenothrin, tetramethrin and piperonyl butoxide. Only the product containing pymethrin had a 100% residual effect after 14 days.

An organochloride wash and an organophosphorus spray produced over 90% mortality after 8 h and 100% mortality in 24 h, in an *in vitro* experiment with adult *Ct. canis*. Both produced 100% mortality of larvae in 24 h.

Management of *Ct. canis* in a colony provides a source for the study. Its persistence on the host means that the regular use of synthetic pyrethroid with residual properties is indicated.

The results of trials did not indicate any development of resistance of *Ct. canis* to the parasiticides tested.

Rolled flea extract contains more hapten than whole flea extract. It will be of greater value for hyposensitization procedures and the study of the tissue response, than whole flea extracts.

PLATELET ACTIVATING FACTOR: A PUTATIVE MEDIATOR OF INFLAMMATION IN EQUINE SWEET-ITCH

A.P. Foster, F. Cunningham and P. Lees *Department of Veterinary Basic Sciences, Royal Veterinary College, North Mymms, Hatfield, Herts, UK*

The effects of platelet activating factor (PAF) on cutaneous inflammatory responses have been compared in clinically normal horses ($n = 6$) and those with sweet-itch ($n = 3$). Wheal volumes were calculated from measurements of skin fold thickness and wheal diameter carried out between 2 and 64 min after intradermal injection of PAF (0.001–1 μg per site; 50 μl volume), vehicle (phosphate buffered saline containing 0.25% equine serum albumin (PBS/ESA)), and histamine (0.22 μg free-base per site), as a positive control. Punch biopsies were taken 1, 2 and 4 h after intradermal injection of 1 μg PAF or PBS/ESA. Cell infiltrates were quantitated histologically.

In normal and sweet-itch horses intradermal injection of 0.1 μg PAF had significantly increased vascular permeability when compared to vehicle, peak responses occurring at 32 min. The vascular responses to PAF were no different in normal and hypersensitive horses. In contrast the permeability response to histamine was significantly reduced in allergic horses when compared to healthy controls (193 ± 15 μl vs 519 ± 60 μl; $p < 0.001$, Student's t test). Furthermore, the mean peak increase in vascular permeability produced by equimolar concentrations of histamine and PAF in normal horses was similar, a result which differs from observations made in other species.

There was no difference between the number of neutrophils accumulating in the dermis of normal and sweet-itch horses in response to 1 μg PAF. Eosinophil, mononuclear and mast cell numbers remained unchanged in both groups throughout the study. However, since ESA has subsequently been found to induce mast cell accumulation, the study is being repeated using PBS alone as the vehicle.

These initial studies show that in normal horses PAF and histamine increase vascular permeability and that in sweet-itch there seems to be a down-regulation of the response to histamine. One possible explanation may be a desensitization due to previous exposure to histamine.

PROTECTION AGAINST UVB DAMAGE TO PORCINE SKIN WITH TOPICAL APPLICATION OF VITAMIN C

D. Darr,[1] T. Manning,[2] S. Dunstan[2] and S Pinnell[1] [1]*Division of Dermatology, Duke University Medical Center, Durham, NC, and* [2]*Cutaneous Pharmacology and Toxicology Center, College of Veterinary Medicine, North Carolina State University, North Carolina, USA*

Ultraviolet (UV) radiation damages skin. The UV effects range from painful, acute sunburn to premature 'aging' of skin and skin cancer. The exact mechanisms of this damage are essentially unknown. With the knowledge that skin damaged by UV radiation may be compared to a skin wound, and hypothesizing that chemically reactive oxygen radicals in the skin might be important aetiologically in inflammatory damage, we have formulated a stable, aqueous solution of *L*-ascorbic acid (a promoter of wound healing and a biological antioxidant) for topical application. Preliminary dermatologic studies have shown that preapplication of this ascorbic acid formulation for several days leads to visible protection from moderate-to-severe sunburn. Other studies have shown that this is not likely a sunscreen effect. Using domestic swine (Yorkshire) we have utilized 'sunburn cell' analysis as well as blood flow (as measured by laser Doppler velocimetry) to quantitate topical vitamin C's protective capability against a UVB insult. By pretreating animals' skin for 1 week, the vitamin C was able to reduce UVB-induced increases in the above parameters by 50% ($p \leq .01\%$; 2–3 MED exposure). Indeed, there is evidence that vitamin C helps protect against the UV damage if only applied after irradiation.

We hypothesize that UV damage, both direct and indirect, results at least in part from the generation of oxygen radicals. Vitamin C is a potent antioxidant, and the ability to increase skin levels of this vitamin pharmacologically, has the potential to help protect against and repair damage due to UV radiation.

JUNCTIONAL EPIDERMOLYSIS BULLOSA (EPITHELIOGENESIS IMPERFECTA) IN FRENCH FOALS

J. M. Gourreau,[1] C. Feillou, M. Morand and A. Alliot *[1]Ministere de l'Agriculture et de la Foret Centre National d'Etudes Vétérinaires et Alimentaires Laboratoire Central de Recherches Vétérinaires, Maison-Alfort, France*

Epitheliogenesis imperfecta is a rare hereditary disorder due to a recessive autosomal gene found in man and several animal species. This paper describes four new cases on draught-horses of two breeds. Signs noted are agenesis of the skin and mucosa, particularly in the limbs and the mouth. In one animal, hooves are lacking. Histological and ultrastructural examinations show separation of the dermo-epidermal junction through the lamina lucida of the basement membrane leaving the intact lamina adherent to the dermis.

Abstracts of Buiatrics Session

DIAGNOSIS OF BOVINE ULCERATIVE MAMILLITIS WHICH APPEARED AT HAUTE-MARNE IN 1988

A. Moussa, J. M. Gourreau, M. Fedida, P. Hermitte, A. Dubois and R. Guerrin
Ministere de l'Agriculture, CNEVA, Laboratoire de Pathologie Bovine, Lyon, France

In early August 1988, first in three localities in the Haute-Marne Department and then within 4 to 5 days, in each of 12 farms, 50–80% dairy cattle developed teat and udder lesions. The disease was characterized by development of vesicles and large ulcers which cicatrized within 3 weeks. The disease propagations stopped by the end of September.

Rapid virological diagnosis by electron microscope examination of scab filtrates revealed the presence of herpesvirus particles. The virus was isolated and identified genetically and serologically as bovine herpesvirus type 2 (BHV-2).

Latterly, seroneutralization in the presence of complement as well as immunofluorescence techniques were used to survey the prevalence of antibodies in cattle sera collected throughout the department; 27 of 120 sera were revealed as positive.

A NEW BOVINE GENODERMATOSIS RESEMBLING EPIDERMOLYSIS BULLOSA SIMPLEX IN MAN

Hugh Bassett *Dept of Veterinary Pathology, Faculty of Veterinary Medicine, University College Dublin, Ballsbridge, Dublin, Ireland*

Bovine epidermolysis, a recently discovered genodermatosis, resembles epidermolysis bullosa simplex of man. The disease, which was first identified in crossbred calves sired by a Simmental bull, is inherited as an autosomal dominant trait. When affected males were experimentally mated with normal unrelated females, bovine epidermolysis was confirmed in ten calves of the 22 calves produced. When affected animals were mated inter-se, four clinically normal calves, two putative affected heterozygotes and two putative affected homozygotes were born.

Clinically, bovine epidermolysis is characterized by an abnormal suseptibility of the skin to trivial trauma.

Stratified squamous keratinizing epithelium of the upper alimentary tract is also affected. Affected heterozygotes show retarded growth, hypotrichosis and breaks in the integrity of the skin. The disease is at its most severe in young calves and its effects moderate as maturity approaches.

Histopathologically, bovine epidermolysis is characterized by a dermo-epidermal separation in which the basement membrane area remains adherent to the dermis. Cytolysis of keratinocytes similar to that seen in the various forms of epidermolysis bullosa simplex of man is evident on ultrastructural examination of experimentally induced lesions.

VACCINATION AGAINST *Dermatophilus congolensis* INFECTION IN RUMINANTS: PROSPECTS FOR CONTROL

S. J. How, D. H. Lloyd and A. B. Sanders *Dept of Veterinary Medicine and Animal Husbandry, Royal Veterinary College, North Mymms, Hatfield, Herts, UK*

Dermatophilus infection in cattle is a major factor limiting cattle husbandry in the humid tropics. Vaccine studies in West Africa have indicated that immunopropylaxis offers the best means of control of this disease but the field efficacy of vaccines has proved disappointing. We have re-evaluated vaccine-induced immunity using a dose response model. In rabbits there is a clear relationship between zoospore challenge dose and the severity of infection. Antigenic differences between strains of *D. congolensis* were also shown to be important. Vaccination increased the minimum infective dose by 10 000-fold and 100-fold respectively for vaccine homologous and heterologous challenges.

Studies in sheep have also demonstrated the importance of energy malnutrition in limiting immunity to *Dermatophilus*. Experimental infections in malnourished animals are prolonged and have altered gross pathology. Both specific and non-specific immunity are affected and the ability to respond to vaccination is impaired. There was a lower minimum infectious dose and lesions were more severe and persisted for longer in malnourished animals.

Further work is required to define the importance of strain difference and immunity in the field. Improved immunity should be possible using vaccines with common protective antigens and by using immunization strategies which avoid vaccination during period of energy malnutrition. In our current work we are evaluating the use of immunostimulatory complex (ISCOM) vaccines. This technique will allow the incorporation of antigens from different *D. congolensis* strains and may provide prolonged and elevated levels of immunity thus avoiding the problems of poor cross-immunity and seasonal periods of malnutrition.

SPORADIC FORMS OF BOVINE DERMATOPHILOSIS IN FRANCE

R. Chermette and J. Bussieras *Service de Parasitologie, Ecole Nationale Vétérinaire d'Alfort, Maison-Alfort, France*

Dermatophilosis due to *Dermatophilus congolensis* is well known in horses and sheep in various parts of France. Sporadic cases were diagnosed in cattle too: in calves in Normandy and northern parts of France and a more extensive form in a herd of Charolais cattle in the department of Indre.

Diagnosis was performed by direct microscopic examination of Giemsa-stained smears of crusts from lesions and sometimes with complementary methods, i.e., experimental inoculation into rabbits and culture on blood-agar.

Dermatophilosis must be now included in the list of the dermatoses possibly encountered in cattle under temperate climate in France. Though less frequently found and less severe than in tropical areas, the infection can be serious sometimes, with generalized crusty lesions leading to death unless adequate antibiotic therapy is carried out.

DISEASES DUE TO PARAPOXVIRUS IN CATTLE

A. Moussa, J. Tektoff, G. Dannacher, J. Espinasse, G. Descours and M. Fedida *Ministere de l'Agriculture, CNEVA, Laboratoire de Pathologie Bovine, Lyon, France*

Bovine papular stomatitis, pseudocowpox thelitis, tail necrotic dermatitis in fattening cattle and necrotic laryngitis represent some clinical manifestations of parapoxvirus infections in cattle. The virus is a member of poxviridae, genus parapox. Virions are in the form of cocoon 250–360 × 140–170 nm. The DNA genome is 140 Kpb in size and 96×10^6 dalton molecular weight. Virus replication takes place entirely in the cytoplasm. Bovine isolated strains studied by the electron microscope showed the presence of 40 nm diameter tubules in the mitochondria and some strains showed other large 80 nm tubules in the nucleolus.

Laboratory diagnosis of parapoxvirus infections can be done rapidly by examination in the electron microscope (EM). Inoculation into susceptible tissue cultures followed 48–72 h later by immunofluorescence using monoclonal antibodies proves a good means for diagnosis especially when virus particle content is too low to be detected by EM.

Serological examinations, using immunofluorescence technique for antibody detection to parapoxvirus, reveals about 95% positive animals. Young calves acquire a passive immunity after ingestion of colostrum.

Animals infected with the parapoxvirus develop a carrier state and can manifest after periods of remission weak-to-moderate disease symptoms. Acquired immunity is of a short duration — 6–8 months. Until now no specific bovine parapoxvirus vaccines are in preparation.

NEW ASPECTS OF PATHOGENESIS AND SKIN DAMAGES IN CATTLE DEMODICOSIS

H. F. Mathes and T. H. Hiepe *Humboldt-Universität Berlin, Sektion Tierproduktion und Veterinarmedizin, Berlin, GDR*

Bovine demodicosis is a parasitic skin disease characterized by chronic folliculitis. Affected cattle show no systemic signs of illness, and production parameters are not altered. There is, however, significant damage to the hide, leading to losses in the leather industry. *Demodex bovis* has been found in nearly all cattle herds in the German Democratic Republic and demodectic nodules have been found in 72% of cattle hides.

The pathogenesis of bovine demodicosis is still not well understood. Based on our experiments, we present a hypothesis concerning the development of nodule formation. The period from follicular invasion to the establishment of a palpable nodule (up to 1 mm in diameter) is about 4 months. The maximum size obtained is 10 mm. The time for regression of a nodule varies from 2–3 weeks to 4 months. In this process secondary bacterial infections seem to play an important role. The leather damage is caused by the presence of different stages of demodectic nodules in the corium. The degree of leather damage depends on the stage of nodule development at the time of slaughter. We distinguish eight main defects on the inner surface — crater at grain deepenings, colour clearings, glitter spots, small gaps, great holes, cicatrices and coarse grain. These defects are seen separately, but in the most cases they overlay each other and so present the various types of damage seen in the leather.

THE FIRST AVIRULENT VACCINE IN CONTROL OF *Trichophyton* INFECTION IN CATTLE IN TURKEY

M. Sahal, H. Y. Imren, N. K. Forku and H. Yardimai *The Veterinary Faculty, Internal Disease Department, University of Ankara, Turkey*

During the winter and spring seasons of 1988 in studies carried out around Ankara and Osmanoik, Corum, an immunogenic lyophilized vaccine prepared from live cultures of the avirulent strain of *Trichophyton verrucosum* (produced by the firm Ivonovic na Hane Bioveta of Czechoslovakia) was given intramuscularly (*M. semitendinosus*) twice, 14 days apart to various breeds of cattle between the ages of 4 weeks and 7 years. This vaccine was tested in 13 cows and 62 calves to investigate its prophylactic effectiveness and in five cows and 41 calves to investigate its therapeutic effectiveness. During the 90 days observational period it was noted that the rate of protection in animals given a prophylactic dose was 98.96% whereas the rate of recovery of the animals given a therapeutic dose was 71.14%.

The results of the prophylactic dose application showed that about 3–4 weeks after the second vaccination there was reliable immunity. Indeed during a year-long observation period, there was no recurrence of the illness.

The vaccine, when given as a therapeutic dose activated the immune system of the organism and ensured recovery within 4–6 weeks of animals with slight or moderate trichophyton lesions and in the regions of the body with lesions the hairs fell out completely. However not much success was obtained in animals with severe lesions.

No side-effects due to the vaccine were observed during this study. The results of the investigation showed that because of its easy application, its ability to break the chain of infection and its effectiveness in successful treatment this vaccine could be used successfully for the eradication of this illness in our country and could replace many other antimycotic drugs. It was also determined that this illness was an important zoonosis in regions where there were infections.

BOVINE NODULAR THELITIS, A STUDY

M. F. Thorel, M. Morand, J. J. Fontaine and J. M. Gourreau *Ministere de l'Agriculture et de la Foret, Centre National d'Etudes Vétérinaries et Alimentaires, Laboratoire Central de Recherches Vétérinaires, Maison-Alfort, France*

The bovine nodular thelitis in dairy cattle is a chronic, enzootic infection. Three stages may be distinguished: growth of nodules within the teat wall (early stage), rupture and ulceration of the nodules and scarring with deformation of the teats. Economically this disease is serious because of the complications of mastitis and the non specific reactions to the intradermal tuberculin test in tuberculosis prevention.

Twenty pathological specimens, udders and teats, were examined. Lesions were located mainly in the lower part of the udder or on the teat and recognized as solid nodules.

These specimens were divided into two parts, the first one for the isolation of mycobacteria and the other for the histopathological examination.

The histopathologic lesions of the teats were of a tuberculoid pattern, characterized by a subacute focal dermatitis with lymphoid cells, macrophages, epitheloid cells and a variable amount of giant cells (Langhans type). The inflammatory infiltrates were mainly perivascular. Sometimes they were found in all the depth of the teat. No necrosis was observed.

The presence of acid-fast bacilli was inconstant. It seems that they were found mainly when giant Langhans cells were numerous.

Three strains of acid fast bacilli have been isolated but only one was identified as *Mycobacterium terrae*, which is a non-pathogen slowly growing non-photochromogenic mycobacteria. The involvement of this organism in tuberculosis-like skin lesions in the bovine udder is discussed.

In conclusion the authors confirm that bovine nodular thelitis in dairy cows is a disease with lesions histologically similar to those of tuberculosis which suggest that an atypical mycobacteria is involved.

CATTLE SUMMER SORES IN THE EAST OF FRANCE

J. Bussieras, R, Chermette, M. Gresset and M. Mass *Service de Parasitologie, Ecole Nationale Vétérinaire, Maison-Alfort, France*

Every year, during the warm season, in the east of France (Jura mountains), some cattle exhibit cutaneous sores associated with severe itching and the presence of countless flies.

These lesions can develop in any part of the body surface, but they are often localized in the fore-hollow of the udder, or on the teats. This last site leads to difficulties in milking, thus increasing the hazard of mastitis.

Parasitological examination of lesions, after excision, allowed us to find nematode larvae, very similar to the third-stage larvae of *Parafilaria bovicola*. However, it was not possible to find adult worms belonging to genus *Parafilaria* in animals originating in this area. Moreover, these larvae are surrounded by a strong eosinophilic reaction, and it seems they do not migrate, but are destroyed locally. The larvae are probably brought by flies but catching, breeding, then dissecting hundreds of cattle flies did not permit the finding of any developing larvae.

Similar lesions are sometimes mentioned in other parts of France. It will be interesting to search there for the presence of nematode larvae in cattle summer sores.

BOVINE DERMATOMYCOSIS IN INDIA

A. Sikdar, S. K. Mitra, P. C. Harbola and G. R. Ghosh *Division of Bacteriology & Mycology, Indian Veterinary Research Institute, Izatnagar UP, India*

Dermatomycosis in man and animals has been reported from prehistoric times throughout the world. In India with hot and humid climatic conditions, the occurrence of these groups of fungal infections are expected to be high. The dermatophytes reported so far in cattle in India are; *T. verruscocum*, *T. mentagrophytes*, *T. rubrum*, *T. violaceum*, *M. terrestre*, *M. canis* and *M. gypseum*. In the present study, a total of 1062 cattle were screened, distributed in different places in Uttar Pradesh. These comprised of three different breeds — Holstein-Friesian Cross, Jersey Cross and Haryana Cross of different ages and of either sex. Young animals were found to suffer more from skin disease which was statistically significant ($p < 0.01$). Dermatophytes recovered from the clinical cases of cattle under the present study were; *M. gypseum*, *T. mentagrophytes*, *T. rubrum* and *T. simii*. Isolation of *T. simii* from cattle appeared to be the first report. Fungal agents other than dermatophytes isolated from the skin scraping were *Alternaria* sp., *Beauveria bassiana*, *Cyrsosporium*, *Keratinophilum*, *Aspergillus* sp., and *Penicillium* sp.

STEPHANOFILARIAL DERMATITIS IN CATTLE OF WEST BENGAL (INDIA)

A. Chakrabarti[1] **and A. Chatterjee**[2] [1]*Dept of Veterinary Medicine and Public Health, Faculty of Veterinary and Animal Sciences, Bidhan Chandra Krishi Viswavidyalaya, Mohanpur, Nadia, West Bengal India* [2]*Moitri Research Laboratory, Calcutta, India*

Stephanofiliarial worms are responsible for producing parasitic dermatitis in cattle, buffaloes and goats. The common site of lesions in cattle is reported to differ with species of the parasite. In India, *Stephanofilaria assamensis* produces lesions in the hump and this condition is widely known as "hump sore". The present communication records some uncommon sites of lesions in cattle reared in this part of the country. Lesions were observed in the teat of a Jersey cow as "teat sore". The lesion was located on the upper third of the teat. One bull had a lesion at the base of the tail as "tail sore". Lesions were recorded at the base of the dew claws described as "leg sore". The lesions were noticed in country breeds as well as exotic breeds. Lesions appeared just around the dew claws, in one or both, fore or hind limbs. It appeared as if the skin of the part had been erased. There was exudation of serum and crust formation. As the lesions advanced, there was swelling and the appearance of granumatous growth. In more advanced cases, the dew claws shed completely leaving behind a crater-like ulcer. Lesions were also noted in the muzzle as "muzzle sore". Initially, papules appeared on the muzzle, which then coalesced and there was formation of crusts due to exudation of serum. There was leukoderma of the surrounding area. It is interesting to note that none of these animals had lesions in the hump which is the preferred site for stephanofilarial lesions in cattle in India. In all the animals, irritation and pruritus were evident. From respective tissues, parasites of the genus *Stephanofilaria* were recorded.

SARCOPTIC MANGE IN THE INDIAN CAMEL

P. M. Raisinghani and D. Kumar *Department of Parasitology, College of Veterinary and Animal Science, Rajasthan Agriculture University, Bikaner, India*

The Indian camel (*Camelus dromedarius*) has acclaimed superiority in India's north west arid and semi-arid belt known as the Thar Desert. India has a camel population of 1.774 million which is 7.8% of the world's population (FAO 1978). Though the camel is a very hardy animal and easily tolerates the rugged climate and extremes of temperature, the scorching heat and stormy weather of the desert and ravages of unprecedented drought, it does suffer from skin diseases. Sarcoptic mange caused by *Sarcoptes scabei* var *cameli* is very prevalent and poses a serious threat to camel health including predisposing it to contract surra.

This paper covers epidemiology, pathology and management of this dreadful skin infection. In 1973 highest (64%) incidence of Sarcoptic mange was in the winter months with the lowest (17.4%) in the summer months. On the basis of 9788 clinical samples analysed during 1978 to 1988, the infection was recorded throughout the year with the maximum record of 51.05 to 62.76% during the months of December, January, February, March and April.

Loss of hair, scab formation, keratinization, proliferation of connective tissue leading to thickening of skin and corrugations were observed due to deep penetration of mites in the skin tissues. It was also found that camel attendants suffered from this infection forming anthropozoonoses. A number of acaricides including Lindane (Lintox 20% EC) have been tried for the control of Sarcoptic mange in camels using 0.05% as deep spray. Recently, Ivermectin was found to be most effective at the dose rate of 200 µg/kg body weight given subcutaneously and repeated after 15 days.

Abstracts of Posters

UNDIFFERENTIATED MASTOCYTOMA

Bärbel Beardi,[1] and Marna Opitz[2] [1]*Tierärztliche Praxis für Hautkrankheiten Veterinärhistologisches Labor, Hannover, FRG;* [2]*Poliklinik für Kleine Haustiere der Universität Berlin, Berlin, FRG*

A case of undifferentiated mastocytoma in an 8-year-old male cocker spaniel and a multicentric lymphosarcoma in an 8-year-old female chow chow are presented, first diagnosied via skin biopsies.

LOW ENERGY LASER TREATMENTS FOR CANINE DERMATOLOGY

J. Bussiéras, Chantal Perraudeau and R. Chermette *Ecole Nationale Vétérinaire, Maison-Alfort, France*

Low power laser rays, as those produced by helium-neon tubes, are said to release energy inside living organisms, with an action of cell stimulation.

In the mammalian skin, they would exert some beneficient effects: antiinflammatory, antipruritic, eutrophic (collagen synthesis, healing).

However, these actions are often questioned, and in some cases the human cures are ascribed to a placebo effect. So it was very interesting to carry out clinical tests in animals, and at the Ecole Nationale Vétérinaire d'Alfort, since 1984, we have used successively two helium-neon laser apparatus (powers respectively 25 and 10 mW).

The case selection was based upon lack of parasitic, fungal, or endocrine aetiology; prevalence of either inflammatory and pruritic symptoms, or cutaneous dystrophy with skin thinning and alopecia; and low extension of the lesion, avoiding a too-long immobilization of animals during treatment.

Thus we treated two major diseases: acral lick dermatitis, which is generally localized on the lower anterior part of one or several legs, and is mainly observed in large breeds (German shepherd, Belgian shepherd, doberman pinscher), and in highly strung animals; also focal alopecia, which typically appears as a non-pruritic hairless circular area, which spreads out after a therapeutic injection, and mainly affects small breeds (Yorkshire terrier, toy poodle, etc.).

Each animal was treated for 10 minutes, once every 2 or 3 days, until a total of about 8 or 10 treatments.

From 1984 to 1989, 63 dogs were treated, 25 of which suffered from lick dermatitis, and 23 others from focal alopecia. The results were often very good, mainly in cases of the two diseases defined above. In cases of focal alopecia, generally a complete hair growth is easily obtained, sometimes after only three or four treatments. In lick dermatitis, 8 to 10 or sometimes 15 treatments were necessary, and it was useful to add topical disinfection (e.g. with chlorhexidine lotions).

The only problem is the high cost of apparatus and scarceness of appropriate cases. This means that treatment is very costly, and the laser may be used for other types of cases (arthrology, rheumatology), and for non-canine cases (feline dermatoses, equine practice, etc.).

HISTOPATHOLOGY OF CELL REGENERATION AFTER AN EXPERIMENTAL SKIN INJURY INDUCED BY MUSTARD GAS

P. Guittin,[1] F. Schorch,[2] J.-J. Fontaine,[2] F. Crespeau[2] and A.-L. Parodi[2] *[1]Centre d'Etudes du Bouchet, Vert-le-petit; [2]Ecole Nationale Vétérinaire, Maisons-Alfort, France*

Experimental skin injury was induced by a single percutaneous dose of mustard gas (bis(2-chloroethyl) sulphide). Sulphur mustard (22 mg/kg) was applied to 1 cm^2 cutaneous site on the back of male rats. Serial histopathological studies were performed from Day 1 to Day 30 posttreatment.

One day after exposure, epidermal necrosis developed and at Day 2, skin ulceration was present and crusts were forming. Figures of epidermal cells regeneration started at Days 5 or 6. They were associated with dermal focal vasodilatation and active polymorphonuclear diapedesis. A scar began at Day 10, the ulcer decreased, keratin markers reappeared and were noted only in stratum spinosum and stratum granulosum. A scar was achieved at Day 30, with acanthosis of epidermis and permanent follicular aplasia.

An infrared laser treatment was applied on this irreversible scar, 2 months after injury. Laser therapy was done during 4 months with three daily local radiations (respectively at 500, 1000 then 2000 Hz) for 3 min each (7 days a week the first 2 months, every 2 days the third month, then every 3 days the fourth month).

This treatment increased dermal vascularization but also induced an abnormal regeneration of epidermis. Scarring and aplasia of hair follicles were persistent.

Mustard gas induced an acute cutaneous injury, followed by an irreversible scar with anormal and persistent acanthosis. These changes were not modified by laser therapy.

A COMPARISON OF THREE LOCAL ANAESTHETIC TECHNIQUES FOR SKIN BIOPSY IN DOGS

Julie I. Headrick, K.L. Thoday and K.W. Head *Royal (Dick) School of Veterinary Studies, Edinburgh, UK*

Local analgesia is commonly used for skin biopsy in dogs. Although several reports document variations in the suitability of different local anaesthetic agents for skin biopsy in humans, no such work has been done in dogs. We now report the results of a study to compare the suitability of three local anaesthetic agents for skin biopsy in dogs. The agents were 1% lignocaine injected subcutaneously, 1% lignocaine with adrenaline injected subtutaneously, and a new, topically active local anaesthetic cream recently marketed for use in humans (EMLA, Astra). The three agents were compared for ease of administration, efficacy of analgesia, side-effects, and any differences in histopathology attributable to the anaesthetic agent.

A total of 25 dogs were biopsied. Three biopsies were taken from each dog, using a different anaesthetic agent for each biopsy. All biopsies were taken and processed identically.

The administration of all three agents was well tolerated by the dogs. Efficacy of analgesia with EMLA was variable, and a possible explanation for this can be derived from the histopathology. Side-effects were noted only with EMLA, but disruption of important histopathological features was noted with both EMLA and 1% lignocaine-adrenaline.

We conclude that 1% lignocaine without adrenaline injected subcutaneously is the analgesic agent of choice for routine skin biopsy in the dog.

PLASMA FATTY ACIDS IN DOGS AND THEIR RESPONSE TO ESSENTIAL FATTY ACID SUPPLEMENTATION

David Horrobin,[1] Sharon Dobbin and Brenda Reynolds [1]*Efamol Vet, Guildford, Surrey, UK*

Plasma essential fatty acid (EFA) levels were measured in normal humans and normal dogs. These were then compared to the EFA levels in subjects with allergic skin disease.

The results show that normal humans and dogs have slightly lower levels of linoleic acid (LA) and slightly higher levels of dihomo-γ linolenic acid (DGLA) and arachidonic acid (AA) than subjects with allergic skin disease.

In human studies, treatment of atopic patients with evening primrose oil (EPO), a rich source of γ (gamma)-linolenic acid (GLA), results in a significant increase in DGLA and a slight increase in AA; GLA is rapidly converted to the antiinflammatory DGLA and then, as in most species, more slowly to AA.

However, in the dog, EPO supplementation of atopic patients results in a slight increase in DGLA and a significant increase in AA. It would appear therefore that the conversion rate of DGLA to AA by the δ-5-desaturase enzyme system is more rapid in the dog than in other species.

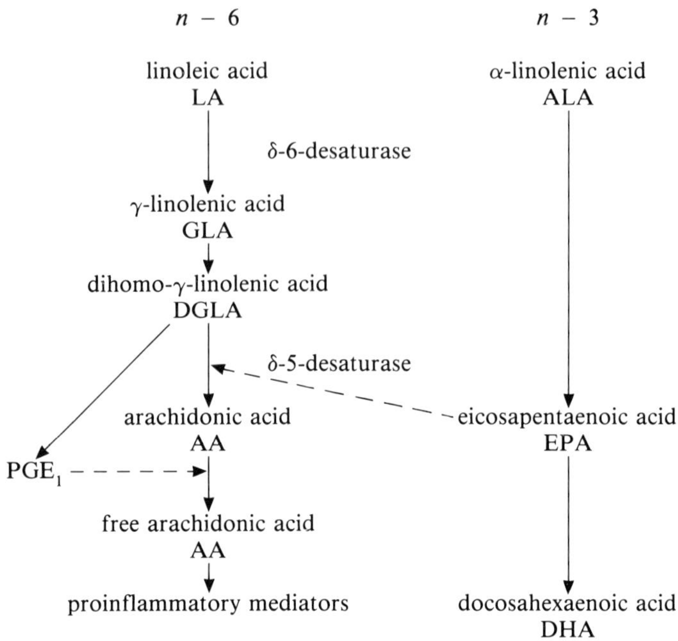

Arachidonic acid is a major component of the phospholipids of all cell membranes and has no adverse affects as long as it stays in that form. However, free AA can readily be converted to a range of proinflammatory substances including 2 series prostaglandins, leukotrienes and thromboxanes.

Dihomo-γ-linolenic acid has highly desirable effects as it is a precursor to antiinflammatory substances such as PGE1 and hydroxy-DGLA. PGE1 inhibits the conversion of AA to proinflammatory free AA and hydroxy & DGLA inhibit the conversion of free AA to the proinflammatory mediators.

Fish oils (FO) contain eicosapentaenoic acid (EPA) which in modest amounts limits the conversion of DGLA to AA and inhibits the formation of proinflammatory metabolites from AA without blocking the production of antiinflammatory metabolites from DGLA. However, high doses of fish oil interfere with the actions of both DGLA and AA.

In humans the δ-5-desaturase enzyme is a rate-limiting step and so human atopic patients show an increased DGLA level following EPO alone.

Because of their efficient δ-5-desaturase enzyme, dogs may have a specific requirement for a small amount of EPA and so an evening primrose oil/fish oil supplement is necessary to ensure the best possible response in dogs with atopic skin disease.

n-3 AND n-6 ESSENTIAL FATTY ACIDS (EFAS) AND THE SKIN

David Horrobin,[1] **Sharon Dobbin and Brenda Reynolds** [1]*Efamol Vet, Guildford, Surrey, UK*

All animals deprived of EFAs develop severe skin disorders with loss of hair, loss of the normal skin permeability barrier and failure of wound healing. There are two types of EFA; the n-6 series derived from linoleic acid (LA) and the n-3 series derived from α-linolenic acid (ALA).

Administration of the n-6 series of EFAs to EFA-deficient animals corrects deficiency signs but n-3 EFAs (derived from fish oil) exacerbate the inflammatory condition of the skin. There is a role for n-3 EFAs in skin disorders, but only as an adjunct to adequate amounts of the n-6 EFAs.

The important EFAs with regard to the skin are γ-linolenic acid (GLA) derived from evening primrose oil, and its immediate metabolite, dihomo-γ-linolenic acid (DGLA). This is converted to arachidonic acid (AA) which is also a necessary constituent of membranes. Arachidonic acid is proinflammatory if released from membranes and converted to proinflammatory prostaglandins, leukotrienes or thromboxanes. Factors affecting release of free AA from the membrane stores include trauma and injury.

The presence of modest amounts of n-3 EFAs as eicosapentaenoic acid (EPA) derived from fish oil, is desirable as it inhibits the conversion of DGLA to AA and the release of AA from the membranes without blocking the conversion of DGLA to its desirable antiinflammatory metabolite PGE_1. However, large amounts of EPA interfere with both DGLA and AA and so may have adverse effects on the skin. Investigators have found that the optimum ratio of evening primrose oil/fish oil for PGE_1 production is approximately 80:20.

Recent work in humans indicates that some LA containing oils may be proinflammatory. For example the LA in safflower oil and corn oils is in a form which may enter a linked enzyme system resulting in an elevation of AA without any corresponding rise in DGLA. EPO provides GLA which appears to enter an enzyme sequence which achieves both affects. This data is supported by a study which showed that the level of urate-induced inflammation was greater in rats fed on normal chow, safflower or fish oil supplemented diets compared with diets supplemented with evening primrose oil.

Therapeutic EFA products must be formulated based on sound biochemical and clinical data in order to maximize efficacy and minimize potential adverse effects of the components.

PATHOLOGY OF CANINE SEBORRHOEIC DERMATITIS AND ASSOCIATED CHANGES IN THYROID

R. Jayaram,[1] S.J. Seshadri,[2] R.N. Sreenivas Gowda[2] and S.K. Vijayasarathi[2]
[1]Department of AH and VS; [2]Department of Veterinary Pathology, Veterinary College, University of Agricultural Sciences, Hebbal, Bangalore, India

Forty-six cases of dermatitis in dogs were studied (27 males; 19 females). Four of them were of sarcoptic mange and the rest, non-parasitic dermatitis.

The gross lesions of sarcoptic mange were in the form of patchy areas of alopecia and erythema in the regions of pinnae, elbow and the hock with also changes of excoriations and encrustations. Histologically marked acanthosis, gradations of hyperkeratosis, formation of keratin plugs, burrows in the keratin layers with presence of mites and microfocal areas of suppuration were the feature. Thyroid glands in three of these cases showed parenchymatous goitre while in the remaining cases, changes of degeneration were noticed. The haematological values showed moderate anaemia while the biochemical findings indicated increase in serum cholesterol and diminished protein-bound iodine values.

Dermatitis of non-parasitic causes were studied under three categories namely generalized lesions; lesions in specific regions and localized lesions. There were nine cases, 25 cases and three cases respectively in these categories. In all cases the gross changes, and changes in histopathology of skin and thyroid, haematological values and values relating to serum cholesterol, protein-bound iodine and alkaline phosphatase were recorded and evaluated.

The changes observed in the thyroid were categorized as those of colloid goitre, parenchymatous goitre, degenerative changes, parafollicular cell hyperplasia and ultimobranchial cyst.

The skin lesions showed varying graduations of alopecia, rough, coarse and bristle-like hairs and abscessations and encrustations. Microscopically epidermal changes consisted of moderate-to-marked acanthosis, with adnexal components cystic or atrophic. Hair follicles characteristically showed cystic dilation with degenerate keratin material or keratin material appearing laminated in a basket weave pattern. There were also changes of inflammatory infiltration and microabscess formations that could be associated with bite injury and secondary infections. The haematological values of moderate anaemia and biochemical values suggested a hypothyroid state.

MANAGEMENT OF EQUINE CUTANEOUS LYMPHOSARCOMA

Janet D. Littlewood and Katherine Whitwell *Animal Health Trust, Newmarket, Suffolk, UK*

Involvement of the skin has been reported in cases of multicentric, alimentary and mediastinal lymphosarcoma in horses. In these cases the clinical course is usually rapid and the disease fatal. However, primary cutaneous lymphosarcoma may occur, without involvement of other organ systems, at least in the early stages of the disease. In contrast to other forms of equine lymphosarcoma, the cutaneous form usually has a chronic time course with animals surviving for prolonged periods, without signs of systemic illness. The cutaneous form was reported to be the most frequently recognized presentation of equine lymphosarcoma encountered by one clinic (Madewell and Theilen, 1987), but other surveys suggest that it is an unusual manifestation. No accounts of cutaneous lymphosarcoma in Britain have been found.

The present report describes a case of cutaneous lymphosarcoma in a cob mare. The mare had a history of multiple subcutaneous nodules which appeared and disappeared over a period of 11 years. The appearance of the nodules seemed to be related to nutritional intake, being coincident with growth of grass or the intake of concentrate food when stabled. A marked deterioration with increase in size of two nodules, accompanied by ulceration and infection, occurred after 'alternative therapy'. Biopsies taken on two occasions, 4 years apart, revealed infiltration of the dermis by small lymphocytes, extending up to but not into the epidermis. No signs of systemic illness were noted. The case was managed by a combination of surgical excision, local infiltration using glucocorticoids and systemic progestagens. All the skin nodules resolved, and the horse remains fit and well and in full work.

REFERENCE

Madewell, B.R. and Theilen, G.H. (1987). In: Theilen, G.H. and Madewell, B.R. (eds) *Veterinary Cancer Medicine* 2nd edn, pp. 431–437. Lea & Febiger, Philadelphia.

SKIN THINNING EFFECTS OF TOPICAL CORTICOSTEROIDS

D. Lubach,[1] M. Kietzmann[2] and V. Itzel-Kietzmann[3] [1]*Hautklinik Linden, Medizinische Hochschule, Hannover;* [2]*Institut für Pharmakologie, Toxikologie und Pharmazie, Tierärztliche Hochschule, Hannover;* [3]*Großburgwedel, FRG*

Corticosteroids are widely used in topical treatment of different skin diseases. Their antiinflammatory, antiproliferative and immunosuppressive action is well known. The treatment is accompanied by different side-effects. In long-term, topical glucocorticoid therapy, skin thinning is the most feared undesired effect. While the decrease of dermal thickness is caused by atrophy, the epidermal thinning is induced by an antiproliferative action. The described study shows the time-dependent development of skin thinning, induced by different dermatocorticosteroids. The thickness of skin fold and epidermis, measured in human beings (forearm) and in mouse tail skin, decreased clearly after topical treatment with βmethasone-17-valerate, clobetasole-17-propionate, diflorasone-17, 21-diacetate and hydrocortisone-17-butyrate. The thymidine triphosphate incorporation rate into DNA of mouse tail epidermis was diminshed also. Only hydrocortisone and alclometasone-17, 21-dipropionate showed moderate effects. The skin thinning was reversible.

Using the mouse tail assay, it seems to be possible to test the skin thinning potentcy of dermatocorticosteroids.

ROLE OF *Amblyomma variegatum* IN THE PATHOGENESIS OF SEVERE CLINICAL DERMATOPHILOSIS

D. Martinez *IEMVT, Pointe-à-Pitre, France*

The association between *Amblyomma variegatum* and dermatophilosis is well known in Africa. In the Caribbean also, a close geographical relationship of the tick and severe forms of the disease have been demonstrated.

Experiments were carried out in Guadeloupe in order to understand the role of *A. variegatum* in the transmission of dermatophilosis and the appearance of severe cases of the disease. Goats from les Saintes islands free of *Amblyomma* and clinical dermatophilosis, were used as experimental animals. They were maintained free of ticks until the start of the experiment. Lack of antidermatophilus antibodies in their sera was confirmed by ELISA. The tick strain used in the experiments were reared in our laboratory for years and fed on goats. The *Dermatophilus congolensis* strain was marked *in vitro* by a genetic resistance to rifampicin.

In order to evaluate the role of vector of *A. variegatum* larvae, nymphs and adults were fed on goats whose skin had been previously covered with a broth culture of marked *D. congolensis*. We succeeded in isolating the bacteria on a selective medium from 12 of 30 male ticks (n = 30), 30 days after their installation on the skin, but not from engorged larvae (n = 30) or nymphs (n = 30). No transstadial transmission could be demonstrated. Moreover, 12 of 30 goats kept free of ticks, either on duckboards or in individual cages became seropositive without lesions of dermatophilosis less than 2 months after their introduction in our stable. Transmission could have occurred either directly by way of a contaminated environment or asymptomatic carriers, or indirectly by insects acting as vectors. Transmission of the bacteria is therefore very effective even without ticks, and animals can remain asymptomatic carriers.

Several observations have shown that *A. variegatum* acts as a starting factor in the clinical disease rather than as vector: extensive fatal dermatophilosis appeared on eight goats scarified with *D. congolensis*, and infested with five or ten male and female ticks, when the three controls without ticks developed only local and transient lesions. Unfortunately, severe forms of the disease cannot be reproduced every time and some factors remain unknown. Goats free of ticks, scarified three times at 6-week intervals, develop a good humoral immunological response to *D. congolensis*. On the other hand, after the first infestation, the antibody level decreases regularly in goats infested with adult ticks supporting the hypothesis of the existence of an immunosuppression induced by the tick saliva or some of its components and responsible for the appearance of clinical dermatophilosis.

TOXIC EPIDERMAL NECROLYSIS SUCCEEDING ERYTHEMA MULTIFORME IN A DOG

D.J. Middleton, D.H. Lloyd, J.R. Rest and E.A. Ferguson *Pathology Department, Royal Veterinary College, North Mymms, Hatfield, Herts, UK*

Erythema multiforme (EM) and toxic epidermal necrolysis (TEN) are uncommon acute dermatoses in the dog. Precipitating factors in both conditions are purported to include infections, adminstration of various drugs or chemicals, neoplasia and connective tissue disorders. The pathogenesis of EM is poorly understood but may be a form of hypersensitivity reaction as, in early lesions in people, C_3 and IgM are demonstrable at the basement membrane and in the walls of superficial dermal blood vessels. Similarly, an immunological reaction involving the epidermis has been postulated in the pathogenesis of TEN which is widely regarded as a severe variant of EM.

Recently, we have identified a dog in which an episode of EM was succeeded after an interval of 5 months by fulminating and fatal TEN. The initial problem manifested as a diffuse, intensely pruritic, erythematous dermatosis with papules and plaques which progressed to exfoliation and ulcerating crusting lesions. On histology, there was epidermal and dermal involvement comprising necrosis of individual keratinocytes at all levels of the epidermis with occasional satellitosis of lyphyocytes and macrophages, hydropic basal cells with a mixed cellular interface dermatitis and a primarily mononuclear cell perivascular dermatitis. Conservative management led to clinical improvement but mild seborrhoea persisted for several months. Then generalized crusting reappeared and rapidly progressed to a painful, ulcerative dermatitis. Histology revealed widespread, full thickness coagulative necrosis of the epidermis including follicular epithelium, with separation at the dermoepidermal junction. Dermal inflammation was minimal apart from areas of ulceration which were secondarily inflamed.

Unfortunately, the factors initiating cutaneous disease in this dog could not be identified with confidence. Occurrence of the unusual conditions of EM and TEN in the one individual is compatible with a pathogenesis involving hypersensitivity or idiosyncratic toxicosis and is consistent with the disorders being part of a clinical and pathological spectrum in the dog.

IMMUNOHISTOCHEMISTRY IN SKIN DISEASE: DIAGNOSTIC VALUE?

S. Mottier and C. von Tscharner *Institute of Animal Pathology, University of Bern, Bern, Switzerland*

As there are well known problems in interpreting immunohistological slides for autoimmune skin disease, we have compared two different methods: peroxydase-antiperoxidase (PAP) and direct immunofluorescence (DIF) on skin biopsies of 30 dogs with autoimmune disease and other inflammatory lesions.

For the DIF method snap frozen or Michel's fixed tissue was incubated with affinity purified FITC conjugated antidog IgG (1/10) after absorption to homogenized normal dog skin. The PAP method was done with formalin fixed and paraffin embedded skin material. As primary antibody we used affinity purified antidog IgG (1/15 000) and an antirabbit IgG (1/20) as link antibody.

With both methods we could find IgG deposits at the basement membrane zone and in the intercellular substance of the epidermis, both in cases of autoimmune disease and other inflammatory lesions.

The staining was often weak and irregular and the basement membrane zone deposits could lead to misdiagnosis. The intercellular pattern was often superficial, localized and related to the inflammatory oedema, or around necrotic keratinocytes.

The advantages and disadvantages of both method are discussed. The great advantage of DIF is that it is a simple, rapid and well established method. Its main disadvantage is the need of special fixation (Michel) or frozen tissue. On the other hand PAP is done on formalin fixed tissue, which permits long time conservation and, therefore, retrospective studies. Counter-staining allows better orientation on the slides and evaluation of the lesions, but it is a more complicated procedure.

In conclusion it can be said that neither DIF nor PAP are good diagnostic tools for autoimmune skin disease without routine histopathology.

COUNTING OF SPECIFIC ANTIBODY FORMING CELLS REVEALS ANTIGENIC DIFFERENCES BETWEEN STRAINS OF *Dermatophilus congolensis*

A.B. Sanders, S.J. How and D.H. Lloyd *Department of Veterinary Medicine and Animal Husbandry, Royal Veterinary College, Hatfield, Herts, UK*

A new method for counting antibody forming cells (AFCs) was used to examine differences in antigenicity between strains of *D. congolensis*.

In this technique semimicrowell tissue culture plates were coated with a mechanically disrupted preparation of *D. congolensis* zoospores. Lymphocytes were obtained either from spleen or peripheral blood, depending of the species under examination and incubated in the coated wells. After removal of the cells themselves the presence of AFCs was revealed by plaques of antibody directed against the bacterial antigens. These antibodies were visualized with an immunogold conjugated antiimmunoglobulin and the reaction was enhanced by silver staining. The plaques were then counted under an inverted microscope.

In one experiment mice were immunized with whole zoospores of a Scottish strain of *D. congolensis* and the number of AFCs directed against antigens from this and from three Caribbean strains were counted. Significantly more AFCs were found to react with antigens from the immunizing strain that with those from the unrelated strains. Polyacrylamide gel electrophoresis (PAGE) analysis of the antigen preparations revealed differences in the protein patterns between the strains, further analysis may reveal if one of these proteins is the major antigenic determinant of *D. congolensis*. The numbers of AFCs were compared with the antibody titres to the same antigens obtained by enzyme linked immunosorbent assay (ELISA). This revealed that the end-point titres were not necessarily linked to the total numbers of AFCs. These results may have implications for the use of seroconversion as a measure of vaccine effectiveness and of resistance to *Dermatophilosis*.

A MULTICENTRE PLACEBO-CONTROLLED PRACTITIONER STUDY TO INVESTIGATE THE EFFECT OF EVENING PRIMROSE OIL IN CANINE ATOPIC DERMATOSIS

D. Scarff,[1] R. Harvey[2] and N. McEwan[3] [1]*The Beaumont Animal Hospital, Camden Town London;* [2]*The Quinton Veterinary Clinic, Coventry;* [3]*The Dermatology Dept., Glasgow Veterinary College, Glasgow, UK*

Previous studies have demonstrated efficacy of evening primrose oil (EPO) in canine atopic dermatosis. This study was designed to investigate the efficacy of EPO supplementation in a multicentre placebo-controlled study in general practice.

Three centres, covering Scotland, the Midlands and South East areas took part in this study between September 1987 and November 1988; 29 dogs of various breeds with a history of atopy and a positive response to a standardized skin test procedure were included. One dog withdrew on placebo because its pruritus exacerbated.

All dogs were given EPO for 12 weeks although randomized into two groups from the start. Between week 12 and 21 one group continued on EPO and the other switched to a matching placebo of olive oil capsules.

In the first 12 weeks, both groups of dogs showed highly significant improvements in scaling, pruritus, erythema, oedema, coat and overall condition as assessed by the veterinarian and compared to baseline improvements.

From weeks 12 to 21 there was no significant difference between placebo and EPO groups although improvement in both groups slowed down reaching a plateau for most parameters. This response is in line with previous human studies in atopic eczema which have shown the presence of a highly significant carry-over effect following EPO supplementation. In human studies this effect continues for at least 12 weeks.

These results in dogs are interesting because they mirror the results of more extensive studies in humans and show that initial improvements in canine atopic dermatosis on high dose EPO therapy are substantial but reach a plateau by 12 weeks. It is likely that maintenance of this plateau response can be achieved by lower dose long-term therapy.

KERATINOCYTE CELL STRAINS DERIVED FROM PLUCKED PIG HAIRS

V.K. Sieber and J.W. Hopewell *CRC Normal Tissue Radiobiology Research Group, Research Institute, Churchill Hospital, Oxford, UK*

Cell strains have been selected from epithelial keratinocytes derived from the follicular epithelium attaching to the outer root-sheath of plucked pig hairs. In comparison with cultures obtained by the conventional methods of disaggregation of biopsy material, this technique represents a simple and non-invasive method for obtaining pure keratinocyte cultures, free from contamination by fibroblasts.

Excised bulbs from aseptically plucked hairs were placed in culture flasks. Following 7 days incubation in culture medium an epithelial colony had migrated from the bulb of $> 20\%$ of the hairs. Following trypsin disaggregation, cell strains have been selected and maintained *in vitro* for up to 20 passages. They were passaged as a single cell suspension and were, therefore, amenable to quantitative analysis. The cell strains were selected and maintained without the necessity for a feeder cell layer which enables biochemical analysis without interference from the metabolic products of the feeder cells. The cells did not appear to be transformed and had a normal karyotype. There were < 5% aneuploid cells in early passage cultures rising to < 20% aneuploid cells following 20 subcultures. The cells were maintained as a monolayer but were capable of stratification. Keratin synthesis was demonstrated by positive immunofluorescence using Miles-Yeda polyclonal antikeratin antiserum. Cell strains cultured without a feeder cell layer had low plating efficiencies (0.1–5.0%) which were not inconsistent with those reported for epithelial keratinocytes maintained with a $3T_3$ feeder cell layer. Enhanced plating efficiencies were found following the use of a lethally irradiated autologous feeder cell layer whilst no significant increase in plating efficiency was found following incubation with a $3T_3$ feeder cell layer. During log-phase growth the doubling time for these cultures was 1.8 days.

CLINICAL FEATURES OF EXPERIMENTALLY INDUCED HYPOTHYROIDISM IN CATS

K.L. Thoday *Royal (Dick) School of Veterinary Studies, Edinburgh, UK*

Despite numerous anecdotal reports, a case of naturally occurring, acquired feline hypothyroidism has never been definitively diagnosed.

Hypothyroidism was induced in two 5-year-old, female, domestic short-haried cats by the intravenous administration of 37 MBq (1 mCi)/kg $Na^{131}I$. To encourage maximal thyroidal uptake of the radioisotope, an iodine deficient diet and deionized water were fed for 5 weeks before, the animals were totally deprived of food for 3 days before and after, and 10 IU TSH were given 24 and 4 h before administration of the radioisotope respectively. Demeanour and appetite were scored daily and meaned to give a weekly result. Other physical parameters (bodyweight, respiratory rate, heart rate, rectal temperature and cutaneous changes) were monitored weekly for 5 weeks before and, after a 4-week period when the cats were deemed too radioactive to handle, for 23 weeks after treatment and then monthly for a further 62 weeks. Detailed clinical monitoring then ceased but skin biopsies were taken from 10 sites during week 119 and ECGs during week 163 of the study.

Confirmation of the hypothyroid state was by determination of the serum TT_4 and TT_3 concentrations before (< 1.3 nmol/l and < 0.10 nmol/l respectively) and 6 h after (< 1.3 nmol/l and < 0.10 nmol/l respectively) the intravenous administration of 0.5 IU/kg bovine TSH (basal reference ranges, T_4: 8.5–46.2 nmol/l; T_3: 0.13–1.27 nmol/l).

Marked lethargy developed by week 17 in both cats, reverted to normal activity at week 40 and continued unchanged. The trend was for the heart rate to be slower after thyroid ablation with bradycardia (< 160 beats per minute) being recorded in both cats after treatment. No ECG abnormalities were noted. From week 18, rectal temperatures were almost continually subnormal, normal temperatures being recorded from each animal on only two occasions. The respiratory rate fluctuated markedly in both animals although the trend was for a lower rate in one after thyroid ablation. There were no significant, long-term changes in appetite and weight gain did not occur.

Skin changes were similar in both cats although always more severe in one. They included dry, brittle hair, failure to groom, dorsal mats, progressive, non-pruritic seborrhoea sicca, bilaterally symmetrical alopecia of the pinnae eventually involving the whole of the distal halves where the skin became hyperpigmented and hyperkeratotic, and focal areas of partial alopecia over the cranio-lateral carpi, caudal hocks and dorsal and lateral tail-base. Hair repeatedly clipped at various sites regrew. Histological changes varied according to the site but included orthokeratotic hyperkeratosis, partial or total apocrine gland atrophy, increased dermal mucin and, from the pinnae, collagen fibres that were swollen, fragmented and had fewer nuclei.

CUTANEOUS LYMPHOMA IN DOGS RESEMBLING MYCOSIS FUNGOIDES IN MAN

M.W. Vroom, W.A. van Vloten, M.A. Wisselink *Faculty of Medicine and Veterinary Medicine of Dermatology, Utrecht, The Netherlands*

Three dogs with skin lesions and with histologic features as seen in cutaneous T-cell lymphoma in man were presented. The skin lesions in the dog developed 3–6 months prior to admission and consisted of nodules and crusted plaques with alopecia all over the body. In one dog, the lesions presented in the gingiva and near the anus. Slightly enlarged lymph nodes were present.

Histological examination of the skin biopsies in all dogs was similar. The epidermis was normal to slightly atrophic and partially ulcerated. In the upper dermis a monomorphic dense cellular infiltrate was present composed of large basophilic lymphoblastic cells. The cells have little-to-moderate cytoplasm and contain a round to oval nucleus with one or more prominent nucleoli. Mitoses were numerous. Scattered between the atypical lymphoblastic cells are small cerebriform mononuclear cells as well as plasma cells and some eosinophils. The abnormal lymphoblastic cells invade the hair follicles and the epidermis forming Pautrier abscesses. In one case the epidermis was almost totally invaded as seen in pagetoid reticulosis. Due to the moderate-to-marked epidermotropism and the cell morphology and the positive T-cell marker staining the skin lesions in these dogs have striking similarities to mycosis fungoides in man.

Subject Index